ANTITHROMBOTIC DRUG THERAPY IN CARDIOVASCULAR DISEASE

For other titles published in this series, go to
www.springer.com/series/7677

ANTITHROMBOTIC DRUG THERAPY IN CARDIOVASCULAR DISEASE

Edited by

ARMAN T. ASKARI, MD
Western Reserve Heart Care, Hudson, OH, USA

A. MICHAEL LINCOFF, MD
The Cleveland Clinic Foundation, Cleveland, OH, USA

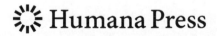 Humana Press

Editors
Arman T. Askari
Western Reserve Heart Care
Hudson, OH 44236
USA
arman.askari64@gmail.org

A. Michael Lincoff
Department of Cardiovascular Medicine
Cleveland Clinic
9500 Euclid Avenue
Cleveland, OH 44195
USA
lincofa@ccf.org

ISBN 978-1-60327-234-6   e-ISBN 978-1-60327-235-3
DOI 10.1007/978-1-60327-235-3
Springer Dordrecht Heidelberg London New York

Library of Congress Control Number: 2009928625

Printed on acid-free paper

Springer is part of Springer Science+Business Media (www.springer.com)

To my wife Jamie and our children Alexa, Amanda, and Jacob and to my parents Ali and Houri for their continued support and understanding.

Arman T. Askari, MD

I would like to recognize the support and patience of my wife Debra and our children Gabrielle, Aaron, and Jacob.

A. Michael Lincoff, MD

Preface

It is now well established that pathologic thrombosis plays a central role in the pathogenesis of acute coronary syndromes (ACS), ischemic complications of percutaneous coronary intervention (PCI), venous thromboembolic disease, and embolic complications of arrhythmias and various cardiomyopathies. Born out of the understanding of the integral role of thrombus formation across the spectrum of cardiovascular diseases is the burgeoning field of antithrombotic therapies. Rigorous investigation of individual or various combinations of the available antithrombotic regimens including fibrinolytic agents, antiplatelet therapies (aspirin, the thienopyridines, glycoprotein IIb/IIIa inhibitors), and anticoagulant therapies (unfractionated heparin, low-molecular-weight heparins, direct thrombin inhibitors, and synthetic factor X inhibitors) has lead to a marked improvement in outcomes for patients with a thrombotic event. Nevertheless, a substantial morbidity and mortality remains associated with these thrombotic events. This realization has fueled the rapid expansion of the available armamentarium to combat pathologic thrombosis.

Antithrombotic Drug Therapy in Cardiovascular Disease will serve as a resource for individuals charged with caring for patients across the spectrum of cardiovascular diseases. This text is a comprehensive, up-to-date overview of the pathophysiology, including the genetics, of arterial and venous thrombosis followed by detailed overviews of the use of antithrombotic therapies for managing patients with various thrombotic disorders. *Antithrombotic Drug Therapy in Cardiovascular Disease*, a compilation of work by thought leaders in the field, is broken down into seven parts which will provide rapid access to various therapies used for each of the major classes of thrombotic disorders commonly encountered by clinicians.

The first part of *Antithrombotic Drug Therapy in Cardiovascular Disease* is comprised of four chapters that will provide a comprehensive overview of the basic principles of thrombosis. Chapters 1 and 2 review the key components of thrombosis, the platelet and the coagulation cascade, respectively. Chapter 3 then develops the link between inflammation, a process demonstrated to be involved in atherogenesis, and thrombosis. Chapter 4 then provides a comprehensive view of the genetics of thrombosis.

Parts II–IV then provide data and clinical recommendations for the use of antithrombotic therapies for common atherothrombotic disorders including stable coronary artery disease (Part II, Chaps. 5 and 6), non-ST-segment elevation (NSTE) ACS (Part III, Chaps. 7–10), and ST-segment elevation myocardial infarction (STEMI) (Part IV, Chaps. 11–13).

Part V provides data and recommendation for the use of various antithrombotic therapies as adjuncts to interventional procedures. Chapter 14 focuses on the use of antithrombotic therapies for PCI, while Chapter 15's focus is on carotid and peripheral interventions. Chapter 16 will provide a detailed review of monitoring of the various antithrombotic therapies in the peri-interventional period.

Part VI focuses on venous thromboembolic diseases. This part of *Antithrombotic Drug Therapy in Cardiovascular Disease* will provide the data necessary to manage patients with deep vein thrombosis (DVT) and pulmonary embolism (PE) in an evidence-based fashion. Chapter 17 focuses on prophylaxis and treatment for patients with DVT/PE. Chapter 18 synthesizes the data on the use of fibrinolysis for PE. Chapter 19 completes the section with a detailed, yet concise overview of the recommended durations of therapy for patients with venous thromboembolic diseases.

The final part of *Antithrombotic Drug Therapy in Cardiovascular Disease* provides detailed overviews of the use of antithrombotic therapies in several clinical conditions commonly encountered in the field of cardiology including atrial fibrillation (Chap. 20), valvular heart disease (Chap. 21), and cardiomyopathy (Chap. 22). Chapter 23 focuses on the pathophysiology and management of heparin-induced thrombocytopenia. Finally, an analysis of the increasingly encountered scenario of aspirin and clopidogrel resistance will be addressed in Chapter 24.

In summary, this textbook will provide detailed, up-to-date data regarding the use of the currently available antithrombotic therapies for commonly encountered clinical situations in cardiology.

Arman T. Askari, MD
A. Michael Lincoff, MD
Cleveland, OH

Contents

Contributors

ZUHEIR ABRAHAMS, MD, PhD • *Department of Cardiovascular Medicine, Cleveland Clinic, Cleveland, OH, USA*

SAIF ANWARUDDIN, MD • *Western Reserve Heart Care, Hudson, OH, USA*

ARMAN T. ASKARI, MD • *Western Reserve Heart Care, Hudson, OH 44236, USA*

JOHN R. BARTHOLOMEW, MD • *Departments of Cardiovascular Medicine and Hematology/ Oncology, Cleveland Clinic, Cleveland, OH, USA*

RICHARD C. BECKER, MD • *Duke Clinical Research Institute, Duke University Medical Center, Durham, NC, USA*

DEEPAK L. BHATT, MD, MPH • *Department of Cardiology, VA Boston Healthcare System, and Integrated Interventional Cardiovascular Program, Brigham and Women's Hospital, Boston, MA, USA*

SORIN J. BRENER, MD • *Division of Cardiology, New York Methodist Hospital, Brooklyn, NY, USA*

IVAN P. CASSERLY, MB, BCH • *Section of Interventional Cardiology, University of Colorado Denver and Health Sciences Center, Aurora, CO, USA; Department of Medicine, Denver Veterans Affairs Medical Center, Denver, CO, USA*

RYAN D. CHRISTOFFERSON, MD • *Department of Cardiovascular Medicine, Cleveland Clinic, Cleveland, OH, USA*

JOHN H. CLEATOR, MD • *Division of Cardiovascular Medicine, Vanderbilt University Medical Center, Nashville, TN, USA*

KRISTOFER DOSH, MD • *Gill Heart Institute, University of Kentucky, Lexington, KY, USA*

MARCUS D. FLATHER, MBBS, FRCP • *Royal Brompton and Harefield NHS Trust, National Heart and Lung Institute, Imperial College, London, UK*

JOHN M. GALLA, MD • *Department of Cardiovascular Medicine, Cleveland Clinic, Cleveland, OH, USA*

J. MICHAEL GAZIANO, MD, MPH • *Divisions of Aging, Cardiology, and Preventive Medicine, Department of Medicine, Brigham and Women's Hospital; Massachusetts Veterans Epidemiology, Research and Information Center, and Geriatric Research, Education, and Clinical Center, Veterans Healthcare System Boston; and Harvard Medical School, Boston, MA, USA*

HITINDER S. GURM, MD • *Division of Cardiovascular Medicine, The University of Michigan, Ann Arbor, MI, USA*

CARMEL M. HALLEY, MD • *Department of Cardiovascular Medicine, Cleveland Clinic, Cleveland, OH, USA*

JAMES E. HARVEY, MD • *Department of Cardiovascular Medicine, Cleveland Clinic, Cleveland, OH, USA*

THOMAS J. HELTON, MD • *Department of Cardiovascular Medicine, Cleveland Clinic, Cleveland, OH, USA*

BRIAN D. HOIT, MD • *Division of Cardiovascular Medicine, University Hospitals Case Medical Center, Cleveland, OH, USA*

SAMIR R. KAPADIA, MD • *Department of Cardiovascular Medicine, Cleveland Clinic, Cleveland, OH, USA*

CLIVE KEARON, MB, MRCPI, FRCPC, PhD • *Department of Medicine, McMaster University, Hamilton, ON, Canada*

PETER KELLY, MD • *Department of Cardiovascular Medicine, Cleveland Clinic, Cleveland, OH, USA*

ESTHER S.H. KIM, MD • *Department of Cardiovascular Medicine, Cleveland Clinic, Cleveland, OH, USA*

MICHAEL S. KIM, MD • *University of Colorado Denver and Health Sciences Center, Aurora, CO, USA*

ALLAN L. KLEIN MD • *Department of Cardiovascular Medicine, Cleveland Clinic, Cleveland, OH, USA*

JINESH KOCHAR, MD, MPH • *Department of Medicine, Medical College of Wisconsin, Milwaukee, WI, USA*

GERALD C. KOENIG, MD, PhD • *Division of Cardiovascular Medicine, The University of Michigan, Ann Arbor, MI, USA*

STAVROS V. KONSTANTINIDES, MD • *Department of Cardiology and Pulmonary Medicine, Georg August University of Goettingen, Goettingen, Germany*

DIPAK KOTECHA, MBChB, MRCP • *Royal Brompton and Harefield NHS Trust, National Heart and Lung Institute, Imperial College, London, UK*

A. MICHAEL LINCOFF, MD • *Department of Cardiovascular Medicine, Cleveland Clinic, 9500 Euclid Avenue Cleveland, OH, 44195, USA*

KANDICE KOTTKE-MARCHANT, MD, PhD • *Department of Clinical Pathology, Cleveland Clinic, Cleveland, OH, USA*

KENNETH W. MAHAFFEY, MD • *Duke Clinical Research Institute, Duke University Medical Center, Durham, NC, USA*

ADRIAN W. MESSERLI, MD • *Cardiac Catheterization Laboratory, St. Joseph's Hospital, Lexington, KY, USA*

ROBERT L. PAGE, PharmD • *University of Colorado Denver and Health Sciences Center, Aurora, CO, USA*

EDWARD F. PLOW, PhD • *Department of Molecular Cardiology, Cleveland Clinic, Cleveland, OH, USA*

MARK ROBBINS, MD • *Division of Cardiovascular Medicine, Vanderbilt University Medical Center, Nashville, TN, USA*

NOAH ROSENTHAL, MD • *Division of Cardiovascular Medicine, University Hospitals Case Medical Center, Cleveland, OH, USA*

MARC S. SABATINE, MD, MPH • *Cardiovascular Division, Brigham and Women's Hospital, Boston, MA, USA*

SVATI H. SHAH, MD, MHS • *Division of Cardiology, Duke Center for Human Genetics, Duke University School of Medicine, Durham, NC, USA*

GEORGE SOKOS, MD • *Department of Cardiovascular Medicine, Cleveland Clinic, Cleveland, OH, USA*

STEVEN STEINHUBL, MD • *Gill Heart Institute, University of Kentucky, Lexington, KY, USA*

TYLER L. TAIGEN, MD • *Department of Cardiovascular Medicine, Cleveland Clinic, Cleveland, OH, USA*

W.H. WILSON TANG, MD • *Department of Cardiovascular Medicine, Cleveland Clinic, Cleveland, OH, USA*

PIERLUIGI TRICOCI, MD, MHS, PhD • *Duke Clinical Research Institute, Duke University Medical Center, Durham, NC, USA*

RORY B. WEINER, MD • *Cardiovascular Division, Brigham and Women's Hospital, Boston, MA, USA*

Part I
Basic Principles

1

Platelets in Arterial Thrombosis

Edward F. Plow and Peter Kelly

CONTENTS

ABSTRACT The central role of the platelet in thrombus formation has been well established. Whereas thrombus formation in some situations may be protective, it can be devastating in others such as in acute coronary syndromes. An understanding of the mechanisms and the molecules involved in platelet-mediated thrombosis is essential in order to be able to devise antiplatelet regimens that may improve patient outcomes and to develop future generations of antithrombotic drugs. This chapter provides a brief summary of the molecules and mechanisms which regulate platelet adhesion and aggregation.

Key words: Adhesion; Aggregation; Platelets; Thrombosis

PLATELETS IN THROMBUS FORMATION

Scenario 1: In an organism with a closed circulatory system, injury to the vasculature can lead to life-threatening exsanguination. To protect the organism, a highly specialized host defense mechanism is evoked to seal the injured blood vessel and limit the extent of blood loss. It is essential that this host defense system be rapidly triggered, be efficient in closing the injured vessel, and be self-limiting to restrict the process to the local site of injury. This scenario describes the modus operandus of the hemostatic response, and the platelet is the primary cellular element of this host defense pathway. Within seconds after injury, platelets within the blood are recruited to the site of injury; they adhere to the injured vessel wall and coalesce with one another to form the plug that limits blood loss and restores homeostasis. Fibrin is also formed locally as a result of activation of the coagulation system and reinforces the platelet-rich thrombus.

From: *Contemporary Cardiology: Antithrombotic Drug Therapy in Cardiovascular Disease*
Edited by: A.T. Askari and A.M. Lincoff (eds.), DOI 10.1007/978-1-60327-235-3_1
© Humana Press, a part of Springer Science+Business Media, LLC 2010

Scenario 2: Injury to the blood vessel occurs as a result of a fissure in an atherosclerotic plaque in a coronary artery. Platelets are again rapidly recruited to the site of injury but the milieu of the ruptured plaque is particularly thrombogenic. Platelet adhesion and aggregation occur robustly, all too robustly. The platelet thrombus continues to grow to the point that it impedes blood flow through the small affected coronary and ultimately can occlude the blood vessel altogether. The consequence of this thrombotic scenario is myocardial infarction.

This chapter provides a brief summary of the molecules and mechanisms which regulate platelet adhesion and aggregation. It is these molecules and the cellular responses which they regulate that are the targets of current and future generations of antithrombotic drugs, and it is these targets that we emphasize. In the interest of brevity, when possible, reviews have been used as references and contain the original citations.

PLATELET ADHESION AND ITS RECEPTORS

The intact endothelium displays a nonadhesive, nonthrombogenic surface to circulating platelets *(1)*. Activation of endothelial cells by inflammatory agonists, particularly in combination with leukocyte stimulation, can result in endothelial-leukocyte conjugates, which, in turn, can recruit platelets to the vessel surface *(2–4)*. However, the primary mechanism for recruitment of platelets to the vessel wall is disruption of the endothelium. Once the endothelium is injured, the exposed subendothelial matrix contains numerous components to which the initial platelets that arrive adhere in order to form the initial sealant of the vessel and support recruitment of many more platelets to form a thrombus. Platelets may encounter many different substrate proteins within the extracellular matrix (ECM), and the platelet surface is endowed with one or more sets of receptors to support adhesion to these ECM proteins.

Platelet-Collagen Interactions

At high shear, which is relevant in small caliber blood vessels and particularly in blood vessels studded with the irregularities of atherosclerotic plaques, exposed collagens become involved prominently in platelet adhesion. Three major receptors systems are implicated in platelet responses to collagen: GPIb-IX-V, GPVI, and integrin $\alpha2\beta1$. These are discussed individually, but they all interact with collagen cooperatively to achieve platelet adhesion.

GPIb-IX-V

This large glycoprotein complex consists of four individual gene products *(5)*; GPIb is composed of a disulfide-linked alpha and beta subunit. Recent data have suggested that the components of the GPIb-IX-V may be present as a 2:2:1 or a 1:2:1 stoichiometric complex on the platelet surface *(6,7)*. All three components of the complex are composed of leucine-rich repeats. GPIbα, with a molecular weight of 135 kDa, is the largest gene product in the complex. It consists of a large extracellular domain that is heavily glycosylated, a single transmembrane domain, and a cytoplasmic tail of 96 amino acids. The extracellular domain is composed of eight leucine-rich repeats. von Willebrand factor (vWF) binding to the extracellular domain of GPIbα mediates indirect tethering of collagen to the platelet surface. vWF possesses a GPIbα-binding site in its A1 domain and collagen-binding sites in its A2 and A3 domains *(6)*. These interactions allow vWF to bridge platelets to subendothelial collagen. Shear is required for the interaction between GPIbα and vWF to be productive *(8–10)*. Flow chambers or other devices that generate shear are needed to demonstrate the role of vWF-GPIb in platelet adhesion to collagen (e.g., *(11)*). This interaction does not result in firm adhesion, but rather slows the platelet on the collagen substrate, leading to platelet rolling. The bleeding complications associated with von Willebrand Disease attest to the biological importance of this interaction.

GPIbα also recognizes several other ligands including thrombin, several proteins of the intrinsic blood coagulation/contact system, and counter-receptors on other cells, including P-selectin and integrin αMβ2, which facilitates conjugate formation between platelets and leukocytes (5,6,12,13). The intracellular domain of GPIbα plays important roles in platelet signaling. It binds directly to the zeta isoform of 14.3.3 and controls the activity of this multifunctional signaling molecule in platelets (14). Signaling pathways influenced by GPIbα engagement include Src family kinases, phospholipase C, phosphoinositol 3-kinase, MAP kinases, Akt, and the nitric oxide-cGMP pathway (15,16). Among the consequences of signaling induced by vWF binding to GPIbα is activation of integrin αIIbβ3 (see later) although this pathway seems to be weak and may require GPVI for optimization (17). The cytoplasmic tail of GPIbα also binds to filamin A, providing a link to the actin-cytoskeleton (18). It is probably loss of such cytoskeletal constraints that gives rise to the giant platelets observed in patients deficient in GPIbα, the Bernard–Soulier Syndrome (BSS) (19).

The GPIbβ (M ~ 25 kDa) is linked to GPIbα via two disulfide bonds. It also is composed of an extracellular, a transmembrane, and short cytoplasmic domain (20). Resident in its cytoplasmic tail is a serine that is a target of phosphorylation, which may regulate vWF-mediated responses (21). GPIX associates noncovalently with the GPIbα/β. It is a relatively small glycoprotein (MW 22 kDa) with a single membrane spanning region. In heterologous cell experiments, significant effects of GPIX on platelet adhesion to collagen are not profound, but a deficiency of GPIX does result in BSS (22,23). Knockout of GPV does not lead to BSS and leads to only a mild hemostatic phenotype, which appears to arise from alterations in clot stability rather than in platelet adhesion (24). GPV is a thrombin substrate, but its cleavage appears to relatively slow and does not appear to be involved in the primary response of platelets to this agonist (25,26).

GPVI

Collagen is a strong platelet aggregation, supporting adhesion, aggregation, and secretion, but GPIbα-collagen-vWF bridging does not efficiently mediate these broad responses. Over the last decade, the concept has emerged that platelet activation by collagen depends primarily upon GPVI (17,27,28). GPVI is a 62-kDa transmembrane glycoprotein. Its extracellular domain is composed of two disulfide-linked Ig-C2–like domains and a mucin-like stalk. There is a single membrane spanning region and a cytoplasmic tail of 51 amino acids. The transmembrane region of GPVI contains an arginine which mediates an association with the Fc receptor-γ (FcRγ). FcRγ contains ITAM motifs in its cytoplasmic tail, domains that are broadly involved in the regulation of signal transduction. Collagen associates with GPVI, but it is the GPVI-FcRγ complex that mediates signaling events in response to collagen. GPVI is restricted to platelets and megakaryocytes, whereas FcRγ is present on a variety of immune cells. If FcRγ is genetically deleted, GPVI is not expressed on platelets (29,30).

The GPVI cytosolic tail contains a proline-rich motif that binds to the SH3 domain of the Src family kinases, Fyn and Lyn (17). Crosslinking of GPVI by ligand binding brings Fyn and Lyn into contact with the FcRγ-chain, leading to phosphorylation of tyrosine residues in its ITAM motif. The tyrosine kinase Syk then binds to the phosphorylated tyrosines and becomes activated via an autophosphorylation mechanism. Activated Syk, in turn, initiates a signaling cascade that involves the adaptors LAT and SLP-76 as well as effector proteins, including phospholipase (PL)Cγ2, phosphoinositide-3 (PI-3) kinase, and small G proteins. PLCγ2 subsequently induces the formation of the second messengers, inositol 1,4,5-trisphosphate (IP$_3$) and 1,2-diacylglycerol (DAG), which releases Ca^{2+} from intracellular stores and activates protein kinase (PK) C, respectively (28,31). Ultimately these events lead to activation of αIIbβ3 and other platelet integrins and platelet secretion. ITAM-dependent signaling is subject to negative regulation by receptors containing ITIM motifs. PECAM-1 is the major ITIM-containing receptor on platelets and may negatively regulate signaling across GPVI. Recent evidence suggests that GPVI may associate with GPIb-IX on platelets, providing a mechanism for their cooperation in platelet adhesion to collagen.

INTEGRIN α2β1

If the primary role of GPIb-IX is to mediate platelet rolling on collagen, and that of GPVI is to induce platelet secretion and activation of αIIbβ3 and other integrins, the primary role of α2β1 is to orchestrate firm adhesion of platelets to the collagen substrate. α2β1 is a member of the integrin family of heterodimeric adhesion receptors. A detailed description of the structure of integrin αIIbβ3 is provided in the section on platelet aggregation and the general features apply to all integrins. The exception is that α2β1 belongs to the group of integrins containing an I-domain inserted into its alpha subunit while αIIbβ3 does not. The I-domain is a segment of about 200 amino acids. In α2β1, and other integrins containing this domain, the I-domain is critical to ligand recognition *(32–34)*. Collagen interacts with the I-domain of α2β1 in a divalent-ion-regulated manner; the interaction is suppressed by calcium and is supported by magnesium *(35)*. Hence, divalent ion availability plays a critical role in regulating the function of the integrin. The contribution of α2β1 in platelet adhesion has been controversial, from assigning it an essential role to no role at all. However, patients who lack functional α2β1 were reported to have a bleeding phenotype *(36)*. Studies in mice lacking GPVI, α2β1 or both receptors have been reported recently *(37)*. These studies suggest roles for both receptors in platelet adhesion under flow conditions and propose a cooperative role for both receptors *(37)*.

Other Adhesion Receptors

Injury to the endothelium or fissures in atherosclerotic plaques may expose a heterogeneous group of ECM proteins in addition to collagen, and the platelet is equipped to adhere to a variety of substrates to establish hemostasis. Major ECM proteins that platelets may encounter include fibronectin, vitronectin, laminin, vWF, fibrin, and thrombospondin. The platelet surface is endowed with receptors for each of these matrix proteins (reviewed in (30,38,39)). Several of these substrates are recognized by members of the integrin family. Fibronectin can mediate platelet adhesion by engaging α5β1 or αIIbβ3. Integrin α5β1 is a broadly distributed fibronectin receptor and can also bind fibrinogen. Vitronectin can interact with αVβ3 or with αIIbβ3 on platelets. αVβ3 is present at only very low levels, 100–500 copies per platelet, and it is likely that recognition of vitronectin as an adhesive substrate is mediated primarily by αIIbβ3. Integrin α6β1 is a laminin receptor. On cells other than platelets, this integrin also recognizes collagen. Studies differ in the extent to which laminin supports platelet responses, and receptors other than α6β1 may mediate platelet responses to this substratum. In addition to its interaction with GPIb-IX, vWF also interacts with integrin αIIbβ3. Fibrin also can engage αIIbβ3; and, hence, fibrin deposition in a developing thrombus can recruit platelets into the thrombus. A tripeptide sequence common to many of the ECM proteins mediates their interaction with many of the integrins. Fibronectin interaction with α5β1, vitronectin interaction with αIIbβ3 and αVβ3, vWF and fibrin interaction with αIIbβ3 can be mediated by the RGD sequences in these ligands. Other sequences within these same ECM proteins also are recognized by these same integrins. Laminins and collagens contain RGD sequences but these are not involved in interaction with α6β1 and α2β1, respectively. However, degradation of these ligands, a common fate of many ECM proteins, can expose their RGD sequences. Thrombospondin-1 (TSP-1), a constituent of the ECM and the major protein secreted from platelets, contains an RGD sequence, which can become available to integrins αIIbβ3 and αVβ3 under circumstances in which the conformation of TSP-1 is reorganized *(40)*. However, a second TSP-1 receptor, CD36, can also mediate recognition of this ligand, leading to signaling events associated with platelet activation *(41,42)*.

AGONIST RECEPTORS

ADP Receptors

Forty-five years ago, ADP was identified as a factor derived from erythrocytes which influenced platelet adhesion to glass *(43)* and induced platelet aggregation *(44)*. However, the molecular structure and identity of the receptors for ADP remained elusive until relatively recently. The ADP receptors on platelets belong to the P2 family, which consists of two classes of membrane receptors: P2X ligand-gated cation channels and G-protein-coupled P2Y receptors *(45)*. ADP activates platelets through three purinergic receptors, P2Y1, P2Y12, and P2X1. The P2X1 cation channel is activated by ATP and the two G-protein-coupled receptors, P2Y1 and P2Y12, are activated by ADP. Of these three receptors, one is coupled to inhibition of adenylyl cyclase through activation of the Gαi subunit, the second is coupled to mobilization of calcium from intracellular stores through activation of the stimulatory Gαq subunit with resultant phospholipase C (PLC) activation, and the third, an ionotropic P2X1 receptor, is coupled to rapid calcium influx.

P2Y1 RECEPTORS

The P2Y1 receptor is widely distributed in many tissues. ADP is its natural agonist, while ATP behaves as an antagonist in platelets *(46)*. About 150 P2Y1 receptor-binding sites are expressed per platelet *(47)*. The Gαq-coupled P2Y1 receptor was the first of the ADP receptors to be cloned *(48)* and consists of 373 amino acids, encoded by a single exon *(49)*. P2Y1 activates the Gαq/phospholipase C pathway leading to generation of second messengers, inositol triphosphate (IP3) and DAG *(50)*. IP3 mobilizes calcium from the intracellular stores while DAG activates the protein kinase C isoforms. This activation leads to platelet shape change *(51)* and contributes to ADP-mediated platelet aggregation and thromboxane A2 generation *(52)*. Platelets from mice deficient in P2Y1 receptor show no shape change or aggregation in response and display mild prolongation in bleeding time *(53,54)*. P2Y1-deficient mice are also resistant to thrombosis induced by agonists like ADP, epinephrine, or collagen *(53–55)*. Also, mouse platelets treated with P2Y1 antagonist MRS2179 display decreased thrombus formation in a ferric chloride-induced vascular injury model *(56)*.

P2Y1 is a high-affinity receptor for ADP, and ATP, 2-chloroATP and 2-MeSATP are competitive antagonists. A number of specific P2Y1 receptor antagonists have been developed which have no effect on the P2Y12 receptor and as such, could be useful therapeutic tools to improve antithrombotic strategies, particularly given the observation that a combination of P2Y1 deficiency and clopidogrel (selective P2Y12 antagonist) treatment confers better thromboresistance than antagonism of the individual ADP receptors *(56)*.

P2Y12 RECEPTORS

The P2Y12 receptor couples to Gαi2. This leads to inhibition of adenylyl cyclase *(57)* and decreasing levels of cAMP. This ADP receptor has been shown to be important for platelet functions very similar to the P2Y1 receptor. In addition, the P2Y12 receptor is also important for potentiation of platelet activation mediated by other physiological agonists including collagen, vWF, and thromboxane A2. P2Y12 stimulation also results in potentiation and amplification of platelet aggregation, procoagulant activity, and dense granule secretion caused by other platelet agonists. Specifically, P2Y12 has been implicated in mediating irreversible aggregation by the protease-activated receptor (PAR)-1 and in playing an integral role in thromboxane- and collagen-mediated aggregation. All these features make P2Y12 a pivotal factor in sustaining platelet aggregation and promoting thrombus growth and stabilization. Coactivation of the P2Y1 and P2Y12 receptors is necessary for normal ADP-induced platelet aggregation (58–60). They are differentially involved in the procoagulant activity of platelets. While both receptors are indirectly involved through their role in platelet P-selectin exposure and in the formation of platelet–leukocyte conjugates leading to leukocyte tissue factor exposure (61,62), P2Y12 is also directly implicated in the exposure of phosphatidylserine at the surface of platelets (55).

P2Y12-deficient mouse platelets aggregate poorly in response to ADP and do not respond to thienopyridine compounds like clopidogrel. These platelets change shape normally indicating that P2Y12 has no role in platelet shape change (63). An in vivo mesenteric artery injury model in P2Y12-deficient mice demonstrated involvement of this receptor in platelet adhesion/activation, thrombus growth, and stability (64). Studies have shown that platelets from patients with P2Y12 receptor deficiency yield a thrombus that is small and loosely packed compared to platelets from normal subjects (65).

Tissue distribution is very limited, although not entirely restricted to platelets, as it is also expressed in brain, endothelial and smooth muscle cells (66). Platelets express approximately 500–800 P2Y12 receptors (47). ADP is the natural agonist of this receptor, while ATP and its triphosphate analogs are antagonists (67,68). Given the potentiating role of P2Y12 in various platelet functions and its limited localization, the P2Y12 receptor has become an enticing target for therapeutic intervention. The search for compounds that target the P2Y12 receptor has led to the development of thienopyridine derivatives that include clopidogrel, ticlopidine (69), and CS747 (70) and prasugrel. The thienopyridine class of P2Y12 antagonists acts as irreversible inhibitors. Thienopyridines, including the active metabolite of clopidogrel, bind covalently to cysteine residues of P2Y12 (71), thus precluding the binding of ADP (72).

P2X1 RECEPTORS

The third component of the platelet P2 receptors involved in ADP recognition is P2X1, the ligand-gated cation channel responsible for the fast calcium entry induced by ATP (73). Seven genes for the P2X receptors have been identified on different chromosomes. Among these, only P2X1 is found in human platelets and megakaryocytes. A characteristic of P2X1 is that it is very quickly desensitized, which hampers study of its function in platelet activation in vitro. However, when desensitization is prevented by addition of a high concentration of apyrase (ATP-diphosphohydrolase, E.C.3.6.1.5.), the selective P2X1 agonist alpha, beta-methylene-ATP ($\alpha\beta$MeATP) induces a rapid calcium influx accompanied by a transient shape change in human platelets (74). Although unable to trigger platelet aggregation by itself, the P2X1 receptor has been shown to participate in collagen- and shear-induced aggregation (75–77).

P2X1 knockout mice show that P2X1 activity is necessary for thrombus formation at high shear (78). These mice have decreased mortality compared to control mice in a laser-induced vessel injury model. These knockout mice appear healthy and have no hemostatic defects and no prolongation of bleeding time. In addition, mouse platelets overexpressing P2X1 show an increase in collagen-induced platelet aggregation, secretion, and ERK2 phosphorylation (79). Finally, the new P2X1 antagonist NF449 [46] has an inhibitory effect on platelet activation and thrombosis in vivo (80). These results suggest that the P2X1 receptor should also be considered as a potential target for antiplatelet strategies, particularly in the setting of severe stenosis where shear forces are very high.

PROTEASE-ACTIVATED RECEPTORS

PARs are G-protein-coupled receptors that mediate the cellular effects of different proteases including thrombin. PARs are activated by proteolytic cleavage of their N-terminal domains which exposes a "tethered ligand" that activates the receptors. PAR-1 was identified first in a search for receptors that could mediate the activation of platelets and other cells by thrombin *(81)*. Now, four PARs have been identified and these are differentially expressed by vascular cells (endothelial cells and vascular smooth muscle cells [VSMCs]), platelets, and other circulating cells. Thrombin activates PAR-1 and PAR-4 and is the main physiological activator of these receptors.

The mechanism of PAR activation and signaling is complex and unusual for several reasons: first, thrombin is an enzyme and, thus, it can activate more than one molecule of the receptor; second, the proteolytic cleavage of the receptor by thrombin is irreversible; third, activated receptors are potentially coupled to different G proteins that signal through multiple signaling pathways and finally, activated PARs are rapidly internalized and targeted to lysosomal degradation. This mechanism involves the phosphorylation of PAR-1 in the C-terminus which triggers membrane translocation and clathrin-mediated internalization for endocytosis *(82)*.

Human platelets express PAR-1 and -4 and either of them can trigger platelet secretion and aggregation *(81,83)*. PAR-1 seems to mediate platelet activation at low thrombin concentrations through a hirudin-like site that acts as a thrombin-binding site *(81)*. PAR-4 lacks the thrombin-binding site but mediates platelet activation at higher thrombin concentrations. In addition, the slow PAR-4 shutoff could be responsible for prolonged thrombin responsiveness in human platelets *(84)*. In addition to PAR activation, thrombin also interacts with GPIbα (see earlier). Platelet activation by thrombin induces shape change, mobilizes P-selectin and CD40L to the platelet membrane, and promotes the release of platelet agonists ADP, serotonin, thromboxane A2, chemokines, and growth factors *(85,86)*.

Human platelets utilize PAR-1 and PAR-4 to respond to thrombin, whereas mouse platelets utilize PAR-3 and PAR-4 *(83)*. Studies in knockout mice reveal that PAR-3 is necessary for mouse platelet activation at low thrombin concentrations. Although PAR-3 itself does not mediate transmembrane signaling, PAR-3 knockout mice are protected against thrombosis as are PAR-4 knockout mice *(87)*. PAR-4 knockout mice appear healthy and platelets from these animals are normal in number and morphology. However, they show markedly prolonged bleeding times, protection against thromboplastin-induced pulmonary embolism, and thrombosis of mesenteric arteries *(87,88)*. PAR-4 activation by thrombin seems to be important to stabilize platelet-platelet aggregates, as has been observed in patients with Hermansky–Pudlak Syndrome, which lack platelet dense granules and have no ADP-autocrine response *(89)*.

Despite the proven efficacy of currently available agents such as aspirin and clopidogrel, antiplatelet therapy remains suboptimal. This has prompted the search for more efficient and safe antiplatelet agents. In this context, strategies to modulate the effects of thrombin through the direct inhibition of PARs have been assessed. Anti-PAR-1 antibodies directed against the thrombin cleavage site have been effective in vitro and in vivo *(90,91)*. Peptide mimetic antagonists that block PARs by competing with the endogenous tethered ligand are currently under investigation. One of these PAR-1 antagonists (RWJ-58259) has been shown to efficiently prevent thrombus formation induced by electrolytic injury in nonhuman primates *(92)*. Blockade of both PAR-1 and PAR-4 with pepducins, cell-penetrating lipopeptides based on the third intracellular loop of PAR-1 and PAR-4, effectively inhibits platelet aggregation *(93)*. Infusion of the anti-PAR-4 pepducin into mice extends bleeding times and protects against systemic platelet activation *(93)*. Studies in animal models have revealed that combined inhibition of both PAR-1 and PAR-4 could be a more appropriate therapeutic strategy to prevent arterial thrombosis than selective monotherapy *(94,95)*. For example, the combination of bivalirudin with novel PAR-4 pepducin effectively inhibits aggregation of human platelets at even high concentrations of thrombin and prevents occlusion of carotid arteries in an animal model *(94)*.

THROMBOXANE A2 RECEPTORS

Thromboxane A2 (TXA2) is one of the bioactive metabolites of arachadonic acid. Cyclooxygenase converts arachadonic acid into prostaglandin endoperoxide H2, which is then further metabolized to TXA2 by thromboxane synthase. TXA2 is released from stimulated platelets and is a potent inducer of platelet aggregation as well as vasoconstriction and bronchoconstriction (96,97). TXA2 exerts its influence on platelet aggregation by interacting with TXA2 receptors on the platelet surface. There are two subtypes of TXA2 receptors, alpha and beta, but its effects in platelets are mediated primarily by the alpha isoform. Thromboxane receptors are seven transmembrane G-protein-coupled receptors as are a number of the agonist receptors on platelets. The transmembrane and extracellular regions of thromboxane receptors are involved in ligand recognition. In addition, separate studies have provided evidence that thromboxane receptors can couple to at least four separate G protein families (98). Consequently, thromboxane receptors can trigger a broad range of cellular responses. In platelets, the TXA2 receptor can couple to $G\alpha$ and $G\alpha_{13}$. $G\alpha_{13}$ is phosphorylated through a PKA-dependent mechanism (98), linking TXA2 receptor signaling to cAMP levels. The long and well-established effectiveness of aspirin as an antiplatelet agent raised the hope that intervention at other sites within the arachondonic acid metabolic pathway or interference with the TXA2 receptor would provide new antithrombotic drugs. TXA2 receptor antagonists were developed throughout the 1980s and 1990s. In preclinical testing in animal models some of these antagonists were found to be protective in models of thromboembolic disease (99). However, such TXA2 receptor antagonists have not yet resulted in the development of effective antiplatelet drugs.

PLATELET AGGREGATION AND ITS RECEPTORS

αIIbβ3

Deficiencies of integrin αIIbβ3, either in humans or in mice, result in a failure of platelets to aggregate in in vitro assays, an absence of thrombus formation in murine models of arterial thrombosis, and in an episodic bleeding syndrome in humans, Glanzmann's thrombasthenia. The contribution of αIIbβ3 to platelet aggregation depends on its capacity to serve as a receptor for adhesive proteins. Occupancy of the integrin by either fibrinogen or vWF supports platelet aggregation (100–102). The ligand repertoire of αIIbβ3 includes still other protein ligands, such as fibronectin and vitronectin, which can support αIIbβ3-mediated platelet adhesion or modulate platelet aggregation but do not themselves have multimeric structures appropriate for bridging platelets together (103).

The essential role of αIIbβ3 in thrombosis and hemostasis served as an impetus for extensive analysis of its structure and function. Dedicated reviews of the structure αIIbβ3 and of integrins in general have been published (100–102,104,105), and only a brief overview is provided here. αIIbβ3 is a typical integrin composed of a noncovalent complex of its αIIb and β3 subunits. The complete amino acid sequences of both subunits and the organization of their genes were determined in the 1980s (106–108). Each subunit can be divided into three regions: a large extracellular region, a single membrane spanning region, and a short cytoplasmic tail. Contacts between subunits occur between all three regions. The large extracellular regions consists of a series of domains that were initially identified in the crystal structure of the αIIbβ3 sister receptor, αVβ3, which shares the same β3 subunit (109,110). Today, several crystal structures of portions of the extracellular domain of αIIbβ3, including complexes with small molecule agonists and antagonists, have been determined (111). Low molecular weight ligands nestle into a groove formed by domains contributed by each subunit: the β-propeller from the αIIb subunit and the A-domain from the β3 subunit. In the β3A-domain, a metal ion bound in a MIDAS motif is critical to function. This metal ion is coordinated by an aspartic acid residue present in the ligand *(112)*. The ability of ligands and antagonists to distinguish between αIIbβ3 and αVβ3 depends upon the "reach" of the bound ligand from the MIDAS cation into the β-propeller of the α subunit *(111)*. Hence, some ligands and antagonists can bind to αIIbβ3, to αVβ3 or to both integrins.

Critical to the function of αIIbβ3 on platelets is its ability to undergo activation. On circulating, unactivated platelets, αIIbβ3 exists in a resting state where it exhibits low affinity for its natural ligands. Hence, platelets can circulate in blood, a rich source of fibrinogen as well as other αIIbβ3 ligands, without occupancy of the receptor and spontaneous aggregation. When a platelet encounters an appropriate agonist, intracellular signaling events are triggered which lead to conversion of αIIbβ3 from its resting to an activated state in which its affinity for ligand increases to the point where receptor occupancy, by fibrinogen and/or other ligands, occurs efficiently and leads to platelet aggregation *(113–115)*. Some of the agonists/receptors which induce αIIbβ3 activation have been discussed earlier and are being actively investigated as antithrombotic drug targets. Other natural agonists can trigger αIIbβ3 activation, particularly in combinations with low or subthreshold doses of ADP *(115)*. Included in this category are epinephrine and serotonin, with platelets expressing the G-protein-coupled receptors that also recognize these agonists.

While the agonist receptors on platelets and the intracellular signaling processes that they elicit are complex, the pathways converge to generate a common *inside-out signal* that changes the cytoplasmic tails and initiates activation of αIIbβ3 *(116)*. As currently envisioned, the cytoplasmic tails of the αIIb and β3 subunits interact with each other through several electrostatic and hydrophobic bonds between their membrane proximal helices. This intersubunit *clasp* maintains the integrin in a resting state. The signaling events from the agonist receptors converge and disrupt the clasp *(117,118)*. This change is sensed in the transmembrane helices of the two subunits, which also are likely to be clasped, and which then undergo an unclasping or a change in registry of their interaction to propagate the inside-out activating signal across the membrane *(119,120)*. In the extracellular region, conformational changes which alter the relationship between the β-propeller and the β3A domain prepare the ligand-binding site to accept macromolecular ligands. A component of this conformational rearrangement may be an unbending of the integrin to bring its ligand-binding site away from the membrane, permitting easier access of large ligands and, once bound, for the ligands to bridge to another platelet *(121,122)*.

The contribution of αIIbβ3 to thrombus formation does not end with its role in binding ligands. Occupancy of αIIbβ3 and other integrins results in their clustering. The consequence of such clustering is to create adhesive patches where platelet cohesive properties are enriched; to recruit, activate, and occupy other αIIbβ3 molecules within the cluster; and to generate *outside-in* signals *(105,123)*. Certain signals can be generated across a single occupied αIIbβ3 but most of the downstream signaling events in platelets require clustering of occupied integrins for transmission. From the standpoint of thrombus formation, such outside-in signals stabilize the thrombus, and interventions, either genetic or pharmacologic that inhibit outside-in signaling, reduce the stability of platelet aggregates in vitro and destabilize thrombi in vivo (e.g., (124)).

Modulators of Platelet Aggregation

An emerging theme of platelet research has been the role of proteins other than αIIbβ3 that modulate platelet aggregation. Antagonism of these molecules may blunt but not necessarily totally suppress platelet aggregation. In principle, such *partial antagonism* of the functional response may limit platelet participation in thrombosis while sparing their hemostatic activity. Thus, interference with the function of these molecules would suppress thrombosis but would not lead to the bleeding complications associated with direct αIIbβ3 antagonists. Included in this group of targets are membrane proteins as well as the soluble ligands that bind to them. One of the first molecules displaying these properties was the growth arrest-specific gene 6, Gas-6. Gas-6 is present in and released from platelet α-granules upon platelet stimulation and aggregation (125). It is a 75-kDa protein which, like several coagulation proteins, contains γ-carboxylated glutamic acids. Gas-6 is a ligand for Axl, Sky, and Mer. These are all transmembrane tyrosine kinases, and all are present on the platelet surface (126). When Gas-6 binds to these receptors, their kinase activities become activated. A downstream target of such activation is phosphorylation of the two tyrosine residues in the cytoplasmic tail of the integrin β3 subunit, which regulate outside-in signaling from the occupied integrin. As a result, thrombus growth and stability is dependent upon Gas-6 and its receptors (125). Platelets from mice deficient in Gas-6 show an initial aggregation response to various agonists but the aggregates are unstable. In vivo, the Gas-6$^{-/-}$ mice are resistant to thrombosis but show normal bleeding times (127). Mice in which the two tyrosine residues in the β3 cytoplasmic tail have been the mutated to phenylalanines, the so-called DiY mice, exhibit a similar phenotype (124). Thus, outside-in signaling may provide multiple targets for dampening thrombosis while sustaining sufficient hemostatic function to avoid bleeding. Several other ligands released from platelets and bound to platelet surface receptors (e.g., CD40L binding to CD40), or membrane proteins involved in homotypic (e.g., PECAM-1 or JAM A and C) or heterotypic (e.g., Eph kinases and ephrins) interactions between platelets have been shown to modulate platelet aggregation. Modulation of platelet response by such molecules has been the subject of recent reviews (128,129). For several of these, deficiencies in mice show their potential to modify thrombosis in vivo.

Another category of platelet proteins that regulate platelet aggregation are ones that affect integrin activation. Talin is a large (220 kDa) and abundant cytoskeletal protein within platelets as well as many other cell types. A substantial body of evidence identifies talin as the final activator of αIIbβ3 and other integrins (130,131). This function depends on binding of talin to the β3 cytoplasmic tail and dissociating the cytoplasmic tail clasp (117,132). Among the evidence that supports this role of talin is the failure of platelets rendered deficient in talin or bearing a mutant αIIbβ3 which does not bind talin, to aggregate (132). Hence, talin and more specifically, the talin-β3 interaction, becomes a potential target for antithrombotic drugs. Recently, our understanding of αIIbβ3 activation has become more complex. Members of the kindlin family of actin-associated proteins have been shown to bind to the β3 cytoplasmic tail but at a different site than talin (29,133,134). Platelets from mice deficient in kindlin-3, one of the three kindlin family members, also fail to aggregate (29). Hence, kindlins also are candidate targets for suppression of platelet responses and thrombosis. Talin and kindlins are widely distributed. Inhibitors of talin and kindlins that could be selectively delivered into platelets or do not have deleterious effects in other cells would need to be developed to exploit these targets.

REFERENCES

1. Marcus AJ, Safier LB. Thromboregulation: multicellular modulation of platelet reactivity in hemostasis and thrombosis. FASEB J. 1993;7:516–522.
2. Diacovo TG, Puri KD, Warnock A, Springer TA, Von Andrian UH. Platelet-mediated lymphocyte delivery to high endothelial venules. Science. 1996;273:252–255.
3. Diacovo TG, Roth SJ, Buccola JM, Bainton DF, Springer TA. Neutrophil rolling, arrest, and transmigration across activated, surface-adherent platelets via sequential action of P-selectin and the β$_2$ integrin CD11b/CD18. Blood. 1996;88:146–157.
4. Coller BS. Binding of abciximab to α$_v$β$_3$ and activated α$_M$β$_2$ receptors: with a review of platelet-leukocyte interactions. Thromb Haemost. 1999;82:326–336.

5. Andrews RK, Gardiner EE, Shen Y, Whisstock JC, Berndt MC. Glycoprotein Ib-IX-V. Int J Biochem Cell Biol. 2003;35:1170–1174.

6. Berndt MC, Shen Y, Dopheide SM, Gardiner EE, Andrews RK. The vascular biology of the glycoprotein Ib-IX-V complex. Thromb Haemost. 2001;86:178–188.

7. Luo SZ, Mo X, Afshar-Kharghan V, Srinivasan S, Lopez JA, Li R. Glycoprotein Ibalpha forms disulfide bonds with 2 glycoprotein Ibbeta subunits in the resting platelet. Blood. 2007;109:603–609.

8. Sixma JJ, van Zanten GH, Saelman EUM, Verkleij M, Lankhof H, Nieuwenhuis HK, et al. Platelet adhesion to collagen. Thromb Haemost. 1995;74:454–459.

9. Ruggeri ZM. Von Willebrand factor, platelets and endothelial cell interaction. J Thromb Haemost. 2003;1:1335–1342.

10. Ruggeri ZM. Role of von Willebrand factor in platelet thrombus formation. Ann Med. 2000;32(Suppl 1):2–9.

11. Sakariassen KS, Aarts PAMM, de Groot PG, Houdijk PM, Sixma JJ. A perfusion chamber developed to investigate platelet interaction in flowing blood with human vessel wall cells, their extracellular matrix, and purified components. J Lab Clin Med. 1983;102:522–535.

12. Lundblad RL, White GC. The interaction of thrombin with blood platelets. Platelets. 2005;16:373–385.

13. Simon DI, Chen ZP, Xu H, Li CQ, Dong JF, McIntire LV, et al. Platelet glycoprotein Ibα is a counterreceptor for the leukocyte integrin Mac-1 (CD11b/CD18). J Exp Med. 2000;192:193–204.

14. Gu M, Xi X, Englund GD, Berndt MC, Du X. Analysis of the roles of 14-3-3 in the platelet glycoprotein Ib-IX-mediated activation of integrin alpha(IIb)beta(3) using a reconstituted mammalian cell expression model. Cell Biol. 1999;147:1085–1096.

15. Ozaki Y, Asazuma N, Suzuki-Inoue K, Berndt MC. Platelet GPIb-IX-V-dependent signaling. J Thromb Haemost. 2005;3:1745–1751.

16. Du X. Signaling and regulation of the platelet glycoprotein Ib-IX-V complex. Curr Opin Hematol. 2007;14:262–269.

17. Nieswandt B, Watson SP. Platelet-collagen interaction: is GPVI the central receptor? Blood. 2003;102:449–461.

18. Fox JEB. Identification of actin-binding protein as the protein linking the membrane skeleton to glycoproteins on platelet plasma membranes. J Biol Chem. 1985;260:11970.

19. Nurden AT. Inherited abnormalities of platelets. Thromb Haemost. 1999;82:468–480.

20. Lopez JA, Chung DW, Fujikawa K, Hagen FS, Davie EW, Roth GJ. The alpha and beta chains of human platelet glycoprotein Ib are both transmembrane proteins containing a leucine-rich amino acid sequence. Proc Natl Acad Sci USA. 1988;85:2135–2139.

21. Bodnar RJ, Gu M, Li Z, Englund GD, Du X. The cytoplasmic domain of the platelet glycoprotein Ibalpha is phosphorylated at serine 609. J Biol Chem. 1999;274:33474–33479.

22. Lanza F, de La SC, Baas MJ, Schwartz A, Boval B, Cazenave JP, et al. A Leu7Pro mutation in the signal peptide of platelet glycoprotein (GP)IX in a case of Bernard-Soulier syndrome abolishes surface expression of the GPIb-V-IX complex. Br J Haematol. 2002;118:260–266.

23. Poujol C, Ramakrishnan V, Deguzman F, Nurden AT, Phillips DR, Nurden P. Ultrastructural analysis of megakaryocytes in GPV knockout mice. Thromb Haemost. 2000;84:312–318.

24. Ni H, Ramakrishnan V, Ruggeri ZM, Papalia JM, Phillips DR, Wagner DD. Increased thrombogenesis and embolus formation in mice lacking glycoprotein V. Blood. 2001;98:368–373.

25. Lanza F, Morales M, de La SC, Cazenave JP, Clemetson KJ, Shimomura T, et al. Cloning and characterization of the gene encoding the human platelet glycoprotein V. A member of the leucine-rich glycoprotein family cleaved during thrombin-induced platelet activation. J Biol Chem. 1993;268:20801–20807.

26. Kahn ML, Diacovo TG, Bainton DF, Lanza F, Trejo J, Coughlin SR. Glycoprotein V-deficient platelets have undiminished thrombin responsiveness and Do not exhibit a Bernard-Soulier phenotype. Blood. 1999;94:4112–4121.

27. Moroi M, Jung SM. Platelet glycoprotein VI: its structure and function. Thromb Res. 2004;114:221–233.

28. Varga-Szabo D, Pleines I, Nieswandt B. Cell adhesion mechanisms in platelets. Arterioscler Thromb Vasc Biol. 2008;28:403–412.

29. Moser M, Nieswandt B, Ussar S, Pozgajova M, Fassler R. Kindlin-3 is essential for integrin activation and platelet aggregation. Nat Med. 2008;14:325–330.

30. Kasirer-Friede A, Kahn ML, Shattil SJ. Platelet integrins and immunoreceptors. Immunol Rev. 2007;218:247–264.

31. Watson SP, Auger JM, McCarty OJ, Pearce AC. GPVI and integrin alphaIIb beta3 signaling in platelets. J Thromb Haemost. 2005;3:1752–1762.

32. Dickeson SK, Santoro SA. Ligand recognition by the I domain-containing integrins. Cell Mol Life Sci. 1998;54:556–566.

33. Emsley J, Knight CG, Farndale RW, Barnes MJ, Liddington RC. Structural basis of collagen recognition by integrin $\alpha_2\beta_1$. Cell. 2000;101:47–56.

34. Smith C, Estavillo D, Emsley J, Bankston LA, Liddington RC, Cruz MA. Mapping the collagen-binding site in the I domain of the glycoprotein Ia/IIa (integrin alpha(2)beta(1)). J Biol Chem. 2000;275:4205–4209.

35. Dickeson SK, Walsh JJ, Santoro SA. Binding of the α_2 integrin I domain to extracellular matrix ligands: structural and mechanistic differences between collagen and laminin binding. Cell Adhes Commun. 1998;5:273–281.

36. Nieuwenhuis HK, Akkerman JWN, Houdijk WPM, Sixma JJ. Human blood platelets showing no response to collagen fail to express surface glycoprotein Ia. Nature. 1985;318:470–472.

37. Chen H, Kahn ML. Reciprocal signaling by integrin and nonintegrin receptors during collagen activation of platelets. Mol Cell Biol. 2003;23:4764–4777.

38. Plow EF. Mechanisms of platelet adhesion. In: Lincoff AM, Topol EJ, editors. Contemporary cardiology: platelet glyco-protein IIb/IIIa inhibitors in cardiovascular disease. Totowa, NJ: Humana; 1999. p. 21–34.

39. Plow EF, Abrams CS. The molecular basis for platelet function. In: Hoffman R, Benz Jr EJ, Shattil SJ, Furie B, Cohen HJ, Silberstein LE, McGlave P, editors. Hematology: Basic Principles and Practice. 4th ed. Philadelphia, PA: Elsevier/ Churchill Livingstone; 2005. p. 1881–1897.

40. Lawler J, Weinstein R, Hynes RO. Cell attachment to thrombospondin: the role of arg-gly-asp, calcium and integrin receptors. J Cell Biol. 1988;107:2351–2361.

41. Asch AS, Silbiger S, Heimer E, Nachman RL. Thrombospondin sequence motif (CSVTCG) is responsible for CD36 binding. Biochem Biophys Res Commun. 1992;182:1208–1217.

42. Dawson DW, Pearce SF, Zhong R, Silverstein RL, Frazier WA, Bouck NP. CD36 mediates the in vitro inhibitory effects of thrombospondin-1 on endothelial cells. J Cell Biol. 1997;138:707–717.

43. Gaarder A, Jonsen J, Laland S, Hellem A, Owren PA. Adenosine diphosphate in red cells as a factor in the adhesiveness of human blood platelets. Nature. 1961;192:531–532.

44. Born GVR. Aggregation of blood platelets by adenosine diphosphate and its reversal. Nature. 1962;194:927–929.

45. Ralevic V, Burnstock G. Receptors for purines and pyrimidines. Pharmacol Rev. 1998;50:413–492.

46. Leon C, Hechler B, Vial C, Leray C, Cazenave JP, Gachet C. The P2Y$_1$ receptor is an ADP receptor antagonized by ATP and expressed in platelets and megakaryoblastic cells. FEBS Lett. 1997;402:26–30.

47. Baurand A, Raboisson P, Freund M, Leon C, Cazenave JP, Bourguignon JJ, et al. Inhibition of platelet function by administration of MRS2179, a P2Y1 receptor antagonist. Eur J Pharmacol. 2001;412:213–221.

48. Ayyanathan K, Webbs TE, Sandhu AK, Athwal RS, Barnard EA, Kunapuli SP. Cloning and chromosomal localization of the human P2Y1 purinoceptor. Biochem Biophys Res Commun. 1996;218:783–788.

49. Ayyanathan K, Naylor SL, Kunapuli SP. Structural characterization and fine chromosomal mapping of the human P2Y1 purinergic receptor gene (P2RY1). Somat Cell Mol Genet. 1996;22:419–424.

50. Offermanns S, Toombs CF, Hu YH, Simon MI. Defective platelet activation in G alpha(q)-deficient mice. Nature. 1997;389:183–186.

51. Jin J, Dasari VR, Sistare FD, Kunapuli SP. Distribution of P2Y receptor subtypes on haematopoietic cells. Br J Pharmacol. 1998;123:789–794.

52. Jin J, Quinton TM, Zhang J, Rittenhouse SE, Kunapuli SP. Adenosine diphosphate (ADP)-induced thromboxane A(2) generation in human platelets requires coordinated signaling through integrin alpha(IIb)beta(3) and ADP receptors. Blood. 2002;99:193–198.

53. Mangin P, Ohlmann P, Eckly A, Cazenave JP, Lanza F, Gachet C. The P2Y1 receptor plays an essential role in the platelet shape change induced by collagen when TxA2 formation is prevented. J Thromb Haemost. 2004;2:969–977.

54. Fabre JE, Nguyen M, Latour A, Keifer JA, Audoly LP, Coffman TM, et al. Decreased platelet aggregation, increased bleeding time and resistance to thromboembolism in P2Y1-deficient mice *Nat*. Nat Med. 1999;5:1199–1202.

55. Leon C, Freund M, Ravanat C, Baurand A, Cazenave JP, Gachet C. Key role of the P2Y(1) receptor in tissue factor-induced thrombin-dependent acute thromboembolism: studies in P2Y(1)-knockout mice and mice treated with a P2Y(1) antagonist. Circulation. 2001;103:718–723.

56. Lenain N, Freund M, Leon C, Cazenave JP, Gachet C. Inhibition of localized thrombosis in P2Y1-deficient mice and rodents treated with MRS2179, a P2Y1 receptor antagonist. J Thromb Haemost. 2003;1:1144–1149.

57. Ohlmann P, Laugwitz KL, Nurnberg B, Spicher K, Schultz G, Cazenave JP, et al. The human platelet ADP receptor activates Gi2 proteins. Biochem J. 1995;312(Pt 3):775–779.

58. Hechler B, Eckly A, Ohlmann P, Cazenave JP, Gachet C. The P2Y1 receptor, necessary but not sufficient to support full ADP-induced platelet aggregation, is not the target of the drug clopidogrel. Br J Haematol. 1998;103:858–866.

59. Savi P, Beauverger P, Labouret C, Delfaud M, Salel V, Kaghad M, et al. Role of P2Y1 purinoceptor in ADP-induced platelet activation. FEBS Lett. 1998;422:291–295.

60. Jin J, Kunapuli SP. Coactivation of two different G protein-coupled receptors is essential for ADP-induced platelet aggregation. Proc Natl Acad Sci USA. 1998;95:8070–8074.

61. Leon C, Ravanat C, Freund M, Cazenave JP, Gachet C. Differential involvement of the P2Y1 and P2Y12 receptors in platelet procoagulant activity. Arterioscler Thromb Vasc Biol. 2003;23:1941–1947.

62. Leon C, Alex M, Klocke A, Morgenstern E, Moosbauer C, Eckly A, et al. Platelet ADP receptors contribute to the initiation of intravascular coagulation Blood. 2004;103:594–600.

63. Foster CJ, Prosser DM, Agans JM, Zhai Y, Smith MD, Lachowicz JE, et al. Molecular identification and characterization of the platelet ADP receptor targeted by thienopyridine antithrombotic drugs. J Clin Invest. 2001;107: 1591–1598.

64. Andre P, Delaney SM, LaRocca T, Vincent D, Deguzman F, Jurek M, et al. P2Y12 regulates platelet adhesion/activation, thrombus growth, and thrombus stability in injured arteries. J Clin Invest. 2003;112:398–406.

65. Remijn JA, Wu YP, Jeninga EH, IJsseldijk MJ, van Willigen G, de Groot PG, et al. Role of ADP receptor P2Y(12) in platelet adhesion and thrombus formation in flowing blood. Arterioscler Thromb Vasc Biol. 2002;22:686–691.

66. Gachet C. Regulation of platelet functions by P2 receptors. Annu Rev Pharmacol Toxicol. 2006;46:277–300.

67. Kauffenstein G, Hechler B, Cazenave JP, Gachet C. Adenine triphosphate nucleotides are antagonists at the P2Y receptor. J Thromb Haemost. 2004;2:1980–1988.

68. Bodor ET, Waldo GL, Hooks SB, Corbitt J, Boyer JL, Harden TK. Purification and functional reconstitution of the human P2Y12 receptor. Mol Pharmacol. 2003;64:1210–1216.

69. Bennett JS. Novel platelet inhibitors. Annu Rev Med. 2001;52:161–184.

70. Sugidachi A, Asai F, Yoneda K, Iwamura R, Ogawa T, Otsuguro K, et al. Antiplatelet action of R-99224, an active metabolite of a novel thienopyridine-type G(i)-linked P2T antagonist CS-747. Br J Pharmacol. 2001;132:47–54.

71. Savi P, Pereillo JM, Uzabiaga MF, Combalbert J, Picard C, Maffrand JP, et al. Identification and biological activity of the active metabolite of clopidogrel. Thromb Haemost. 2000;84:891–896.

72. Ding Z, Kim S, Dorsam RT, Jin J, Kunapuli SP. Inactivation of the human P2Y12 receptor by thiol reagents requires interaction with both extracellular cysteine residues, Cys17 and Cys270. Blood. 2003;101:3908–3914.

73. Mahaut-Smith MP, Tolhurst G, Evans RJ. Emerging roles for P2X1 receptors in platelet activation. Platelets 2004;15:131–144.

74. Rolf MG, Brearley CA, Mahaut-Smith MP. Platelet shape change evoked by selective activation of P2X1 purinoceptors with alpha, beta-methylene ATP. Thromb Haemost. 2001;85:303–308.

75. Hechler B, Lenain N, Marchese P, Vial C, Heim V, Freund M, et al. A role of the fast ATP-gated P2X1 cation channel in thrombosis of small arteries in vivo. J Exp Med. 2003;198:661–667.

76. Oury C, Toth-Zsamboki E, Thys C, Tytgat J, Vermylen J, Hoylaerts MF. The ATP gated P2X1 ion channel acts as a positive regulator of platelet responses to collagen. Thromb Haemost. 2001;86:1264–1271.

77. Cattaneo M, Marchese P, Jacobson KA, Ruggeri Z. New insights into the role of P2X1 in platelet function. Haematologica. 2002;87:13–14.

78. Oury C, Kuijpers MJ, Toth-Zsamboki E, Bonnefoy A, Danloy S, Vreys I, et al. Overexpression of the platelet P2X1 ion channel in transgenic mice generates a novel prothrombotic phenotype. Blood. 2003;101:3969–3976.

79. Paul BZ, Vilaire G, Kunapuli SP, Bennett JS. Concurrent signaling from Gαq and Gαi-coupled pathways is essential for agonist-induced αVβ3 activation on human platelets. J Thromb Haemost. 2003;1:814–820.

80. Hechler B, Magnenat S, Zighetti ML, Kassack MU, Ullmann H, Cazenave JP, et al. Inhibition of platelet functions and thrombosis through selective or nonselective inhibition of the platelet P2 receptors with increasing doses of NF449 [4, 4', 4'', 4'''-(carbonylbis(imino-5, 1, 3-benzenetriylbis-(carbonylimino)))t etrakis-benzene-1, 3-disulfonic acid octasodium salt]. J Pharmacol Exp Ther. 2005;314:232–243.

81. Vu TK, Hung DT, Wheaton VI, Coughlin SR. Molecular cloning of a functional thrombin receptor reveals a novel proteolytic mechanism of receptor activation. Cell. 1991;64:1057–1068.

82. Trejo J, Altschuler Y, Fu HW, Mostov KE, Coughlin SR. Protease-activated receptor-1 down-regulation: a mutant HeLa cell line suggests novel requirements for PAR1 phosphorylation and recruitment to clathrin-coated pits. J Biol Chem. 2000;275:31255–31265.

83. Kahn ML, Zheng YW, Huang W, Bigornia V, Zeng D, Moff S, et al. A dual thrombin receptor system for platelet activation. Nature. 1998;394:690–694.

84. Shapiro MJ, Weiss EJ, Faruqi TR, Coughlin SR. Protease-activated receptors 1 and 4 are shut off with distinct kinetics after activation by thrombin. J Biol Chem. 2000;275:25216–25221.

85. Brass LF. Thrombin and platelet activation. Chest. 2003;124:18S–25S.

86. Wu CC, Hwang TL, Liao CH, Kuo SC, Lee FY, Teng CM. The role of PAR4 in thrombin-induced thromboxane production in human platelets. Thromb Haemost. 2003;90:299–308.

87. Weiss EJ, Hamilton JR, Lease KE, Coughlin SR. Protection against thrombosis in mice lacking PAR3. Blood. 2002;100: 3240–3244.

88. Sambrano GR, Weiss EJ, Zheng YW, Huang W, Coughlin SR. Role of thrombin signalling in platelets in haemostasis and thrombosis. Nature. 2001;413:74–78.

89. Covic L, Singh C, Smith H, Kuliopulos A. Role of the PAR4 thrombin receptor in stabilizing platelet-platelet aggregates as revealed by a patient with Hermansky-Pudlak syndrome. Thromb Haemost. 2002;87:722–727.

90. Brass LF, Vassallo RR Jr, Belmonte E, Ahuja M, Cichowski K, Hoxie JA. Structure and function of the human platelet thrombin receptor. Studies using monoclonal antibodies directed against a defined domain within the receptor N terminus. J Biol Chem. 1992;267:13795–13798.

91. Cook JJ, Sitko GR, Bednar B, Condra C, Mellott MJ, Feng DM, et al. An antibody against the exosite of the cloned thrombin receptor inhibits experimental arterial thrombosis in the African green monkey. Circulation. 1995;91:2961–2971.

92. Derian CK, Damiano BP, Addo MF, Darrow AL, D'Andrea MR, Nedelman M, et al. Blockade of the thrombin receptor protease-activated receptor-1 with a small-molecule antagonist prevents thrombus formation and vascular occlusion in nonhuman primates. J Pharmacol Exp Ther. 2003;304:855–861.

93. Covic L, Misra M, Badar J, Singh C, Kuliopulos A. Pepducin-based intervention of thrombin-receptor signaling and systemic platelet activation. Nat Med. 2002;8:1161–1165.

94. Leger AJ, Jacques SL, Badar J, Kaneider NC, Derian CK, Andrade-Gordon P, et al. Blocking the protease-activated receptor 1-4 heterodimer in platelet-mediated thrombosis. Circulation. 2006;113:1244–1254.

95. Wu CC, Teng CM. Comparison of the effects of PAR1 antagonists, PAR4 antagonists, and their combinations on thrombin-induced human platelet activation. Eur J Pharmacol. 2006;546:142–147.

96. Shankar H, Kahner B, Kunapuli SP. G-protein dependent platelet signaling – perspectives for therapy. Curr Drug Targets. 2006;7:1253–1263.

97. Murugappan S, Shankar H, Kunapuli SP. Platelet receptors for adenine nucleotides and thromboxane A2. Semin Thromb Hemost. 2004;30:411–418.

98. Huang JS, Ramamurthy SK, Lin X, Le Breton GC. Cell signalling through thromboxane A2 receptors. Cell Signal. 2004;16:521–533.

99. Dogne JM, Hanson J, de Leval X, Pratico D, Pace-Asciak CR, Drion P, et al. From the design to the clinical application of thromboxane modulators. Curr Pharm Des. 2006;12:903–923.

100. Plow EF, Byzova T. The biology of glycoprotein IIb-IIIa. Coron Artery Dis. 1999;10:547–551.

101. Plow EF, Shattil SJ. Integrin αIIbβ3 and platelet aggregation. In: Colman RW, Hirsh J, Marder VJ, Clowes AW, George JN, editors. Hemostasis and thrombosis: basic principles and clinical practice. 4th ed. Philadelphia, PA: Lippincott Williams & Wilkins; 2001. p. 479–491.

102. Bennett JS. Structure and function of the platelet integrin alphaIIbbeta3. J Clin Invest. 2005;115:3363–3369.

103. Plow EF, Haas TA, Zhang L, Loftus J, Smith JW. Ligand binding to integrins. J Biol Chem. 2000;275:21785–21788.

104. Hato T, Ginsberg MH, Shattil SJ. Integrin αIIbβ3. In: Michelson AD, editor. Platelets. San Diego, CA: Academic; 2002. p. 105–116.

105. Shattil SJ, Newman PJ. Integrins: dynamic scaffolds for adhesion and signaling in platelets. Blood. 2004;104: 1606–1615.

106. Heidenreich R, Eisman R, Surrey S, Delgrosso K, Bennett JS, Schwartz E, et al. Organization of the gene for platelet glycoprotein IIb. Biochemistry. 1990;29:1232–1244.

107. Fitzgerald LA, Steiner B, Rall SCJ, Lo SS, Phillips DR. Protein sequence of endothelial glycoprotein IIIa derived from a cDNA clone. Identity with platelet glycoprotein IIIa and similarity to "integrin". J Biol Chem. 1987;262: 3936–3939.

108. Zimrin AB, Gidwitz S, Lord S, Schwartz E, Bennett JS, White GC II, et al. The genomic organization of platelet glycoprotein IIIa. J Biol Chem. 1990;265:8590–8595.

109. Xiong JP, Stehle T, Diefenbach B, Zhang R, Dunker R, Scott DL, et al. Crystal structure of the extracellular segment of integrin alpha Vbeta3. Science. 2001;294:339–345.

110. Xiong JP, Stehle T, Zhang R, Joachimiak A, Frech M, Goodman SL, et al. Crystal structure of the extracellular segment of integrin alpha Vbeta3 in complex with an Arg-Gly-Asp ligand. Science. 2002;296:151–155.

111. Xiao T, Takagi J, Coller BS, Wang JH, Springer TA. Structural basis for allostery in integrins and binding to fibrinogen-mimetic therapeutics. Nature. 2004;432:59–67.

112. Xiong JP, Stehle T, Goodman SL, Arnaout MA. Integrins, cations and ligands: making the connection. J Thromb Haemost. 2003;7:1642–1654.

113. Marguerie GA, Plow EF, Edgington TS. Human platelets possess an inducible and saturable receptor specific for fibrinogen. J Biol Chem. 1979;254:5357–5363.

114. Bennett JS, Vilaire G. Exposure of platelet fibrinogen receptors by ADP and epinephrine. J Clin Invest. 1979;64: 1393–1401.

115. Marguerie GA, Plow EF. The fibrinogen dependent pathway of platelet aggregation. Ann NY Acad Sci. 1983;408: 556–567.

116. Ginsberg MH, Du X, Plow EF. Inside-out integrin signaling. Curr Opin Cell Biol. 1992;4:766.

117. Vinogradova O, Velyvis A, Velyviene A, Hu B, Haas TA, Plow EF, et al. A structural mechanism of integrin αIIbβ3 "inside-out" activation as regulated by its cytoplasmic face. Cell. 2002;110:587–597.

118. Ma YQ, Qin J, Plow EF. Platelet integrin αIIbβ3 : activation mechanisms. J Thromb Haemost. 2007;5:1345–1352.

119. Partridge AW, Liu S, Kim S, Bowie JU, Ginsberg MH. Transmembrane domain helix packing stabilizes integrin alphaIIbbeta3 in the low affinity state. J Biol Chem. 2005;280:7294–7300.

120. Luo BH, Carman CV, Takagi J, Springer TA. Disrupting integrin transmembrane domain heterodimerization increases ligand binding affinity, not valency or clustering. Proc Natl Acad Sci USA. 2005;102:3679–3684.

121. Takagi J, Petre BM, Walz T, Springer TA. Global conformational rearrangements in integrin extracellular domains in outside-in and inside-out signaling. Cell. 2002;110:599–611.

122. Shimaoka M, Takagi J, Springer TA. Conformational regulation of integrin structure and function. Annu Rev Biophys Biomol Struct. 2002;31:485–516.

123. Shattil SJ. Signaling through platelet integrin alpha IIb beta 3: inside-out, outside-in, and sideways. Thromb Haemost. 1999;82:318–325.

124. Phillips DR, Nannizzi-Alaimo L, Prasad KS. Beta3 tyrosine phosphorylation in alphaIIbbeta3 (platelet membrane GP IIb-IIIa) outside-in integrin signaling. Thromb Haemost. 2001;86:246–258.

125. Maree AO, Jneid H, Palacios IF, Rosenfield K, MacRae CA, Fitzgerald DJ. Growth arrest specific gene (GAS) 6 modulates platelet thrombus formation and vascular wall homeostasis and represents an attractive drug target. Curr Pharm Des. 2007;13:2656–2661.

126. Gould WR, Baxi SM, Schroeder R, Peng YW, Leadley RJ, Peterson JT, et al. Gas6 receptors Axl, Sky and Mer enhance platelet activation and regulate thrombotic responses. J Thromb Haemost. 2005;3:733–741.

127. Angelillo-Scherrer A, de Frutos P, Aparicio C, Melis E, Savi P, Lupu F, et al. Deficiency or inhibition of Gas6 causes platelet dysfunction and protects mice against thrombosis. Nat Med. 2001;7:215–221.

128. Brass LF, Zhu L, Stalker TJ. Minding the gaps to promote thrombus growth and stability. J Clin Invest. 2005;115:3385–3392.

129. Brass LF, Jiang H, Wu J, Stalker TJ, Zhu L. Contact-dependent signaling events that promote thrombus formation. Blood Cells Mol Dis. 2006;36:157–161.

130. Tadokoro S, Shattil SJ, Eto K, Tai V, Liddington RC, de Pereda JM, et al. Talin binding to integrin β tails: a final common step in integrin activation. Science. 2003;302:103–106.

131. Ratnikov BI, Partridge AW, Ginsberg MH. Integrin activation by talin. J Thromb Haemost. 2005;3:1783–1790.

132. Wegener KL, Partridge AW, Han J, Pickford AR, Liddington RC, Ginsberg MH, et al. Structural basis of integrin activation by talin. Cell. 2007;128:171–182.

133. Shi X, Ma YQ, Tu Y, Chen K, Wu S, Fukuda K, et al. The mitogen inducible gene-2 (Mig-2)-integrin interaction strengthens cell-matrix adhesion and modulates cell motility. J Biol Chem. 2007;282:20455–20466.

134. Ma YQ, Qin J, Wu C, Plow EF. Kindlin-2 (Mig-2): a co-activator of beta3-integrins. J Cell Biol. 2008;181(3):439–446.

2 The Role of Coagulation in Arterial and Venous Thrombosis

Kandice Kottke-Marchant

CONTENTS

ABSTRACT The coagulation cascade is integral to the hemostatic process and serves to limit the amount of blood loss during trauma. However, derangements in this process can result in venous thrombosis and contribute to the development of arterial atherothrombotic disease. Indeed, in arterial thrombosis, the effects of thrombin may extend far beyond coagulation activation and play an important role in activation of a wide variety of cells and the inflammatory processes. Venous thrombosis and arterial thrombotic diseases have traditionally been thought of as separate processes; however, they share many similarities in pathophysiology and risk factors. The activation of the coagulation cascade underlies both arterial and venous thrombosis, and biological triggers, such as inflammation, prothrombotic microparticles, and endothelial activation provide a plausible link between the two.

Key words: Coagulation cascade; Mechanism; Pathophysiology; Platelets; Thrombosis

INTRODUCTION

Hemostasis and thrombosis are related processes involving the coagulation system, platelets, endothelial cells, and the vascular wall. Indeed, Rudolf VIrchow, in the 1800s, postulated a triad of causes for thrombin formation: changes in the composition of blood, alterations in the vessel wall, and disruption of blood flow *(1)*. Physiological hemostasis occurs as a protective response to vascular injury; exposure of blood components to subendothelial proteins stimulates activation of platelets and production of the key coagulation enzyme thrombin leading to formation of a fibrin meshwork *(2,3)*. This process prevents

From: *Contemporary Cardiology: Antithrombotic Drug Therapy in Cardiovascular Disease*
Edited by: A.T. Askari and A.M. Lincoff (eds.), DOI 10.1007/978-1-60327-235-3_2
© Humana Press, a part of Springer Science+Business Media, LLC 2010

excessive bleeding or exsanguination after vascular injury or trauma. On the other hand, thrombosis can be considered "hemostasis in the wrong place and at the wrong time" *(4)*, with dysregulation of one or more elements of the hemostatic system contributing to formation of a platelet-fibrin thrombus that often occludes blood vessels, leading to pathologic complications *(5)*. If the thrombus occurs in the arterial system, distal ischemia can lead to acute coronary syndromes, myocardial infarctions, stroke, and peripheral extremity necrosis. Thrombus formation in the venous system, typically deep venous thrombosis, leads to local tissue congestion and decreased venous blood return, but dislodged thromboemboli may result in the potentially devastating complications of pulmonary infarction or, paradoxically, stroke.

CLINICAL MANIFESTATIONS OF ARTERIAL AND VENOUS THROMBOSIS

Thrombosis in the arterial system typically occurs superimposed on vascular abnormalities that are the result of other diseases, such as atherosclerosis or vasculitis *(6,7)*. Arterial atherosclerotic plaques are well known to liberate prothrombotic and inflammatory substances, such as oxidized lipids *(8)*, and express procoagulant molecules such as tissue factor *(9)*. While coagulation activation is undoubtedly involved in arterial thrombosis, platelet activation plays a crucial role, as described in Chap. 1, and antiplatelet drugs are the predominant pharmacologic therapy for this class of disorders *(10)*.

Arterial thrombosis in this setting, leading to vascular occlusion, can result in vascular-bed-specific pathologies. Coronary artery occlusion results in acute coronary syndromes or myocardial infarction, while cerebrovascular occlusion results in thrombotic stroke, and occlusion of peripheral arteries leads to peripheral arterial disease and gangrene. Paradoxical embolism of a venous thrombus through a patent foramen ovale may also lead to cerebrovascular thrombosis *(11)*.

In contrast to arterial thrombosis, venous thrombotic disorders are not usually associated with underlying vascular pathologies. Instead, venous thrombosis is associated with venous stasis or congenital dysregulation of coagulation proteins or natural anticoagulants *(12)*. Deep vein thrombi, most often involving the veins of the lower extremities, may dislodge and result in embolism to the pulmonary vasculature, with segmental pulmonary infarction and an attendant high morbidity rate *(13)*. Prolonged atrial fibrillation is often complicated by thrombosis of the atrial appendages. While multifactorial, stasis is a contributing factor in thrombosis observed with atrial fibrillation, the role of the coagulation system is highlighted by success with targeted anticoagulant therapies *(14,15)*.

While a direct clinical link between arterial and venous thrombosis has not been demonstrated, atherosclerosis and venous thromboembolic disease share similar risk factors, such as age, obesity, diabetes mellitus, and the metabolic syndrome *(16)*. The activation of the coagulation cascade underlies both arterial and venous thrombosis, and biological triggers, such as inflammation, prothrombotic microparticles, and endothelial activation provide a plausible link between the two. Some disorders, such as the antiphospholipid antibody syndrome (APS) and heparin-induced thrombocytopenia (HIT), have clear clinical associations with both arterial and venous thrombosis *(17)*. The thrombosis in HIT, for example, is thought to be multifactorial, with platelet activation, endothelial activation, and thrombin generation all contributing to the pathophysiology *(18)*. In the following sections, the physiology of coagulation and its regulation will be described, followed by a discussion of coagulation-associated risk factors for both arterial and venous thrombosis.

COAGULATION PHYSIOLOGY

The coagulation system, together with endothelial cells and platelets, is responsible for maintaining blood in a fluid state, but, when activated, rapidly results in development of a fibrin clot by conversion of the plasma protein, fibrinogen, to the polymer fibrin by the key enzyme, thrombin *(2,3)* (See Fig. 1).

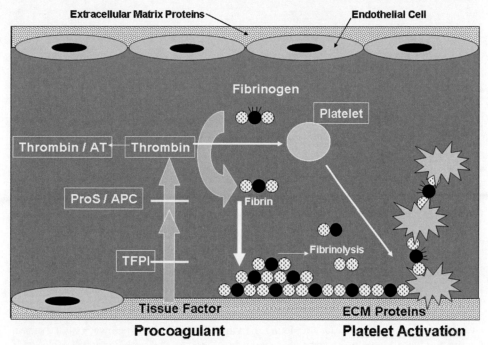

Fig. 1. The elements of the hemostatic system, with the relationship between endothelial cells, the vascular wall, coagulation, coagulation inhibitors, and platelet activation. *AT* antithrombin, *ProS* protein S, *APC* activated protein C, *TFPI* tissue factor pathway inhibitor, *ECM* extracellular matrix.

In addition to production of fibrin, thrombin has wide reaching functions that range from platelet activation to stimulation of endothelial cells, vascular smooth muscle cells (VSMC), monocytes, T lymphocytes, and fibroblasts, so the production and inhibition of thrombin is tightly regulated *(19,20)*.

The coagulation system comprises proenzymes that typically reside in the intravascular space in an inactivated state together with cofactors, cations, and cell-associated phospholipid. Coagulation can be activated by two principal mechanisms, the intrinsic and the extrinsic pathways that converge to produce thrombin by the common pathway through a series of inter-related enzymatic reactions *(21,22)* (See Fig. 2). These classical pathways form the basis of the two most frequently performed coagulation tests, the prothrombin time (PT), which measures the extrinsic and common pathways; and the activated partial thromboplastin time (APTT), which measures the intrinsic and common pathways. However, the physiologic activation of coagulation in vivo is not so segregated, with the initiation phase occurring through tissue factor exposed during vascular injury leading to a subsequent propagation phase and further amplification of the process by thrombin, due to activation of factors, V, VIII, XI *(23)*.

The Intrinsic Pathway

One mechanism of coagulation activation is the intrinsic pathway, so called because its components, factors XII, XI, IX, VIII, prekallikrein (PK), and high molecular weight kininogen (HMWK), are all plasma proteins and are "intrinsic" to the lumen of the blood vessel *(24)*. The intrinsic pathway can be activated when factor XII undergoes autoactivation to factor XIIa on a negatively charged surface through a process called "contact activation" *(25,26)* (See Fig. 3). Negatively charged surfaces

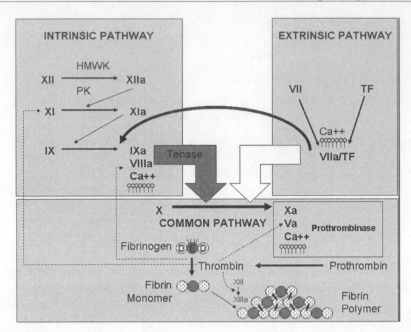

Fig. 2. Diagram of the coagulation cascade, depicting the intrinsic and extrinsic pathways of activation. The extrinsic pathway of activation is started with exposure of tissue factor (TF), coupled with factor VIIa that leads to the activation of factor X. The intrinsic pathway is started by the contact activation factors (factor XII, high molecular weight kininogen (HMWK), and prekallikrein (PK)) with eventual activation of factor X by the tenase complex (factors IXa, VIIIa, calcium (Ca++), and phospholipid). Activated factor X (Xa) participates in the prothrombinase complex (factor Xa, Va, Ca++, phospholipids) for the conversion of prothrombin to thrombin, which converts fibrinogen to fibrin monomer. Fibrin then polymerizes and is crosslinked by factor XIIIa. Further activation of coagulation is fostered by thrombin's activation of factors V, VIII, and XI.

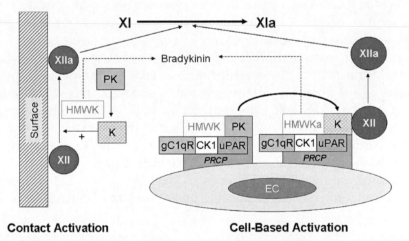

Fig. 3. The contact activation and cell-based activation pathways of the intrinsic factors. Negatively charged surfaces can activate the contact activation factors. Activation of factor XII leads to conversion of prekallikrein (PK) to kallikrein (K), facilitated by the cofactor high molecular weight kininogen (HMWK), with kallikrein further stimulating the activation of factor XII. Activated factor XII subsequently activates factor XI. The intrinsic pathway can also be activated in a cell-based process. HMWK-PK binds to a cell-based receptor complex, which includes a binding protein for the globular head domains of complement component C1q, designated gC1qR, cytokeratin 1 (CK1) and urokinase plasminogen activator receptor (u-PAR). Prolylcarboxypeptidase (PRCP) bound to the complex activates PK to form plasma kallikrein, resulting in factor XII activation.

include the artificial reagents in the APTT assay, such as kaolin, celite, and silica, which explains the dependence of the APTT on the contact activation factors. However, the intrinsic pathway can be activated in vivo by substances such as articular cartilage, endotoxin, L-homocysteine, and the developing thrombus (27,28).

Activation of factor XII leads to conversion of PK to kallikrein, facilitated by the cofactor HMWK, with kallikrein further stimulating the activation of factor XII (27). Activated factor XII subsequently activates factor XI, with factor XIa activating factor IX. Factor IXa, together with factor VIIIa, phospholipids, and calcium form the tenase complex that activates factor X.

The intrinsic pathway can also be activated in a cell-based process, as the components can assemble on endothelial cells, platelets, and granulocytes (27,29). HMWK-PK binds to a cell-based receptor complex, which includes a binding protein for the globular head domains of complement component C1q, designated gC1qR, cytokeratin 1 (CK1) and urokinase plasminogen activator receptor (u-PAR) (27) (See Fig. 3). Prolylcarboxypeptidase (PRCP) bound to the complex activates PK to form plasma kallikrein, resulting in factor XII activation (30). Apart from activation of factor XI, this complex is involved in other physiologic activities through formation of bradykinin, which participates in fibrinolysis activation and the production of antiplatelet molecules, nitric oxide and prostacyclin, from endothelial cells (27).

The role of the contact activation factors, XII, HMWK, and PK, has traditionally been discounted in physiological hemostasis, as patients with deficiencies of these proteins do not manifest a bleeding diathesis (31). Studies have shown that factor IX is principally activated not by the contact factors but by the tissue factor/factor VIIa complex, as described later, and physiologic hemostasis is thought to proceed principally through that extrinsic pathway (32). However, recent studies with factor XI and XII knockout mice have indicated that deficiency of these factors may impair formation of occlusive thrombi in arterial injury models and may be attractive targets for new antithrombotic agents (26,28,33).

The Extrinsic Pathway

The so-called Extrinsic Pathway of coagulation, comprising tissue factor and factor VII, is activated by tissue injury or cellular activation and is likely the primary mechanism for in vivo hemostasis (2,34). Tissue factor, complexed with activated factor VIIa in the presence of calcium and phospholipids, activates coagulation through conversion of factor X to Xa and also through activation of factor IX to IXa (35) (See Fig. 4).

Tissue factor is an intrinsic membrane glycoprotein expressed on many vascular wall cells, such as smooth muscle cells, pericytes, and fibroblasts (34,36). Constitutively expressed cell-based tissue factor can be exposed to the blood following vascular injury, but tissue factor expression can also be induced on vascular endothelial cells and leukocytes by thrombin and inflammatory stimuli (34,37,38). This induction is well described for monocytes, but also may occur in neutrophils and eosinophils and is thought to play a role in the thrombotic consequences of disseminated intravascular coagulation and sepsis (37,39). Activation of many cells leads to production of minute membrane-bound microparticles, which may be a source of circulating tissue factor activity (40). Platelets may also play a role, as recent studies have shown that platelets can be stimulated to produce TF mRNA and synthesize TF protein (34,41).

Fibrin Formation and Common Pathway Activation

The purpose of coagulation is the formation of an insoluble fibrin polymer as a hemostatic plug. To this end, the transformation of plasma-based fibrinogen to crosslinked fibrin is accomplished by several mechanisms and is tightly regulated.

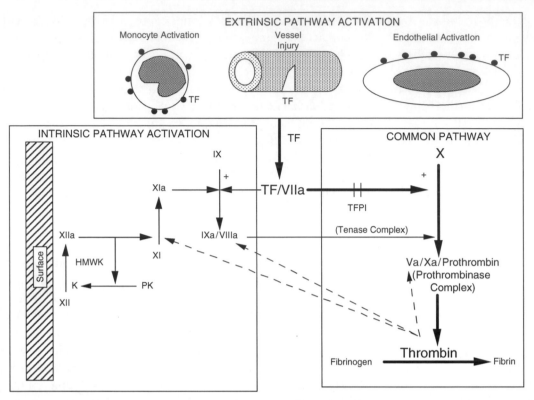

Fig. 4. Sources of tissue factor (TF) in the activation of coagulation. Tissue factor is expressed by many vascular wall cells and is exposed upon vascular injury. It can also be expressed during activation of endothelial cells and leukocytes, such as monocytes. Various cells, from endothelial cells to leukocytes and smooth muscle cells can produce small membrane-bound vesicles, called microparticles, that may express tissue factor. Tissue factor/factor VIIa is involved in the activation of coagulation through direct activation of factor X, but this is inhibited by tissue factor pathway inhibitor (TFPI). Tissue factor/factor VIIa can also activate factor IX, which leads to factor X activation through the tenase complex.

Fibrinogen is a large plasma protein that is a dimer composed of two mirror-image groups of three polypeptide chains, the Aα, Bβ, and γ chains *(42)* which are held together by a group of central disulfide bonds. Fibrinogen has a trinodular structure, with the central disulfide bonded area forming the central E domain, and the flanking polypeptides forming two lateral D domains *(43)* (See Fig. 2). The serine protease thrombin cleaves off small fibrinopeptides from the Aα and Bβ chains, converting fibrinogen to fibrin monomer. Binding sites in the central region of the fibrin monomer, termed A-knobs and B-knobs, are exposed. This allows the "knobs" on one monomer to bind to γC and βC "holes" in the D domains in another monomer in a half-staggered overlap pattern, facilitating noncovalent assembly into a fibrin protofibril polymer *(44,45)*. The protofibrils then associate laterally into bundles that form thicker fibers. Concurrent with the conversion of fibrinogen to fibrin, thrombin catalyzes the activation of factor XIII, a transglutaminase enzyme that stabilizes the fibrin polymer by forming covalent crosslinks between γ chains in the D domains of adjacent fibrin molecules *(46)*.

Thrombin, which plays a key role in the formation of fibrin and its crosslinking, is a serine protease that is formed from prothrombin by the action of factor Xa and the prothrombinase complex, a phospholipid membrane-based complex consisting of factors Xa and Va together with calcium *(20)*. Thrombin has many functions apart from fibrin formation and is associated with propagation of coagulation through activation of factors V and VIII, thus accelerating the activity of the prothrombinase and tenase complexes, respectively *(47)* (Fig. 2). Thrombin is further involved with amplification of coagulation through its direct activation of factor XI. Indeed, individuals with factor XI deficiency typically only have bleeding when large amounts of thrombin are formed, such as during surgical procedures *(48)*.

Thrombin, through a series of G-coupled protease-activated receptors (PARs), also activates platelets and other cells, such as endothelial cells and monocytes *(19)*. Upregulation of PARs in smooth muscle cells is thought to play a key role in the pathogenesis of atherosclerosis and restenosis *(49)*. Due to its wide-ranging effects, the activity of thrombin is closely regulated, as discussed later.

The activation of thrombin requires the action of factor Xa, another serine protease, in the prothrombinase complex resulting in cleavage of a peptide fragment, prothrombin fragment F1 + 2, from prothrombin *(50)*. The formation of active factor Xa from the proenzyme factor X is considered the start of the common pathway and can be triggered by both tissue factor/factor VIIa from the extrinsic pathway and by the tenase complex (factors IXa, VIIIa, calcium, and phospholipids) from the intrinsic pathway *(2)*. Having two separate mechanisms for factor Xa activation is thought to be associated with two temporal stages of blood coagulation *(32,51)*, the initiation and propagation stages. In the initiation stage, factor X is initially activated by tissue factor/factor VIIa. This produces small amounts of thrombin, which activates factors V and VIII, leading to further thrombin production *(47)*. After initiation, an inhibitor, tissue factor pathway inhibitor (TFPI), downregulates the ability of tissue factor/VIIa to activate factor X *(52)*. Coagulation then enters the propagation phase, directing the activity of tissue factor/VIIa toward activation of factor IXa, resulting in a switch of the primary activation of factor X to be via the intrinsic pathway tenase complex *(51)*. Further thrombin production leads to the activation of factor XIa, which amplifies the propagation phase further.

Lessons from Studying In Vivo Coagulation Activation

Most studies that have been used to define the coagulation process have been performed in vitro, often with highly purified single protein components. While these have helped delineate the processes involved, they may not necessarily indicate the relative importance of coagulation factors in hemostasis, hemorrhage, or thrombosis *(145)*. For example, the processes of hemostasis and thrombosis may differ, as in vivo studies have shown defective thrombus formation in the absence of factors XII and XI, while patients with factor XII deficiency do not display a hemostatic defect *(26,28)*. The clinical phenotype for deficiency of factors VIII and IX is hemophilia, a significant bleeding disorder, so this helps to indicate the importance of factor X activation by the tenase complex compared to tissue factor/VIIa. Contrary to the dogma that tissue factor is extrinsic to the blood vessel lumen, circulating tissue factor-bearing microparticles have been shown to be involved with in vivo thrombus development *(53)*. It has been shown from in vivo studies that platelet thrombus formation and fibrin formation may occur more simultaneously than sequentially, and other studies question the crucial role of platelet membrane phospholipids in the formation of fibrin *(54,55)*. While these studies may challenge the classical paradigm of coagulation and its relationship with platelets, they also serve to underscore the complex and inter-related nature of the hemostatic process.

REGULATION OF COAGULATION

Coagulation activation involves numerous proteins and amplification steps, so its activation and propagation is closely regulated. The activities of thrombin and tissue factor, in particular, have several well-studied inhibitors and/or regulatory mechanisms. These regulatory mechanisms are of clinical significance, as defective regulation due to congenital inhibitor deficiency may lead to clinical thrombosis, while pharmacologic use of the inhibitors has successfully controlled thrombosis. The endothelial cells that line the blood vessels also are able to regulate the function of many aspects of hemostasis from coagulation to platelet activation to fibrinolysis

Regulation of Tissue Factor

Classically, since tissue factor was thought only to exist in locations extrinsic to the blood vessel lumen, regulation of tissue factor activity has been thought to involve primarily vessel injury with exposure of constitutively expressed tissue factor to flowing blood. While this process is undoubtedly involved, other mechanisms for regulation of tissue factor exposure and activity likely play a role. Tissue factor can exist in an encrypted, inactive form, or a decrypted, active form; decryption may involve conformational or disulfide bonding changes *(56,57)*. The major regulation of tissue factor/factor VIIa activity is through tissue factor pathway inhibitor β (TFPIβ), a Kunitz-type proteinase inhibitor *(52)*. TFPIβ forms a quaternary complex with tissue factor, factors VIIa and Xa; the factor Xa within the complex is deactivated, but binding to adjacent tissue factor/factor VIIa prevents further factor X activation *(38,58)*. TFPI may also further downregulate coagulation by causing TF-expressing cells to internalize cell surface TF/factor VIIa complexes *(59)*. The importance of TFPI as a hemostatic regulator is highlighted by the embryonic lethality due to hemorrhage observed in TFPI knockout mice *(60)*.

Regulation of Thrombin

The activity of thrombin is closely regulated by several direct and indirect mechanisms; these involve antithrombin, a direct-acting inhibitor, or take advantage of thrombin's proteolytic activities through the activation of protein C. Several naturally occurring thrombin inhibitory molecules have been developed by blood-sucking insects or envenoming snakes. One such molecule, hirudin, is a very potent direct thrombin inhibitor (DTI); OTIs have been developed as successful commercial antithrombotic agents, highlighting the importance of regulating endogenous thrombin activity *(61)*.

Antithrombin (formerly called Antithrombin III) is a serine protease inhibitor that is a direct inhibitor of thrombin and other serine proteases *(2,20)*. The reactive site loop (P1–P17) of antithrombin includes a scissile P_1-P_1' (Arg393-Ser394) bond that resembles the substrate for thrombin and other serine proteases *(62,63)*. Once thrombin cleaves the bond, the protease is covalently linked to the P1 residue and an inactive thrombin/antithrombin complex is formed (See Fig. 5). The ability of antithrombin to inhibit thrombin is accelerated approximately 1000-fold by heparin binding to arginine residues in the D-helix of antithrombin, with a resultant conformational change of the P1-P17 loop and exposure of the P1-P1' reactive center *(64,65)*. The inactivated thrombin/antithrombin complex dissociates from heparin, allowing heparin to bind to another antithrombin molecule and catalyze the inactivation of yet more thrombin. In vivo, the luminal surface of endothelial cells is rich in heparan sulfate; bound antithrombin is thus maintained in an active conformation, ready to facilitate the rapid inactivation of thrombin.

Another thrombin regulatory mechanism is the thrombomodulin/protein C system, a multimolecular system that regulates blood coagulation, principally through the proteolytic degradation of activated factors V (fVa) and VIII (fVIIIa) *(20,66,67)* (See Fig. 5). Thrombin binds to an endothelial cell receptor, thrombomodulin, via the anion-binding exosite *(68)* and through conformational changes leads to a change in thrombin's substrate specificity from fibrinogen to protein C with activation of protein C *(69)*. Protein C interacts with the thrombomodulin/thrombin complex by binding to endothelial cell protein C receptor (EPCR), which appears to be an important step in physiological protein C activation *(70)*. In addition to activating protein C, the thrombomodulin/thrombin complex also is able to

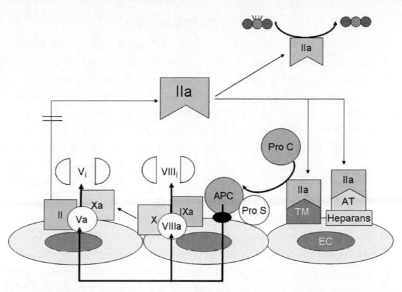

Fig. 5. Inhibition of thrombin. Thrombin (Factor IIa) is inhibited by antithrombin (AT) bound to heparans on endothelial surfaces. It is also regulated by binding to thrombomodulin (TM) on endothelial cells, where it converts protein C (Pro C) to activated protein C (APC). APC is a protease that degrades factors Va and VIIIa, thus decreasing further thrombin production.

activate thrombin activatable fibrinolysis inhibitor (TAFI), which results in inhibition of fibrin degradation and may also have a broad anti-inflammatory role *(71,72)*. Activated protein C is released from the EPCR, and combines with protein S, another vitamin K-dependent factor, on endothelial or platelet phospholipid surfaces *(66,67)*. This activated protein C complex is able to degrade factors Va and VIIIa, thus slowing the procoagulant drive *(2)*.

Protein Z System

Another inhibitory mechanism of the coagulation system has been described, namely the protein Z system. Protein Z is a vitamin-K dependent protein, with an inhibitor, known as protein Z-dependent protease inhibitor (ZPI) *(73)*. ZPI has been shown to inhibit factor Xa in a process that requires protein Z, calcium, and phospholipids *(74)*. ZPI has further been shown to inhibit factors XIa and IXa in a mechanism not requiring protein Z, calcium, or phospholipids *(75,76)*. This inhibitory mechanism has been shown to play a role in hemostasis from in vitro studies and mouse models, but the role of ZPI and protein Z as an anticoagulant system in humans remains to be fully elucidated *(73)*.

Role of Endothelium

Endothelial cells are involved in many aspects of coagulation regulation. As indicated earlier, heparan sulfate and thrombomodulin are involved in inhibition of thrombin activity. Endothelial cells also inhibit platelet function through release of nitric oxide and prostacyclin and have profibrinolytic function through release of tissue plasminogen activator (tPA) *(77)*. However, when activated by thrombin or inflammatory cytokines, endothelial cells can facilitate coagulation through expression of tissue factor, expression of procoagulant lipids, release of procoagulant microparticles, downregulation of thrombomodulin, and release of von Willebrand factor *(78)*.

Role of Microparticles

Microparticles are minute membrane-bound vesicles released from cell membranes by an exocytosis process *(79)*. They have been shown to arise from a wide variety of cells, including endothelial cells, platelets, monocytes, and erythrocytes *(80)*. Microparticles are released from the surface of cells following apoptosis or activation; the release can be stimulated by a wide variety of agonists, such as cytokines, thrombin, and endotoxin, but also physical stimuli such as shear stress or hypoxia *(79,81)*. During the formation of microparticles, membrane asymmetry is lost, with an exposure of anionic phospholipids, for example, phosphatidyl serine, to the external microparticle membrane *(82)*. This provides a binding site for coagulation complexes, such as the tenase and prothrombinase complexes. Because microparticles arise from the cell membrane, their protein antigen composition is characteristic of their cell of origin and can be used to identify their source.

Circulating microparticles may contribute to the support of coagulation and development of thrombosis or may have anticoagulant properties, depending on their number and cell of origin or the producing stimuli. The microparticle's anionic phospholipid surface has been shown to support thrombin generation through assembly of procoagulant complexes, and may be associated with clinical procoagulant states and other diseases *(83,84,146)*. Tissue factor can be expressed by microparticles' release by some cell types and may further contribute to their procoagulant activity *(38,85)*. Depending on their cell surface antigens, microparticles may also contribute to the recruitment of cells to developing thrombi. For example, monocyte microparticles expressing tissue factor and P selectin glycoprotein ligand-1 have been shown to bind to endothelial cells and platelets and to accumulate with the developing thrombus *(86)*. However, not all microparticles are necessarily procoagulant. Microparticles arising from endothelial cells have been shown to have anticoagulant properties in some circumstances, with increased expression of TFPI and expression of activated protein C *(79,87)*.

Elevated microparticle levels have been described in many cardiovascular and thrombotic disorders and are often reported to correlate with clinical events *(79–81)*. However, until the laboratory methods for quantifying and characterizing microparticles are more standardized, their use as a diagnostic or prognostic tool will be limited *(79,88)*.

Interaction Between Coagulation and Platelet Activation

A striking feature of the hemostatic system is the degree of redundancy and interdependence of the activation and regulatory processes involved. Not only are there multiple ways for coagulation to become activated, but there are also numerous and bidirectional associations between the coagulation system and platelets.

The coagulation system supports platelet activation and function in several ways. Thrombin is a potent activator of platelets through activation of PARs *(19,89)*. Fibrinogen provides the bridge for platelet-platelet aggregation through its bivalent binding to the platelet glycoprotein IIb/IIIa (α_{IIb}/β_3) receptor *(90)*. Von Willebrand factor, a hemostatic protein released from endothelial cells, supports both platelet adhesion under shear and platelet aggregation *(91)*.

On the other hand, activated platelets play a vital procoagulant role that serves as a link between platelet function and coagulation activation *(92)*. Platelet membrane phospholipids undergo a rearrangement during activation with a transfer of phosphatidyl serine from the inner table to the outer table of the platelet membrane, providing a binding site for phospholipid-dependent coagulation complexes that activate both factor X and prothrombin. Additionally, the GPIb/V/IX complex is thought to participate in activation of factors XI and XII. The platelet alpha granules release many procoagulant factors during platelet activation, including fibrinogen, von Willebrand factor, and factor V.

COAGULATION DYSREGULATION IN ARTERIAL AND VENOUS THROMBOSIS

The pathophysiology of arterial thrombotic diseases, mainly centered around cardiovascular atherosclerotic sequelae, is largely considered distinct from that of venous thrombotic disorders, such as deep vein thrombosis (DVT). Inflammation, the metabolic syndrome, lipid dysregulation, endothelial dysfunction, and platelet activation are characteristics of arterial thrombotic syndromes. Dysregulation of the coagulation system is thought to play a major role in the pathophysiology of venous thrombosis, highlighted by the well-described association between deficiency of the natural anticoagulants and venous thrombosis *(93)*. However, evaluation of the risk factors for both disorders shows some similarities, particularly age and obesity, and there is some evidence that patients with venous thrombosis have a higher risk of cardiovascular disease *(94,95)*. Indeed, some disorders such as antiphospholipid antibodies and HIT are complicated by both arterial and venous thrombosis, suggesting a unifying mechanism.

Coagulation Dysregulation and Venous Thromboembolic Disease

Venous thrombosis typically manifests as a DVT, usually in the lower extremities, or as a pulmonary embolism (PE) due to embolization of the thrombus to the pulmonary vasculature. A combination of vascular stasis and coagulation dysregulation is thought to be principally involved in the pathophysiology of venous thrombosis, as there is usually little underlying vascular pathology. However, inflammatory and fibrinolytic mechanisms and production of tissue factor-bearing microparticles may contribute *(96)*. Venous thrombosis is relatively common, with an average annual incidence rate of 121.5 per 100,000 person-years in the USA and is the third most prevalent cardiovascular disease after coronary artery disease and stroke *(97)*. The risk factors for venous thrombosis have been well studied and include both acquired and congenital risk factors (See Table 1). In general, venous thrombosis is considered a multifactorial or multigenetic disease, with the combination of more than one risk factor increasing the risk of developing venous thrombosis *(98)*.

CONGENITAL THROMBOPHILIA

Recognition of familial tendencies for thrombosis initially led to a search for genetic abnormalities in the coagulation system. The genetic abnormalities first to be described in association with thrombophilia were mutations leading to loss-of-function of natural anticoagulants, such as antithrombin, protein C, or protein S *(99–101)*. These disorders are rare and heterozygous individuals have an increased risk for venous thromboembolism. In addition, elevated plasma levels of several coagulation proteins, including fibrinogen, factors VIII, IX, and XI, have been described to be associated with an increased risk of venous thrombosis *(102)*. Furthermore, genetic polymorphisms associated with venous thrombosis and arterial vascular disease have been found in many of the procoagulant proteins, including prothrombin, fibrinogen, factors V, VII, XI, and XIII *(103,147)*. Polymorphisms of EPCR, Z Protein inhibitor, fibrinolytic proteins, and enzymes in the transsulfuration pathway leading to high homocysteine levels have also been described, but their association with venous thrombotic disease is not well established. The following discussion will concentrate on the two most well-described venous thrombotic risk factors, Factor V Leiden and the prothrombin G20210A mutation

FACTOR V LEIDEN

Patients resistant to the activity of APC were described by Dahlback in 1993 *(104)*, and the molecular basis for this defect was shown to be a point mutation in the factor V gene located on chromosome 1 (1691G-A), which was called Factor V Leiden (FVL) *(105)*. The FVL mutation results in an arginine-glutamine substitution at amino acid 506 (Arg506Gln), the site of the first molecular cleavage of factor Va by APC. This results in diminished activated protein C cleavage of factor Va and continued formation of thrombin by the prothrombinase complex (i.e., APC resistance).

The FVL mutation is fairly common in the Caucasian population with a frequency of 2–15%, but is uncommon in African blacks and Asians *(106,107)*. The mutation is detected in up to 40% of patients with venous thrombosis *(103)*. FVL alone imparts approximately a five to eightfold increased risk for venous thrombosis in heterozygotes and 80-fold in homozygotes *(108,109)*. Clinical studies have shown FVL to be a risk factor for deep venous thrombosis, pulmonary embolism, cerebral vein thrombosis, and superficial thrombophlebitis *(110)*.

PROTHROMBIN G20210A

Due to the central role of thrombin, increased prothrombin levels are a likely risk factor for venous thrombosis. In studying patients from families with unexplained thrombophilia, Poort et al. identified a G-A transition at nucleotide 20210 in the 3′-untranslated portion of the prothrombin gene in 5 of 28 patients *(111)*. The mutation is associated with increased levels of functionally normal prothrombin, with heterozygotes having a level about 50% higher than unaffected individuals *(111)*. Prothrombin G20210A results in elevated prothrombin levels and a two to fivefold increased risk of venous thrombosis *(108,111)*

ACQUIRED THROMBOPHILIA

Venous thrombosis is predominantly a disease of the aging, with the annual incidence increasing rapidly after age 45 to approximately 1,000 per 100,000 person-years by age 80 *(112)*. Other acquired risk factors associated with venous thrombosis include malignancy, obesity, surgery, trauma, immobilization, central venous catheters, prior venous thrombosis, pregnancy, and hormone therapy *(112,113)* (See Table 1). Apart from age, malignancy has the strongest association with venous thrombosis, with 20% of venous thromboembolic events occurring in the setting of malignancy, most commonly with malignant brain tumors and cancer of the ovary, pancreas, colon, stomach, lung, and kidney *(112,114)*. There has been a great deal of recent press regarding an increased risk of thrombosis associated with long-haul airplane travel, and epidemiologic studies have shown approximately a two to fourfold increased risk *(115)*.

Two acquired risk factors for thrombosis, APS and HIT, merit discussion, as they are autoimmune-based disorders and are associated clinically with both venous and arterial thrombosis *(17)*. HIT is a syndrome associated with thrombocytopenia and thrombosis developing approximately 5–14 days following heparin therapy *(18)*. The inciting antigen in HIT is thought to be heparin/platelet factor 4 *(116)*, with complexes of antibodies/heparin/platelet factor 4 binding to the FcγIIa receptor on platelets and endothelial cells, triggering platelet and endothelial activation with release of prothrombotic microparticles *(117)*. In the APS, the antigen is variable, but is typically a protein associated with phospholipid membranes or cardiolipin; common antigens include β2-glycoprotein I and prothrombin *(118)*, resulting in laboratory detection of anticardiolipin antibodies, anti-β2 glycoprotein I antibodies and/or the lupus anticoagulant. The APS is associated clinically with arterial thrombosis, venous thrombosis, and pregnancy complications in the setting of persistence of antiphospholipid antibodies for more than twelve weeks *(119)*. The mechanism of thrombosis in patients with APS is still a matter of debate, but proposed mechanisms include platelet activation through binding b2 glycoprotein I, disruption of the Annexin V anticoagulant shield, and upregulation of endothelial cell tissue factor activity *(17,120,121)*. Since both APS and HIT involve activation of platelets, coagulation, and endothelial cells, it is not surprising that both populations of patients demonstrate similar indicators of a hypercoagulable and inflammatory state, including increased thrombin generation, markers of platelet activation, endothelial cell dysfunction, and increased microparticles *(17,79,122–124)*.

Table 1

Risk factors associated with venous thrombosis

Acquired	*Inherited*
Major surgery	Factor V Leiden
Trauma, accidental and surgical	Prothrombin gene mutation G20210A
Solid and hematopoietic malignancies	Antithrombin deficiency
Cancer therapies	
Central venous catheters	Protein C deficiency
Limb immobilization	Protein S deficiency
Hip, knee replacement	
Prolonged cast or splinting	
Stroke	
Bed ridden due to acute illness:	Hyperhomocysteinemia*
Cardiopulmonary disease	FVIII activity*
Infectious disease	*Hereditary and environment contributions
Inflammatory disease	
Malignancy	
Antiphospholipid antibody syndrome	Dysfibrinogenemia
Heparin-induced thrombocytopenia	
Paroxysmal nocturnal hemaglobinuria	
Disseminated intravascular coagulation/sepsis	
Inflammatory bowel disease	
Advancing age, especially >50	
Obesity	
Pregnancy, oral contraceptives, hormone replacement therapies	
Long-haul airline travel	Controversial:
	Factors IX and XI
	Plasminogen deficiency
	Hypofibrinolysis
	PAI-1 4G/5G mutation
	ZPI deficiency
	Factor XIII polymorphisms
	Endothelial protein C receptor
	Thrombomodulin

References: *(107,116,117)*

The Role of Coagulation in Arterial Disease

LINKS BETWEEN COAGULATION AND ATHEROSCLEROSIS

Atherogenesis is a complex process involving endothelial cells, VSMC, macrophages, platelets, lipids, the inflammatory system, and cytokines that leads to the development of lipid-rich atherosclerotic plaques that result in vascular stenosis *(9,125,126,148)*. Ongoing inflammation steers cellular proliferation and extracellular matrix production toward apoptosis, matrix degradation, and accumulation of necrotic material *(9,126)*. Further disruption of a plaque made vulnerable by inflammation often leads to an acute thrombosis and vascular occlusion, due to platelet thrombus formation *(127–129)*. Increased tissue factor expression by cells within the ruptured plaque can lead to coagulation activation, thrombin activation, and fibrin formation *(23)*. If vascular occlusion does not occur with subclinical rupture, repetitive plaque rupture, thrombosis, and cellular proliferation lead to further luminal narrowing *(130)*. The crucial role of both platelets and coagulation in the pathogenesis of acute coronary atherothrombosis is shown by the success of pharmacologic intervention with antiplatelet and anticoagulant drugs *(131,132)*.

Tissue factor plays several roles in atherogenesis. Many cells within the atherosclerotic plaque express tissue factor *(23)*. That tissue factor may play a role in pathogenesis of plaque-associated thrombosis is shown by animal studies demonstrating inhibition of thrombosis by treatment with recombinant-activated factor VII or TFPI *(133,134)*. In addition, circulating tissue factor associated with cellular microparticles may also play a role in atherothrombosis. Procoagulant microparticles have been shown to be elevated in patients with acute coronary syndromes compared to patients with stable angina *(79,135)*. However, other reports indicate that endothelial microparticles observed in acute myocardial infarction may have an anticoagulant phenotype, through expression of TFPI and activated protein C *(87)*. An observation of increased levels of leukocyte-derived microparticles in subclinical atherosclerosis suggests a predictive value for microparticle measurement *(84,136)*. While the role of circulating microparticles in atherothrombosis is not firmly established, drugs such as statins, which have been shown to decrease microparticle release, may play an additional role in treatment of coronary disease *(137)*.

Thrombin generation certainly plays a role in atherothrombosis through its stimulation of fibrin production, but it has been shown to be an integral regulator as well due to its ability to activate platelets, and mediate inflammatory signals to macrophages, smooth muscle cells and endothelial cells *(9,19,149)*. Thrombin, through action on endothelial PARs-1 and -2, stimulates expression of leukocyte adhesion molecules and secretion of proinflammatory chemokines such as monocyte chemotactic protein-1, platelet-derived growth factor (PDGF), IL-6 and IL-8 *(9,138)*. Thrombin may also play a role in matrix remodeling due to its ability to stimulate endothelial production of matrix metalloproteinases *(139)*. Further coagulation effects of thrombin on endothelial cells include release of von Willebrand factor, factor VIII, and tPA *(19)*. Smooth muscle cells also express PAR-1 and -2, and thrombin may stimulate their proliferation, production of growth factors, production of extracellular matrix proteins, and expression of tissue factor *(9,140)*. Thrombin activation of platelets through PAR-3 and -4 not only leads to platelet activation, but also to secretion of inflammatory mediators (PDGF, platelet factor 4, RANTES) and expression of CD40 ligand, that serves to attract leukocytes and activate them *(141)*. As discussed previously, thrombin's protease activity is usually short lived due to many inhibitory mechanisms. However, there is some evidence that thrombin may be sequestered in atherosclerotic lesions, resulting in persistent thrombin activity with consequent cellular effects and vascular remodeling *(19)*.

ROLE OF THROMBOPHILIA RISK FACTORS IN ARTERIAL THROMBOSIS

Thrombophilia risk factors, as described earlier, are typically associated with an increased risk of venous thrombosis as most risk factors are due to increased function of coagulation proteins or decreased function of the natural anticoagulants. There is, however, a modest association between some of the thrombophilia risk factors with arterial thrombotic disease *(142)*, especially in younger individuals or in association with oral contraceptive use. The association between factor V Leiden and myocardial infarction has been studied in several large meta-analyses, with an overall modestly increased relative risk of MI in factor V Leiden carriers of 1.17 (95% CI 1.08–1.28) *(143)*. Data from a meta-analysis of prothrombin G20210A and MI showed an increased odds ratio of 1.28 that was nonsignificant (95% CI, 0.94–1.73) *(144)*. Despite single case reports, prospective studies have not shown an association between deficiency of antithrombin, protein C, or protein S and MI *(142)*.

SUMMARY

The coagulation proteins have a vital role in the hemostatic process, defending the body from exsanguination during trauma. However, it is clear that dysregulation of the coagulation system can variously lead to venous thrombosis and contribute to the development of arterial atherothrombotic disease. Indeed, in arterial thrombosis, the effects of thrombin may extend far beyond coagulation activation and play an important role in activation of a wide variety of cells and the inflammatory processes. Venous thrombosis and arterial thrombotic diseases have traditionally been thought of as separate processes; however, they share many similarities in pathophysiology and risk factors. The activation of the coagulation cascade underlies both arterial and venous thrombosis, and biological triggers, such as inflammation, prothrombotic microparticles, and endothelial activation provide a plausible link between the two.

REFERENCES

1. Virchow R (1856) Phlogose und thrombose in Gefasystem. Staatsdruckeri, Gesammelte Abhandlungen zur Wissenschaftlichen Medizin, Frankfurt
2. Dahlback B (2000) Blood coagulation. Lancet 355:1627–1632
3. Mann KG (1999) Biochemistry and physiology of blood coagulation. Thromb Haemost 82:165–174
4. Macfarlane RG (1977) Haemostasis: introduction. Br Med Bull 33:183–185
5. Colman RW (2006) Are hemostasis and thrombosis two sides of the same coin? J Exp Med 203:493–495
6. Badimon L, Chesebro JH, Badimon JJ. Thrombus formation on ruptured atherosclerotic plaques and rethrombosis on evolving thrombi. Circulation 1992;86(upplIII):III-74 – III-85.
7. Badimon L, Vilahur G (2007) Platelets, arterial thrombosis and cerebral ischemia. Cerebrovasc Dis 24(Suppl 1):30–39
8. Fruhwirth GO, Loidl A, Hermetter A (2007) Oxidized phospholipids: from molecular properties to disease. Biochim Biophys Acta 1772:718–736
9. Croce K, Libby P (2007) Intertwining of thrombosis and inflammation in atherosclerosis. Curr Opin Hematol 14(1):55–61
10. Lange RA, Hillis LD (2004) Antiplatelet therapy for ischemic heart disease. N Engl J Med 350:277–280
11. Montessuit M, Pretre R, Bruschweiler I, Faidutti B (1997) Screening for patent foramen ovale and prevention of paradoxical embolus. Ann Vasc Surg 11(2):168–172
12. Rosendaal FR (1999) Venous thrombosis: a multicausal disease. Lancet 353:1167–1173
13. Tapson VF (2008) Acute pulmonary embolism. N Engl J Med 358:1037–1052
14. Hughes M, Lip GY: Guideline Development Group, National Clinical Guideline for Management of Atrial Fibrillation in Primary and Secondary Care, National Institute for Health and Clinical Excellence. Stroke and thromboembolism in atrial fibrillation: a systematic review of stroke risk factors, risk stratification schema and cost effectiveness data. Thromb Haemost. 2008;99:295-304
15. Tan KT, Lip GY (2003) Atrial fibrillation: should we target platelets or the coagulation pathway? Card Electrophysiol Rev 7:370–371
16. Pradoni P (2007) Links between arterial and venous disease. J Intern Med 262:341–350
17. Hoppensteadt DA, Walenga JM (2008) The relationship between the antiphospholipid syndrome and heparin-induced thrombocytopenia. Hematol Oncol Clin North Am 22:1–18
18. Warkentin TE (2007) Heparin-induced thrombocytopenia. Hematol Oncol Clin North Am 21:589–607
19. Martorell L, Martinez-Gonzalez J, Rodriguez C, Gentile M, Calvayrac O, Badimon L (2008) Thrombin and protease-activated receptors (PARs) in atherothrombosis. Thromb Haemost 99:305–315
20. Lane DA, Philippou H, Huntington JA (2005) Directing thrombin. Blood 106:2605–2612
21. Macfarlane RG (1964) An enzyme cascade in the blood clotting mechanism, and its function as a biochemical amplifier. Nature 202:498–499
22. Davie EW, Ratnoff OD (1964) Waterfall sequence for intrinsic blood clotting. Science 145:1310–1312
23. Mackman N (2004) Role of tissue factor in hemostasis, thrombosis, and vascular development. Artioscler Thromb Vasc Biol 24:1015–1022

24. Sainz PRA, Colman RA (2007) Fifty years of research on the plasma kallikrein-kinin system: from protein structure and function to cell biology and in-vivo pathophysiology. Thromb Haemost 98:77–83
25. Wiggins RC, Cochran CG (1979) The autoactivation of rabbit Hageman factor. J Exp Med 150:1122–1133
26. Gailani D, Tenne T (2007) Intrinsic pathway of coagulation and arterial thrombosis. Arterioscler Thromb Vasc Biol 27:2507–2513
27. Schmaier AH, McCrae KR (2007) The plasma kallikrein-kinin system: its evolution from contact activation. J Thromb Haemost 5:2323–2329
28. Renne T, Pozgajova M, Gruner S, Schuh K, Pauer HU, Burfeind P, Gailani D, Nieswandt B (2005) Defective thrombus formation in mice lacking coagulation factor XII. J Exp Med 280:28572–28580
29. Motta G, Rojkjaer R, Hasan AAK, Cines DB, Schmaier AH (1998) High molecular weight kininogen regulates prekallikrein assembly and activation on endothelial cells: a novel mechanism for contact activation. Blood. 91:516–528
30. Shariat-Madar Z, Mahdi F, Schmaier AH (2002) Identification and characterization of prolylcarboxypeptidase as an endothelial cell prekallikrein activator. J Biol Chem 277:17962–17969
31. Kaplan AP (1996) Intrinsic coagulation, thrombosis, and bleeding. Blood 87:2090
32. Butenas S, van't Veer C, Mann KG (1997) Evaluation of the initiation phase of blood coagulation using ultrasensitive assays for serine proteases. J Biol Chem 272:21527–21533
33. Gailani D, Renne T (2007) The intrinsic pathway of coagulation: a target for treating thromboembolic disease. J Thromb Haemost 5:1106–1112
34. Mackman N, Tilley RE, Key NS (2007) Role of the extrinsic pathway of blood coagulation in hemostasis and thrombosis. Arterioscler Thromb Vasc Biol 27:1687–1693
35. Mann KG, van't Veer C, Cawthern K, Butenas S (1998) The role of the tissue factor pathway in initiation of coagulation. Blood Coagul Fibrinolysis 9:S3–S7
36. Fleck RA, Rao LVM, Rapaport SI, Varki N (1990) Localization of human tissue factor antigen by immunostaining with monospecific, polyclonal anti-human tissue factor antibody. Thromb Res 57:765–781
37. Osterud B (1998) Tissue factor expression by monocytes: regulation and pathophysiological roles. Blood Coagul Fibrinolysis 9(Suppl 1):9–14
38. Monroe DM, Key NS (2007) The tissue factor-factor VIIa complex: procoagulant activity, regulation, and multitasking. J Thromb Haemost 5:1097–1105
39. Franco RF, de Jonge E, Dekkers PEP, Timmerman JJ, Spek CA, van Deventer SJH, van Deursent P, van Kerkhoff L, van Gemen B, ten Cate H, van der Poll T, Reitsma PH (2000) The in vivo kinetics of tissue factor messenger RNA expression during human endotoxemia: relationship with activation of coagulation. Blood 96:554–559
40. Aras O, Shet A, Bach RR, Hysjulien JL, Slungaard A, Hebbel RP, Escolar G, Jilma B, Hey NS (2004) Induction of microparticle- and cell-associated intravascular tissue factor in human endotoxemia. Blood 103:4545–4553
41. Panes O, Matus V, Saez CG, Quiroga T, Pereira J, Mezzano D (2007) Human platelets synthesize and express functional tissue factor. Blood 109:5242–5250
42. McKee PA, Rogers LA, Marler E, Hill RL (1966) The subunit polypeptides of human fibrinogen. Arch Biochem BIophys 116:271–279
43. Hantgan RR, Lord ST (2006) Fibrinogen structure and physiology. In: Colman RW, Marder VJ, Clowes AW, George JN, Goldhaber SZ (eds) Hemostasis and thrombosis. Basic principles and clinical practice, 5th edn. Lippincott Williams and Wilkins, Philadelphia, PA, pp 285–316
44. Weisel JW (1986) Fibrin assembly. Lateral aggregation and the role of the two pairs of fibrinopeptides. Biophys J 50:1079–1093
45. Yang Z, Mochalkin I, Doolittle RF (2000) A model of fibrin formation based on crystal structures of fibrinogen and fibrin fragments complexed with synthetic peptides. Proc Natl Acad Sci USA 97:14156–14161
46. Chen R, Doolittle RF (1969) Identification of the polypeptide chains involved in the cross-linking of fibrin. Proc Natl Acad Sci USA 63:420–427
47. Brummel KE, Paradis SG, Butenas S, Mann KG (2002) Thrombin functions during tissue factor-induced blood coagulation. Blood 100:148–152
48. Salomon O, Steinberg DM, Seligshon U (2006) Variable bleeding manifestations characterize different types of surgery in patients with severe factor XI deficiency enabling parsimonious use of replacement therapy. Haemophilia 12:490–493
49. Barnes JA, Singh S, Gomes AV (2004) Potease activated receptors in cardiovascular function and disease. Mol Cell Biochem 26:227–239
50. Tracy PB, Eide LL, Mann KG (1985) Human prothrombinase complex assembly and function on isolated peripheral blood cell population. J Biol Chem 260:2119–2124

51. Butenas S, Orfeo T, Brummel-ziedins KE, Mann KG (2007) Tissue factor in thrombosis and hemorrhage. Surgery 142:S2–S14

52. Baugh RJ, Broze GJ Jr, Krishnaswamy S (1998) Regulation of extrinsic pathway factor Xa formation by tissue factor pathway inhibitor. J Biol Chem 273:4378–4386

53. Gross PL, Furie BC, Merrill-Skoloff G, Chou J, Furie B (2005) Leukocyte-versus microparticle-mediated tissue factor transfer during arteriolar thrombus development. J Leukoc Biol 78:1318–1326

54. Furie B, Furie BC (2007) In vivo thrombus formation. J Thromb Haemost 5(Suppl 1):12–17

55. Falati S, Gross P, Merrill-Skoloff G, Furie BC, Furie B (2002) Real-time in vivo imaging of platelets, tissue factor and fibrin during arterial thrombus formation in the mouse. Nat Med 8:1175–1181

56. Dietzen DJ, Page KL, Tetzloff TA (2004) Lipid rafts are necessary for tonic inhibition of cellular tissue factor procoagulant activity. Blood 103:3038–3044

57. Chen VM, Ahamed J, Versteeg HH, Berndt MC, Ruf W, Hogg PJ (2006) Evidence for activation of tissue factor by an allosteric disulfide bond. Biochemistry 45:12020–12028

58. Broze GJ Jr, Warren LA, Novotny WF, Higuchi DA, Girard JJ, Miletich JP (1988) The lipoprotein-associated coagulation inhibitor that inhibits the factor VII-tissue factor complex also inhibits factor Xa: insight into its possible mechanism of action. Blood 71:335–343

59. Iakhiaev A, Pendurthi UR, Voigt J, Ezban M, Vijaya Mohan Rao L (1999) Catabolism of factor VIIa bound to tissue factor in fibroblasts in the presence and absence of tissue factor pathway inhibitor. J Biol Chem 274:36995–37003

60. Huang ZF, Higuchi D, Lasky N, Broze GJ Jr (1997) Tissue factor pathway inhibitor gene disruption produces intrauterine lethality in mice. Blood 90:944–951

61. Wong CK, White HD (2007) Direct antithrombins: mechanisms, trials, and role in contemporary interventional medicine. Am J Cardiovasc Drugs 7:249–257

62. Carrell RW, Evans DLI, Stein H (1991) Mobile reactive centre of serpins and the control of thrombosis. Nature 353:576–579

63. Carrell RW, Perry DJ (1996) The unhinged antithrombins. Brit J Haematol 93:253–257

64. Jin L, Abrahams JP, Skinner R et al (1997) The anticoagulant activation of antithrombin by heparin. Proc Natl Acad Sci USA 94:14683–14688

65. Huntington JA, Olson ST, Fan B, Gettins PGW (1996) Mechanism of heparin activation of antithrombin. Evidence for reactive center loop preinsertion with expulsion upon heparin binding. Biochemistry 35:8495–8503

66. Kottke-Marchant K, Comp P (2002) Laboratory issues in diagnosing abnormalities of protein C, thrombomodulin and endothelial cell protein C receptor. Arch Pathol Lab Med 126:1337–1348

67. Dahlback B (1995) The protein C anticoagulant system: inherited defects as basis for venous thrombosis. Thromb Res 77:1–43

68. Sadler JE, Lentz SR, Sheehan JP, Tsiang M, Wu Q (1993) Structure-function relationships of the thrombin-thrombomodulin interaction. Haemostasis 23:183–193

69. Ye J, Esmon NL, Esmon CT, Johnson AE (1991) The active site of thrombin is altered upon binding to thrombomodulin: two distinct structural changes are detected by fluorescence, but only one correlates with protein C activation. J Biol Chem 266:23016–23021

70. Taylor FB Jr, Peer GT, Lockhart MS, Ferrell G, Esmon CT (2001) Endothelial cell protein C receptor plays an important role in protein C activation in vivo. Blood 97:1685–1688

71. Bajzar L, Morser J, Nesheim M (1996) TAFI, or plasma procarboxypeptidase B, couples the coagulation and fibrinolytic cascade through the thrombin-thrombomodulin complex. J Biol Chem 271:16603–16608

72. Myles T, Nishimura T, Yun TH, Nagashima M, Morser J, Patterson AJ, Pearl RG, Leung LL (2003) Thrombin activatable fibrinolysis inhibitor. A potential regulator of vascular inflammation. J Biol Chem 278:51059–51067

73. Corral J, Gonzalez-Conejero R, Hernandez-Esponosa D, Vicent V (2007) Protein Z/Z-dependent protease inhibitor (PZ/ZPI) anticoagulant system and thrombosis. Br J Haematol 137:99–108

74. Han X, Fiehler R, Broze GJ Jr (1998) Isolation of a protein Z-dependent plasma protease inhibitor. Proc Natl Acad Sci USA 95:9250–9255

75. Han X, Fiehler R, Broze GJ Jr (2000) Characterization of the protein Z-dependent protease inhibitor. Blood 96:3049–3055

76. Heeb MJ, Cabral KM, Ruan L (2005) Down-regulation of factor IXa in the factor Xase complex by protein Z-dependent protease inhibitor. J Biol Chem 280:33819–33825

77. Verhamme P, Hoylaerts MF (2006) The pivotal role of the endothelium in haemostasis and thrombosis. Acta Clin Belg 61:213–219

78. Schouten M, Wiersinga WJ, Levi M, van der Poll T (2008) Inflammation, endothelium, and coagulation in sepsis. J Leukoc Biol 83:536–545

79. Lynch SF, Ludlam CA (2007) Plasma microparticles and vascular disorders. Brit J Haematol 137:36–48
80. Piccin A, Murphy W, Smith O (2007) Circulating microparticles: pathophysiology and clinical implications. Blood Rev 21:157–171
81. van Wijk MJ, Van Bavel E, Sturk A, Niuwland R (2003) Microparticles in cardiovascular diseases. Cardiovasc Res 59:277–287
82. Zwaal RFA, Schroit AJ (1997) Pathophysiologic implications of membrane phospholipid asymmetry in blood cells. Blood 89:1121–1132
83. Pereira J, Alfaro G, Goycoolea M, Quiroga T, Ocqueteau M, Massardo L, Perez C, Saez C, Panes O, Matus V, Mezzano D (2006) Circulating platelet-derived microparticles in systemic lupus erythematosus. Association with increased thrombin generation and procoagulant state. Thromb Haemost 95:94–99
84. Ardoin SP, Shanahan JC, Pisetsky DS (2007) The role of microparticles in inflammation and thrombosis. Scand J Immunol 66:159–165
85. Kushak RI, Nestoridi E, Lambert J, Selig MK, Ingelfinger JR, Grabowski EF (2005) Detached endothelial cells and microparticles as sources of tissue factor activity. Thromb Res 116:409–419
86. del Conde I, Shrimpton CN, Thiagarajan P, Lopez JA (2005) Tissue-factor-bearing microvesicles arise from lipid rafts and fuse with activated platelets to initiate coagulation. Blood 106:1604–1611
87. Steppich B, Mattisek C, Sobczyk D, Kastrati A, Schomig A, Ott I (2005) Tissue factor pathway inhibitor on circulating microparticles in acute myocardial infarction. Thromb Haemost 93:35–39
88. Hugel B, Zobairi F, Freyssinet JM (2004) Measuring circulating cell-derived microparticles. J Thromb Haemost 2:1846–1847
89. Lundblad RL, White GC II (2005) The interaction of thrombin with blood platelets. Platelets 16:373–385
90. Suehiro K, Smith JW, Plow EF (1996) The ligand recognition specificity of beta3 integrins. J Biol Chem 271:10365–10371
91. Reininger AJ, Heijnen HF, Schumann H, Specht HM, Schramm W, Ruggeri ZM (2006) Mechanism of platelet adhesion to von Willebrand factor and microparticle formation under high shear stress. Blood 107:3537–3545
92. Kottke-Marchant K, Corcoran G (2006) The laboratory diagnosis of platelet disorders: an algorithmic approach. Arch Pathol Lab Med 126:133–146
93. Rosendaal FR (1997) Risk factors for venous thrombosis: prevalence, risk and interaction. Semin Hematol 34:171–187
94. Prandoni P (2007) Venous thromboembolism and atherosclerosis: is there a link? J Thromb Haemost 5(Suppl 1):270–275
95. Prandoni P, Bilora F, Marchiori A, Bernardi E, Petrobelli F, Lensing AWA, Prins MH, Girolami A (2003) An association between atherosclerosis and venous thrombosis. N Engl J Med 348:1435–1441
96. Wakefield TW, Myers DD, Henke PK (2008) Mechanisms of venous thrombosis and resolution. Arterioscler Thromb Vasc Biol 28:387–391
97. Silverstein MD, Heit JA, Mohr DN, Petterson TM, O'Fallon WM, Melton JL III (1998) Trends in the incidence of deep vein thrombosis and pulmonary embolism: a 25 year population-based study. Arch Intern Med 158:585–593
98. Seligsohn U, Zivelin A (1997) Thrombophilia as a multigenic disorder. Thromb Haemost 78:297–301
99. Egeberg O (1965) Inherited antithrombin III deficiency causing thrombophilia. Thromb Diath Haemorrh 13:516–530
100. Griffin JH, Evatt B, Zimmerman TS, Kleiss AJ, Wideman C (1981) Deficiency of protein C in congenital thrombotic disease. J Clin Invest 68:1370–1373
101. Comp PC, Nixon RR, Cooper MR, Esmon CT (1984) Familial protein S deficiency is associated with recurrent thrombosis. J Clin Invest 74:2082–2088
102. Nossent AY, Eikenboom JCJ, Bertina RM (2007) Plasma coagulation factor levels in venous thrombosis. Semin Hematol 44:77–84
103. Kottke-Marchant K (2002) Genetic polymorphisms associated with venous and arterial thrombosis – an overview. Arch Pathol Lab Med 126:295–304
104. Dahlback B, Carlsson M, Svensson PJ (1993) Familial thrombophilia due to a previously unrecognized mechanism characterized by poor anticoagulant response to activated protein C. Proc Natl Acad Sci USA 90:1004–1008
105. Bertina RM, Koeleman BPC, Koster T, Rosendaal FR, Dirven RJ, de Ronde H, van der Velden PA, Reitsma PH (1994) Mutation in blood coagulation factor V associated with resistance to activated protein C. Nature 369:64–67
106. Hoerl HD, Tabares A, Kottke-Marchant K (1996) The diagnosis and clinical manifestations of activated protein C resistance: a case report and review of the literature. Vasc Med 1:275–280
107. Rees DC, Cox M, Clegg JB (1995) World distribution of factor V Leiden. Lancet 345:1133–1134
108. Bertina RM (1997) Factor V Leiden and other coagulation risk factor mutations affecting thrombotic risk. Clin Chem 43:1678–1683

109. Segers K, Dahlback B, Nicolaes GA (2007) Coagulation factor V and thrombophilia: Background and mechanisms. Thromb Haemost 98:530–542

110. Bertina RM (1999) Molecular risk factors for thrombosis. Thromb Haemost 82:601–609

111. Poort SR, Rosendaal FR, Reitsma PH, Bertina RM (1996) A common genetic variation in the 3'-untranslated region of the prothrombin gene is associated with elevated plasma prothrombin levels and an increase in venous thrombosis. Blood 88:3698–3703

112. Heit JA (2006) Epidemiology of venous thromboembolism. In: Colman RW, Marder VJ, Clowes AW, George JN, Goldhaber SZ (eds) Hemostasis and thrombosis. Basic principles and clinical practice, 5th edn. Lippincott Williams and Wilkins, Philadelphia, PA, pp 1227–1233

113. Olson JD, Eby C. Thrombophilia and Arterial and Venous Thrombosis in Adults. In: An Algorithmic Approach to Hemostasis Testing. K. Kottke-Marchent, Ed., CAP Press, Chicago, Chapter 17, October 29, 2008

114. Heit JA, O'Fallon WM, Petterson TM, Lohse CM, Silverstein MD, Mohr DN, Melton LJ III (2002) Relative impact of risk factors for deep vein thrombosis and pulmonary embolism: a population-based study. Arch Intern Med 162:1245–1248

115. Kuipers S, Schreijer AJ, Annegieter SC, Buller HR, Rosendaal FR, Middeldorp S (2007) Travel and venous thrombosis: a systematic review. J Intern Med 262:615–634

116. Greinacher A, Potzsch B, Amiral J, Dummel V, Eichner A, Mueller-Eckhardt C (1994) Heparin-associated thrombocytopenia: isolation of th antibody and characterization of a multimolecular PF4-heparin complex as the major antigen. Thromb Haemost 71:247–251

117. Warkentin TE, Hayward CPM, Boshkov LK, Santos AV, Sheppard JA, Bode AP, Kelton JG (1994) Sera from patients with heparin-induced thrombocytopenia generate platelet-derived microparticles with procoagulant activity: an explanation for the thrombotic complications of heparin-induced thrombocytopenia. Blood 84:3691–3699

118. Lim W, Crowther MA (2007) Antiphospholipid antibodies: a critical review of the literature. Curr Opin Hematol 14:494–499

119. Miyakis S, Lockshin MD, Atsumi T et al (2006) International consensus statement on an update of the classification criteria for definite antiphospholipid syndrome (APS). J Thromb Haemost 4:295–306

120. Kaburaki J, Kuwana M, Yamamoto M, Kawai S, Ikeda Y (1997) Clinical significance of anti-annexin V antibodies in patients with systemic lupus erythematosus. Am J Hematol 54:209–213

121. Brandt JT (1991) The effects of lupus anticoagulant on the expression of tissue factor activity by cultured endothelial cells. Thromb Haemost 65:673

122. Mak K-H, Kottke-Marchant K, Brooks LM, Topol EJ (1998) In vitro efficacy of platelet glycoprotein IIb/IIIa antagonist in blocking platelet function in plasma of patients with heparin-induced thrombocytopenia. Thromb Haemost 80:989–993

123. Walenga JM, Michal K, Hoppensteadt D et al (1999) Vascular damage correlates between heparin induced thrombocytopenia and the antiphospholipid antibody syndrome. Clin Appl Thromb Hemost 5(Suppl 1):S76–S84

124. Dignat-George F, Camoin-Jau L, Sabatier F, Arnoux D, Anfosso F, Bardin N, Veit V, COmbes V, Gentile S, Moal V, Sanmarco M, Sampol J (2004) Endothelial microparticles: a potential contribution to the thrombotic complications of the antiphospholipid syndrome. Thromb Haemost 91:667–673

125. Hansson GK, Libby P (2006) The immune response in atherosclerosis: a double-edged sword. Nat Rev Immunol 6:508–519

126. Libby P (2002) Inflammation in atherosclerosis. Nature 420:868–874

127. Weyrich A, Cipollone F, Mezzetti A, Zimmerman G (2007) Platelets in atherothrombosis: new and evolving roles. Curr Pharm Des 13:1685–1691

128. Davies MJ (1997) The composition of coronary artery plaques. N Engl J Med 336:1312–1314

129. Nesto RW, Waxman S, Mittleman MA et al (1998) Angioscopy of culprit coronary lesions in unstable angina pectoris and correlation of clinical presentation with plaque morphology. Am J Cardiol 81:225–228

130. Burke AP, Kolodgie FD, Farb A, Weber DK, Malcom GT, Smialek J, Virmani R (2001) Healed plaque ruptures and sudden coronary death: evidence that subclinical rupture has a role in plaque progression. Circulation 103:934–940

131. Cohen M, Demers C, Gurfinkel EP, Turpie AG, Fromell GJ, Goodman S, Langer A, Califf RM, Fox KA, Premmereur J, Bigonzi F (1997) A comparison of low molecular weight heparin with unfractionated heparin for unstable coronary artery disease. N Engl J Med 337:447–452

132. The PURSUIT Trial Investigators (1998) Inhibition of platelet glycoprotein IIb/IIIa with eptifibatide in patients with acute coronary syndromes. N Engl J Med 339:436–443

133. Chi L, Gibson G, Peng YW, Bouwley R, Brammer D, Rekhter M, Chen J, Leadley R (2004) Characterization of a tissue factor/factor VIIa-dependent model of thrombosis in hypercholesterolemia rabbits. J Thromb Haemost 2:85–92

134. Asada Y, Hara S, Tsuneyoshi A, Hatakeyama K, Kisanuki A, Marutsuka K, Sato Y, Kamikubo Y, Sumiyoshi A (1998) Fibrin-rich and platelet-rich thrombus formation on neointima: recombinant tissue factor pathway inhibitor prevents fibrin formation and neointimal development following repeated balloon injury of rabbit aorta. Thromb Haemost 80:506–511

135. Bernal-Mizrachi L, Jy W, Jimenez JJ, Pastor J, Maro LM, Horstman LL, de Marchena E, Ahn YS (2003) High levels of circulating endothelial microparticles in patients with acute coronary syndromes. Amer Heart J 145:962–970

136. Chironi G, Simon A, Hugel B, Del Pino M, Gariepy J, Freyssinet JM, Tedgui A (2006) Circulating leukocyte-derived microparticles predict subclinical atherosclerosis burden in asymptomatic subjects. Arterioscler Thromb Vasc Biol 26:2775–2780

137. Tramontano AF, O'Leary J, Black AD, Muniyappa R, Cutaia MV, El-Sherif N (2004) Statin decreases endothelial microparticle release from human coronary artery endothelial cells: implication for the Rho-kinase pathway. Biochem Biophy Res Commun 320:34–38

138. Minami T, Sugiyama A, Wu SQ et al (2004) Thrombin and phenotypic modulation of the endothelium. Arterioscler Thromb Vasc Biol 24:41–53

139. Duhamel-Clerin E, Orvain C, Lanza F et al (1997) Thrombin receptor-mediated increase of two matrix metalloproteinases, MMP-1 and MMP-3, in human endothelial cells. Arterioscler Thromb Vasc Biol 17:1931–1938

140. Wu SQ, Aird WC (2005) Thrombin, TNF-alpha and LPS exert overlapping but nonidentical effects on gene expression in endothelial cells and vascular smooth muscle cells. Am J Physiol Heart Circ Physiol 289:H873–H885

141. Gawaz M, Langer H, May AE (2005) Platelets in inflammation and atherogenesis. J Clin Invest 115:3378–3384

142. de Moerloose P, Boehlen F (2007) Inherited thrombophilia in arterial disease: a selective review. Semin Hematol 44:106–113

143. Ye Z, Liu EHC, Higgins JPT, Keavney BD, Lowe GDO, Collins R et al (2006) Seven haemostatic gene polymorphisms in coronary disease: meta-analysis of 66, 155 cases and 91, 307 controls. Lancet 367:651–658

144. Kim RJ, Becker RC (2003) Assocation between factor V Leiden, prothrombin G20210A and methylenetetrahydrofolate reductase C677T mutations and events of the arterial circulatory system: a meta-analysis of published studies. Am Heart J 146:948–957

145. Bodary PF, Eitzman DT (2009) Animal models of thrombosis. Curr Opin Hematol [epub ahead of print]

146. Chironi GN, Boulanger CM, Simon A, Dignat-George F, Freyssinet JM, Tredgui A (2009) Endothelial microparticles in diseases. Cell Tissue Res 335(1):143–51

147. Reiner AP, Lange LA, Smith NL, Zakai NA, Cushman M, Folsom AR (2009) Common hemostasis and inflammation gene variants and venous thrombosis in older adults from the Cardiovascular Health Study. J Thromb Haemost [epub ahead of print]

148. Libby P (2009) Molecular and celluar mechanisms of the thrombotic complications of atherosclerosis. J Lipid Res 50 Suppl:S352-7

149. Kastl SP, Speidl WS, Katsaros KM, Kaun C, Rega G, Assadian A, Hagmueller GW, Hoeth M, de Martin R, Ma Y, Mauer G, Huber K, Wojta J (2009) Thrombin induces the expression of oncostatin M via AP-1 activation in human macrophages: a link between coagulation and inflammation. Blood [epub ahead of print]

3   The Link Between Inflammation and Thrombosis

John H. Cleator and Mark Robbins

CONTENTS

ABSTRACT Atherosclerosis is an inflammatory disease. This fact is now strongly supported by clinical, basic, and pathological research which has caused an evolution in thought concerning the evaluation and treatment of acute coronary syndromes (ACS). The initial insult is endothelial injury and subsequent dysfunction via the deleterious effects of the known cardiac risk factors such as oxidized LDL, hyperglycemia, hypertension, hyperhomocystinemia, and smoking. Irrespective of the cause of endothelial damage, the resultant activation and proliferation of inflammatory cells, smooth muscle cells, and generation of cytokines and growth factors lead to the progression of atherosclerosis. The presence and extent of inflammation, procoagulant state and composition of the atherosclerotic plaque have been strongly associated with an increased risk of future cardiac events. Thus, the perpetuation of the inflammatory response likely plays a pivotal role in the pathobiology and vulnerability of the atherosclerotic plaque. Inflammatory markers once thought to be passive observers are now being investigated as active participants in the progression of atherosclerosis and therefore targets for future pharmacologic intervention.

Key words: CAD; Thrombosis; Inflammation; ACS; Adhesion Molecules; Chemokines; Cytokines; C reactive protein; MPO; Interleukins; von Willebrand factor; P-selectin; Serum amyloid A; A2 Phospholipases; Tumor necrosis factor-α; NF-κB; HMG-CoA reductase inhibitors; PPAR agonists; Aspirin; Cyclooxygenase-2; Protease-activated receptors; Thrombin receptor antagonist

From: *Contemporary Cardiology: Antithrombotic Drug Therapy in Cardiovascular Disease*
Edited by: A.T. Askari and A.M. Lincoff (eds.), DOI :10.1007/978-1-60327-235-3_3
© Humana Press, a part of Springer Science+Business Media, LLC 2010

PATHOBIOLOGY OF INFLAMMATION, ATHEROSCLEROSIS, AND ACS

Endothelial Function

The endothelium lies in a critical location between the remaining vascular wall and the circulating blood, thereby functioning as the pivotal barrier that protects the arterial wall from injury. This critical monolayer of cells is pluripotential, carrying out the following functions; *(1)* provision of a nonthrombotic surface; *(2)* maintenance of vascular tone through the production and release of nitric oxide (NO), prostacyclin, and endothelin; *(3)* regulation of growth factors and cytokines; *(4)* provision of a nonadherent surface for leukocytes and platelets; and *(5)* the modification of lipoproteins as they transverse its permeable barrier *(5)*. Injury to this monolayer plays a key role in the initiation and progression of the atherosclerotic lesion by increasing adhesive cell surface glycoproteins, adherence, migration, and activation of leukocytes, and smooth muscle cells, production of cytokines, chemokines, and growth factors, as well as the reversal from an antithrombotic to a prothrombotic state *(1–4,7,9–12)* (Fig. 1).

Adhesion Molecules

Cell-cell interactions are a vital component in the pathogenesis of inflammation and propagation of atherosclerosis. Collectively known as cell adhesion molecules, three distinct families exist (selectins, integrins, and the immunoglobulin superfamily) each with its own specific role in the inflammatory process. The process entails tethering and rolling of leukocytes on the activated endothelium, leukocyte activation, and ultimately firm adhesion and transendothelial migration along a chemotactic gradient generated by mediators of inflammation *(13,14)*.

Selectins are expressed on the cell surface of leukocytes (L-selectin), platelets (P-selectin), and endothelial cells (E-selectin). Upon activation from inflammatory cytokines, mainly tumor necrosis factor-α (TNF-α) and IL-1, cell surface expression of each selectin is enhanced *(15–17)*. This process is vital in the early phase of inflammation mediating leukocyte recruitment and transient endothelial

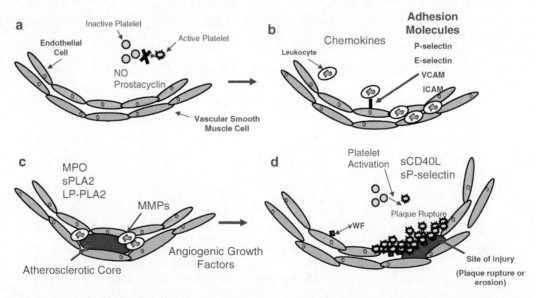

Fig. 1. Schematic of the protective role the endothelium in preventing the progression of atherosclerosis.

cell to leukocyte interactions (tethering and rolling phase). The subsequent steps of firm adhesion and migration of leukocytes are predominantly mediated through the following: (1) interaction of integrins (leukocyte function associated antigen-1 [LAF-I], macrophage antigen-1 [MAC-I], very late activation antigen-4 [VLA-4] and GPIIbIIIa receptor), (2) the immunoglobulin superfamily (VCAM-1, VCAM-2, and ICAM-1), and (3) potent stimulation by inflammatory cytokines and chemokines including IL-1, IL-4, IL-8, TNF-α, INF-ψ, and chemotactic protein-1 (13,14). In addition to the cell adhesion molecules on endothelial cells, leukocytes, and platelets, ICAM-1 and VCAM-1 are expressed on smooth muscle cells (18). The interaction between leukocytes and smooth muscle cells contributes to smooth muscle cell migration and proliferation, cellular composition of the atherosclerotic plaque, and an increased expression of monocyte tissue factor mRNA (18,19). An additional component that ties inflammation and the prothrombotic state (1,2,4,7,9) involves the adhesion of activated platelets to the endothelium through the P-selectin-GPIIbIIIa receptor interactions with s ubsequent platelet aggregation and thrombus formation (20).

Growing evidence supports that the presence of increased cell adhesion molecules in serum or vascular tissue may reflect ongoing active vascular remodeling due to persistent inflammation. Elevated serum levels of the soluble form of the VCAM-1 receptor (sVCAM-1) have been associated with the extent of atherosclerosis in patients with peripheral vascular disease (21). In patients with coronary artery disease, elevated levels of the soluble ICAM-1 (SICAM-1) have been found to be inversely proportional to HDL levels and associated with the presence of other coronary risk factors, unstable angina, myocardial infarction, and importantly to increased risk of future myocardial infarction in apparently healthy men (22,23). Immunohistochemical evaluation of coronary atherectomy tissue has shown P-selectin but not E-selectin, or ICAM-1 was expressed significantly greater in the setting of unstable angina vs. stable angina (24). This reflects an augmented response between an endothelial cell adhesion molecule and the activated platelet linking thrombus formation and unstable coronary syndromes. Elevated levels of soluble P-selectin have as well been shown to predict cardiovascular events in a prospective study of healthy women (25).

Cellular and Humoral-Mediated Response

MONOCYTES AND MACROPHAGES

Monocytes, the circulating precursors of tissue macrophages, are essential in the progression of atherosclerosis and are found in all stages of atherosclerotic lesions (3,26). Their recruitment and infiltration through the endothelium into the intima is tightly coupled to the humoral activity of the T-lymphocyte. The colocalization of CD4+ T-cells and macrophages and the abundant expression of HLA 11 molecules in atherosclerotic lesions is strong evidence for the role of cell-mediated immunity in the development and progression of atherosclerosis. Population size of CD14dimCD 16a+ peripheral blood monocytes has been shown to correlate with degree of hypercholesterolemia and is dramatically reduced with lipid-lowering therapy (27). This phenotypic expression, in contrast to other phenotypes of monocytes, is shown to express high levels of inflammatory cytokines such as TNF-α whereas the anti-inflammatory IL-10 is low or absent. In addition, these cells are further characterized by an upregulation of cell surface adhesion molecules, suggesting an increased capacity for cell to cell interactions (28).

The degree of macrophage infiltration has been shown to distinguish between unstable and stable coronary lesions. The preferential localization of macrophages in high-flow shoulder regions of the atherosclerotic plaque correlates with areas at highest risk for plaque instability. In contrast to controls, infiltrates of CD68-positive macrophages and CD3- and CD8-positive T-cells were statistically associated with the severity and frequency of superficial plaque inflammation and rupture *(29–31)*. This plaque instability, in part, stems from metalloproteinase (MMP-1 and MMP-2) production and release by activated macrophages within the inflamed atherosclerotic plaque *(32)*. (Fig. 1C)

Antigen-presenting macrophages induce T-cell activation and result in inflammatory amplification through T-cell release of TNF-α, and INF-γ, further activating macrophages, platelets, and smooth muscle cells *(33)*. Levels of the main specific immune markers CD4+ and CD3+/DR+ T-cells, IL-2, and IgM have all been reported to be higher in unstable than in stable angina patients *(34)*. In addition, a higher percentage of IL-2 receptor positive T-lymphocytes in culprit lesions of patients with acute coronary syndromes indicates recent activation and amplification of the immune response within plaques. These findings support the concept that a burst of inflammatory products could initiate or accelerate the onset of an acute coronary event *(35)*.

MAST CELLS

Mast cells have been recently identified to inhabit the vulnerable shoulder regions of the atherosclerotic plaque and to be associated with plaque erosion and rupture *(36,37)*. The population size of mast cells in artherectomy tissue correlates with the clinical severity of coronary syndromes. Their presence in the adventitia of ruptured plaques has led to the postulate that histamine release may provoke coronary spasm and contributes to the onset of myocardial infarction *(38,39)*. Mast cells have a primary role in the perpetuation of the inflammatory response in atherosclerosis, characterized by the production of TNF-α and neutral proteases (tryptase and chymase) *(40,41)*. TNF-α stimulates macrophages and smooth muscle cells to produce two prometalloproteinases - prostromelysin and procollagenase. Subsequent activation of these prometalloproteinases by mast cell produced tryptase and chymase leading to fibrous cap degradation and plaque destabilization *(42)*.

NEUTROPHILS

As previously discussed, macrophages and T lymphocytes are the predominant cellular components of local inflammation within the atherosclerotic plaque. Neutrophils, although found sparsely in atherosclerotic plaques, play an integral part in the acute inflammatory response to tissue injury and have been implicated as a major factor in tissue damage in response to ischemia and reperfusion *(43)*. TNF-α, IL-8, IL-6, platelet-activating factor, and leukotrienes enhance neutrophil recruitment to ischemic and reperfused myocardium by augmenting cell adhesion molecule expression. The extent of accumulation has also been correlated to the degree of tissue injury *(44,45)*. A systemic activation of neutrophils has been reported in patients with angiographically documented coronary artery disease as compared with normal controls providing further proof for a chronic systemic inflammatory state in patients with atherosclerosis *(46)*.

PLATELETS

Recent discoveries have led investigators to believe that platelets are critical constituents that tie in both inflammation and thrombosis. The presence of serologic markers of platelet activation is well established in the setting of an ACS *(47–49)*. Inflammatory cytokines induce the translocation of the cell adhesion molecule P-selectin to the surface of the platelet membrane, facilitating interactions among platelets, endothelial cells, and monocytes. Monocyte expression of tissue factor is induced by P-selectin and may be an initiator of thrombosis in areas of vascular injury *(50)*.

An initial step to answer the question of whether platelet activation is a result of or results in the development of an ACS was reported by Furman et al. *(51)*. In a flow cytometric analysis patients with stable coronary artery disease were shown to not only have increased levels of circulating activated platelets with enhanced P-selectin expression, but also to have an increased propensity to form monocyte-platelet aggregates *(51)*. Additional evidence to implicate platelets as inflammatory mediators is their expression of CD40L. This transmembrane protein found on constituents of both cellular and humoral components of the inflammatory system is structurally related to TNF-α. CD40L is rapidly expressed by activated platelets and induces the expression of chemokines and cell adhesion molecules by endothelial cells thus provoking cell attraction, activation, and migration into the arterial wall *(52)*.

Chemokines and Cytokines

CHEMOKINES

Chemokines consist of a family of chemotactic cytokines involved in leukocyte trafficking and activation. Chemokines initiate signaling via chemokine G protein–coupled receptors, which then activates cellular integrins leading to reorganization of the cytoskeleton. More recently, this ever-expanding family has been implicated in platelet activation and thrombus formation *(53)*. In addition, a large number of chemokines have been suggested to play a role in mediating the progression of atherosclerosis *(54)*. Some of the key chemokines involved in thrombogenicity and atherosclerosis are listed in Table 1. One of the more prominent chemokines is Monocyte chemoattractant Protein-1 (MCP-1) or CCL2. MCP-1 is a chemokine that induces monocyte migration to sites of inflammation. MCP-1 inhibition has been shown to attenuate left ventricular remodeling and failure after experimental myocardial infarction *(55)*. Further, increased levels of MCP-1 in the coronary sinus have been found to correlate to extent of coronary atherosclerosis *(56)*. Elevated levels of MCP-1 in the sera of patients enrolled in the OPUS-TIMI-16 trial were associated with an increased risk of death or MI independent of traditional risk factors *(57)*.

Table 1
The role of select chemokines in thrombosis and atherosclerosis

Name/common name	Cell of origin	Target cell	Experimental effect on thrombosis	Experimental effect on atherosclerosis	Clinical effect of increased levels
CCL2/MCP-1	Monocytes, endothelial cells	Monocytes, T cells, eosinophils, basophils and platelets	Recruits leukocytes and inflammatory response *(200)*	Reduction in Double KO LDLR-/-, MCP-1-/- *(201)*	Correlated with extent of CAD and MACE *(57)*
CCL5/rantes	T cells, platelets	T cells, eosinophils, basophils, NK cells	Recruits monocytes on inflamed endothelial cells *(202)*	Reduction in LDLR-/- and with RANTES antagonist *(203)*	Correlated with MACE *(204,205)*
CXCL7/NAP-2	Platelets, monocytes	Neutrophils	Recruits Monocytes, mobilizes calcium *(206,207)*	?	Associated in stable and USA *(208)*
CX3CR1/ fractalkine	Endothelial cells	Endothelial cell, platelets, and monocytes	Activates platelets and is located in atherosclerotic lesions *(209)*	Reduction in double KO ApoE-/-, CX3CR1-/- *(210)*	?

TUMOR NECROSIS FACTOR-α

TNF-α is a pleiotropic proinflammatory cytokine with a wide range of effects that extend across a spectrum of pathologic conditions. Present in atherosclerotic lesions *(58)*, TNF-α, appears to be one of the most important influences on the progression of atherosclerosis. Its upregulation is known to mediate and amplify a multitude of interactions resulting in progressive inflammation, plaque destabilization, and prothrombotic tendencies *(59–67)* (Table 2). Treatment with a chimeric mAb to TNF-α has been shown to suppress inflammation and improve patient well-being in rheumatoid arthritis (RA). Administration of anti-TNF-α, Ab has also been associated with the rapid downregulation of a spectrum of cytokines (IL-6), cytokine inhibitors (TNF receptors p75 and p55), and acute-phase proteins (amyloid A, haptoglobin, and fibrinogen) *(68)*. This potent suppression of markers and mediators of inflammation may have tremendous potential in preventing progression of atherosclerosis.

INTERLEUKINS

IL-6 and IL-1Ra (K-1 receptor antagonist) not only have been shown to be elevated in the setting of ACS, but also are associated with increased risk of in-hospital events *(69)*. IL-6, produced by a variety of inflammatory cell types, has been shown to remain elevated up to 4 weeks after a myocardial infarction. Its properties increase fibrinogen and PAI-1, promote adhesion of neutrophils and myocytes during myocardial reperfusion, and produce a negative inotropic effect on the myocardium *(70–74)*. Elevated levels of IL-6 in subjects with unstable angina (FRISC-II study) were associated with higher 6- and 12-month mortality which was additive and independent of troponin levels *(75)*. Pannitteri et al. *(76)* reported that levels of IL-8 not only are elevated in the setting of acute myocardial infarction but also that they precede the levels of IL-6 and parallel the kinetics of CPK. IL-8 is a powerful trigger for firm

Table 2
The predictive value of CRP in ACS

Trial	Patient characteristics	Outcome associated with elevated CRP	Ref
MONICA (MONItoring of trends and determinants in CArdiovascular diseases) Study	Healthy men	MI or sudden cardiac death	*(211)*
Physician's Health Study	Healthy men	Predictive of first MI	*(212)*
Woman's Health Study	Healthy women	Any vascular event and combined CVA or MI	*(213)*
Gasparadone et al.	Stable Angina/ Elective PCI	12-month follow-up cumulative event rate	*(214)*
Liuzzo et al.	Preinfarction UA	Preinfarction CRP levels higher than unheralded MI	*(215)*
Biassicci et al.	UA (without myocardial injury)	Recurrent coronary instability and MI	*(216)*
Milazzo et al.	CABG	New ischemic events	*(217)*
European Concerted Action on Thrombosis and Disabilities (ECAT) Angina Pectoris Study	UA	Predictive of future coronary events	*(218–220)*
Fragmin during Instability in Coronary Artery Disease (FRISC)	UA		*(6)*
TIMI-11a	UA and NSTEMI	14-day mortality	*(221)*
Anzai et al.	STEMI	Worse prognosis	*(131)*
Tommasi et al.	First MI	Cardiac death	*(8)*

adhesion of monocytes to vascular endothelium. In addition, it may play a potential atherogenic role by inhibiting local inhibitors of metalloproteinases in atherosclerotic plaques and by stimulation of smooth muscle cell migration (77,78). IL-4 and IL-13 have been shown to enhance the ability of activated human monocytes to oxidize LDL, thus potentiating its toxic effects (79). OxLDL induces IFN-γ production by T-helper-1-like cells, which is known to inhibit local collagen synthesis by smooth muscle cells, stimulate expression of tissue factor and CD40, and selectively induce MCP-I (80,81). Many other cytokines have been implicated in immunity, inflammation, thrombosis, and angiogenesis (82).

CD40 AND CD4OL

CD40 is a phosphorylated 49-kDa glycoprotein expressed on B-lymphocytes, fibroblasts, monocytes, platelets, epithelial cells, and endothelial cells (83). CD40L, also named CD154 or gp39, belongs to the TNF family of cytokines. The presence of CD40 and CD40L has been found in human atheroma, and their association is implicated with expression of cell adhesion molecules, cytokines, matrix metalloproteinases, and tissue factor (52,83). Anti-CD40L has been shown to regulate autoimmune diseases such as lupus nephritis, skin and cardiac allograft rejection, and multiple sclerosis in experimental models (84–86). Mach et al. (87) reported a reduction in aortic atherosclerotic lesion size, fewer T-lymphocytes and macrophages, and a decreased presence of cell adhesion molecules in atheroma in cholesterol-fed mice lacking the LDL receptor when treated with anti-CD40L antibody (87). Aukrust et al. (88) reported elevated levels of CD40-CD40L in patients with angina pectoris, as well as higher concentrations in patients with more unstable syndromes as compared to stable angina. The authors concluded that presence of CD40-CD40L may have a pathologic role in plaque destabilization and the development of ACS (88)

Nuclear Transcription Factors

NF-κB

NF-κB is a transcription factor located in the cytoplasm of many cells as an inactive complex associated with a specific class of inhibitory proteins, called IKB. This complex binds and prevents nuclear translocation and DNA binding of NF-κB (89). In response to inflammatory stimuli IKB is eventually degraded and NF-κB is released and transported to the nucleus. In the nuclei, NF-κB can initiate and regulate early response gene transcription by binding to promoter or enhancer regions (90). NF-κB is known to regulate or be regulated by genes involved in every aspect of the proinflammatory cascade (91,92). TNF-α and IL-1 are two important inducers, contributing to a positive feedback loop for NF-κB activation. As a consequence, there is a continuous upregulation of cytokines and perpetuation of inflammation (90). NF-κB has been implicated in a variety of inflammatory diseases, such as allograft rejection, RA, asthma, and inflammatory bowel disease (91). In RA, NF-κB is overly expressed in synovial tissue, associated with surface expression of cell adhesion molecules, production of cytokines, and upregulation of the inducible isoform of cyclooxygenase (COX-2). These processes are identical to those found in atherosclerotic lesions (91).

NF-κB activity is enhanced by known cardiac risk factors such as VLDL, OxLDL, hyperglycemia, and elevated levels of angiotensin II. On the contrary, its activity is inhibited by HMG-CoA reductase inhibitors, antioxidants, and gallates (phenolic compounds found abundantly in red wine) (93–98). Ritchie (99) reported data showing that NF-κB is activated in patients with unstable angina without evidence of myonecrosis and is therefore potentially linked in plaque disruption. Immunosuppression with glucocorticoids, gold, cyclosporin, FK506, and, importantly, aspirin and salicylates is known to inhibit NF-κB. Kopp et al. (100) demonstrated that aspirin inhibits NF-κB activity by preventing the degradation of IKB, while Weber et al. (101) established aspirin's ability to inhibit TNF-α-stimulated NF-κB activity.

PPAR

Peroxisomal proliferator-activated receptors (PPARs), including PPAR-α, PPAR-γ, and PPAR-8, are a group of nuclear transcription factors which play a key role in adipogenesis and lipid metabolism *(102)*. PPAR modulation of the development and progression of atherosclerosis has been substantiated by research that appears to link its activity with the regulation of inflammation and plaque stability through their interactions with macrophages, endothelial cells, smooth muscle cells, and metalloproteinases. Ricote et al. *(103)* found PPAR-γ to be upregulated in activated macrophages and to inhibit gelatinase B, nitric oxide synthase, and scavenger receptors. OxLDL has been shown to induce PPAR-γ expression in macrophages, resulting in monocyte differentiation and enhanced uptake in OxLDL *(104,105)*. Marx et al. *(106)* reported elevated levels of PPAR-γ expression on monocytes in human atherosclerotic lesions as compared to normal controls. Furthermore, PPAR-y stimulation leads to a concentration-dependent decrement in monocyte-derived metalloproteinase activity. Finally, PPAR-α and γ have been implicated in the induction of macrophage apoptosis through inhibition of NF-κB antiapoptotic pathways *(107)*. Endothelial cells also appear to be under the influence of PPARs by the regulation of leukocyte-endothelial cell interactions. Jackson et al. *(108)* demonstrated an inhibitory effect of stimulated PPAR on endothelial cell expression of VCAM-1. In addition, stimulated PPAR-α has been shown to inhibit TNF-α-mediated endothelial cell VCAM-1 expression, COX-2 expression, IL-1 induced production of IL-6, and thrombin-induced endothelial-1 production *(109–111)*.

Key stimulatory PPAR ligands are naturally occurring prostaglandins, as well as synthetic antidiabetic and antilipidemic drugs. Gemfibrozil, a fenofibrate and stimulator of PPAR-α, has been shown to dramatically reduce IL-1-induced production of IL-6, expression of COX-2 in human smooth muscle cells, and cardiovascular events in patients with low HDL levels. Importantly, this reduction in cardiovascular events was independent of LDL levels *(111,112)*. Troglitazone, an insulin sensitizer and PPAR-γ ligand, demonstrates a range of anti-inflammatory and potential plaque-stabilizing activities such as PPAR-γ induced inhibition of macrophage metalloproteinases *(106)*.

Currently, the complex activities of PPARs and their ligands are not completely understood, although ligands with positive effects on lipid lowering (fenofibrates) and glycemic control (troglitazone) would suggest that these transcriptional factors are clinically beneficial and mainly antiatherogenic.

Other Mediators

Myeloperoxidase

Myeloperoxidase (MPO) is a heme protein produced by leukocytes that has been shown to convert LDL into an atherogenic form, activate metalloproteinases, and catalytically consume nitric oxide causing vasoconstriction all of which affects the stability of atherosclerotic plaques, *(113,114)*. Zhang et al. found an association between MPO levels and the risk of CAD in a case control study comparing patient with and without angiographic documented CAD *(115)*. The relationship between MPO and ACS was again demonstrated when it was shown that neutrophil MPO content was reduced across the right and left coronary vascular bed in patients with ACS *(116)*. This finding suggested that widespread neutrophil activation may play a role in the development of ACS. Indeed, a single measurement of MPO in a prospective study of patients presenting with chest pain, independently predicted risk of MI *(117)*. In addition, elevated MPO levels significantly predicted risk of death or MI in a prospective study of patient with ACS independent of established biomarkers *(118)*. More recently, elevated MPO levels were found to predict future risk of CAD in a cohort of healthy individuals *(119)*.

A2 PHOSPHOLIPASES

A2 Phospholipases (PLA_2) is responsible for cleaving phospholipids into free fatty acids and lyso-phospholipids which are then metabolized and generate multiple inflammatory mediators. Secretory PLA_2 ($sPLA_2$) increases the atherogenic properties of LDL particles by promoting LDL oxidation *(120)*. Elevated levels of $sPLA_2$ in patients presenting with unstable angina have been associated with an increased risk of events spanning a 2-year period. *(121)*. Further studies, including subjects from the Global Registry of Acute Coronary Events (GRACE) study, demonstrated that elevated levels of circulating $sPLA_2$ were associated with an increased risk of death or MI *(122)*. The related lipoprotein-associated A2 ($Lp-PLA_2$) has also been associated with increased cardiovascular risk in West of Scotland Coronary Prevention Study (WOSCOPS) trial and was found to be predictive independent from other risk factors such as C-reactive protein (CRP) *(123)*.

ANGIOGENIC GROWTH FACTORS

A number of growth factors that affect angiogenesis have been associated with ACS. Vascular endothelial growth factor (VEGF) regulates endothelial cell proliferation permeability and survival and has been shown to enhance atherosclerosis plaque progression in animal models *(124)*. In the CAPTURE (c7E3 Fab Anti-Platelet Therapy in Unstable Refractory Angina) study, VEGF levels at presentation independently predicted adverse events in patients with ACS at 72 hours *(120)*. Placental growth factor (PGF) is a member of the VEGF family and is expressed in many types of inflammatory cells *(125)*. Similarly, measurement of PGF was also included in the CAPTURE trial and elevated PGF levels also independently predicted adverse events at 72 hours *(126)*. Hepatocyte growth factor (HGF) is a growth factor with angiogenic activity that was shown to be elevated 1 month after MI specifically in the territory of the infarction *(127)*. Elevated levels of HGF have been associated with a more robust collateral circulation at the time of coronary angiography and predict improved outcomes after ACS *(120)*. Accordingly, elevated levels of HGF in the CAPTURE study correlated with a reduced rate of adverse events at 72 hours *(120)*.

It is clear that further study is needed to clarify the role of angiogenic growth factors in risk stratification in ACS, as well as their potential in pharmacological intervention.

The discussion underscores the vast trafficking, redundancy, and interplay of the cytokine system. Each mediator, though, must work through specific receptors which ultimately regulate gene expression of proteins vital to the potentiation and regulation of the inflammatory cascade.

MARKERS AND MEDIATORS OF INFLAMMATION

C-Reactive Protein and Serum Amyloid A

Although many markers of inflammation have been associated with adverse cardiovascular outcome, CRP has been evaluated in every clinical phase of coronary disease. It therefore provides a superlative avenue to thoroughly discuss the prognostic significance of inflammatory markers in cardiovascular disease. CRP is an acute-phase reactant whose concentration in blood rises dramatically in response to nonspecific inflammatory stimuli. It has been convincingly linked to cardiovascular disease, initially in sera of patients after acute myocardial infarction and recently in the wall of human coronary arteries possibly linking its presence directly with the development of atherosclerosis *(128–131)*. Multiple studies conducted in the spectrum of ACS have identified CRP to be associated with either future cardiac events or a worse prognosis (Table 1). Ex vivo studies have recently introduced the concept that detecting heat release by inflammatory cells within an atherosclerotic plaque may predict future instability and rupture *(132)*. Stefanadis et al. *(133)*, using a thermography catheter, demonstrated heterogeneity in heat production of 20%, 40%, and 67% in atherosclerotic plaques of patients with stable angina, unstable angina, and acute myocardial infarction, respectively. Most importantly there was a significant correlation between thermal heterogeneity and baseline CRP *(133)*.

More conclusive evidence that chronic, indolent inflammation plays a principal role in the development and progression of atherosclerosis has come from the long-term follow-up of patients with no known atherosclerotic disease but increased levels of CRP (Table 1). In a prospective study in a cohort of initially healthy women, the value of fibrinogen (measured with an immunoassay) was added to measurement of HsCRP. The investigators concluded that baseline measurements of fibrinogen coupled with CRP provided additive values in predicting incident CVD *(134)*.

CRP is well accepted as an indirect cardiovascular risk factor as it reflects inflammation related to coronary vessel pathogens, extent of atherosclerosis, myocardial necrosis, myocardial ischemia, and activity of circulating proinflammatory cytokines *(135)*. The question remains what if any direct role CRP plays in the development of atherosclerosis. Direct evidence supporting CRP's role in the pathogenesis of atherosclerosis is its presence in the arterial wall that predicts severity of atherosclerosis as well as its ability to bind to damaged membranes and lipids and activate complement *(136–139)*. More recently, CRP has been suggested to play a more direct role in atherothrombosis involving the endothelium, platelets, leukocytes, as well as vascular smooth muscles cells *(55,140,141)* (Fig. 2). Evidence now suggests that CRP may possess procoagulant activity, as it has been shown to decrease tPA (tissue plasminogen activator activity) in human aortic endothelial cells, while increasing PAI-1 (plasminogen activator inhibitor) levels *(142,143)*. CRP has also been demonstrated to inhibit endothelial nitric oxide synthase (eNOS) *(144,145)* and prostacyclin activity *(144)* thus, promoting a prothrombotic state. Tissue factor (TF) can also be altered by CRP, as increased synthesis of TF on monocytes has been demonstrated by CRP exposure *(139)*. Further evidence suggests that CRP promotes platelet adhesion to bovine endothelial cells mediated via upregulation of P-selectin *(146)*. In addition, CRP has been demonstrated to promote monocyte-platelet aggregation that is calcium dependent and mediated via P-selectin glycoprotein ligand-1 binding *(147)*. CRP has also been shown to upregulate angiotensin type 1 receptors in vascular smooth muscle, increase vascular smooth

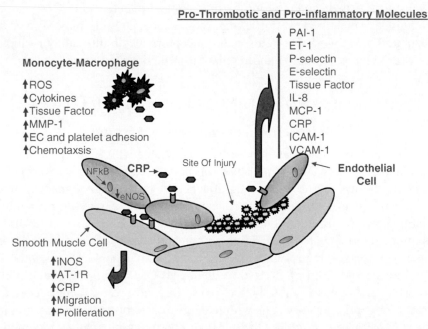

Fig. 2. The potential causative role of CRP in the pathogenesis of atherosclerosis and ACS.

muscle cell migration and proliferation, as well as neointima formation *(148)*. Despite the increasing recognition of the role of inflammation in ACS, the latest 2007 guidelines for treatment of UA/NSTEMI have not recommended measuring CRP until further validated and investigated *(149)*.

Serum Amyloid A (SAA) is an acute-phase reactant primarily produced by the liver that has well known role in the pathogenesis of Alzheimer's disease. However, it has been increasingly recognized that SAA may play a role in ACS. At high levels SAA displaces apolipoprotein A-1 (ApoA-1) yielding fractions containing SAA, lipid poor ApoA-1, and lipoprotein-free SAA. This lipid-poor form has many proinflammatory actions one of which is the induction of monocyte Tissue factor *(150)*.

THE FUTURE OF INFLAMMATION CONTROL IN ACS

Aspirin

Aspirin, initially thought of mainly as an antiplatelet drug in the battle with atherosclerotic heart disease, is becoming more recognized for its anti-inflammatory properties. In addition to aspirin's COX-1 and weak COX-2 activity, the inhibition of NF-κB activity is achieved by inhibiting both the degradation of IKB and the effects of TNF-α. Clinical evidence to support aspirin's anti-inflammatory role has been reported by Ridker et al *(151)*. Aspirin reduced first MI in the Physicians Health Study, and this effect was directly related to the baseline CRP level *(151)*.

HMG-CoA Reductase Inhibitors (Statins)

HMG-CoA reductase inhibitors have been shown to dramatically reduce cardiovascular mortality and morbidity. Sacks et al. found the reduction in events was not linear with the reduction of LDL cholesterol below 125 mg/dL *(152)*. More recently aggressive stain treatment has been associated with a further reduction of adverse cardiovascular events *(153)*, *(154)*. In addition, intensive statin therapy has also been shown to decrease CRP levels after ACS *(153,155)*. In an analysis of the Cholesterol and Recurrent Events (CARE) trial, Ridker et al. *(156)* reported a significant 22% drop in CRP over a 5-year period in those treated with pravastatin vs. placebo. Interestingly, CRP rose even in the placebo-treated arm which realized a reduction in LDL cholesterol.

Evidence continues to mount suggesting an anti-inflammatory role for HMG-CoA reductase inhibitors as these agents have been shown to alter regulation of DNA transcription, regulate natural-killer-cell cytotoxicity, inhibit platelet-derived growth factor-induced DNA synthesis, and decrease macrophage production of metalloproteinases *(156–159)*. Additionally the clinical finding that the administration of atorvastatin to statin naïve patients undergoing PCI (started 7 days before the procedure) reduced subsequent myocardial infarction suggests that the short-term effects of statins may not be solely attributed to their ability to lower lipids *(160)*. These findings have led some investigators to hypothesize that the early benefits of statin therapy could be attributed to HMG-CoA reductase inhibitors pleiotropic actions including its anti-inflammatory effects. A less recognized action of blockade of HMG-CoA reductase that may explain their acute beneficial affects is their ability to reduce prenylation of the small GTP-binding proteins Rho and Ras. The proteins when prenylated, translocate to the cell membrane where they initiate signaling cascades involved in regulating transcription and stabilization of eNOS (Fig. 3). Aggressive statin dosing would therefore be expected to inhibit inflammation via reduced prenylation and a decrease in LDL. In the A Study To Evaluate the Effect of Rosuvastatin on Intravascular Ultrasound-Derived Coronary Atheroma Burden (ASTEROID) trial, aggressive treatment with the most potent statin, rosuvastatin, resulted in a 53% reduction of LDL (baseline LDL level of 130–60 mg/dL) as well as decreased coronary atheroma burden as assessed by IVUS *(161)*.

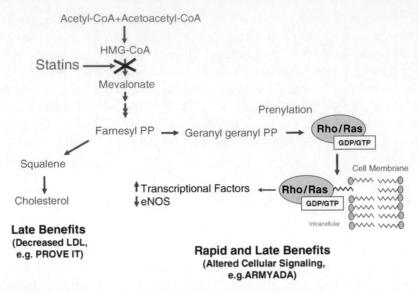

Fig. 3. The mechanistic action of the early and late benefits of statin therapy.

ACE Inhibitors

Angiotensin II (AII) has a myriad of effects on vascular tissue promoting the development of atherosclerosis. For example, AII promotes vasoconstriction, inflammation, plaque instability, thrombosis, and vascular remodeling *(162)*. ACE inhibitors have recently been demonstrated to possess potent anti-inflammatory properties that may explain their regulating effects on atherosclerotic-driven endpoints. As ACE Inhibitors block the formation of AII, it is not surprising that they have been shown to exhibit antiproliferative and antimigratory effects on smooth muscle cells and leukocytes, restore endothelial function, modulate platelet effects, and promote endogenous fibrinolysis *(163)*. More recently, ACE inhibition has been shown to decrease angiotensin-II-Induced monocyte adhesion to endothelial cells *(164)* and chemokine release *(165)*. The Heart Outcomes Prevention Evaluation (HOPE) study reported a dramatic and significant decrease in cardiovascular death, MI, and stroke in patients treated with the ACE inhibitor ramipril vs. placebo *(166)*. In addition, multiple studies (The Fourth International Study of Infarct Survival (ISIS-4), Gruppo Italiano per lo Studio della Sopravvivenza nell'Infarto Miocardico (GISSI-3), The Trandolapril Cardiac Evaluation (TRACE) study group, and Survival of Myocardial Infarction Long-term Evaluation (SMILE) study) have demonstrated that other ACE inhibitors besides ramipril have decreased mortality in patient with cardiovascular disease *(167)*. These findings strongly suggest the beneficial effects of ACE inhibition are more than can be expected from blood pressure control alone.

Thrombin Receptor Antagonists

Thrombin displays a diverse range of effects in vascular cells that functionally connects tissue damage to both hemostatic and inflammatory responses *(168,169)* (Fig. 4). Thrombin is the key effector of the coagulation cascade and converts fibrinogen to fibrin which is essential for laying the meshwork for clot formation. Thrombin also provides positive feedback by converting inactive coagulation factors into their active state, thereby generating more thrombin. Many of the cellular effects of thrombin are initiated via activation of a family of protease-activated receptors (PARs) which are coupled to heterotrimeric G proteins. Recently, initial studies with an antagonist to PAR-1, named thrombin

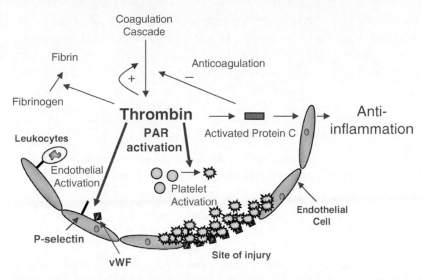

Fig. 4. The role of protease-activated receptors in mediating the cellular proinflammatory effects of thrombin.

receptor antagonists (TRA), have shown promise in patients undergoing PCI. PARs are unique among G protein–coupled receptors (GPCRs) in that they are activated by thrombin through proteolytic generation of a tethered ligand. The ability of the tethered ligand to initiate transmembrane signaling through intramolecular binding has hampered the generation of potent antagonists to these receptors; partly because thrombin's proteolytic cleavage of PAR is irreversible and the tethered ligand cannot diffuse from the receptor. PAR1 activation in endothelial cells leads to cell proliferation, attachment of polymorphonuclear cells, and increased permeability, which are important steps in the inflammatory cascade. An agent that would selectively block the inflammatory and thrombotic effects of thrombin by selectively blocking PAR activation, without altering the protective Activated protein C (APC) pathway or inhibiting fibrin generation (bleeding) would potentially have a more desirable risk/benefit ratio. Thus far, four PARs have been cloned (PAR1, PAR2, PAR3, and PAR4). Endothelial cells express both PAR1 and PAR2, while PAR3 transcripts have been found at considerably lower levels when compared to PAR1 in endothelial cells *(170)*. Human platelets contain both PAR1 and PAR4 *(171)*. Thrombin stimulates PAR-1 and PAR-3, while trypsin/tryptase and coagulation proteases upstream of thrombin (e.g., tissue factor/VIIa complex, factor Xa, and the cognate ternary complex) stimulate PAR2 *(172)*. PAR2 plays a pivotal, yet undefined role, in inflammation and ischemia with evidence for both pro- and anti-inflammatory roles *(172)*. The new oral PAR1 antagonist, (TRA) SCH 530348, was not associated with an increase in minor or major bleeding in patients undergoing PCI when TRA was added to standard antiplatelet therapy. In addition, TRA was associated with a strong trend toward reducing ischemic events by 46%. Based on the mounting information the FDA has granted fast-track designation for a Phase III clinical trial with enough power to establish the effectiveness of TRA for the reduction of ischemic events.

　　Thrombin stimulation of preformed von Willebrand factor (vWF) and P-selectin from Weibel-Palade bodies (WPB) in endothelial cells links inflammation and atherosclerosis *(173)*. Secreted vWF in turn facilitates platelet aggregation at sites of vascular injury promoting thrombosis. This finding supports evidence that elevated levels of vWF predict adverse outcomes in acute coronary syndromes *(174–176)*. In addition to thrombin's role in mediating coagulation and inflammation, thrombin also possesses antithrombotic activity at low concentrations *(177)*. The paradoxical antithrombotic activity of thrombin partly stems from the ability of thrombin in the presence of thrombomodulin to activate

Protein C, which is a potent anticoagulant that inactivates the coagulation cascade. APC also possess anti-inflammatory activity or protective effects and has been demonstrated to be essential for the maintenance of pregnancy *(178)* in addition to blocking apoptosis in ischemic brain endothelium *(179)*. The antithrombotic, anti-inflammatory, and profibrinolytic activity of Recombinant APC is used therapeutically to lessen the negative outcomes of severe infection (sepsis) *(180,181)*.

Inhibition of Cell-to-Cell Interaction

Treatment strategies available based on the inhibition of cell-to-cell interactions have shown promise in the treatment of chronic inflammatory diseases and recently coronary artery disease *(13,182)*. This should not be surprising given the marked similarities that exist between the pathophysiology of inflammatory diseases, such as RA and atherosclerosis. ASA and other NSAIDS affect the expression and function of cell adhesion molecules, and have been shown to inhibit many phases of the adhesion cascade *(18)*. Direct antagonism via monoclonal antibodies and selectin-blocking agents against ICAM-1 and L-selectin has been shown to reduce neutrophil accumulation and myocardial injury in experimental animal studies *(183,184)*. Recently, a novel oral small-molecule inhibitor of P-selectin not only decreased thrombus formation, but also reduced inflammation in a baboon model of venous thrombosis *(185)*. The question then arises if inhibition of P-selectin can inhibit arterial thrombus formation. In P-selectin knockout mice, inhibition of P-selectin reduced inflammation in an arterial aneurysm model has been observed *(186)* as well as decreased atherosclerosis when P-selectin knockout mice were crossed with apo-E deficient mice *(187)*. This would support the hypothesis that inhibiting P-selectin in an arterial model would reduce thrombus formation. New approaches using antisense oligonucleotides to inhibit mRNA translation for cell adhesion molecule expression, and inhibition of gene expression by synthetic DNA molecules and triplex-forming oligonucleotides have shown conceptual promise in animal studies *(13)*.

CLOSING THOUGHTS AND CAUTIONARY ACCOUNTS FROM PREVIOUS ANTI-INFLAMMATORY STRATEGIES

Logic and intuition would suggest that inhibiting inflammation should reduce the severity and burden of ACS. Unfortunately, not all strategies to reduce inflammation have realized a positive clinical outcome. Although investigators have demonstrated that administration of prednisone resulted in significant reductions in restenosis after bare-metal stent implantation (restenosis is influenced by inflammation) *(188)*, its administration to patients after a myocardial infarction resulted in expansion of infarcts and led to deleterious outcomes *(189)*.

Another example illustrating our ever-expanding knowledge base involves the selective cyclooxygenase 2 inhibitors. COX-2 is felt to be the principal isoform that participates in inflammation and has been found to be widely expressed in atherosclerotic tissue *(190,191)*. Evidence exists that suggested COX-2 inhibition may be beneficial with respect to endothelial cell function in a population of patients with CAD *(191,192)*. Furthermore, when COX-2 knockout mice are crossed with LDL-receptor mice, the development of atherosclerosis is accelerated *(193)*. This once formed the basis for considering the use of COX-2 inhibitors in patients with CAD *(194)*. However, withdrawal of the COX-2 inhibitor Rofecoxib secondary to evidence of increased risk of cardiovascular events in patients taking this selective COX-2 inhibitor in both the VIGOR (Vioxx GI Outcomes Research) study and APPROVe (Adenomatous Polyp PRevention On Vioxx) study trials challenges this line of thinking *(195,196)*. Subsequent studies have shown similar, although not as striking, effects with Celecoxib *(197)*. The underlying pathological basis for these effects appears to be secondary to increased production of thromboxane with an accompanying decreased production of prostacyclin *(162)*, therefore altering the balance favoring platelet activation. In addition, fenofibrates and insulin sensitizers such as troglitazone are stimulators of PPAR receptors and have received attention for their anti-inflammatory and antiatherogenic potential. However, a recent meta-analysis suggests that rosiglitazone, a selective PPAR-γ agonist, increased the risk of MI and death from cardiovascular cause *(198)*, resulting in a safety alert from the FDA.

Prevention of reperfusion injury in patients presenting with ACS by inhibiting leukocyte adhesion was reported from the HALT MI study. There was no significant reduction in infarct size and unfortunately a significant increase in infection rates in those randomized to a high dose of the CDll/CDI8 inhibitor *(199)*. This trial underscores the careful balance needed between adequate anti-inflammatory control and clinically significant immunosuppression.

While atherosclerosis is an inflammatory disease the mentioned examples underscores the vast pitfalls that exist when targeting specific inflammatory mediators. Treatment of atherosclerosis as an inflammatory disease should therefore first focus on those proven pathogens known to initiate and propagate this disease, such as hypercholesterolemia, hypertension, diabetes, and smoking. Caution must be warranted when targeting specific anti-inflammatory mediators as improper modulation can have unperceived and deleterious effects as has been realized thus far with the COX-2 inhibitors and PPAR agonist.

REFERENCES

1. Alexander RW (1994) Inflammation and coronary artery disease. N Engl J Med 331:468–469
2. Ross R, Glomset JA (1976) The pathogenesis of atherosclerosis (first of two parts). N Engl J Med 295:369–377
3. Ross R (1993) The pathogenesis of atherosclerosis: a perspective for the 1990s. Nature 362:801–809
4. Ross R (1999) Atherosclerosis – an inflammatory disease. N Engl J Med 340;115–126
5. Ross R (1986) The pathogenesis of atherosclerosis an update. N Engl J Med 314:488–500
6. Toss H, Lindahl B, Siegbahn A, Wallentin L (1997) Prognostic influence of increased fibrinogen and C-reactive protein levels in unstable coronary artery disease. FRISC Study Group. Fragmin during instability in coronary artery disease. Circulation 96:4204–4210
7. Liuzzo G, Biasucci LM, Gallimore JR et al (1994) The prognostic value of C-reactive protein and serum amyloid a protein in severe unstable angina. N Engl J Med 331:417–424
8. Tommasi S, Carluccio E, Bentivoglio M et al (1999) C-reactive protein as a marker for cardiac ischemic events in the year after a first, uncomplicated myocardial infarction. Am J Cardiol 83:1595–1599
9. Biasucci LM, Liuzzo G, Caligiuri G et al (1996) Temporal relation between ischemic episodes and activation of the coagulation system in unstable angina. Circulation 93:2121–2127
10. Bhagat K (1998) Endothelial function and myocardial infarction. Cardiovasc Res 39:312–317
11. Kinlay S, Selwyn AP, Libby P, Ganz P (1998) Inflammation, the endothelium, and the acute coronary syndromes. J Cardiovasc Pharmacol 32(Suppl 3):S62–S66
12. Noll G, Luscher TF (1998) The endothelium in acute coronary syndromes. Eur Heart J 19(Suppl C):C30–C38
13. Gonzalez-Amaro R, Diaz-Gonzalez F, Sanchez-Madrid F (1998) Adhesion molecules in inflammatory diseases. Drugs 56:977–988
14. Petruzzelli L, Takami M, Humes HD (1999) Structure and function of cell adhesion molecules. Am J Med 106:467–476
15. Frenette PS, Wagner DD (1996) Adhesion molecules – part II: blood vessels and blood cells. N Engl J Med 335:43–45
16. Frenette PS, Wagner DD (1996) Adhesion molecules – part 1. N Engl J Med 334:1526–1529
17. Springer TA (1990) Adhesion receptors of the immune system. Nature 346:425–434
18. Braun M, Pietsch P, Schror K, Baumann G, Felix SB (1999) Cellular adhesion molecules on vascular smooth muscle cells. Cardiovasc Res 41:395–401
19. Marx N, Neumann FJ, Zohlnhofer D et al (1998) Enhancement of monocyte procoagulant activity by adhesion on vascular smooth muscle cells and intercellular adhesion molecule-1-transfected Chinese hamster ovary cells. Circulation 98:906–911

20. Phillips DR, Charo IF, Parise LV, Fitzgerald LA (1988) The platelet membrane glycoprotein IIb-IIIa complex. Blood 71:831–843

21. De Caterina R, Basta G, Lazzerini G et al (1997) Soluble vascular cell adhesion molecule-1 as a biohumoral correlate of atherosclerosis. Arterioscler Thromb Vasc Biol 17:2646–2654

22. Ridker PM, Hennekens CH, Roitman-Johnson B, Stampfer MJ, Allen J (1998) Plasma concentration of soluble intercellular adhesion molecule 1 and risks of future myocardial infarction in apparently healthy men. Lancet 351:88–92

23. Rohde LE, Hennekens CH, Ridker PM (1999) Cross-sectional study of soluble intercellular adhesion molecule-1 and cardiovascular risk factors in apparently healthy men. Arterioscler Thromb Vasc Biol 19:1595–1599

24. Tenaglia AN, Buda AJ, Wilkins RG et al (1997) Levels of expression of P-selectin, E-selectin, and intercellular adhesion molecule-1 in coronary atherectomy specimens from patients with stable and unstable angina pectoris. Am J Cardiol 79:742–747

25. Ridker PM, Buring JE, Rifai N (2001) Soluble P-selectin and the risk of future cardiovascular events. Circulation 103:491–495

26. Gown AM, Tsukada T, Ross R (1986) Human atherosclerosis. II. Immunocytochemical analysis of the cellular composition of human atherosclerotic lesions. Am J Pathol 125:191–207

27. Schmitz G, Herr AS, Rothe G (1998) T-lymphocytes and monocytes in atherogenesis. Herz 23:168–177

28. Frankenberger M, Sternsdorf T, Pechumer H, Pforte A, Ziegler-Heitbrock HW (1996) Differential cytokine expression in human blood monocyte subpopulations: a polymerase chain reaction analysis. Blood 87:373–377

29. Boyle JJ (1997) Association of coronary plaque rupture and atherosclerotic inflammation. J Pathol 181:93–99

30. Moreno PR, Falk E, Palacios IF, Newell JB, Fuster V, Fallon JT (1994) Macrophage infiltration in acute coronary syndromes. Implications for plaque rupture. Circulation 90:775–778

31. Dirksen MT, van der Wal AC, van den Berg FM, van der Loos CM, Becker AE (1998) Distribution of inflammatory cells in atherosclerotic plaques relates to the direction of flow. Circulation 98:2000–2003

32. Shah PK, Falk E, Badimon JJ et al (1995) Human monocyte-derived macrophages induce collagen breakdown in fibrous caps of atherosclerotic plaques. Potential role of matrix-degrading metalloproteinases and implications for plaque rupture. Circulation 92:1565–1569

33. Hansson GK, Jonasson L, Seifert PS, Stemme S (1989) Immune mechanisms in atherosclerosis. Arteriosclerosis 9:567–578

34. Caligiuri G, Liuzzo G, Biasucci LM, Maseri A (1998) Immune system activation follows inflammation in unstable angina: pathogenetic implications. J Am Coll Cardiol 32:1295–1304

35. van der Wal AC, Piek JJ, de Boer OJ et al (1998) Recent activation of the plaque immune response in coronary lesions underlying acute coronary syndromes. Heart 80:14–18

36. Kaartinen M, Penttila A, Kovanen PT (1994) Accumulation of activated mast cells in the shoulder region of human coronary atheroma, the predilection site of atheromatous rupture. Circulation 90:1669–1678

37. Kovanen PT, Kaartinen M, Paavonen T (1995) Infiltrates of activated mast cells at the site of coronary atheromatous erosion or rupture in myocardial infarction. Circulation 92:1084–1088

38. Kaartinen M, van der Wal AC, van der Loos CM et al (1998) Mast cell infiltration in acute coronary syndromes: implications for plaque rupture. J Am Coll Cardiol 32:606–612

39. Laine P, Kaartinen M, Penttila A, Panula P, Paavonen T, Kovanen PT (1999) Association between myocardial infarction and the mast cells in the adventitia of the infarct-related coronary artery. Circulation 99:361–369

40. Irani AA, Schechter NM, Craig SS, DeBlois G, Schwartz LB (1986) Two types of human mast cells that have distinct neutral protease compositions. Proc Natl Acad Sci USA 83:4464–4468

41. Kaartinen M, Penttila A, Kovanen PT (1996) Mast cells in rupture-prone areas of human coronary atheromas produce and store TNF-alpha. Circulation 94:2787–2792

42. Hibbs MS, Hoidal JR, Kang AH (1987) Expression of a metalloproteinase that degrades native type V collagen and denatured collagens by cultured human alveolar macrophages. J Clin Invest 80:1644–1650

43. Takeshita S, Isshiki T, Ochiai M et al (1997) Systemic inflammatory responses in acute coronary syndrome: increased activity observed in polymorphonuclear leukocytes but not T lymphocytes. Atherosclerosis 135:187–192

44. Dreyer WJ, Smith CW, Michael LH et al (1989) Canine neutrophil activation by cardiac lymph obtained during reperfusion of ischemic myocardium. Circ Res 65:1751–1762

45. Smith EF 3rd, Egan JW, Bugelski PJ, Hillegass LM, Hill DE, Griswold DE (1988) Temporal relation between neutrophil accumulation and myocardial reperfusion injury. Am J Physiol 255:H1060–H1068

46. Kassirer M, Zeltser D, Prochorov V et al (1999) Increased expression of the CD11b/CD18 antigen on the surface of peripheral white blood cells in patients with ischemic heart disease: further evidence for smoldering inflammation in patients with atherosclerosis. Am Heart J 138:555–559

47. Fuster V, Badimon L, Badimon JJ, Chesebro JH (1992) The pathogenesis of coronary artery disease and the acute coronary syndromes (2). N Engl J Med 326:310–318

48. Fuster V, Badimon L, Badimon JJ, Chesebro JH (1992) The pathogenesis of coronary artery disease and the acute coronary syndromes (1). N Engl J Med 326:242–250
49. Fitzgerald DJ, Roy L, Catella F, FitzGerald GA (1986) Platelet activation in unstable coronary disease. N Engl J Med 315:983–989
50. Celi A, Pellegrini G, Lorenzet R et al (1994) P-selectin induces the expression of tissue factor on monocytes. Proc Natl Acad Sci USA 91:8767–8771
51. Furman MI, Benoit SE, Barnard MR et al (1998) Increased platelet reactivity and circulating monocyte-platelet aggregates in patients with stable coronary artery disease. J Am Coll Cardiol 31:352–358
52. Henn V, Slupsky JR, Grafe M et al (1998) CD40 ligand on activated platelets triggers an inflammatory reaction of endothelial cells. Nature 391:591–594
53. Lambert MP, Sachais BS, Kowalska MA (2007) Chemokines and thrombogenicity. Thromb Haemost 97:722–729
54. Braunersreuther V, Mach F, Steffens S (2007) The specific role of chemokines in atherosclerosis. Thromb Haemost 97:714–721
55. Jialal I, Devaraj S, Venugopal SK (2004) C-reactive protein: risk marker or mediator in atherothrombosis? Hypertension 44:6–11
56. Serrano-Martinez M, Palacios M, Lezaun R (2003) Monocyte chemoattractant protein-1 concentration in coronary sinus blood and severity of coronary disease. Circulation 108:e75
57. de Lemos JA, Morrow DA, Sabatine MS et al (2003) Association between plasma levels of monocyte chemoattractant protein-1 and long-term clinical outcomes in patients with acute coronary syndromes. Circulation 107:690–695
58. Horrevoets AJ, Fontijn RD, van Zonneveld AJ, de Vries CJ, ten Cate JW, Pannekoek H (1999) Vascular endothelial genes that are responsive to tumor necrosis factor-alpha in vitro are expressed in atherosclerotic lesions, including inhibitor of apoptosis protein-1, stannin, and two novel genes. Blood 93:3418–3431
59. Rus HG, Niculescu F, Vlaicu R (1991) Tumor necrosis factor-alpha in human arterial wall with atherosclerosis. Atherosclerosis 89:247–254
60. Ahmad M, Theofanidis P, Medford RM (1998) Role of activating protein-1 in the regulation of the vascular cell adhesion molecule-1 gene expression by tumor necrosis factor-alpha. J Biol Chem 273:4616–4621
61. Morisaki N, Xu QP, Koshikawa T, Saito Y, Yoshida S, Ueda S (1993) Tumour necrosis factor-alpha can modulate the phenotype of aortic smooth muscle cells. Scand J Clin Lab Invest 53:347–352
62. Weber C, Draude G, Weber KS, Wubert J, Lorenz RL, Weber PC (1999) Downregulation by tumor necrosis factor-alpha of monocyte CCR2 expression and monocyte chemotactic protein-1-induced transendothelial migration is antagonized by oxidized low-density lipoprotein: a potential mechanism of monocyte retention in atherosclerotic lesions. Atherosclerosis 145:115–123
63. Barks JL, McQuillan JJ, Iademarco MF (1997) TNF-alpha and IL-4 synergistically increase vascular cell adhesion molecule-1 expression in cultured vascular smooth muscle cells. J Immunol 159:4532–4538
64. Libby P, Sukhova G, Lee RT, Galis ZS (1995) Cytokines regulate vascular functions related to stability of the atherosclerotic plaque. J Cardiovasc Pharmacol 25(Suppl 2):S9–S12
65. Galis ZS, Muszynski M, Sukhova GK et al (1994) Cytokine-stimulated human vascular smooth muscle cells synthesize a complement of enzymes required for extracellular matrix digestion. Circ Res 75:181–189
66. Rajavashisth TB, Xu XP, Jovinge S et al (1999) Membrane type 1 matrix metalloproteinase expression in human atherosclerotic plaques: evidence for activation by proinflammatory mediators. Circulation 99:3103–3109
67. Dosquet C, Weill D, Wautier JL (1995) Cytokines and thrombosis. J Cardiovasc Pharmacol 25(Suppl 2):S13–S19
68. Charles P, Elliott MJ, Davis D et al (1999) Regulation of cytokines, cytokine inhibitors, and acute-phase proteins following anti-TNF-alpha therapy in rheumatoid arthritis. J Immunol 163:1521–1528
69. Biasucci LM, Liuzzo G, Fantuzzi G et al (1999) Increasing levels of interleukin (IL)-1Ra and IL-6 during the first 2 days of hospitalization in unstable angina are associated with increased risk of in-hospital coronary events. Circulation 99:2079–2084
70. Miyao Y, Yasue H, Ogawa H et al (1993) Elevated plasma interleukin-6 levels in patients with acute myocardial infarction. Am Heart J 126:1299–1304
71. Kushner I, Ganapathi M, Schultz D (1989) The acute phase response is mediated by heterogeneous mechanisms. Ann N Y Acad Sci 557:19–29 discussion 29-30
72. Bevilacqua MP, Schleef RR, Gimbrone MA Jr, Loskutoff DJ (1986) Regulation of the fibrinolytic system of cultured human vascular endothelium by interleukin 1. J Clin Invest 78:587–591
73. Youker K, Smith CW, Anderson DC et al (1992) Neutrophil adherence to isolated adult cardiac myocytes. Induction by cardiac lymph collected during ischemia and reperfusion. J Clin Invest 89:602–609
74. Finkel MS, Oddis CV, Jacob TD, Watkins SC, Hattler BG, Simmons RL (1992) Negative inotropic effects of cytokines on the heart mediated by nitric oxide. Science 257:387–389

75. Lindmark E, Diderholm E, Wallentin L, Siegbahn A (2001) Relationship between interleukin 6 and mortality in patients with unstable coronary artery disease: effects of an early invasive or noninvasive strategy. JAMA 286:2107–2113
76. Pannitteri G, Marino B, Campa PP, Martucci R, Testa U, Peschle C (1997) Interleukins 6 and 8 as mediators of acute phase response in acute myocardial infarction. Am J Cardiol 80:622–625
77. Gerszten RE, Garcia-Zepeda EA, Lim YC et al (1999) MCP-1 and IL-8 trigger firm adhesion of monocytes to vascular endothelium under flow conditions. Nature 398:718–723
78. Yue TL, McKenna PJ, Gu JL, Feuerstein GZ (1993) Interleukin-8 is chemotactic for vascular smooth muscle cells. Eur J Pharmacol 240:81–84
79. Folcik VA, Aamir R, Cathcart MK (1997) Cytokine modulation of LDL oxidation by activated human monocytes. Arterioscler Thromb Vasc Biol 17:1954–1961
80. Edgington TS, Mackman N, Brand K, Ruf W (1991) The structural biology of expression and function of tissue factor. Thromb Haemost 66:67–79
81. Nie Q, Fan J, Haraoka S, Shimokama T, Watanabe T (1997) Inhibition of mononuclear cell recruitment in aortic intima by treatment with anti-ICAM-1 and anti-LFA-1 monoclonal antibodies in hypercholesterolemic rats: implications of the ICAM-1 and LFA-1 pathway in atherogenesis. Lab Invest 77:469–482
82. Mantovani A, Garlanda C, Introna M, Vecchi A (1998) Regulation of endothelial cell function by pro- and anti-inflammatory cytokines. Transplant Proc 30:4239–4243
83. Mach F, Schonbeck U, Libby P (1998) CD40 signaling in vascular cells: a key role in atherosclerosis? Atherosclerosis 137(Suppl):S89–S95
84. Mohan C, Shi Y, Laman JD, Datta SK (1995) Interaction between CD40 and its ligand gp39 in the development of murine lupus nephritis. J Immunol 154:1470–1480
85. Larsen CP, Elwood ET, Alexander DZ et al (1996) Long-term acceptance of skin and cardiac allografts after blocking CD40 and CD28 pathways. Nature 381:434–438
86. Gerritse K, Laman JD, Noelle RJ et al (1996) CD40-CD40 ligand interactions in experimental allergic encephalomyelitis and multiple sclerosis. Proc Natl Acad Sci USA 93:2499–2504
87. Mach F, Schonbeck U, Sukhova GK, Atkinson E, Libby P (1998) Reduction of atherosclerosis in mice by inhibition of CD40 signalling. Nature 394:200–203
88. Aukrust P, Muller F, Ueland T et al (1999) Enhanced levels of soluble and membrane-bound CD40 ligand in patients with unstable angina. Possible reflection of T lymphocyte and platelet involvement in the pathogenesis of acute coronary syndromes. Circulation 100:614–620
89. Baeuerle PA (1998) IkappaB-NF-kappaB structures: at the interface of inflammation control. Cell 95:729–731
90. Mercurio F, Manning AM (1999) Multiple signals converging on NF-kappaB. Curr Opin Cell Biol 11:226–232
91. Lee JI, Burckart GJ (1998) Nuclear factor kappa B: important transcription factor and therapeutic target. J Clin Pharmacol 38:981–993
92. Barnes PJ, Karin M (1997) Nuclear factor-kappaB: a pivotal transcription factor in chronic inflammatory diseases. N Engl J Med 336:1066–1071
93. Massi-Benedetti M, Federici MO (1999) Cardiovascular risk factors in type 2 diabetes: the role of hyperglycaemia. Exp Clin Endocrinol Diabetes 107(Suppl 4):S120–S123
94. Dichtl W, Nilsson L, Goncalves I et al (1999) Very low-density lipoprotein activates nuclear factor-kappaB in endothelial cells. Circ Res 84:1085–1094
95. Brand K, Eisele T, Kreusel U et al (1997) Dysregulation of monocytic nuclear factor-kappa B by oxidized low-density lipoprotein. Arterioscler Thromb Vasc Biol 17:1901–1909
96. Kranzhofer R, Browatzki M, Schmidt J, Kubler W (1999) Angiotensin II activates the proinflammatory transcription factor nuclear factor-kappaB in human monocytes. Biochem Biophys Res Commun 257:826–828
97. Yerneni KK, Bai W, Khan BV, Medford RM, Natarajan R (1999) Hyperglycemia-induced activation of nuclear transcription factor kappaB in vascular smooth muscle cells. Diabetes 48:855–864
98. Bustos C, Hernandez-Presa MA, Ortego M et al (1998) HMG-CoA reductase inhibition by atorvastatin reduces neointimal inflammation in a rabbit model of atherosclerosis. J Am Coll Cardiol 32:2057–2064
99. Ritchie ME (1998) Nuclear factor-kappaB is selectively and markedly activated in humans with unstable angina pectoris. Circulation 98:1707–1713
100. Kopp E, Ghosh S (1994) Inhibition of NF-kappa B by sodium salicylate and aspirin. Science 265:956–959
101. Weber C, Erl W, Pietsch A, Weber PC (1995) Aspirin inhibits nuclear factor-kappa B mobilization and monocyte adhesion in stimulated human endothelial cells. Circulation 91:1914–1917
102. Plutzky J (1999) Atherosclerotic plaque rupture: emerging insights and opportunities. Am J Cardiol 84:15J–20J

103. Ricote M, Li AC, Willson TM, Kelly CJ, Glass CK (1998) The peroxisome proliferator-activated receptor-gamma is a negative regulator of macrophage activation. Nature 391:79–82
104. Nagy L, Tontonoz P, Alvarez JG, Chen H, Evans RM (1998) Oxidized LDL regulates macrophage gene expression through ligand activation of PPARgamma. Cell 93:229–240
105. Tontonoz P, Nagy L, Alvarez JG, Thomazy VA, Evans RM (1998) PPARgamma promotes monocyte/macrophage differentiation and uptake of oxidized LDL. Cell 93:241–252
106. Marx N, Sukhova G, Murphy C, Libby P, Plutzky J (1998) Macrophages in human atheroma contain PPARgamma: differentiation-dependent peroxisomal proliferator-activated receptor gamma(PPARgamma) expression and reduction of MMP-9 activity through PPARgamma activation in mononuclear phagocytes in vitro. Am J Pathol 153:17–23
107. Chinetti G, Griglio S, Antonucci M et al (1998) Activation of proliferator-activated receptors alpha and gamma induces apoptosis of human monocyte-derived macrophages. J Biol Chem 273:25573–25580
108. Jackson SM, Parhami F, Xi XP et al (1999) Peroxisome proliferator-activated receptor activators target human endothelial cells to inhibit leukocyte-endothelial cell interaction. Arterioscler Thromb Vasc Biol 19:2094–2104
109. Marx N, Sukhova GK, Collins T, Libby P, Plutzky J (1999) PPARalpha activators inhibit cytokine-induced vascular cell adhesion molecule-1 expression in human endothelial cells. Circulation 99:3125–3131
110. Delerive P, Martin-Nizard F, Chinetti G et al (1999) Peroxisome proliferator-activated receptor activators inhibit thrombin-induced endothelin-1 production in human vascular endothelial cells by inhibiting the activator protein-1 signaling pathway. Circ Res 85:394–402
111. Staels B, Koenig W, Habib A et al (1998) Activation of human aortic smooth-muscle cells is inhibited by PPARalpha but not by PPARgamma activators. Nature 393:790–793
112. Rubins HB, Robins SJ, Collins D et al (1999) Gemfibrozil for the secondary prevention of coronary heart disease in men with low levels of high-density lipoprotein cholesterol. Veterans Affairs High-Density Lipoprotein Cholesterol Intervention Trial Study Group. N Engl J Med 341:410–418
113. Nicholls SJ, Hazen SL (2005) Myeloperoxidase and cardiovascular disease. Arterioscler Thromb Vasc Biol 25:1102–1111
114. Hazen SL (2004) Myeloperoxidase and plaque vulnerability. Arterioscler Thromb Vasc Biol 24:1143–1146
115. Zhang R, Brennan ML, Fu X et al (2001) Association between myeloperoxidase levels and risk of coronary artery disease. JAMA 286:2136–2142
116. Buffon A, Biasucci LM, Liuzzo G, D'Onofrio G, Crea F, Maseri A (2002) Widespread coronary inflammation in unstable angina. N Engl J Med 347:5–12
117. Brennan ML, Penn MS, Van Lente F et al (2003) Prognostic value of myeloperoxidase in patients with chest pain. N Engl J Med 349:1595–1604
118. Baldus S, Heeschen C, Meinertz T et al (2003) Myeloperoxidase serum levels predict risk in patients with acute coronary syndromes. Circulation 108:1440–1445
119. Meuwese MC, Stroes ES, Hazen SL et al (2007) Serum myeloperoxidase levels are associated with the future risk of coronary artery disease in apparently healthy individuals: the EPIC-Norfolk Prospective Population Study. J Am Coll Cardiol 50:159–165
120. Heeschen C, Dimmeler S, Hamm CW, Boersma E, Zeiher AM, Simoons ML (2003) Prognostic significance of angiogenic growth factor serum levels in patients with acute coronary syndromes. Circulation 107:524–530
121. Kugiyama K, Ota Y, Sugiyama S et al (2000) Prognostic value of plasma levels of secretory type II phospholipase A2 in patients with unstable angina pectoris. Am J Cardiol 86:718–722
122. Mallat Z, Steg PG, Benessiano J et al (2005) Circulating secretory phospholipase A2 activity predicts recurrent events in patients with severe acute coronary syndromes. J Am Coll Cardiol 46:1249–1257
123. Packard CJ, O'Reilly DS, Caslake MJ et al (2000) Lipoprotein-associated phospholipase A2 as an independent predictor of coronary heart disease. West of Scotland Coronary Prevention Study Group. N Engl J Med 343:1148–1155
124. Celletti FL, Waugh JM, Amabile PG, Brendolan A, Hilfiker PR, Dake MD (2001) Vascular endothelial growth factor enhances atherosclerotic plaque progression. Nat Med 7:425–429
125. Autiero M, Luttun A, Tjwa M, Carmeliet P (2003) Placental growth factor and its receptor, vascular endothelial growth factor receptor-1: novel targets for stimulation of ischemic tissue revascularization and inhibition of angiogenic and inflammatory disorders. J Thromb Haemost 1:1356–1370
126. Heeschen C, Dimmeler S, Fichtlscherer S et al (2004) Prognostic value of placental growth factor in patients with acute chest pain. JAMA 291:435–441
127. Yasuda S, Goto Y, Baba T et al (2000) Enhanced secretion of cardiac hepatocyte growth factor from an infarct region is associated with less severe ventricular enlargement and improved cardiac function. J Am Coll Cardiol 36:115–121

128. Zimmermann-Gorska I, Kujawa H, Drygas J (1972) Studies of acute phase reactants in myocardial infarction. Pol Med J 11:779–785
129. Jain VC (1968) An evaluation of C-reactive protein test in acute myocardial infarction. Indian Heart J 20:16–21
130. Zhang YX, Cliff WJ, Schoefl GI, Higgins G (1999) Coronary C-reactive protein distribution: its relation to development of atherosclerosis. Atherosclerosis 145:375–379
131. Anzai T, Yoshikawa T, Shiraki H et al (1997) C-reactive protein as a predictor of infarct expansion and cardiac rupture after a first Q-wave acute myocardial infarction. Circulation 96:778–784
132. Casscells W, Hathorn B, David M et al (1996) Thermal detection of cellular infiltrates in living atherosclerotic plaques: possible implications for plaque rupture and thrombosis. Lancet 347:1447–1451
133. Stefanadis C, Diamantopoulos L, Vlachopoulos C et al (1999) Thermal heterogeneity within human atherosclerotic coronary arteries detected in vivo: a new method of detection by application of a special thermography catheter. Circulation 99:1965–1971
134. Mora S, Rifai N, Buring JE, Ridker PM (2006) Additive value of immunoassay-measured fibrinogen and high-sensitivity C-reactive protein levels for predicting incident cardiovascular events. Circulation 114:381–387
135. Lagrand WK, Visser CA, Hermens WT et al (1999) C-reactive protein as a cardiovascular risk factor: more than an epiphenomenon? Circulation 100:96–102
136. Toschi V, Gallo R, Lettino M et al (1997) Tissue factor modulates the thrombogenicity of human atherosclerotic plaques. Circulation 95:594–599
137. Pepys MB, Rowe IF, Baltz ML (1985) C-reactive protein: binding to lipids and lipoproteins. Int Rev Exp Pathol 27:83–111
138. Volanakis JE (1982) Complement activation by C-reactive protein complexes. Ann N Y Acad Sci 389:235–250
139. Cermak J, Key NS, Bach RR, Balla J, Jacob HS, Vercellotti GM (1993) C-reactive protein induces human peripheral blood monocytes to synthesize tissue factor. Blood 82:513–520
140. Mazer SP, Rabbani LE (2004) Evidence for C-reactive protein's role in (CRP) vascular disease: atherothrombosis, immuno-regulation and CRP. J Thromb Thrombolysis 17:95–105
141. Paffen E, DeMaat MP (2006) C-reactive protein in atherosclerosis: a causal factor? Cardiovasc Res 71:30–39
142. Singh U, Devaraj S, Jialal I (2005) C-reactive protein decreases tissue plasminogen activator activity in human aortic endothelial cells: evidence that C-reactive protein is a procoagulant. Arterioscler Thromb Vasc Biol 25:2216–2221
143. Devaraj S, Xu DY, Jialal I (2003) C-reactive protein increases plasminogen activator inhibitor-1 expression and activity in human aortic endothelial cells: implications for the metabolic syndrome and atherothrombosis. Circulation 107:398–404
144. Venugopal SK, Devaraj S, Jialal I (2003) C-reactive protein decreases prostacyclin release from human aortic endothelial cells. Circulation 108:1676–1678
145. Verma S, Wang CH, Li SH et al (2002) A self-fulfilling prophecy: C-reactive protein attenuates nitric oxide production and inhibits angiogenesis. Circulation 106:913–919
146. Yaron G, Brill A, Dashevsky O et al (2006) C-reactive protein promotes platelet adhesion to endothelial cells: a potential pathway in atherothrombosis. Br J Haematol 134:426–431
147. Danenberg HD, Kantak N, Grad E, Swaminathan RV, Lotan C, Edelman ER (2007) C-reactive protein promotes monocyte-platelet aggregation: an additional link to the inflammatory-thrombotic intricacy. Eur J Haematol 78:246–252
148. Wang CH, Li SH, Weisel RD et al (2003) C-reactive protein upregulates angiotensin type 1 receptors in vascular smooth muscle. Circulation 107:1783–1790
149. Anderson JL, Adams CD, Antman EM et al (2007) ACC/AHA 2007 guidelines for the management of patients with unstable angina/non ST-elevation myocardial infarction: a report of the American College of Cardiology/American Heart Association Task Force on Practice Guidelines (Writing Committee to Revise the 2002 Guidelines for the Management of Patients With Unstable Angina/Non ST-Elevation Myocardial Infarction): developed in collaboration with the American College of Emergency Physicians, the Society for Cardiovascular Angiography and Interventions, and the Society of Thoracic Surgeons: endorsed by the American Association of Cardiovascular and Pulmonary Rehabilitation and the Society for Academic Emergency Medicine. Circulation 116:e148–e304
150. Cai H, Song C, Endoh I et al (2007) Serum amyloid A induces monocyte tissue factor. J Immunol 178:1852–1860
151. Ridker PM, Cushman M, Stampfer MJ, Tracy RP, Hennekens CH (1997) Inflammation, aspirin, and the risk of cardiovascular disease in apparently healthy men. N Engl J Med 336:973–979
152. Sacks FM, Ridker PM (1999) Lipid lowering and beyond: results from the CARE study on lipoproteins and inflammation. Cholesterol and recurrent events. Herz 24:51–56
153. Cannon CP, Braunwald E, McCabe CH et al (2004) Intensive versus moderate lipid lowering with statins after acute coronary syndromes. N Engl J Med 350:1495–1504
154. Schwartz GG, Olsson AG, Ezekowitz MD et al (2001) Effects of atorvastatin on early recurrent ischemic events in acute coronary syndromes: the MIRACL study: a randomized controlled trial. JAMA 285:1711–1718

155. Kinlay S, Schwartz GG, Olsson AG et al (2003) High-dose atorvastatin enhances the decline in inflammatory markers in patients with acute coronary syndromes in the MIRACL study. Circulation 108:1560–1566

156. Ridker PM, Rifai N, Pfeffer MA et al (1998) Inflammation, pravastatin, and the risk of coronary events after myocardial infarction in patients with average cholesterol levels. Cholesterol and Recurrent Events (CARE) Investigators. Circulation 98:839–844

157. Vaughan CJ, Murphy MB, Buckley BM (1996) Statins do more than just lower cholesterol. Lancet 348:1079–1082

158. McPherson R, Tsoukas C, Baines MG et al (1993) Effects of lovastatin on natural killer cell function and other immunological parameters in man. J Clin Immunol 13:439–444

159. Bellosta S, Via D, Canavesi M et al (1998) HMG-CoA reductase inhibitors reduce MMP-9 secretion by macrophages. Arterioscler Thromb Vasc Biol 18:1671–1678

160. Pasceri V, Patti G, Nusca A, Pristipino C, Richichi G, Di Sciascio G (2004) Randomized trial of atorvastatin for reduction of myocardial damage during coronary intervention: results from the ARMYDA (Atorvastatin for Reduction of MYocardial Damage during Angioplasty) study. Circulation 110:674–678

161. Nissen SE, Nicholls SJ, Sipahi I et al (2006) Effect of very high-intensity statin therapy on regression of coronary atherosclerosis: the ASTEROID trial. JAMA 295:1556–1565

162. Krotz F, Schiele TM, Klauss V, Sohn HY (2005) Selective COX-2 inhibitors and risk of myocardial infarction. J Vasc Res 42:312–324

163. Cheng JW, Ngo MN (1997) Current perspective on the use of angiotensin-converting enzyme inhibitors in the management of coronary (atherosclerotic) artery disease. Ann Pharmacother 31:1499–1506

164. Soehnlein O, Schmeisser A, Cicha I et al (2005) ACE inhibition lowers angiotensin-II-induced monocyte adhesion to HUVEC by reduction of p65 translocation and AT 1 expression. J Vasc Res 42:399–407

165. Schmeisser A, Soehnlein O, Illmer T et al (2004) ACE inhibition lowers angiotensin II-induced chemokine expression by reduction of NF-kappaB activity and AT1 receptor expression. Biochem Biophys Res Commun 325:532–540

166. Yusuf S, Sleight P, Pogue J, Bosch J, Davies R, Dagenais G (2000) Effects of an angiotensin-converting-enzyme inhibitor, ramipril, on cardiovascular events in high-risk patients. The Heart Outcomes Prevention Evaluation Study Investigators. N Engl J Med 342:145–153

167. Dzau VJ, Bernstein K, Celermajer D et al (2002) Pathophysiologic and therapeutic importance of tissue ACE: a consensus report. Cardiovasc Drugs Ther 16:149–160

168. Coughlin SR (2000) Thrombin signalling and protease-activated receptors. Nature 407:258–264

169. Jamieson GA (1997) Pathophysiology of platelet thrombin receptors. Thromb Haemost 78:242–246

170. Schmidt G, Selzer J, Lerm M, Aktories K (1998) The Rho-deamidating cytotoxic necrotizing factor 1 from *Escherichia coli* possesses transglutaminase activity. J Biol Chem 273:13669–13674

171. Camerer E, Huang W, Coughlin SR (2000) Tissue factor- and factor X-dependent activation of protease-activated receptor 2 by factor VIIa. Proc Natl Acad Sci USA 97:5255–5260

172. Coughlin SR, Camerer E (2003) PARticipation in inflammation. J Clin Invest 111:25–27

173. Cleator JH, Zhu WQ, Vaughan DE, Hamm HE (2006) Differential regulation of endothelial exocytosis of P-selectin and von Willebrand factor by protease-activated receptors and cAMP. Blood 107:2736–2744

174. Ruggeri ZM (2003) Von Willebrand factor, platelets and endothelial cell interactions. J Thromb Haemost 1:1335–1342

175. Montalescot G, Philippe F, Ankri A et al (1998) Early increase of von Willebrand factor predicts adverse outcome in unstable coronary artery disease: beneficial effects of enoxaparin. French investigators of the ESSENCE trial. Circulation 98:294–299

176. Collet JP, Montalescot G, Vicaut E et al (2003) Acute release of plasminogen activator inhibitor-1 in ST-segment elevation myocardial infarction predicts mortality. Circulation 108:391–394

177. Hanson SR, Griffin JH, Harker LA, Kelly AB, Esmon CT, Gruber A (1993) Antithrombotic effects of thrombin-induced activation of endogenous protein C in primates. J Clin Invest 92:2003–2012

178. Isermann B, Sood R, Pawlinski R et al (2003) The thrombomodulin-protein C system is essential for the maintenance of pregnancy. Nat Med 9:331–337

179. Cheng T, Liu D, Griffin JH et al (2003) Activated protein C blocks p53-mediated apoptosis in ischemic human brain endothelium and is neuroprotective. Nat Med 9:338–342

180. McCoy C, Matthews SJ (2003) Drotrecogin alfa (recombinant human activated protein C) for the treatment of severe sepsis. Clin Ther 25:396–421

181. Bernard GR, Ely EW, Wright TJ et al (2001) Safety and dose relationship of recombinant human activated protein C for coagulopathy in severe sepsis. Crit Care Med 29:2051–2059

182. Davis LS, Kavanaugh AF, Nichols LA, Lipsky PE (1995) Induction of persistent T cell hyporesponsiveness in vivo by monoclonal antibody to ICAM-1 in patients with rheumatoid arthritis. J Immunol 154:3525–3537

183. Buerke M, Weyrich AS, Zheng Z, Gaeta FC, Forrest MJ, Lefer AM (1994) Sialyl Lewisx-containing oligosaccharide attenuates myocardial reperfusion injury in cats. J Clin Invest 93:1140–1148
184. Silver MJ, Sutton JM, Hook S et al (1995) Adjunctive selectin blockade successfully reduces infarct size beyond thrombolysis in the electrolytic canine coronary artery model. Circulation 92:492–499
185. Myers DD Jr, Wrobleski SK, Longo C et al (2007) Resolution of venous thrombosis using a novel oral small-molecule inhibitor of P-selectin (PSI-697) without anticoagulation. Thromb Haemost 97:400–407
186. Hannawa KK, Cho BS, Sinha I et al (2006) Attenuation of experimental aortic aneurysm formation in P-selectin knock-out mice. Ann N Y Acad Sci 1085:353–359
187. Burger PC, Wagner DD (2003) Platelet P-selectin facilitates atherosclerotic lesion development. Blood 101:2661–2666
188. Versaci F, Gaspardone A, Tomai F et al (2002) Immunosuppressive therapy for the prevention of restenosis after coronary artery stent implantation (IMPRESS Study). J Am Coll Cardiol 40:1935–1942
189. Roberts R, DeMello V, Sobel BE (1976) Deleterious effects of methylprednisolone in patients with myocardial infarction. Circulation 53:I204–I206
190. Baker CS, Hall RJ, Evans TJ et al (1999) Cyclooxygenase-2 is widely expressed in atherosclerotic lesions affecting native and transplanted human coronary arteries and colocalizes with inducible nitric oxide synthase and nitrotyrosine particularly in macrophages. Arterioscler Thromb Vasc Biol 19:646–655
191. Schonbeck U, Sukhova GK, Graber P, Coulter S, Libby P (1999) Augmented expression of cyclooxygenase-2 in human atherosclerotic lesions. Am J Pathol 155:1281–1291
192. Bogaty P, Brophy JM, Noel M et al (2004) Impact of prolonged cyclooxygenase-2 inhibition on inflammatory markers and endothelial function in patients with ischemic heart disease and raised C-reactive protein: a randomized placebo-controlled study. Circulation 110:934–939
193. Sessa WC (2004) eNOS at a glance. J Cell Sci 117:2427–2429
194. Linton MF, Fazio S (2004) Cyclooxygenase-2 and inflammation in atherosclerosis. Curr Opin Pharmacol 4:116–123
195. Bombardier C, Laine L, Reicin A et al (2000) Comparison of upper gastrointestinal toxicity of rofecoxib and naproxen in patients with rheumatoid arthritis. VIGOR Study Group. N Engl J Med 343:1520–1528 2 p following 1528
196. Bresalier RS, Sandler RS, Quan H et al (2005) Cardiovascular events associated with rofecoxib in a colorectal adenoma chemoprevention trial. N Engl J Med 352:1092–1102
197. Solomon SD, McMurray JJ, Pfeffer MA et al (2005) Cardiovascular risk associated with celecoxib in a clinical trial for colorectal adenoma prevention. N Engl J Med 352:1071–1080
198. Nissen SE, Wolski K (2007) Effect of rosiglitazone on the risk of myocardial infarction and death from cardiovascular causes. N Engl J Med 356:2457–2471
199. Faxon DP, Gibbons RJ, Chronos NA, Gurbel PA, Sheehan F (2002) The effect of blockade of the CD11/CD18 integrin receptor on infarct size in patients with acute myocardial infarction treated with direct angioplasty: the results of the HALT-MI study. J Am Coll Cardiol 40:1199–1204
200. Humphries J, McGuinness CL, Smith A, Waltham M, Poston R, Burnand KG (1999) Monocyte chemotactic protein-1 (MCP-1) accelerates the organization and resolution of venous thrombi. J Vasc Surg 30:894–899
201. Gu L, Okada Y, Clinton SK et al (1998) Absence of monocyte chemoattractant protein-1 reduces atherosclerosis in low density lipoprotein receptor-deficient mice. Mol Cell 2:275–281
202. Mause SF, von Hundelshausen P, Zernecke A, Koenen RR, Weber C (2005) Platelet microparticles: a transcellular delivery system for RANTES promoting monocyte recruitment on endothelium. Arterioscler Thromb Vasc Biol 25:1512–1518
203. Veillard NR, Kwak B, Pelli G et al (2004) Antagonism of RANTES receptors reduces atherosclerotic plaque formation in mice. Circ Res 94:253–261
204. Nomura S, Uehata S, Saito S, Osumi K, Ozeki Y, Kimura Y (2003) Enzyme immunoassay detection of platelet-derived microparticles and RANTES in acute coronary syndrome. Thromb Haemost 89:506–512
205. Parissis JT, Adamopoulos S, Venetsanou KF, Mentzikof DG, Karas SM, Kremastinos DT (2002) Serum profiles of C-C chemokines in acute myocardial infarction: possible implication in postinfarction left ventricular remodeling. J Interferon Cytokine Res 22:223–229
206. Walz A, Baggiolini M (1990) Generation of the neutrophil-activating peptide NAP-2 from platelet basic protein or connective tissue-activating peptide III through monocyte proteases. J Exp Med 171:449–454
207. Holt JC, Yan ZQ, Lu WQ, Stewart GJ, Niewiarowski S (1992) Isolation, characterization, and immunological detection of neutrophil-activating peptide 2: a proteolytic degradation product of platelet basic protein. Proc Soc Exp Biol Med 199:171–177
208. Smith C, Damas JK, Otterdal K et al (2006) Increased levels of neutrophil-activating peptide-2 in acute coronary syndromes: possible role of platelet-mediated vascular inflammation. J Am Coll Cardiol 48:1591–1599

209. Kowalska MA, Ratajczak MZ, Majka M et al (2000) Stromal cell-derived factor-1 and macrophage-derived chemokine: 2 chemokines that activate platelets. Blood 96:50–57

210. Teupser D, Pavlides S, Tan M, Gutierrez-Ramos JC, Kolbeck R, Breslow JL (2004) Major reduction of atherosclerosis in fractalkine (CX3CL1)-deficient mice is at the brachiocephalic artery, not the aortic root. Proc Natl Acad Sci USA 101:17795–17800

211. Koenig W, Sund M, Frohlich M et al (1999) C-Reactive protein, a sensitive marker of inflammation, predicts future risk of coronary heart disease in initially healthy middle-aged men: results from the MONICA (Monitoring Trends and Determinants in Cardiovascular Disease) Augsburg Cohort Study, 1984 to 1992. Circulation 99:237–242

212. Ridker PM, Glynn RJ, Hennekens CH (1998) C-reactive protein adds to the predictive value of total and HDL cholesterol in determining risk of first myocardial infarction. Circulation 97:2007–2011

213. Ridker PM, Buring JE, Shih J, Matias M, Hennekens CH (1998) Prospective study of C-reactive protein and the risk of future cardiovascular events among apparently healthy women. Circulation 98:731–733

214. Gaspardone A, Crea F, Versaci F et al (1998) Predictive value of C-reactive protein after successful coronary-artery stenting in patients with stable angina. Am J Cardiol 82:515–518

215. Liuzzo G, Baisucci LM, Gallimore JR et al (1999) Enhanced inflammatory response in patients with preinfarction unstable angina. J Am Coll Cardiol 34:1696–1703

216. Biasucci LM, Liuzzo G, Grillo RL et al (1999) Elevated levels of C-reactive protein at discharge in patients with unstable angina predict recurrent instability. Circulation 99:855–860

217. Milazzo D, Biasucci LM, Luciani N et al (1999) Elevated levels of C-reactive protein before coronary artery bypass grafting predict recurrence of ischemic events. Am J Cardiol 84:459–461 A9

218. Haverkate F, Thompson SG, Pyke SD, Gallimore JR, Pepys MB (1997) Production of C-reactive protein and risk of coronary events in stable and unstable angina. European Concerted Action on Thrombosis and Disabilities Angina Pectoris Study Group. Lancet 349:462–466

219. Verheggen PW, de Maat MP, Cats VM et al (1999) Inflammatory status as a main determinant of outcome in patients with unstable angina, independent of coagulation activation and endothelial cell function. Eur Heart J 20:567–574

220. Biasucci LM, Vitelli A, Liuzzo G et al (1996) Elevated levels of interleukin-6 in unstable angina. Circulation 94:874–877

221. Morrow DA, Rifai N et al (1998) C-reactive protein is a potent predictor of mortality independently of and in combination with troponin T in acute coronary syndromes: a TIMI 11A substudy. Thrombolysis in myocardial infarction. J Am Coll Cardiol 31:1460–1465

4 The Genetics of Thrombosis

Svati H. Shah and Richard C. Becker

CONTENTS

ABSTRACT Coagulation and hemostasis are the result of a complex interplay of platelets, coagulation factors, and fibrinolytic proteins. Genetic variants underlying these factors may contribute to derangement of this coordinated system, resulting in abnormal coagulation or fibrinolysis and subsequent thrombosis. Human pathologic thrombosis remains a complex, heterogeneous disease. The advent of advanced genetic and molecular technologies has facilitated an explosion of studies of genetics of human thrombotic disease, resulting in several advances in our understanding of such disorders.

Key words: Genetics; Platelets; Thrombosis, Thromboembolism

INTRODUCTION

Coagulation and hemostasis are the result of a complex interplay of platelets, coagulation factors, and fibrinolytic proteins. Genetic variants underlying these factors may contribute to derangement of this coordinated system, resulting in abnormal coagulation or fibrinolysis and subsequent thrombosis. However, until 1990 only three single-gene disorders had been identified for risk of human venous thromboembolism (VTE): antithrombin, protein C and protein S deficiencies, which in combination occur in only about 15% of families with familial thrombosis. Furthermore, few (if any) genetic variants had been reproducibly associated with arterial thrombotic risk. Concomitant with the publication

From: *Contemporary Cardiology: Antithrombotic Drug Therapy in Cardiovascular Disease*
Edited by: A.T. Askari and A.M. Lincoff (eds.), DOI 10.1007/978-1-60327-235-3_4
© Humana Press, a part of Springer Science+Business Media, LLC 2010

of the first complete draft sequence of the human genome (Human Genome Project *(1)*), the advent of advanced genetic and molecular technologies has facilitated an explosion of studies of genetics of human thrombotic disease, resulting in several advances in our understanding of such disorders. However, human pathologic thrombosis remains a complex, heterogeneous disease. We review herein the currently available knowledge of the genetics of human thrombosis, but there remains a large amount of unexplained variation in the genetic, molecular, and clinical manifestations of this disease.

Evidence For a Genetic Basis To Thrombosis

To begin to unravel the underlying genetic architecture of thrombosis, one must first establish that a genetic basis exists. Heritability is defined as the proportion of the total phenotypic variation within a population that is attributable to genetic variance. Twin studies have suggested that coagulation is hereditary. For example, de Lange and colleagues performed a study of 1,002 female twins, 149 monozygotic twin pairs, and 325 dizygotic twin pairs to assess heritability of levels of coagulation factors *(2)*. They found that genetic factors were responsible for 41–75% of the variation in fibrinogen, factor VII, factor VIII, plasminogen activator, factor XIII A-subunit and B-subunit, and von Willebrand factor. Factor XIII showed the highest heritability (82%) and factor XII demonstrated the lowest heritability (38%). Further supporting a genetic basis to these coagulation proteins, they also found a higher correlation for all of these coagulation factors in monozygotic as compared with dizygotic twins *(2)*. Another study evaluated heritability of hemostatic proteins in 130 monozygotic and 155 dizygotic older same-sex twins (73–94 years of age), participating in the Longitudinal Study of Aging of Danish Twins *(3)*. They found that the heritability of hemostatic factors varied from 33% (D-dimer) to as high as 71% (thrombin activatable fibrinolysis inhibitor), suggesting that age has only a modest effect on hemostatic proteins. In the Genetic Analysis of Idiopathic Thrombosis (GAIT) study, investigators estimated an additive genetic heritability of 60% for thrombosis *(4)*. These studies suggest that genes represent the largest casual mechanism in the underlying pathophysiology of thrombosis, greater than that observed in other common diseases.

The Evolutionary Basis of Coagulation

In mammals, the complex network of integrated biochemical events leading to coagulation is composed primarily of five proteases (factor II or prothrombin; factors VII, IX, X; and protein C), which interact with five cofactors (tissue factor, factors VIII and V, thrombomodulin, and membrane proteins) to generate fibrin *(5)*. Interestingly, data from protein structure, gene, and sequence analysis suggest that coagulation regulatory proteins may have emerged greater than 400 million years ago from duplication and diversification of just two gene structures: a vitamin K-dependent serine protease with an epidermal growth factor (EGF)-like domain (common to factors VII, IX, and X, and protein C), and a second domain structure common to factors V and VIII *(5)*. Prothrombin, also a vitamin-K dependent serine protease, contains kringle domains rather than EGF domains, which suggests a replacement during gene duplication and exon shuffling *(6)*. Thrombin has active-site amino acid residues that distinguish it from other serine proteases, supporting its position as the ancestral blood enzyme *(7)*. Furthermore, there is evidence that local duplication and/or translocation may have contributed to the evolution of multigene families residing on disparate chromosomal regions *(8)*. The coagulation genome itself in mammals probably evolved from invertebrate or early vertebrate species, where the corresponding genes (i.e., orthologs) for primary coagulant and fibrinolytic proteins have been shown to have homology to mammalian genes *(9)*.

In evolutionary terms, however, hemostasis is a relatively recent addition *(10)*; it first arose in vertebrates at the time of development of a closed, high pressure circulatory system *(11)*. Concomitantly, there was a need for a system that could respond rapidly with hemostasis, since even a minor injury could cause lethal bleeding. However, the system needed to be tightly regulated to avoid a potentially lethal excessive response *(10)*. Evolutionary forces have thus led to the highly integrated hemostatic system characterized by many interconnected pathways with an underlying architecture of many genes. In fact, genetic mutations have been identified in nearly every component of the hemostatic system *(10)*.

THE GENETICS OF COAGULATION AND THROMBOSIS IN HUMANS

The publication of the completed draft sequence of the entire human genome as part of the Human Genome Project promises to revolutionize medical science and care of patients *(12)*. Although the human genome is 99% similar across all individuals, there exist at least two million locations along the human genome where single nucleotide changes differentiate humans, so-called single nucleotide polymorphisms (SNPs), which occur in genes and between genes (intergenic). A polymorphism is a change in the sequence of a normal gene that is relatively abundant in a population (>1%), whereas a mutation is a change in the sequence of a normal gene that is less common. Recent advances in human genetics have shown that such seemingly minor variations account not only for human heterogeneity, but also for the underlying predisposition to human disease *(13,14)*.

Linkage Analysis To Define Genetics Of Thrombosis

Refining which SNPs or other variations may be accounting for disease involves carefully conducted studies where the disease "phenotype" (the outward manifestation of the underlying genetics) is well characterized. In human genetics, there are two main types of studies that evaluate the relationship between genetic polymorphisms and disease: linkage analysis and association studies. Linkage analyses investigate the cosegregation of DNA markers with disease in families and allow an unbiased examination of the entire genome. Linkage studies are more technically challenging, as they rely on ascertainment of related individuals, but are important in uncovering novel genes underlying clinical phenotypes. Often, linkage studies are utilized to identify and narrow genomic regions, within which association studies are then done to further examine mutations or polymorphisms in candidate genes residing within these "linked" genomic regions. For example, several linkage studies have been performed to evaluate genes for arterial thrombosis, specifically coronary artery disease (CAD) and myocardial infarction (MI) *(15–18)*, from which several susceptibility genes have been identified for CAD/MI risk *(17,19,20)*. In VTE, investigators from the GAIT study have performed linkage analysis for VTE and plasma levels of thrombotic factors, revealing several regions and genes as susceptibility candidates for VTE risk *(21,22)*.

In addition to identifying genetic variants predisposing to a given binary trait, linkage analysis can be used to identify genetic loci underlying variability of quantitative traits, so-called quantitative trait locus (QTL) analysis. The genetic study of quantitative traits has many advantages over studies based on the presence or absence of a disease. For example, many diseases are defined in terms of an underlying quantitative liability scale, with these intermediate factors residing closer to the underlying etiologic gene and thereby potentially providing a stronger genetic signal *(22)*. This study design has been successful in elucidating the genetic architecture underlying several thrombotic factors. For example, the GAIT study has performed QTL analysis for several thrombosis-related quantitative traits, revealing multiple genomic regions and genes underlying the variability of plasma thrombotic factor levels. Table 1 reviews QTLs that have been identified from thrombosis-related quantitative traits.

Table 1
Quantitative trait loci (QTL) identified for thrombosis/hemostasis related traits
(Adapted from Blangero et al. (21) and Soria et al. (22))

Trait	Linkage odds (LOD) score[a]	Genomic location of QTL	Gene
Factor XII coagulant activity/thrombosis (398)	11.73	5q35	F12
Factor II coagulant activity/thrombosis (132)	4.70	11p11	F2
Activated protein C ratio/Factor VIII coagulant activity/thrombosis (399)	4.50	18p11	Unidentified
Histidine-rich glycoprotein (400)	4.17	3q27	HRG
Free protein S (401)	4.07	1q32	Unidentified
P-selectin (402)	3.81	15q26	Unidentified
Factor XII coagulant activity (398)	3.53	10p13	Unidentified
Von Willebrand factor (403)	3.46	9q34	ABO blood group
Protein C (404)	3.69	16q23	NQO1
Factor VIII (405)	4.44	5/11	Unidentified
Homocysteine (406)	3.01	11q23	NNMT
Fibrinogen (407)	3.12	14q11	Unidentified
Activated protein C ratio (399)	3.05	1q24	F5
Tissue factor pathway inhibitor (408)	3.52	2q	TFPI

[a]A measure of the strength of linkage of that genomic region to the trait

HRG histidine-rich glycoprotein; TFPI Tissue factor pathway inhibitor gene

Association Studies In Genetics Of Thrombosis

Although linkage analysis has proven to be successful in mapping rare, high-risk genetic variants, association analysis of unrelated individuals is thought to be a more powerful tool for mapping modest-risk genetic variants that contribute to complex disease. This is because increased patterns of allele sharing between family members can make it difficult to identify subtle disease-related variants using linkage. Ancestral recombination between unrelated individuals resulting in smaller shared regions compared to those of family members makes it easier to detect modest genetic association effects given a sufficient density of genetic markers (23). Association studies rely primarily on assessing frequencies of genetic mutations in unrelated individuals based on clinical phenotypes (i.e., "case-control" studies). These studies work under the assumption that genetic variants are either related directly to the phenotype, or are closely linked to a causative variant for the phenotype. Although population stratification (spurious association due to underlying differences in race/ethnicity or other factors) is always a concern in association studies, careful selection of a control population can obviate this problem (24). Hundreds of association studies have been published detailing many candidate genes for venous and arterial thrombotic risk; a review of the most relevant and reproducible variants is presented later. Furthermore, the Human Genome Project has facilitated the development of new approaches for association mapping of complex diseases. N Studies of the simultaneous assessment of hundreds of thousands of SNPs across the human genome ("Genome-Wide Association Studies" or GWAS) are emerging, identifying novel markers for thrombotic phenotypes. For example, a recently published GWAS has identified an SNP associated with MI in multiple populations (25).

Regardless of the type of study, one must be careful when interpreting human genetic studies. Save for a handful of reproducible variants, the studies of genes for venous and/or arterial thrombosis are characterized by inconsistent and often irreproducible results. Hence, one must bear in mind issues of power, study design, case/control selection, potential confounders, and population stratification when

Table 2
Causes of inherited thrombophilia
(Adapted from WHO Bulletin (27))

Acquired
    Antithrombin deficiency
    Protein C deficiency
    Protein S deficiency
    APC-R/Factor V Leiden
    Dysfibrinogenemia
    Thrombomodulin
Acquired/inherited
    Hyperhomocysteinemia
    Elevated factor VIII
    Elevated fibrinogen
Potentially inherited
    Plasminogen deficiency
    Heparin cofactor II deficiency

conducting and interpreting genetic studies. Furthermore, the reported genetic variant may in fact be in linkage disequilibrium (i.e., genetically linked to) a different variant which in fact is the functional mutation resulting in disease. Finally, thrombosis is typical of a complex, heterogeneous disease, characterized by the strong influence of environmental factors; gene with modest effects, variable penetrance and difficult to characterize modes of inheritance; as well as gene–environment and gene–gene interactions.

Until 1990, only three single-gene disorders had been identified for risk of VTE: antithrombin, protein C and protein S deficiencies, which occur only in about 15% of families with familial thrombosis and only in a small proportion of all patients with VTE (26), and are inherited in an autosomal dominant manner. The remaining 85% of families in whom a genetic predisposition cannot be identified spurred application of genetic and epidemiologic tools to research in familial thrombophilia, resulting in several advances in our understanding of familial thromboembolic disorders. A list of potential factors causing hereditary thrombosis is presented in Table 2 (27). However, these factors only represent the presence of an inherited factor that predisposes to thrombosis, but requires interaction of other factors (acquired or inherited) to produce the clinical disorder. There are several such genetic and environmental factors that have been identified as risk factors for arterial and/or VTE (Table 3).

GENETIC VARIANTS IMPLICATED IN VENOUS THROMBOTIC DISORDERS

The pathophysiology of VTE has at its core the interaction of acquired factors such as age, obesity, prolonged immobilization, surgery, pregnancy, oral contraceptives and cancer, in the setting of a genetic predisposition to disease. In fact, one or more predisposing factors are identified in approximately 80% of patients, with inherited thrombophilia being identified in 24–37% of unselected patients with DVT (28–30) and in the majority of patients with familial thrombosis (28). Table 4 summarizes the risk and incidence of a first episode of VTE with various risk factors. These genetic disorders can be divided pathophysiologically into two main categories, either due to decreased levels of antithrombotic proteins (i.e., antithrombin III deficiency, protein C or S deficiency, factor V Leiden) or the result of increased levels of prothrombotic proteins (i.e., prothrombin G20210A).

Table 3

Risk factors predisposing to thromboembolism (Adapted from Andreotti and Becker *(358)*)

	Venous	*Arterial*
Inherited	Genetic polymorphisms of the hemostatic system (Factor V Leiden, Prothrombin G20210A, Gain-of-Function variants of Factors VIII, IX, XI)	Gene polymorphisms of the hemostatic system (Factor V Leiden, Prothrombin G20210A, Gain-of-function variants of fibrinogen, factor VII, plasminogen activator inhibitor type-1, glycoprotein IIIa (Leu33Pro)
	Deficiencies of antithrombin, proteins C and S	Family history of arterial thrombosis
	Dysfibrinogenemia	Homocysteinurias
	Family history of VTE	Congenital dyslipidemias
	Homocysteinurias and MTHFR C677T variant	
	Varicose veins	
Physiologic	Pregnancy, puerperium	Male gender (if before 65 years of age)
	Aging	Aging
Environmental	Surgery, trauma, immobilization	Smoking, cocaine use
	Oral contraceptives, hormone replacement therapy	Oral contraceptives, hormone replacement therapy
	HIT	HIT
	Antifibrinolytic agents, prothrombin complex concentrates	Antifibrinolytic agents, prothrombin complex concentrates
	Endotoxemia	Thienopyridine-related TTP
Other	Previous VTE	Previous arterial thrombosis
	Behcet's disease, other vasculitis	Atherosclerosis, vasculitis
	Malignancy	Malignancy
	Congestive heart failure, nephrotic syndrome	Congestive heart failure, renal failure
	Antiphospholipid antibodies	Antiphospholipid antibodies, SLE, RA
	Polycythemia vera, essential thrombocythemia	Polycythemia vera, essential thrombocythemia
	Obesity	Atrial fibrillation
	Paroxysmal nocturnal hemoglobinuria	Hypercholesterolemia, metabolic syndrome and its components
		Sickle cell anemia, macroglobulinemia

HIT heparin-induced thrombocytopenia; *TTP* thrombotic purpura; *SLE* systemic lupus erythematosis; *RA* rheumatoid arthritis

Factor V Leiden is the most common genetic cause of VTE, with the prothrombin gene mutation, deficiencies in protein S, protein C, and antithrombin accounting for most of the remaining cases (Table 5). The most studied and clinically relevant genetic variants for VTE risk are discussed in detail as follows and summarized in Table 6.

Antithrombin III Deficiency

In 1965, Egeberg discovered the first genetic predisposition to VTE, namely that of antithrombin deficiency *(31)*. Antithrombin (also known as heparin cofactor I) is a major component of the coagulation cascade synthesized in the liver, is an inhibitor of thrombin, and is one of the most important physiological regulators of fibrin formation. Heparin, one of the most common clinically used anticoagulants, works via augmentation of antithrombin's inhibitory activity on thrombin. Egeberg described

Table 4
Risk and incidence of a first episode of venous thrombosis (Adult subjects only. Reproduced with permission from UpToDate; data from Leiden Thrombophilia Study)

Condition/risk factor(s)	Relative risk	Incidence, percent per year
Normal	1	0.008
Hyperhomocysteinemia (MTHFR 677T mutation)	2.5	0.02
	1	–
Prothrombin gene mutation	2.8	0.02
Oral contraceptives	4	0.03
Factor V Leiden (heterozygous)	7	0.06
Oral contraceptives plus heterozygous factor V Leiden	35	0.29
Factor V Leiden (homozygous)	80	0.5 to 1.0

Table 5
Prevalence of Factor V leiden and prothrombin gene mutations in various populations
(Adapted from Seligsohn, et al. (161) and Federici et al. (357))

Variant	General population (%)	Unselected patients with VTE (%)	Selected patients[a] with VTE (%)	Relative risk for VTE
Factor V Leiden (heterozygote)	4.8	18.8% (heterozygotes)	40.0%	~3–7 (heterozygotes); 50–100 (homozygotes)
Prothrombin G20210A (heterozygote)	2.7	~7%	16%	~2–5 (heterozygotes)
Antithrombin III deficiency	0.02–0.04	~1	?	~20–50
Protein C deficiency	0.2–0.5	~2–5	?	7–10
Protein S deficiency	0.1–1	~1–3	?	~2
MTHFR C677T	5–15	15–20 (homozygotes)	?	2–3 (homozygotes)

[a]Selected patients, age less than 50 years with a family history of venous thrombosis, a history of recurrent event, and the absence of acquired risk factors except pregnancy or the use of oral contraceptives

low antithrombin and low heparin cofactor activity in a family heavily burdened with VTE and identified the genetic predisposition to be transmitted in an autosomal dominant fashion. Antithrombin III deficiency has since been shown to be a heterogeneous disorder and as such, is currently subclassified into two categories. Type I antithrombin deficiency is characterized by reduced function of immunologic and functional antithrombin. Type II is characterized by a variant antithrombin molecule with a defect in its reactive site (type II RS), in the heparin-binding site (type II HBS), or multiple functional defects (type II PE (pleiotrophic effects)) (32,33). Interestingly, there is also heterogeneity in clinical presentation by subtype, with type II HBS having the lowest risk for VTE (34). Conversely, type I defects are more prevalent among thrombophilic families.

The antithrombin gene resides on chromosome 1q23-25 and is composed of seven coding regions; more than 100 different mutations have been identified with several mutations leading to antithrombin III deficiency. Type I antithrombin deficiency is due to one of several genetic mutations, most often interfering with protein synthesis. Patients with type II HBS usually have mutations at the amino-terminal end of the molecule (35) resulting in approximately 50% of normal plasma antithrombin-heparin

Table 6
Genetic variants implicated in venous thrombotic disorders

Gene	Variant	Function	Phenotype
Factor V	(1) Factor V Leiden (R506Q) (2) Factor V R2 (H1299R)	Incompletely characterized *(85)*	Venous thromboembolism *(98,99)*; miscarriages *(104)*, obstetrical complications *(409)*
Prothrombin	G20210A		DVT, PE *(136–140)*
Platelet activator inhibitor-1 (PAI-1)	4G/5G promoter		Portal vein thrombosis *(410)*
Estrogen receptor beta	1730A>G		DVT *(411)*
JAK2	V617F		Budd-Chiari, portal, splanchnic and mesenteric vein thrombosis, catastrophic intra-abdominal thrombosis (reports inconsistent) *(412–414)*
Endothelial protein C receptor	(1) Haplotype 1 (H1, tagged by rs9574) (2) Haplotype 3 (H3) (3) Haplotype 4 (H4) (4) 4600AG, 4678CC *(126)*		VTE; VTE in carriers of Factor V Leiden *(124–128)*
Factor XIIIA	Val34Leu	Changes FXIII activation rate and fibrin structure/function	DVT, MI, CVA *(8,232,358,415,416)*
Fibrinogen Aα	Thr312Ala	Changes fibrin structure/ function and FXIII crosslinking	Pulmonary embolism *(417)*
Thrombomodulin	Several missense mutations	Various	VTE *(183–186)*
Tissue-factor pathway inhibitor (TFPI)	Pro151Leu	Unknown	VTE (contradictory reports) *(181,182)*

cofactor activity measurements. Patients with type II RS generally have mutations near the thrombin-binding site at the carboxy terminal end of the molecule. Type II PE also involves a mutation at the carboxy terminal end of the antithrombin molecule resulting in conformational changes in the protein. This includes the first reported antithrombin genetic variant, Budapest, which consists of a proline to leucine replacement at residue 429 *(36,37)*.

Estimates of the prevalence of antithrombin deficiency in the general population range from one in 2,000–5,000 *(38)* to as high as one in 500 *(39)*. The majority of patients with antithrombin deficiency identified in these studies did not have VTE or a familial history of thrombosis. The prevalence of hereditary antithrombin deficiency is ~0.5–1% in patients presenting with a first thrombotic event *(29)*. In a Spanish study of over 2,000 consecutive patients with VTE, 12.9% were found to have an anticoagulant protein deficiency (7.3% protein S, 3.2% protein C, and 0.5% antithrombin) *(29)*. Clinically, approximately 55% of patients with type I and type II RS present with VTE *(40,41)*, with a much lower incidence of 6% in patients heterozygous for type II HBS *(34)*. In another study, the lifetime probability of developing VTE in carriers of antithrombin III deficiency mutations was 8.1

times higher compared to those with no defect *(42)*. The lifetime probability in protein S deficiency was 8.5 times higher, for protein C 7.3 times higher, and for factor V Leiden, 2.2 times higher. In patients with protein C, protein S, or antithrombin deficiency, 80% of patients have their first thrombotic event prior to age 40, and 32–62% of thrombotic events occur in the presence of other risk factors such as surgery, immobilization, or pregnancy, with the highest prevalence of these risk factors occurring in activated protein C resistance (APCR) *(33)*. Patients with antithrombin deficiency are at particularly high risk during pregnancy with a 37–44% incidence of thrombosis during pregnancy and puerperium, which is more than that seen in protein C or protein S deficiency (12–19%); or in APCR (28%) *(43,44)*. Overall, antithrombin-, protein-C-, or protein-S-deficient individuals account for 22% of venous thrombosis that complicates surgery, with no difference in type of deficiency or type or surgical procedure. Approximately 60% of patients with antithrombin deficiency and VTE suffer from recurrent thrombotic episodes. Homozygous forms of antithrombin deficiency are rare and result in severe, early-onset thrombosis, which is often arterial *(45)*. Arterial thrombosis is rare in antithrombin deficiency but has been reported *(46)*.

Diagnosis of type I antithrombin III deficiency is done using immunoassays which quantify antithrombin antigen. Type II deficiencies require functional assays of antithrombin activity. The antithrombin-heparin cofactor assay measures the ability of heparin to bind lysyl residues on antithrombin and catalyzes neutralization of coagulation enzymes such as thrombin and factor Xa. All four types of antithrombin deficiencies can be diagnosed with this assay in combination with an immunoassay and, therefore, it is felt to be the best single screening test for antithrombin deficiency *(47)*. This assay should be performed when the patient is not receiving heparin, and ideally, at least 2 weeks after completing oral anticoagulant therapy (Table 10).

The clinical management of patients with antithrombin III deficiency with an acute VTE event is in general the same as those without the deficiency; however, resistance to heparin can be a clinical concern. In fact, the majority of patients with clinical heparin resistance are antithrombin deficient *(18,19)*. Such patients require large doses of heparin for therapeutic anticoagulation, due in part to the action of heparin further lowering antithrombin levels by approximately 30%. Antithrombin concentrate can be used safely and effectively in such settings *(50,51)*. Antithrombin concentrate is prepared from pooled normal human plasma and is administered over a 10–20 min period. Antithrombin concentrate can be considered in patients with unusually severe thrombosis, those who develop recurrent thrombosis despite adequate anticoagulation, or in those with difficulty achieving adequate anticoagulation *(52)*. However, the use of antithrombin concentrate has not been studied in a randomized, controlled trial.

Protein S Deficiency

Protein C and S deficiencies were first discovered in the 1980s *(53,54)*. Protein S is a vitamin-K-dependent plasma glycoprotein that functions as a nonenzymatic cofactor to activated protein C in the degradation of Factors Va and VIIIa. Thrombin and Factor Xa cleave protein S, rendering it inactive *(55)*. Protein S circulates in a free form with activated protein C cofactor activity; and a bound form with no activated protein C cofactor activity *(56)*. Protein S deficiency is predominantly inherited as an autosomal dominant trait, and heterozygous individuals are at risk of recurrent VTE *(53)*. There are three subtypes of protein S deficiency as defined by total and free protein S concentrations and activated protein C cofactor activity. In type I protein S deficiency, the genetic defect results in a reduction of total protein S antigen as well as protein S activity. In the more rare type II protein S deficiency, there is normal protein S antigen, but a functionally abnormal protein S molecule with reduced protein S functional activity. In type III protein S deficiency, there is normal total protein S antigen, but reduced free protein S antigen and activity *(57)*.

The protein S gene is structurally complex and has a pseudogene (a segment of DNA that resembles a gene, but cannot be transcribed) with high homology which has made genetic analysis more complicated. The 5' end of the gene shows high homology with other vitamin-K-dependent proteins. Interestingly, only about 50–60% of patients with protein S deficiency have identified genetic mutations *(58,59)*. The majority of genetic variants causing type I protein S deficiency are SNPs and insertions and deletions with at least 33 unique variants identified *(27)*. Four different mutations have been identified that cause type II protein S deficiency *(60,61)*, including two in the propeptide, one in the EGF domain and one in the second EGF domain. Reports have suggested that type I and type III protein S deficiency may be phenotypic variants of the same genotype *(62,63)*. For example, in one study of French patients with low free protein S, 82% of patients in whom mutations could be identified had a Ser460Pro SNP *(58)*, also known as protein S Heerlen *(64)*. However, in this same study, this SNP had the same frequency in patients with thrombosis as in the general population; hence, its association with increased thrombotic risk remains to be clarified. The prevalence of familial protein S deficiency in the general population is approximately 0.03–0.13% *(65)* with a prevalence of 7.3% in patients with VTE *(29)*. The absolute risk of thrombosis in patients with protein S deficiency has been estimated at 8.5 times higher as compared with individuals with no defect *(42)*. Homozygous protein S deficiency is rare and associated with neonatal purpura fulminans *(66)*. Although reports of arterial thrombosis in patients with protein S deficiency are published *(67)*, larger studies have not confirmed a role in arterial thrombosis *(68)*. Clinical diagnosis of protein S deficiency relies on a functional and immunoassay (Table 10), and as with antithrombin III deficiency, testing for the underlying genetic variant is not clinically indicated.

Protein C Deficiency

Protein C, a vitamin-K-dependent plasma glycoprotein is the precursor of the serine-proteinase-activated protein C (APC), which subsequently inactivates coagulation factors Va and VIIIa, an effect enhanced by protein S. Interestingly, APC has anti-inflammatory activities and protects endothelial barrier function in reactions mediated by the endothelial protein C receptor (EPCR) *(69)*. Protein C deficiency is a heterogeneous disorder inherited in an autosomal dominant fashion, and two subtypes have been identified *(70)*. In the more common type I protein C deficiency, there is reduction both in protein C activity and in protein C antigen, and is characterized by marked phenotypic variability. In type II protein C deficiency, there is evidence of an abnormal protein C molecule but with normal protein C antigen. The gene for protein C is located on chromosome 2 and is closely related to the gene for factor IX *(71)*. More than a hundred different genetic mutations have been associated with the two subtypes *(72)*. There appears to be the presence of a founder effect in Dutch families with type I deficiency *(73)*.

The prevalence of heterozygous protein C deficiency ranges from 1 in 200–500 in a healthy population *(74)*, increasing to 2–5% in a population of patients with VTE *(29)*. Clinically, protein C deficiency presents as VTE, neonatal purpura fulminans (primarily in homozygous or double heterozygous newborns), warfarin-induced skin necrosis, and has also been linked to fetal loss *(75)*. Warfarin-induced skin necrosis is an infrequent complication induced by a transient hypercoagulable state; the initiation of warfarin leads to a decrease in protein C anticoagulant activity, with more pronounced effects when doses greater than 10 mg of warfarin daily are used. Arterial thrombosis has not been consistently associated with protein C deficiency, though there have been reports of nonhemorrhagic stroke in young adults *(76)*. Homozygous protein C deficiency can cause purpura fulminans (caused by thrombosis of small vessels), occurring soon after birth or in the first year of life; or can result in milder manifestations similar to those with heterozygous deficiency *(77)*. The median age-of-onset of

VTE in protein C deficiency is 45 years in unselected patients and 30 years in members of thrombophilia families (78). Recurrent VTE develops in 60% of carriers with VTE. The absolute risk of thrombosis in patients with protein C deficiency is about sevenfold higher than that of normal subjects (42,79). However, there is marked variability in families with protein C deficiency, suggesting factors other than that explained by the genetic defect. One such risk factor for higher risk of VTE is presence of a second thrombotic defect, especially factor V Leiden. For example, a review of four studies revealed that 75% of family members who carried two defects suffered VTE, compared with 10–30% of carriers of only one defect (80).

Protein C deficiency is diagnosed by a variety of immunologic and functional assays (47). Patients with a protein C level <55% of normal likely have a genetic abnormality, whereas levels between 55 and 65% are either due to a deficient state or represent lower limits of normal (81). Warfarin therapy reduces functional and immunologic measurements of protein C. If it is not possible to stop anticoagulation, i.e., due to severity of the thrombotic tendency, individuals can be studied while anticoagulated with heparin using protein C antigen level testing. When treating an acute VTE event in patients with known protein C deficiency, oral anticoagulation should be started only after full heparinization is achieved. Further, to avoid warfarin-induced skin necrosis, the initial dose of warfarin should be low and then increased slowly until therapeutic. In patients with heterozygous protein C deficiency and a history of warfarin-induced skin necrosis, supplemental administration of protein C should be considered until a stable warfarin dose is achieved (82).

Activated Protein C Resistance (Factor V Leiden)

Dahlbäck and colleagues discovered APCR in 1993 (83) and it is responsible for 20–30% of cases of VTE. Plasma is diagnosed as "APC resistant" if addition of exogenous APC fails to prolong its clotting time in an activated partial thromboplastin time (aPTT) assay (83). Factor V is a plasma glycoprotein cofactor; during coagulation, factor V is converted to factor Va by meizothrombin and/or factor Xa. Furthermore, factor V is a cofactor in the inactivation of factor VIIIa by activated protein C. Approximately 90% of cases of VTE due to APC resistance are due to an SNP in the Factor V gene (G to A at position 1691 in exon 10), resulting in an arginine to glutamine in amino acid 506, also known as Factor V Leiden (84). Factor V Leiden is the most common cause of VTE, accounting for 40–50% of cases. The underlying molecular mechanism by which Factor V Leiden causes APCR is still under biochemical investigation. Factor Va Leiden has been shown to be inactivated more slowly by APC than normal factor Va, resulting in increased coagulation (85). Furthermore, factor V Leiden results in decreased anticoagulation by leading to lack of cleavage of factor V at position 506, which would normally serve as a cofactor with APC in degradation in factors VIIIa and Va. APC resistance can also be caused by the Factor V R2 (H1299R) mutation. The rare R306T (Factor V Cambridge (86)) and R306G (Factor V Hong Kong (87)) affect the APC cleavage site at Arg306, conferring only mild APC resistance (88). Factor V Liverpool (Ile359Thr) results in poor APC cofactor activity for the inactivation of factor VIIIa, as well as reduced APC mediated inactivation of factor Va (89).

Factor V Leiden has a prevalence of up to 6% in Caucasians, but is much lower in African and Asian populations (90). In Europeans, the mutation is found in up to 50% of familial thrombotic disorders (84). A study of over 4,000 subjects in the Physicians' Health Study and Women's Health Study found carrier frequencies in Caucasians of 5.3%, in Hispanic Americans of 2.2%, in Native Americans of 1.25%, in African-Americans of 1.2%, and in Asian Americans of 0.45% (91). It appears that the mutation originated approximately 30,000 years ago based on haplotype analyses suggesting evidence for a founder effect (92).

The transmission is autosomal dominant. This mutation is associated with a significant increase in thrombotic risk and is found in 20% of patients with thrombophilia (up to 50% in selected patients, i.e., those with a family history of thrombosis) *(84,93,94)*. There is evidence that this variant (balanced with the prothrombin 202010A) may reflect a selective advantage in heterozygotes, offering benefits for reducing blood loss associated with giving birth and trauma *(95)*, decreased risk of intracranial hemorrhage *(96)*, and protecting against blood loss after cardiac surgery *(97)*. Factor V R2 has not been shown to be associated with an increased risk of VTE, but has been shown to increase Factor V Leiden-related thrombosis risk in individuals doubly heterozygous at these mutations *(98,99)*. Factor V Liverpool has been associated with an increased risk of VTE *(89)*. Factor V Cambridge and factor V Hong Kong do not appear to be associated with thrombosis *(100)*.

The clinical manifestations of factor V Leiden include DVT, pulmonary embolism *(101)*, as well as cerebral *(102)*, mesenteric, and portal vein thrombosis, and may play a role in recurrent fetal loss *(103)*. In addition, factor V Leiden has been associated with other obstetric complications including pre-eclampsia, fetal growth restriction, and abruption placenta *(104)*; however, these associations need further validation. Interestingly, it appears that the lifetime risk of VTE and the severity of VTE are less in patients heterozygous for factor V Leiden when compared with patients with the less common thrombophilias *(42)*. Factor V Leiden may be associated with increased risk of recurrent VTE; however, data are conflicting *(105)*. Factor V Leiden does not appear to be associated with risk of arterial thrombosis: most studies, including two meta-analyses, have been unable to find a significant increase in the prevalence of factor V Leiden in patients with myocardial infarction and stroke *(106,107)*. However, an increased risk of arterial thrombosis may be confined to young female smokers who carry factor V Leiden *(108,109)*.

Patients with VTE who have other thrombotic defects such as protein C, protein S, or antithrombin deficiency, and prothrombin gene mutations have an increased prevalence of factor V Leiden, with the presence of two defects increasing the thrombotic risk in family members up to threefold in comparison with the risk of a single defect *(110,111)*. In a review of case-control studies of factor V Leiden and prothrombin G20210A, patients doubly heterozygous for the two mutations had a fourfold increase in risk of VTE compared with patients heterozygous only for the factor V Leiden mutation (odds ratio 4.9 vs. 20.0) *(112)*. The risk of VTE has been found to be increased threefold in first-degree relatives who are carriers of factor V Leiden if factor VIII levels are ≥150 IU/dL *(113)* and also increased in patients with concomitant factor V deficiency *(114)*. Patients with non-O blood types have a two to four times increased risk of VTE in both heterozygous and homozygotes for factor V Leiden *(115)*. Patients with concomitant factor V Leiden and hyperhomocysteinemia have an increased risk of VTE *(116)*. Further, as shown in Table 4, the risk of VTE is increased with concomitant use of oral contraceptives, hormone replacement therapy, or pregnancy *(117,118)* Other concomitant clinical factors may also increase VTE risk in the presence of factor V Leiden: a prospective study of almost 10,000 Danish patients found that VTE risk in patients heterozygous or homozygous for factor V Leiden increases with age, smoking, and increasing body mass index (BMI) *(119)*.

Other Forms of Activated Protein C Deficiencies

APCR can also occur in the absence of a genetic mutation in factor V, for example, in patients with cancer, which may contribute to the increased thrombotic incidence in these patients *(120)*; however, the clinical utility of diagnosing this type of APC resistance is unclear. APC resistance can also be acquired in those using oral contraceptives or hormone replacement therapy *(121)*. In addition to mutations in the Factor V gene, activated protein C deficiencies can result from other genetic mutations. The EPCR is a type I transmembrane protein highly expressed on the endothelium of large vessels *(122)*, enhancing the rate of protein C activation *(123)*. Several polymorphisms in the EPCR gene have been associated with venous and arterial thrombosis by affecting the coupling of protein C to the EPCR, resulting in an alteration of APC generation *(124)*. Four haplotypes have been found in the EPCR gene (H1, H2, H3, H4), which have been associated with VTE, but with varying results. The H3 haplotype has been associated with an increased risk of VTE (OR: 1.8) *(125)*, though other studies have found no increased risk *(126,127)*. The H1 haplotype, which is tagged by the SNP 4678 G/C (aka rs9574), has been associated with decreased risk of VTE (OR: 0.59) *(126)*, and with decreased risk of VTE in carriers of the Factor V Leiden mutation (OR: 0.31) *(128)*. Another study evaluated two SNPs in exon 4 of the EPCR gene and found that the 4600AG genotype had significantly higher soluble EPCR levels than the AA genotype, though it was not associated with VTE risk, but that the 4678CC genotype was associated with decreased VTE risk (OR: 0.61) *(126)*. Further, a 23-bp insertion in exon 3 was shown to be a risk factor for atherothrombotic disease *(129)*; however, a subsequent study failed to confirm that association *(130)*. Further studies are necessary to establish the importance of the EPCR gene in thrombotic disease.

Prothrombin 20210A

Prothrombin (aka factor II), is the precursor to thrombin, is vitamin K dependent, and plays a key role in the conversion of fibrinogen to fibrin. In 1996, Poort et al. described the prothrombin 20210A mutation in an investigation of patients with a personal and family history of VTE and in healthy controls: 18% of patients with VTE had the substitution (adenine for guanine at position 20210) compared with an only 1% prevalence in healthy controls *(131)*. These investigators subsequently conducted a population-based, case-control study which revealed that 6.2% of consecutive patients with a first DVT carried the G20210A allele as compared with 2.3% of age- and sex-matched control subjects. They further found that a higher level of prothrombin activity itself was associated with increased risk of VTE and individuals with one copy of the A allele had significantly higher mean prothrombin levels as compared with individuals with the GG genotype *(131)*. More recent reports have found little correlation between this mutation and plasma prothrombin levels. One study did show a highly significant LOD score between the G20210A mutation and a QTL for prothrombin activity, and further, that simultaneously accounting for association with the variant completely eliminated the linkage signal suggesting that G20210A is a functional polymorphism *(132)*.

G20210A represents the second most frequent prothrombotic genetic polymorphism, and like Factor V Leiden, the transmission is autosomal dominant. The prevalence of this mutation varies widely geographically. In whites, the prevalence varies from 0.7 to 6.5% *(133–135)* with an overall prevalence in one study of 11 centers in nine countries of 2% *(134)*, and is very rare in black and Asian populations. Carriers of this mutation have a threefold increased risk of VTE *(131)*. Many subsequent reports have confirmed the role of prothrombin 20210A in risk of DVT and PE, with odds ratios ranging from 2.0 to 5.0 *(136–140)*. For example, in the Leiden Thrombophilia Study, 6.2% patients with DVT had the G20210A variant compared with 2.3% of healthy matched controls *(131)*, with a 2.8-fold independently increased risk of VTE across sexes and age groups. Given its strong role in risk of VTE, studies have investigated the role of this polymorphism in recurrent thrombotic events with some studies showing no association *(141)* and one meta-analysis suggesting association with recurrent DVT (OR: 1.72; 95% CI: 1.27–2.31) *(105)*. Carriers of this mutation may also have an increased risk of VTE in the setting of pregnancy, with one study showing that 31% of pregnant or postpartum women with VTE carried the mutation as compared with 4.2% of controls without VTE (OR: 10.2; 95% CI: 4.0–25.9) *(142)*. Prothrombin G20210A has also been shown to be a risk factor for cerebral venous thrombosis with a gene-environment effect concentrated in patients using oral contraceptives *(143)*.

As mentioned previously, given the high frequency of many of the genetic variants associated with predilection to thrombosis, a number of studies have evaluated whether the coinheritance of two or more defects increases the likelihood of thrombosis and have found this to be the case. For example, one study compared the prothrombin G20210A allele in individuals with a history of VTE and found that 5% of patients carried both factor V Leiden and the prothrombin variant, higher than the expected population frequency of 0.1% *(144)*. In a study of neonatal thrombosis, there was a very high prevalence of concurrent factor V Leiden and prothrombin G201210A mutation *(145)*. A pooled analysis of eight case-control studies found that the odds ratio for risk of VTE was 20.0 for double heterozygotes (i.e., patients with both the prothrombin G20210A and factor V Leiden mutations), as compared with 3.8 to 4.9 in patients with only the prothrombin or factor V Leiden mutations *(112)*. Of patients with VTE, 2.2% were double heterozygotes, 12% were factor V Leiden heterozygotes only, and 23% were prothrombin G20210A heterozygotes only. These results have been replicated in other studies *(133,136,144,146,147)*. In fact, many investigators now believe that the prothrombin variant is not sufficient in and of itself to predispose to VTE. To study this, investigators examined 281 patients referred for thrombosis in Italy and found that risk of VTE associated with this variant was significant only in the subset of patients with additional risk factors *(147)*.

The role of the prothrombin G20210A mutation in arterial thrombosis is controversial, with most studies showing no association or showing association only in the presence of another known risk factor *(137,148–155)*. For example, one study found weak association of the mutation with heart disease in young women (OR: 4.0), but when the variant was present in conjunction with smoking or a metabolic risk factor (obesity, hypertension, hyperlipidemia, or diabetes), the risk of heart disease increased to 34–43-fold increased risk *(155)*. Another study showed similar results in men with MI; patients who smoke and have metabolic risk factors in combination with the genetic variant had a higher risk of MI compared with noncarriers with the same risk factors *(150)*. The prothrombin G20210A variant has also been evaluated in relation to risk of ischemic stroke with similarly conflicting data. Most studies have shown no association *(137,152,156)*, but one study in 72 young patients with no traditional risk factors found a 3.8-fold risk of ischemic stroke associated with the heterozygous mutation *(157)*.

There have been very few descriptions of individuals homozygous for prothrombin G20210A; these have shown marked variation in the clinical manifestation ranging from ischemic stroke *(157)* to no clinical manifestations *(158)*. Other mutations have been identified in the prothrombin gene including C20209T and A19911G, with varying reports about their association with VTE risk *(159,160)*. Tables 4.4 and 4.5 detail the prevalence of Factor V Leiden and prothrombin gene mutations in different populations, illustrating its relative abundance in patients with VTE *(161)*. In summary, these studies suggest that the prothrombin G20210A variant may be a VTE susceptibility variant, but with significant contributions from other genetic, molecular, and clinical risk factors.

Hyperhomocysteinemia

Homocystinuria is a rare autosomal recessive hereditary disease resulting in extremely high plasma and urine homocysteine concentrations and clinical manifestations including thromboembolic disease and premature atherosclerosis. In contrast to this very rare condition, 5–7% of the population manifests less marked plasma homocysteine elevations *(162)*, and evidence suggests that moderate hyperhomocysteinemia is a risk factor for VTE and atherosclerosis *(163)*. There are several mechanisms by which hyperhomocysteinemia may play a role in thrombotic risk. A recent study in apolipoprotein-E-deficient mice suggests that hyperhomocysteinemia results in endothelial dysfunction and subsequent accelerated carotid artery thrombosis *(164)*. Another study in mice suggests that susceptibility to arterial thrombosis with hyperhomocysteinemia may involve oxidative stress and impairment of the protein C anticoagulant pathway *(165)*. In addition to nutritional deficiencies, certain medications *(166)*, chronic kidney failure, and cigarette smoking *(167)*, genetics have been shown to cause elevations in plasma homocysteine concentrations. MTHFR (5,10-methylenetetrahydrofolate reductase) is an enzyme that catalyzes the conversion of homocysteine to methionine. The thermolabile T allele of the *MTHFR* gene SNP C677T results in an amino acid change from alanine to valine in the *MTHFR* gene, reducing its efficiency by half, and is associated with elevated homocysteine levels in individuals with low folate intake *(168)*. The prevalence of the mutation is 5–14% in a general population *(169)*. Although it appears that hyperhomocysteinemia is a risk factor for VTE *(163)* and recurrent VTE *(170)*, there are conflicting results about the prothrombotic role of the C677T polymorphism (reviewed in Ray et al. *(171)*). Regardless, this mutation plays much less of a role than the 20210A and Factor V Leiden mutations in thrombosis risk.

The *MTHFR* C677T variant has also been implicated to a variable degree in arterial thrombosis. In a meta-analysis of greater than 11,000 individuals homozygous for the thermolabile variant of *MTHFR* and over 12,000 matched controls enrolled in 40 observational studies, patients with the TT genotype had moderate but statistically significant increased risk of coronary heart disease as compared with controls (OR: 1.16; 95% CI: 1.05–1.28) *(172)*. Another meta-analysis suggested international geographic variations in risk conferred by the *MTHFR* variant, with no association in North American, European, and Australian populations, but evidence of a relationship in Middle Eastern and Asian populations *(173)*. One explanation for this heterogeneity may be due to differences in folate status: the North American studies were conducted where there was greater use of vitamin B and folate supplementation or fortification. Hence, it appears that the effect of the *MTHFR* variant has minimal effect on risk of cardiovascular disease in populations with adequate folate levels.

Lupus Anticoagulant/Antiphospholipid Antibodies

The antiphospholipid syndrome is defined by the clinical manifestation of venous or arterial thrombosis, recurrent fetal loss, or thrombocytopenia coupled with the presence in the serum of at least one type of antiphospholipid antibody. Lupus anticoagulants are one of a group of antiphospholipid antibodies and are common in patients with the antiphospholipid syndrome. They are associated with thromboembolism, recurrent spontaneous abortion, and thrombocytopenia *(174)* but lupus anticoagulants are also present in 1–5% of healthy individuals. Relatives of probands with antiphospholipid antibody syndrome are more likely to have aPL, and there is a strong association between aPL and HLA types *(175,176)*. Therefore, studies have attempted to identify genetic variants that may interact with, or operate in the background of, antiphospholipid antibodies. One study found that the P-selectin Pro715 allele was not present in patients with lupus anticoagulant who suffered arterial thrombosis (but was slightly more frequent in patients with VTE), whereas the CA repeat polymorphism in the 3′-noncoding region of CD154 was associated with risk of development of arterial thrombosis *(177)*. The authors suggest that these genetic variants can differentiate between risk of venous and arterial thrombosis in patients with lupus anticoagulant. Studies have also shown that the concurrent presence of other genetic mutations including factor V Leiden, the prothrombin G20210A mutation, and APCR increases the risk of antiphospholipid-associated VTE *(178,179)*. Further studies of the genetics of this disease are necessary.

Other Genetic Factors Associated with VTE

Tissue-factor pathway inhibitor (TFPI) plays a major role in the inhibition of the extrinsic coagulation pathway *(180)*. The Pro15Leu SNP in *TFPI* has been shown to be a risk factor for VTE *(181)*; however, subsequent studies did not confirm this association *(182)*. Thrombomodulin, a component of the protein C anticoagulant pathway, is a transmembrane protein synthesized by endothelial cells and acts as a receptor for thrombin and as cofactor of thrombin in the activation of protein C. Several missense mutations in the thrombomodulin gene have been identified in patients with VTE *(183–186)*; however, the relationship between these variants and risk of VTE remains unclear. Variants in the thrombomodulin gene have also inconsistently been associated with coronary heart disease and/or MI *(187–195)*. A recently published large-scale study of genetic variants in DVT found variants within several genes to be associated with DVT in three case-control datasets, including *CYP4V2, SERPINC1, GP6 (196)*. Further studies of these various genetic variants are necessary to establish their role in VTE risk.

Laboratory Assays and Diagnostic Testing for Hereditary VTE

Table 10 presents an overview of the various laboratory assays for the more commonly tested genetic thrombophilias. The primary screening tests for APC resistance are aPTT-based assays. In such, the aPTT is done with and without a standardized amount of APC. The two generated clotting times are then converted to an APC ratio which is compared to the normal range or by normalizing to the APC resistance ratio from normal pooled plasma. This test is not valid in patients receiving anticoagulants, in patients with a baseline abnormal aPTT due to other coagulation defects, and has not been validated in patients with acute thrombotic events or pregnant women *(197)*. In second-generation functional assays, patient plasma is diluted in a sufficient volume of factor-V-deficient plasma, and then an aPTT-based assay or a tissue factor-dependent factor V assay is performed *(198)*. This assay can be performed in patients receiving anticoagulants and in those with abnormal baseline aPTT due to other coagulation defects. Factor V Leiden specifically can be detected by a genetic test in DNA extracted from peripheral blood mononuclear cells to detect the substitution of A for G at nucleotide 1691 in the factor V gene, which results in the Arg506Gln mutation in the factor V protein and hence loss of an MnlI cleavage site *(84)*.

Similarly, the G20210A gene mutation is usually identified in DNA extracted from peripheral blood mononuclear cells using PCR-based methods. Plasma prothrombin assays are not diagnostic for this mutation. For diagnosis of hyperhomocysteinemia, there are sensitive assays that allow quantification of total plasma homocysteine concentrations. Normal values range from 5 to 15 µmol/L, with moderate hyperhomocysteinemia defined as 15–30 µmol/L, intermediate defined as 30–100 µmol/L, and severe hyperhomocysteinemia defined as >100 µmol/L *(199)*. However, identification of the *MTHFR* genotype is not cost effective and the clinical utility is uncertain.

GENETIC VARIANTS IN ARTERIAL THROMBOTIC DISORDERS

The clinical manifestations of arterial thrombosis are diverse. For example, acute thrombosis at the site of a ruptured, lipid-rich atherosclerotic plaque is thought to be the precipitating event underlying development of acute MI, ischemic stroke, or peripheral arterial disease (PAD) *(200)*. Given that almost half of all thrombotic events occur in patients without traditional cardiovascular risk factors *(201)*, there have been extensive efforts in elucidating novel risk factors, including genetic risk factors, for arterial thrombosis (reviewed in Voetsch and Loscalzo *(202)*). Hundreds of genetic variants have been implicated in CAD and arterial thrombotic risk, and an exhaustive review is beyond the scope of this chapter. An overview of the most relevant and validated prothrombotic genetic variants is presented in Table 7. Overall, few (if any) genetic variants contribute significantly to risk of arterial thrombotic disorders and in general, clinical testing of these variants is not indicated except in certain subgroups of patients (summarized as follows and in Fig. 1).

Table 7
Genetic factors implicated in arterial thromboembolism

Gene	Variant	Function (if known)	Phenotype
Fibrinogen β	(1) BcI (2) Arg448Lys (3) −455G/A	(1) Increases fibrinogen level (2) Alters nuclear protein binding; changes fibrin structure/function (3) Increased transcription of β-fibrinogen (206)	MI, atheroma progression, lacunar infarcts (207–215) (conflicting results)
Fibrinogen α	Thr312Ala	Results in more extensive a-chain crosslinking and thicker clot fibers (216)	Poststroke mortality in pts with Afib (217,219); venous thromboembolism (218)
Factor VII	(1) Arg353Gln(2) Hypervariable region 4 (HVR4)	Higher levels of factor VII	MI
Factor XIIIA	Val34Leu	Changes FXIII activation rate and fibrin structure/function	MI (8,358)
Fibrinogen Aα	Thr312Ala	Changes fibrin structure/function and FXIII crosslinking	Atrial fibrillation (417)
Thrombomodulin	Ala455Val, Ala25Thr, −33 G/A	Unknown	MI, CAD, though reports inconsistent (187–195)
GPIIIa	Leu33Pro (PlA2)	Results in conformational change in disulfide loop important for fibrinogen binding (418)	CAD, stroke, MI, venous thrombosis (237–242,418)
Glycoprotein Ia-IIa (α2β1 integrin)	C807T	Affects α2β1 integrin density on platelets and collagen receptor activity (259,260)	MI and stroke, particularly in young patients (263–265), results contradictory (266,267)
Glycoprotein Ib-V-IX	(1) HPA-2 (C3550T), VNTR (2) Kozak sequence (T/C dimorphism at nucleotide -5)	(1) Poorly defined (2) More efficient mRNA translation and increased levels of Ibα receptor on platelet surface (Afshar-Kharghan V. 186)	(1) MI and stroke, results contradictory (242,251–256) (2) MI (258)
Plasminogen activator inhibitor-1 (PAI-1)	4G/5G promoter indel	4G allele associated with higher PAI-1 levels	CAD, MI (270–274,278), dialysis access thrombosis (interaction with TGF-β1 haplotype) (419)
Tissue-type plasminogen activator (t-PA)	(1) 311-bp Alu indel in intron 8 (2) −7351C/T (3) rs7007329-rs8178750 haplotype	Associated with t-PA release	(1–2) MI (280,284,285), ischemic stroke (286) (3) Ischemic stroke (420)

(continued)

Table 7
(continued)

Gene	Variant	Function (if known)	Phenotype
Thrombin-activatable fibrinolysis inhibitor (TAFI)	Ala147Thr	Associated with plasma TAFI antigen levels	Angina, MI (289,290)
MTHFR	677 C/T	Leads to thermo liability of the enzyme	CAD, MI, stroke (292,293,421)
Endothelial nitric oxide synthase (eNOS)	(1) VNTR in intron 4 and 13 (2) Promoter SNPs (−786 T/C, −922 A/G, −1468 T/A)	(1) Unknown (2) −786 T/C results in reduction in eNOS promoter activity	(1) MI, CAD (298) (2) Coronary spasm, reduced cerebral blood flow, CAD, endothelial dysfunction (299–302)
P-selectin	PSGL-1	VNTR	Coronary stent thrombosis (422)
IL-6	(1) −572G C (2) −174G C		(1) Ischemic stroke (308) (2) MI, stroke, CAD (423–425)
Von Willebrand factor (vWF) (426)	1798 C/G		Coronary artery disease, advanced atherosclerosis
Factor V	Factor V Leiden		Conflicting results: MI, ischemic stroke, peripheral vascular disease (109,145,220–223)
Prothrombin	G20210A		Controversial and conflicting association with MI (137,148–155,427), ischemic stroke (137,152,156,157), cryptogenic stroke (428), peripheral vascular disease
MTHFR	C677T		MI, ischemic stroke, peripheral vascular disease (172,220,291–294)
Fucosyltransferase 3	T59G		Atherothrombotic disease (429)
Tissue factor	I1208D	Lower levels of circulating tissue factor (D allele) (235)	Protective against VTE, no association with coronary disease (235)
Paraoxonase	Various	Various	Coronary artery disease, MI (303,305–307)
ALOX5AP/LTA4	Various	Involved in leukotriene pathway	Coronary artery disease, MI (17,430)
CDKN2A/CDKN2B	Several SNPs adjacent to CDKN2A/CDKN2B genes	Unknown	Coronary artery disease, MI (25,309)
Endothelial protein C receptor (EPCR)	23-bp insertion in exon 3	Unknown	Atherothrombotic disease, reports contradictory (129,130)

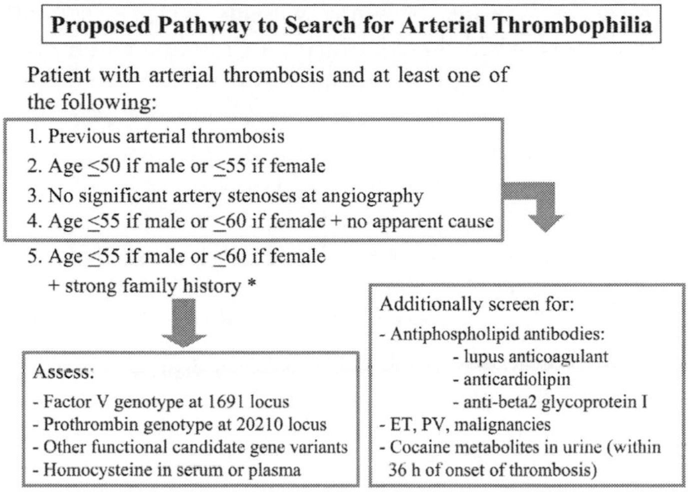

Fig. 1. Proposed criteria for the selection of patients in whom it may be justified to perform testing for underlying thrombophilic conditions (Factor V Leiden, prothrombin G20210A, and MTHFR C677T mutations) (Reproduced with permission from Andreotti et al. *(358)*).

Genetic Variants In Hemostatic System Genes

FIBRINOGEN

Fibrinogen is the precursor of fibrin and fibrinogen levels influence platelet aggregation. Elevated fibrinogen levels have been associated with MI, stroke, and PAD *(203,204)*, with a meta-analysis showing an overall twofold increased risk of cardiovascular disease in healthy and high-risk subjects *(205)*. Genetic factors are estimated to contribute to approximately 50% of variability in fibrinogen levels *(202)*. Variants in the genes encoding the three pairs of fibrinogen polypeptide chains (α, β, and γ) have been studied in relation to arterial thrombotic risk, with most studies focusing on variants within the gene encoding β-fibrinogen: −148C/T, −455G/A (*Hae*III), *Bcl*I (in 3′ untranslated region), and −854G/A. The −455G/A and BclI variants are in linkage disequilibrium (i.e., are correlated) with each other. The AA genotype of the −455G/A SNP has been associated with 10% higher fibrinogen levels compared with the GG genotype *(202)*. Studies have further shown that the A allele binds less well to a putative repressor protein complex, resulting in increased fibrinogen-β chain transcription *(206)*. However, the association between this fibrinogen gene variant and risk of arterial thrombosis remains unclear, with some studies showing an association and others showing none *(207–213)*. A systematic review of the association of this SNP revealed that homozygosity for the −455A allele was marginally protective against acute MI (OR: 0.66; 95% CI: 0.44–0.99) *(214)*; but in another study, this allele was associated with a 2.5-fold increase in risk of multiple cerebral lacunar infarcts but not with large-artery strokes *(215)*. A variant in the α-fibrinogen gene Thr312Ala results in more extensive α-chain crosslinking and thicker fibers with clot formation *(216)*, and has been shown to be associated with mortality rates after stroke *(217)* and VTE *(218)*. However another study showed no association with risk of MI *(219)*. These widely conflicting results suggest there is little if any role for fibrinogen variants in thrombotic disorder risk.

FACTOR V LEIDEN AND PROTHROMBIN G20210A

The Factor V Leiden and prothrombin G20210A SNPs have been examined for association with arterial thrombotic disorders in numerous studies (reviewed in a meta-analysis by Kim and Becker

2003 *(220)*), most showing negative results even in very young age-of-onset individuals *(221)*. Studies showing a positive association between these variants include association of factor V Leiden with ischemic stroke, especially in women *(222)* and in children *(223)*; and association between pro-thrombin 20210 with stroke in children *(223)*. In a meta-analysis of more than 17,000 patients, the association between these inherited gene mutations and arterial ischemic events was modest (Factor V Leiden OR: 1.21 (95% CI: 0.99–1.49); prothrombin G20210A OR: 1.32 (95% CI: 1.03–1.69)), with subgroup analyses of patients less than 55 years old and of women showing slightly stronger association overall *(145,220)*. Both the factor V Leiden and the prothrombin mutations show evidence for a gene–environment interaction with smoking, resulting in a 32-fold higher risk of MI in female smokers who carry Factor V Leiden *(109)*, and a greater than 40-fold increase in risk of MI in young female smokers who carry the prothrombin 20210A allele *(155)*. Such gene–environment interactions were subsequently confirmed in studies of men *(150,224)*.

Therefore, in the general population unlike risk of VTE these polymorphisms do not appear to be associated with arterial thrombotic risk, though may be risk factors in select populations (i.e., in women and/or children) and in select circumstances, i.e., in combination with smoking or other cardiovascular risk factors. The underlying reason for this difference in arterial vs. venous thrombotic risk is reviewed in a meta-analysis by Kim and Becker *(220)*: VTE is most strongly influenced by the presence of activated coagulation proteases leading to thrombin generation *(225)*, and therefore an intact system for intrinsic vascular resistance to thrombosis (such as provided by activated protein C, antithrombin, and TFPI) is necessary. In contrast, arterial thrombosis occurs at sites of arterial wall injury in the background of activated endothelial cells, monocytes, and platelet aggregates *(226)*, and this environment is minimally influenced by small decreases in the function or level of the vascular surface anticoagulant system *(220)*. Young patients may be the exception, where the underlying mechanism of MI, stroke, or PVD is a primary thrombotic event, whereas in older individuals, chronic atherosclerotic disease and its risk factors are primary.

OTHER COAGULATION PROTEINS AND ARTERIAL THROMBOSIS RISK

Given the role of factor VII in the initiation of coagulation, the factor VII gene has been of interest in understanding arterial thrombosis. Factor VII levels have been inconsistently associated with CAD *(204,227)*, and polymorphisms in the factor VII gene account for approximately 30% of the variability in factor VII levels *(202)*. The most commonly studied variants are the Arg353Gln SNP in exon 8 and the hypervariable region 4 (HVR4) that involves a 37-basepair repeat in intron 7 of the factor VII gene. It appears that these polymorphisms have a functional effect on factor VII levels, though the relative influence of each remains to be clarified fully *(202,227)*. The 353GlnGln and the HVR4 H7H7 genotypes have been associated with a significant decrease in the risk of MI *(228)*; however, other studies have failed to replicate this finding *(229–231)*, suggesting that the association between factor VII genetic variants and arterial thrombotic disease is small at best. Factor XIII stabilizes fibrin clot. Studies have reported an association between a polymorphism in the A subunit of factor XIII (Val34Leu) and arterial thrombotic risk, with the 34Leu allele being protective against MI and stroke (reviewed by Ariens and colleagues *(232)*). This SNP influences the transglutaminase activity of FXIII and homozygosity for the mutation is associated with increased enzyme activity *(233)*.

Plasma thrombomodulin levels have been associated with increased risk of MI *(234)*. Two polymorphisms in the thrombomodulin gene have shown to be associated with MI (Ala455Val *(192)* and Ala25Thr *(187)*). The Ala455Val SNP has been associated with a sixfold increased risk of coronary heart disease in blacks *(195)*. The 25Thr allele of the Ala25Thr SNP has been found to be more prevalent in male MI patients, with a higher risk (6.5-fold increase) in young patients and in the presence of additional metabolic risk factors or smoking *(75,187)*. However, this finding was not confirmed in two subsequent studies *(193,194)*. A third variant in the thrombomodulin gene, −33 G/A in the promoter region, has been shown to influence plasma soluble thrombomodulin levels and is associated with a 1.8-fold increased risk of coronary heart disease in Chinese and with carotid atherosclerosis in young patients *(191)*. Further validation and functional studies are necessary before the role of the thrombomodulin gene in arterial thrombotic risk can be established.

Tissue factor, the major initiator of the blood coagulation cascade, has been investigated in relation to genetic risk of thrombotic disease. Sequencing of the promoter region of the TF gene revealed six novel polymorphisms, and the 1208D allele was found to be associated with lower levels of circulating tissue factor and concomitantly was protective against VTE, though did not influence risk of coronary thrombotic risk *(235)*.

Genetic Variants In Platelet Surface Receptors

Several variants within genes coding for surface membrane glycoproteins have been associated with arterial thrombotic diseases. Glycoproteins are integral to adhesion of platelets to exposed extracellular matrix components and for platelet–platelet interactions. Probably the most studied genetic variant is the Leu33Pro SNP within the GPIIIa subunit (aka integrin β3) of the GPIIb/IIIa complex, with the 33Pro allele commonly referred to as PlA2 (and the 33Leu allele responsible for the PlA1 epitope). The PlA2 allele occurs with a frequency of 0.11–0.15 in whites and 0.08 in blacks; however, it is nearly absent in Asians *(236)*. The first report of the association of this SNP with acute MI was published by Weiss and colleagues, who reported the strongest risk in patients less than 60 years of age (relative risk: 6.2) *(237)*. Several subsequent studies confirmed the association of this variant with MI and/or stroke *(238,239)*; however, the majority have not *(240,241)*. One study showed a 1.8-fold increase in risk in individuals with at least one copy of the PlA2 allele *(242)*, with evidence for a gene–environment interaction with smoking. Studies of platelet function in humans have found that Pro33-positive subjects have shorter bleeding times, enhanced thrombin generation, and enhanced prothrombin consumption as compared with Pro33-negative subjects *(243–245)*. A larger study of 1,422 subjects from the Framingham Offspring Study found that platelets from individuals with the Pro33 allele required less epinephrine to induce platelet aggregation and/or ADP *(246)*. Hence, it appears that the Pro33 polymorphism of glycoprotein IIIa alters human platelet aggregation, adhesion, and secretion, perhaps through the mechanism of increased signaling and cytoskeletal changes, leading to stabilization of platelet–platelet and/or platelet–extracellular matrix interactions *(236)*. Another variant that has been studied in the GPIIb-IIIa gene is the Ile843Ser polymorphism that has been shown to be associated with increased risk of MI in young women in the presence of other risk factors *(247)*, but other studies have shown negative results *(248,249)*.

Genetic variants in other glycoproteins have been inconsistently associated with CAD and stroke, including a Thr145Met SNP (aka HPA-2) and a variable number of tandem repeats (VNTR) in a 39-bp segment of the GPIbα subunit. Each repeat in the VNTR results in the addition of 13 amino acids to the protein, and it is thought that this modifies the distance between the vWF-binding domain and the platelet surface. The VNTR and the HPA-2 are in tight linkage disequilibrium *(250)*. These polymorphisms have been shown to be associated with arterial thrombotic diseases, though results are contradictory *(242,251–256)*, and hence the contribution of these GP Ibα gene variants to arterial thrombosis remains unclear. More recently, a T/C variant at nucleotide-5 located in the translation initiation codon of the GpIbα gene (the Kozak sequence) has been shown to be associated with more efficient mRNA translation and increased levels of the Ibα receptor on the platelet surface *(257)*, and has been shown to be protective against for MI in young women *(258)*.

Integrin $\alpha2\beta1$ (ITGA2, aka glycoprotein Ia-IIa) is one of the platelet collagen receptors, and studies have shown that the 807T allele in this gene is associated with higher levels of integrin $\alpha2\beta1$ *(259)*, correlating with a greater rate of platelet attachment to surfaces coated with collagen type I *(260)*. The T allele of the variant modulates platelet aggregation and clopidogrel antiplatelet effects, suggesting it may contribute to increased thrombotic risk *(261)*. For example, the T allele has been associated with a 1.6-fold increased risk of MI with stronger association in younger patients *(262)*. Other studies have also found the 807T allele to be associated with MI and stroke *(263–265)*, especially in young patients, though reports have been contradictory *(266,267)*. This SNP is in tight linkage disequilibrium with a second ITGA2 SNP (G873A) and with other variations in the same gene *(259,260)*.

Genetic Variants In The Fibrinolytic System

Increased levels of tissue-type plasminogen activator (t-PA, the primarily endothelium-derived activator of the fibrinolytic system) and plasminogen activator inhibitor-1 (PAI-1, the major inhibitor of t-PA), as well as variants within the genes encoding both of these proteins, have been associated with arterial thrombosis risk *(227)*. The most studied variant in the PAI-1 gene is the 4G/5G insertion/ deletion polymorphism located in the promoter of the gene. The 4G allele has been associated with elevated PAI-1 plasma levels *(268)* and increased mRNA transcription *(269)*. Several studies have shown that carriers of the 4G allele have an elevated risk of MI, CAD, and stroke *(270–274)*; however, larger studies have failed to confirm this association *(275–277)*. A meta-analysis of this variant shows an overall slight increase in the risk of MI in carriers of the 4G allele (OR: 1.2), primarily in high-risk subgroups *(278)*.

The most studied t-PA variant is a 311-basepair Alu insertion/deletion that influences release rates of total t-PA *(279)* and has been associated with a 50% increase in risk of MI in one study *(280)*, though later studies did not validate this finding *(281,282)*. Further work to identify other variants in the t-PA gene yielded discovery of the −7351 promoter polymorphism which, like the Alu polymorphism, is associated with t-PA release after stress *(283)*, suggesting that decreased local release of tPA but not systemic levels may increase risk of arterial thrombosis *(283,284)*. Subsequent studies have found that carriers of the −7531T allele have up to a 3.1-fold increased risk of MI *(284,285)* and the SNP is also associated with ischemic stroke (OR: 1.9; 95% CI: 1.01–3.6) *(286)*. Given that this SNP is in linkage disequilibrium with the Alu polymorphism, but is located within an Sp1-binding site, it is more likely the functional variant within this gene accounting for thrombotic risk.

Thrombin-activatable fibrinolysis inhibitor (TAFI) is involved in fibrinolysis regulation; it removes lysine and arginine residues from fibrin and hence decreases plasminogen binding to its surface *(287)*. Elevated TAFI levels have been associated with DVT *(288)* and CAD *(289)*, and several variants within the TAFI gene have been associated with plasma TAFI levels. Only one variant, the Ala147Thr SNP, has been associated with arterial thrombotic risk, with individuals with the 147 Thr/Thr genotype having an almost threefold increase in relative risk of angina *(289)*; however, in another study, the 147 Thr allele was protective against MI *(290)*. Further studies of these genes in arterial thrombosis are necessary.

Other Mechanisms Of Genetic Risk For Arterial Thrombosis

In addition to the defined genes in key pathways integral to hemostasis and thrombolysis, genes residing in pathways associated with endothelial dysfunction (and associated platelet activation and thrombosis) have also been associated with arterial thrombotic risk. Probably the most well-studied such genetic variant is the 677 C/T SNP in the *MTHFR* gene, homozygosity of which is the most common genetic cause of mild-to-moderate hyperhomocysteinemia. Elevated levels of homocysteine are an independent risk factor for atherosclerosis, MI, and stroke *(291)*. Studies of the 677 C/T SNP have shown that this variant is associated with a greater than threefold increase in risk of CAD and stroke, although results of other studies have been inconsistent (reviewed by Fletcher and colleagues *(292)*). A meta-analysis showed that individuals homozygous for the T allele had higher fasting homocysteine levels than heterozygous or normal individuals; however, of the 12 studies included, only four reported an association between the TT genotype and increased cardiovascular risk *(293)*. Two larger meta-analyses corroborated these findings, with the overall odds ratio modestly significant at 1.16–1.20 *(172,220)*. Hence, it appears that this SNP confers only a modest risk of arterial thrombosis. Further studies have suggested the existence of a gene–environment interaction between the 677 C/T SNP and folate levels: homocysteine levels are only elevated in individuals homozygous for this variant when plasma folate concentrations are low *(294)*.

Variants within the endothelial nitric oxide synthase (*eNOS*) gene have been studied with regard to arterial thrombotic risk. NO is produced by endothelium and serves as a smooth muscle relaxant and regulator of vascular tone, as well as inhibiting activation and aggregation of platelets *(295)*. Endothelial dysfunction dependent on NO is an integral first step in atherosclerosis and thrombosis initiation. The variable nucleotide tandem repeat (VNTR) in intron 4 of the eNOS gene has been shown to be associated with MI *(296)*, though this has not been replicated in other populations *(297)*. Another VNTR in intron 13 has been associated with a 2.2-fold increase in CAD risk *(298)*. Several promoter SNPs have been variably associated with cardiovascular disease including coronary spasm, CAD, and endothelial dysfunction *(299–302)*.

Serum paraoxonase activity is reduced in patients with acute MI *(303)*, and two coding SNPs in the paraoxonase (PON1) gene independently influence PON1 activity (Gln192Arg and Leu55Met) *(304)*. However, studies evaluating the association of PON1 polymorphisms and cardiovascular disease have shown conflicting results *(303, 305–307)*. Other variants in genes such as plasma glutathione peroxidase (GPx-3), connexin 37, P-selectin, and in the NADPH oxidase system have been shown to be associated with arterial thrombotic diseases (reviewed in Voetsch and colleagues *(202,304)*), as has an SNP in the interleukin-6 (IL6) gene which was significantly associated with both ischemic stroke and intracerebral hemorrhage *(308)*. Finally, as noted previously, genome-wide association studies have identified a variant on chromosome 9p as a susceptibility variant for CAD and MI *(25,309)*.

GENETIC BASIS FOR RELATIONSHIP BETWEEN ARTERIAL AND VENOUS THROMBOTIC RISK

Thromboembolic arterial diseases and VTE are clinically considered to represent separate disease entities. Further, they differ physiologically, with arterial thrombi being composed mainly of platelets (white clots), while venous thrombi are composed primarily of red blood cells and fibrin (so-called red clots) *(310)*. Recently, attention has been paid to the possible relationships between arterial disease and VTE risk. Risk factors for both diseases overlap: age, obesity, estrogen use, or pregnancy, etc. Observational studies have found associations between arterial thrombotic risk factors such as metabolic syndrome *(311)*, diabetes *(312)*, waist circumference and smoking *(313)*, and development of VTE, and between statin use and lower incidence of VTE *(314)*. VTE has also been associated with subclinical atherosclerosis: one study found that patients with a prior history of VTE had a higher risk of carotid plaque on ultrasound imaging *(315)* and another found a higher incidence of coronary artery calcium in patients with idiopathic VTE than in matched controls without VTE *(316)*. However, two subsequent large observational trials found no relationship between the presence of subclinical atherosclerosis and subsequent VTE risk *(317,318)*.

Studies have also suggested an increased risk of development of subsequent arterial thrombotic events after VTE *(319,320)*. For example, one prospective study of 1,919 consecutive patients followed prospective after a first episode of VTE followed for a median of 4 years found that patients with idiopathic VTE had a 60% higher risk of suffering from at least one episode of arterial thrombotic events as compared with patients with secondary VTE *(321)*, suggesting the presence of a common risk factor contributing to a shared prothrombotic state. While factor V Leiden, prothrombin G20210A, and APCR have been associated with both VTE and arterial thrombotic risk as outlined earlier, further studies are necessary to understand the possible genetic factors underlying risk of subsequent arterial thrombosis in patients with a history of VTE.

PHARMACOGENOMICS

Clinical trials of antithrombotic therapies have shown improved patient outcomes across a broad range of thrombotic disorders. However, not all patients respond similarly and favorably to antithrombotic agents. Further, few clinical factors have been identified that significantly influence this heterogeneity. Pharmacogenomics holds promise in furthering the field of "personalized medicine," where a health care provider would use genomic testing to help identify the ideal treatments and medicine(s) for an individual patient. Candidate genes evaluated in pharmacogenomic studies can influence metabolism of a drug by modifying drug metabolizing enzymes *(322)* (pharmacodynamics); affect binding of a drug to target proteins (pharmacokinetics); or affect absorption, distribution, excretion, and targeting to the site of action and thus affect the final pharmacological response to a drug *(323)*; or, genetic variants could influence effectiveness of a drug by affecting the level or function of the target of the treatment *(324)*. Table 8 details pharmacogenetic studies of commonly used antiplatelet agents in cardiovascular disease (modified from Marin and colleagues *(324)*).

Pharmacogenetics of Resistance To Antiplatelet Agents

Many variants have been evaluated in relationship to aspirin in hopes of further understanding the phenomenon of so-called aspirin resistance. Previous reports suggested the prevalence of aspirin resistance to be 5–40%, depending on the assay and population studied *(325,326)*. Genetic variants related to potential platelet hyper-reactivity, collagen sensitivity, and platelet–red cell interaction have been studied in an attempt to understand heterogeneity of aspirin response. The most studied polymorphism is the PlA variant in the glycoprotein IIIa gene (resulting in Pro33Leu substitution). There are several reports suggesting that this variant may account for differences in aspirin-induced effects *(243,327,328)*, with carriers of the PlA2 allele requiring a higher dose of aspirin to reach the same antiplatelet aggregation effect as individuals homozygous for the PlA1 genotype *(327)*. Individuals with the PlA2 variant also have increased risk for cardiovascular thrombosis *(245,319,320,327,329)*, as well as increased risk of worse outcomes after percutaneous coronary interventions (PCI) *(330–332)*. Furthermore, this polymorphism appears to modulate antiplatelet effects induced by the thienopyridine derivative clopidogrel, commonly used as an adjunctive antithrombotic treatment after acute coronary syndromes and after PCI with stenting. Specifically, reduction in platelet activation induced by clopidogrel was significantly attenuated in carriers of the PlA2 polymorphism as compared with individuals homozygous for the PlA1 genotype *(333)*. Investigators have also studied pharmacogenetic effects of this polymorphism with glycoprotein IIb/IIIa receptor inhibitors, antiplatelet drugs used in high-risk patients with acute coronary syndromes especially those undergoing early PCI *(334)*; however, results of these studies have been inconsistent and controversial. It appears that glycoprotein IIb/IIIa inhibitors are less efficient in platelet inhibition in carriers of the PlA2 allele

Table 8

Pharmacogenetic studies of commonly used antiplatelet, anticoagulant, and fibrinolytic medications in cardiovascular disease (Modified from Marin and colleagues (324))

Gene	Genetic variant	Medication	Functional effect	Clinical effect
Glycoprotein IIIa	PlA (Pro33Leu)	(1) Aspirin (243,245,327,328, 330–332,431)	(1) PlA2 allele requires higher dose of aspirin	(1) Increased thrombotic risk, worse outcome after angioplasty/stent
		(2) Clopidogrel (333)	(2) Less reduction of platelet aggregation with clopidogrel	(2) No data
		(3) Ticlopidine (330,331)	(3) Inconsistent data	(3) Inconsistent data
		(4) Intravenous glycoprotein IIb/IIIa inhibitors (243,335,338,432,433)	(4) Inconsistent data	(4) Inconsistent data
		(5) Oral glycoprotein IIb/ IIIa inhibitors (434)	(5) Related to an adverse interaction	(5) SNP associated with absence of clinical benefit
COX-1	C50T (435)	Aspirin	Associated with higher levels of thromboxane	No data
COX-2	G765C (435)	Aspirin	Associated with higher reduction of thromboxane levels after aspirin treatment	No data
Glycoprotein Ia	C807T	(1) Aspirin (266,327,328,435)	(1) Associated with differential expression on platelet surface	(1) No association
		(2) Clopidogrel (436)	(2) T allele associated with increased platelet reactivity	(2) No data
ADP subtype receptor	P2Y$_{11}$	(1) Aspirin (437)	(1) Less reduction of platelet aggregation after aspirin	(1) No data
		(2) Clopidogrel (333,456)	(2) No consistent functional changes	(2) No data
Fc γ	RIIa-R-H131	Unfractionated heparin (438,439)	Controversial data	Controversial data
Cytochrome p450	CYP2CP (Ile359Leu)	Coumadin (343,345, 347–349)	Less enzymatic activity	Confers unstable anticoagulant response, associated with bleeding complications
Factor VII	−323 Indel	Coumadin (340,440)	Reduced factor VII coagulation activity	Increased diurnal variation of INR
Factor XIII	Val34Leu	Fibrinolytics (232,339,340,440)	Related to different resistance of clot	Fibrinolysis less efficient

(243,335), however, these data are difficult to analyze independent of potential effects of aspirin *(324)*. Other genetic variants with potential pharmacogenetic interactions with aspirin, clopidogrel, and glycoprotein IIb/IIIa inhibitors are reviewed in Table 8.

Pharmacogenetics of Fibrinolytic Therapies

Few studies have evaluated pharmacogenetics in fibrinolytic medication therapy for acute MI. Similar to other clinical scenarios, few clinical factors have been identified that account for interindividual heterogeneity in the response to thrombolytic therapy *(336)*. Studies evaluating the role of genetic variants for further explaining this heterogeneity have been performed, but have shown no association *(336–338)*. One study has suggested that the Val34Leu polymorphism in the factor XIII gene may be associated with resistance to fibrinolytic therapy, with individuals carrying the Leu34 allele having significant less efficient fibrinolysis than those with the Val/Val genotype *(339,340)*.

Pharmacogenetics of Warfarin

Probably the most well-studied and consistent pharmacogenetic association in thrombosis is with the anticoagulant warfarin, a vitamin K antagonist used widely in the management of a wide variety of venous and arterial thrombotic disorders. The response to coumadin is dependent on several clinical factors including sex, age, diet, and interacting drugs *(341)*; however, significant unexplained interindividual variability in response to coumadin still exists, resulting in potential predisposition to thrombotic or bleeding complications *(342)*. Studies have shown that genetic variations in the hepatic enzyme that metabolizes the potent isomer S-warfarin, cytochrome P450 2C9, are associated with individual variation in therapeutic dose requirements and risk of bleeding *(343–345)*. Two genetic variants in this cytochrome reduce its enzymatic activity, CYP2C9*2 (Arg144Cys) and CYP2C9*3 (Ile359Leu) *(346)*. The CYP2C9*3 variant has been associated with lower coumadin dose requirements, higher frequency of excessive anticoagulation at initiation of coumadin therapy, and bleeding complications *(343,345–349)*. A recent study of 297 patients starting warfarin therapy found that compared with patients with the non-A/non-A haplotype, patients with the A/A haplotype of VKORC1 had a decreased time to first INR within therapeutic range and to first INR greater than 4.0 *(350)*. Further, both the CYP2C9 genotype and the VKORC1 haplotype had a significant influence on the necessary warfarin dose after the first 2 weeks of therapy. A recent clinical trial randomized 206 patients to standard dosing following an empirical protocol versus pharmacogenetic-guided dosing including three genetic variants (CYP2C9*2, CYP2C9*3, and VKORC1 C1173T) and age, sex, and weight *(351)*. Patients were followed for up to 3 months. Results revealed that the pharmacogenetic-guided dosing more accurately approximated stable doses of warfarin ($P < 0.001$), resulting in smaller and fewer dosing changes and INRs. However, there was no significant difference in the primary endpoint of percent out-of-range INRs. Therefore, pharmacogenetic-guided dosing may show promise of improving accuracy and efficiency of warfarin dose initiation; larger clinical trials are ongoing and hopefully will be able to further address the usefulness of genetic variants on clinical endpoints.

CLINICAL CONSIDERATIONS IN INHERITED THROMBOTIC DISORDERS

Clinical Manifestations of Hereditary Thrombotic Disorders

Clinically, as is seen with other genetic disorders, patients with inherited thrombotic disorders tend to manifest disease at an earlier age, experience recurrent events, have familial clustering of thrombosis, and may have thrombosis in atypical sites. The most common manifestation of inherited thrombosis is deep venous thrombosis of the lower extremities, accounting for 90% of thrombotic events *(33)*. More unusual sites of thrombosis include mesenteric or cerebral veins which account for less than 5% of events (and are even rarer in patients with APC resistance). The presence of an inherited thrombophilia increases risk of recurrence and is even higher in the presence of more than one mutation, which may be seen with the more common mutations (factor V Leiden, prothrombin 20210, MTHFR), or in mutations existing in the homozygous or double heterozygous forms *(352)*. The risk of recurrent arterial thrombosis is affected by several clinical variables such as age, vascular bed, coexisting disease in other vascular beds, concomitant risk factors, use and effectiveness of existing treatments, and presence of a defined thrombophilia.

Screening Considerations

The Centers for Disease Control and Prevention, Office of Genomics and Disease Prevention has stressed the importance of collecting a detailed family history *(353)*. This is a simple, cheap, and frequently underutilized tool for assessing risk for common diseases. Testing for an underlying inherited thrombophilia is not indicated in asymptomatic populations, nor in general is it indicated in individuals with a family history of thrombosis. This is primarily because testing would not change management of these patients given lack of data justifying risks of long-term or permanent prophylactic anticoagulation in an asymptomatic patient *(354–356)*. Recommendations for testing of first-degree relatives of a patient with thrombosis with an identified inherited thrombophilia are variable; testing can be considered after careful discussion with the patient and the family. These family members could then be educated about precautions and symptoms, as well as considered for prophylactic therapy in the setting of high-risk situations. Testing should also be considered in women with recurrent unexplained fetal loss after 9 weeks in the presence of placental ischemia/infarction and/or maternal vessel thrombosis.

In patients presenting with a VTE, further evaluation and testing should be considered in the following individuals: age <50 years; thrombosis at unusual sites (cerebral, mesenteric, hepatic, or portal veins); recurrent VTE; VTE with a strong family history of thrombotic disease; and in women with recurrent miscarriages and/or puerperal complications *(161)* (summarized in Table 9). Testing for arterial or venous thrombotic events can be performed during hospitalization and even during the initial stages of a thrombotic episode, and should occur concurrently with evaluation for acquired thrombophilia (i.e., malignancy, systemic disorders, etc.). Table 10 details methods for different types of the more commonly used thrombosis risk tests (adapted from Federici et al. *(357)*). GeneTests (http://www.genetests.org), a National Institutes of Health-funded medical genetics information resource developed for healthcare providers and researchers, also provides extensive information on genetic testing and its use in diagnosis and management, detailing both clinical and research laboratories available for specific genetic testing.

Further clinical testing for an underlying thrombophilic condition in patients presenting with arterial thrombosis should be considered in the presence of at least one of the following: (1) recurrent thromboembolic events; (2) young age (≤50 years of age in males; ≤55 years if female); (3) lack of significant arterial stenosis at angiography; (4) age ≤55 years in males or ≤60 years if female and no apparent cause (i.e., lack of traditional cardiovascular risk factors, systemic illnesses, malignancies, offending drugs); or (5) age ≤55 years in males or ≤60 years in females and a strong family history of thrombosis *(358)* (Fig. 1).

Cost effectiveness is an issue when considering genetic testing, incorporating both cost of the testing and the cost associated with long-term anticoagulation. For example, some studies of the factor V Leiden variant suggest that it is not cost effective to test in patients with a first DVT *(359)* or in

Table 9
Current recommendations for screening for thrombophilia in VTE (Reproduced with permission from up to date (modified from Bauer (365)))

Recommended screening for thrombophilia
The following recommendations concerning which conditions should be tested for are based on a characterization
  of the patient as either "strongly" or "weakly" thrombophilic:
Strongly thrombophilic:
First idiopathic venous thrombosis before 50 years of age OR
History of recurrent thrombotic episodes OR
First-degree relative(s) with documented thromboembolism before age 50
Weakly thrombophilic:
First episode of idiopathic venous thromboembolism at age <50 years AND
Negative family history of thromboembolism

Condition tested for:	Strongly thrombophilic	Weakly thrombophilic
Activated protein C resistance	Yes	Yes
Prothrombin mutation	Yes	Yes
Antiphospholipid antibodies	Yes	Yes
Antithrombin deficiency	Yes	No
Protein C deficiency	Yes	No
Protein S deficiency	Yes	No

pregnant women *(360)*. A simulation study based on risk in 60-year-old men did show that screening and prolonged prophylaxis for factor V Leiden carriers is cost effective *(361)*, especially in combination with testing for the prothrombin G20210A variant *(362)*. However, the authors note that testing would not be cost effective in populations where the prevalence of carriers is low; if the risk of a major bleed is high; or in which the risk of recurrent DVT is low.

Implications For Treatment

INITIAL TREATMENT OF VTE

The management of acute venous or arterial thrombosis in patients with inherited thrombophilia in general is the same as with other patients, with a few exceptions:

1. In patients with antithrombin III deficiency, antithrombin concentrate can be used safely and effectively in the setting of acute VTE *(50,51)*. Antithrombin concentrate can be considered in patients with unusually severe thrombosis, those who develop recurrent thrombosis despite adequate anticoagulation, or in those with difficulty achieving adequate anticoagulation *(52)*. However, the use of antithrombin concentrate in such scenarios has not been studied in a randomized, controlled trial.
2. In patients with protein C deficiency, oral anticoagulation should be started only after full heparinization is achieved. Further, to avoid warfarin-induced skin necrosis, the initial dose of warfarin should be low and then increased slowly until therapeutic.

LONG-TERM ANTICOAGULATION

In inherited thrombophilias, genetic testing can assist in determining susceptibility to recurrent events, treatment duration, and whether to perform testing in related family members. Unfortunately, in the setting of long-term management of patients with inherited risk factors who have had a VTE (or patients exposed to increased risk with surgery or pregnancy), in most cases randomized trials

Table 10
Methods for testing for common thrombosis risk tests (Modified from Federici et al. (357))

Thrombophilic condition	Laboratory test	Method	Can be performed while on anticoagulants?	
			Heparin	Coumadin
Protein C deficiency	Protein C activity	Functional, immunoassay	No (if anticoagulation cannot be stopped, protein C antigen levels can be tested while on heparin)	No
APC resistance/factor V Leiden	(1) APC resistance ratio	(1) Clotting time (with and without APC)	(1) No	(1) No
	(2) Second-generation coagulation based assay	(2) Clotting time	(2) Yes	(2) Yes
	(3) Factor V Leiden mutation testing	(3) DNA mutation testing	(3) Yes	(3) Yes
Protein S deficiency	Protein S activity	Functional, immunoassay	No	No
Antithrombin III deficiency	Antithrombin III activity	Functional (antithrombin-heparin cofactor assay). Immunoassay	No	Ideally wait until 2 weeks after anticoagulants stopped
Prothrombin G20210A	Prothrombin G20210A mutation	DNA mutation test	Yes	Yes
Hyperhomocysteinemia	Homocysteine	HPLC, ELISA	Yes	Yes
MTHFR C677T variant	MTHFR C677T variant	DNA mutation test	Yes	Yes

have not been performed making it difficult to establish guidelines for management of patients with a genetic variant and thrombosis. Patients with VTE and an inherited thrombophilia are usually treated with oral anticoagulants for a minimum of 6–12 months with a goal INR of 2.0–3.0. Long-term treatment following this period is dependent on the number of recurrences and the number of genetic defects found. These decisions are complicated by the fact that risk of recurrence varies depending on the genetic defect.

In patients with factor V Leiden, long-term (indefinite) oral anticoagulation should be considered in those with recurrent VTE, multiple thrombophilic disorders, coexistent risk factors (i.e., prolonged immobility), and in patients who are homozygous for the mutation. Long-term anticoagulation is not indicated in all patients after first DVT who are heterozygous for factor V Leiden as shown in several studies *(363,364)*, including the Leiden Thrombophilia study of patients with a first DVT where the risk of recurrent VTE was similar in patients with and without an underlying inherited thrombophilic defect *(364)*. For other inherited thrombophilias, in general, long-term (i.e., indefinite) anticoagulation is not indicated except in the setting of (1) recurrent spontaneous thromboses (or one spontaneous thrombosis in the case of antithrombin III deficiency or antiphospholipid syndrome); (2) one spontaneous life-threatening thrombosis; (3) one spontaneous thrombosis at an unusual site (i.e., mesenteric or cerebral vein); or (4) one spontaneous thrombosis in the setting of more than one inherited genetic defect *(146,362,365)*.

MANAGEMENT OF PREGNANCY

Anticoagulation in pregnant women with a known inherited thrombophilic defect is controversial and should be considered on an individual-by-individual basis. Small, observational studies have suggested that prophylactic antithrombotic therapy is beneficial in such women *(366,367)*, and one randomized trial has shown benefit *(368)*. In this study, 160 women heterozygous for factor V Leiden or prothrombin G20210A mutations, or with protein S deficiency, who had had one unexplained pregnancy loss after 10 weeks of gestation were randomized to aspirin (100 mg daily) or low-molecular-weight heparin from 8 to 37 weeks of gestation. They found that women treated with enoxaparin had a higher live birth rate than those treated with aspirin (86.3% vs. 28.8%; OR: 15.5 (95% CI: 7–34), as well as higher birth weights and lower rate of fetal growth restriction. Therefore, women with high-risk thrombophilia (antithrombin III deficiency, factor V Leiden or prothrombin G20210A homozygotes, or compound heterozygotes for factor V Leiden and prothrombin) should be considered for treatment with prophylactic dose anticoagulation with heparin during pregnancy and postpartum. In the setting of high-risk thrombophilia and a personal or strong family history of VTE, therapeutic dose anticoagulation with heparin should be considered. Women with lower risk thrombophilia (heterozygous factor V Leiden or prothrombin G20210A, protein C or S deficiency) should be managed depending on their personal history of thrombotic events; if they have a personal history of thrombotic events, they should be considered for prophylaxis during pregnancy and postpartum.

OTHER MANAGEMENT CONSIDERATIONS

In general, oral contraceptives should not be started or continued after a thrombotic episode regardless of the presence of an inherited thrombophilic defect. Women with a family history of multiple thromboses (especially those occurring at a younger age) should be cautioned about the significant danger of oral contraceptive use. Testing for hereditary thrombophilias may be useful in this group to help in decision making about contraceptive use *(369)*. Women heterozygous for factor V Leiden should be discouraged against use of oral contraceptives, though it is not an absolute contraindication.

COMPLEX DISEASE GENETICS

Until the mid- to late 1990s, textbooks listed only a small number of single-gene defects associated with thrombosis. The focus was primarily on Mendelian genetics, where there were single genes with strong effects and predictable patterns of inheritance and high penetrance. Methods for identifying such genes have been used to identify Mendelian diseases of the hemostatic system, with results primarily in disorders of bleeding as opposed to disorders of thrombosis. For example, there exists a rare inherited bleeding disorder, combined deficiency of factors V and VII (F5F8D), where patients show a marked reduction in plasma levels of factors V and VIII. The gene underlying this disorder (*LMAN1*) was identified using family-based genetic analyses *(370,371)*. The gene for the rare disease familial thrombotic thrombocytopenic purpura (TTP) was also identified using similar methods in rare patients with the disorder *(372)*.

However, the publication of the completed draft sequence of the human genome (Human Genome Project *(1)*) and the rapid development of genomic technologies have served to expand the focus of human genetics beyond Mendelian traits to a deeper understanding of complex disease genetics. In contrast to Mendelian genetics, complex genetic diseases are usually characterized by multiple genes, each with modest effects, potentially unclear modes of inheritance, lower penetrance, and are the result of a complex interplay of gene–gene and gene–environment interactions. Thrombotic disorders have many of these characteristics. The diagnosis and therapy of most inherited thrombotic and hemorrhagic disorders is made more complex by the presence of incomplete penetrance and variable expressivity *(10)*.

Gene–Environment Interactions

As reviewed under individual genetic variants, there are several known gene–environment interactions for risk of thrombotic disease. For example, in individuals who are heterozygous for the Factor V Leiden variant, oral contraceptive use or being post partum conferred an additional relative risk of 6.0, increasing to a relative risk of 60 if the individuals also carried the prothrombin 202010A variant *(373)*. Another study has clearly shown an incrementally increased risk of thromboembolism in carriers of this variant who smoked and were overweight *(119)*. Interactions have been shown between factor V Leiden, smoking, and increased risk of stroke *(108)*; and between prothrombin G20210A carriership and use of hormone replacement therapy in risk of MI in postmenopausal women *(374)*.

VASCULAR-BED SPECIFIC FACTORS

One can view the local vascular bed as an environment, which may interact with the underlying genetic architecture of a given individual to result in disease. For example, it is a well-recognized feature of thrombophilias that there is focal and vascular-bed-specific expression of thrombosis. This suggests that local regulatory pathways and intrinsic vessel-determined responses to prothrombotic stimuli are in play *(375)*. Studies have shown that endothelial cells from different vascular beds exhibit distinct phenotypes, including differences in signaling pathways *(376)*; mitosis rates *(377)*; growth responses *(378)*; and in expression of nitric oxide synthase, von Willebrand factor, and tissue-type plasminogen activator *(379–382)*. Furthermore, relationships between vascular endothelial cells and surrounding tissues may be important in site-specific responses to prothrombotic stimuli *(183,379,383,384)*. Clinically, this can manifest with site-specific thrombotic complications (Table 11) *(375)*. Therefore, screening, diagnostic testing, and management should include consideration of a patient/vascular-bed-specific approach rather than a more generalized strategy.

Table 11

Factors in vascular bed-specific thrombosis (Reproduced with permission from Edelberg et al. (375))

	Organ bed				
	Heart	*Lung*	*Spleen*	*Kidney*	*Brain*
Clinical disorders/ associated syndromes	Myocardial infarction, acute coronary syndromes	Pulmonary hypertension, pulmonary embolism/ infarction	Splenic infarction	Nephropathy, renal thrombosis	Stroke
Clinically associated factors	Activated factor IX peptide, Factor XIIa, Fibrinogen, Plasminogen activator inhibitor-1, Tissue-type plasminogen activator antigen, von Willebrand factor	Fibrinopeptide A, Hereditary spherocytosis, Soluble thrombomodulin	Protein C Sickle cell anemia	Factor V Leiden, Homocysteine, Plasminogen activator inhibitor-1 4G/4G	Antithrombin III, Factor V Leiden, Homocysteinuria

Gene–Gene Interactions

As reviewed earlier, given the high frequency of many of the genetic variants associated with predilection to thrombosis, a number of studies have evaluated and confirmed that the coinheritance of two or more defects increases the likelihood of thrombosis, including factor V Leiden and Protein C *(385)*, factor V Leiden and antithrombin *(386)*, factor V Leiden and protein S deficiency *(111)*, and others *(387)*. For example, one study compared the prothrombin G20210A allele in individuals with a history of VTE and found that 5% of patients carried both factor V Leiden and the prothrombin variant, higher than the expected population frequency of 0.1% *(144)*. Another study evaluated simultaneously the effects of variants covering four thrombosis genes (factor V, intercellular adhesion molecular 1 (ICAM1), protein C, and thrombomodulin) with cardiovascular disease risk *(388)*. They found that several combinations of variants within these genes were associated with cardiovascular events, suggesting that variants may act in combination to increase risk. Another study of five functional hemostatic polymorphisms found an interaction of factor XIII and prothrombin polymorphisms in risk of premature MI *(389)*. In individuals with anticardiolipin antibodies, there appears to exist an incremental risk of thrombotic events as the number of concomitant risk factors increases (i.e., factor V Leiden, MTHFR C677T, prothrombin 20210A, etc.), with an odds ratio of 1.46 per each additional prothrombotic risk factor *(390)*. These reports highlight that thrombosis is a complex genetic trait and is a polygenic disorder. Continued advances in human genetics will most likely highlight more gene–gene and gene–environment interactions in venous and arterial thrombosis.

Beyond Genetics

TRANSCRIPTOMICS

In this era of complex disease genetics, evaluation and understanding of processes distal to DNA are vital for dissecting the complex interplay between genes, and between genes and environment, to result in health and disease. Transcriptomics refers to large-scale gene-expression profiling which allows simultaneous detection of thousands of different genes on one single "chip." Application of such technology to thrombotic disorders is demonstrated by a study performed at Duke University where Potti et al. *(391)* examined gene-expression profiles in patients with anticardiolipin antibodies and identified expression "signatures" composed of 50 genes whose expression patterns were able to discriminate and predict those who would suffer subsequent thrombotic events in these patients (Fig. 2). Hence, these technologies hold promise in developing novel diagnostic tools for determining which patients may be at risk and potentially intervening prior to a clinical event. For example, the Bloodomics project at Cambridge University has as its primary objective to discover genetic markers within platelets that predict arterial thrombotic risk *(392)*.

PROTEOMICS

There exists significant structural homology among coagulation factors. For example, in a study of a group of healthy subjects participating in the Leiden Thrombophilia Study *(393)*, investigators found clustering of plasma concentrations of vitamin-K-dependent factors (II, VII, IX, X); of factors XI and XII; and factors V and VIII clustered with fibrinogen and D-dimer. The anticoagulant factors (proteins C and S, antithrombin III) clustered together *(393)*. These results of several independent clusters suggest that the basis for individual fluctuations in plasma levels may lie outside the genes coding for these factors. Thus, evaluating the coagulation and fibrinolytic pathways behind DNA is important; gene sequences cannot fully predict the complex structure of proteins, nor their function or dysfunction. For example, regulation of proteins occurs beyond the level of DNA through post-translational modification and protein–protein interactions. Proteomics has therefore emerged as a

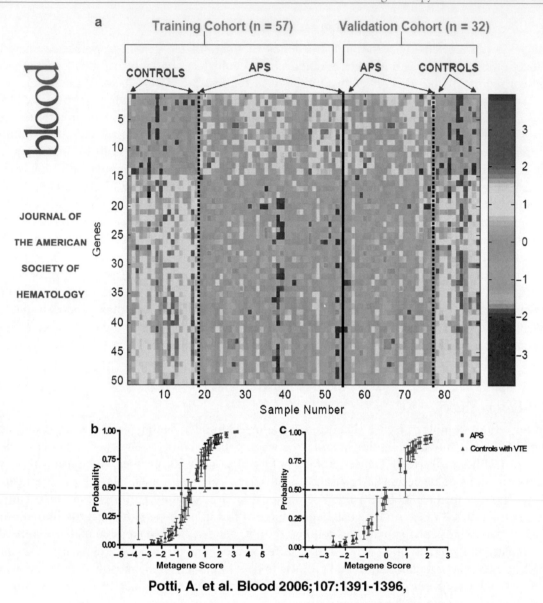

Potti, A. et al. Blood 2006;107:1391-1396,

Fig. 2. Gene-expression profiles that classify and predict APS phenotype.

key component of the molecular characterization of complex diseases, and is defined as the identification and functional characterization of the full complement of proteins expressed by complex biological systems. Furthermore, post-translational modification of proteins may be involved in the pathogenesis and clinical manifestation of thrombophilias. For example, if thrombomodulin is oxidized at methionine residue 388, its capacity to downregulate coagulation is reduced (through activated protein C), but its capacity to inhibit fibrinolysis is unchanged (through thrombin activatable fibrinolysis inhibitor) *(394)*. Modification of the amino acid side chain of apoprotein B on low-density lipoprotein results in its oxidation and renders it prothrombotic *(395)*. A study has shown correlation between the oxidative state of plasma proteins and several markers of thrombin generation and activity *(396)*. Advancing technological platforms including mass spectrometry have facilitated high-throughput proteomic evaluation of plasma and serum. With the use of such technologies, we will be able to further understand the role of known coagulation proteins and potentially novel proteins in thrombotic risk.

Considerations In Genomic Studies

With the increasing use of emerging genomic technologies in thrombotic disease research, clinicians and researchers must be aware of potential pitfalls and issues in conducting and interpreting such studies. Over the past decade hundreds of association studies have been published for association of genetic variants with thrombotic risk though few have been consistently replicated. Positive associations can be the result of a true association, but can also be due to type I error (observing an association when one does not exist, for example, if one evaluates several variants, a proportion will be positively associated purely by chance); differing phenotype definitions; linkage disequilibrium (where the genetic variant is linked to the true etiologic variant); confounders; or population stratification (spurious association due to underlying differences in race/ethnicity or other factors). These considerations need to be carefully addressed in association studies. Investigators should also evaluate a given candidate gene systematically, assessing both known functional and nonfunctional variants, and should consider potential gene–gene and gene–environment interactions. The functional significance of associated genetic variants should then be assessed to understand and further confirm the etiologic role of the variant. Reviews of such issues in conduction genetic studies have been published (397). Studies of transcriptomics and large-scale proteomics must pay careful attention to the analytic issues prompted by analysis of tens of thousands of variables usually with small sample sizes. Integration of the different platforms is vital to fully understanding thrombotic risk in a "systems biology" approach, but provides further analytic challenge. Finally, the clinical relevance of these studies must be evaluated, including consideration of whether the genetic variant (or gene-expression profile, protein, etc.) adds to what is known from clinical factors; whether testing would lead to a change in patient management; and attention to cost effectiveness of testing. In particular, carefully conducted clinical trials showing utility of testing for genomic markers are necessary prior to initiating widespread testing in clinical practice. Only with such diligence will genomic research in thrombotic diseases lead to the eventual goal of "personalized medicine" where genes, gene expression, and other molecular information are used in conjunction with clinical information to stratify disease or select specific medications and/or therapies to benefit one particular individual.

CONCLUSIONS

Herein we have reviewed the current state of the genetics of thrombosis. The past decade has spurred an explosion of studies of the genetic basis of complex diseases such as venous and arterial thrombosis. Coupled with great strides in molecular technologies, the next decade holds much promise for further understanding of the underlying genetic and molecular architecture of thrombosis risk.

REFERENCES

1. International Human Genome Sequencing Consortium (2001) Initial sequencing and analysis of the human genome. Nature 409:860–921
2. de Lange M, Snieder H, Ariens RA et al (2001) The genetics of haemostasis: a twin study. Lancet 357:101–105
3. Bladbjerg EM, de Maat MP, Christensen K et al (2006) Genetic influence on thrombotic risk markers in the elderly – a Danish twin study. J Thromb Haemost 4:599–607

4. Souto JC, Almasy L, Borrell M et al (2000) Genetic susceptibility to thrombosis and its relationship to physiological risk factors: the GAIT study. Genetic Analysis of Idiopathic Thrombophilia. Am J Hum Genet 67:1452–1459

5. Davidson CJ, Tuddenham EG, McVey JH (2003) 450 million years of hemostasis. J Thromb Haemost 1:1487–1494

6. Doolittle RF (1993) The evolution of vertebrate blood coagulation: a case of Yin and Yang. Thromb Haemost 70: 24–28

7. Krem MM, Di Cera E (2002) Evolution of enzyme cascades from embryonic development to blood coagulation. Trends Biochem Sci 27:67–74

8. Abi-Rached L, Gilles A, Shiina T et al (2002) Evidence of en bloc duplication in vertebrate genomes. Nat Genet 31:100–105

9. Hanumanthaiah R, Day K, Jagadeeswaran P (2002) Comprehensive analysis of blood coagulation pathways in teleostei: evolution of coagulation factor genes and identification of zebrafish factor VIIi. Blood Cells Mol Dis 29:57–68

10. Ginsburg D (2005) Identifying novel genetic determinants of hemostatic balance. J Thromb Haemost 3:1561–1568

11. Jiang Y, Doolittle RF (2003) The evolution of vertebrate blood coagulation as viewed from a comparison of puffer fish and sea squirt genomes. Proc Natl Acad Sci U S A 100:7527–7532

12. Collins FS, McKusick VA (2001) Implications of the Human Genome Project for medical science. JAMA 285: 540–544

13. Cargill M, Altshuler D, Ireland J et al (1999) Characterization of single-nucleotide polymorphisms in coding regions of human genes. Nat Genet 22:231–238

14. Halushka MK, Fan J-B, Bentley K et al (1999) Patterns of single-nucleotide polymorphisms in candidate genes for blood-pressure homeostasis. Nat Genet 22:239–247

15. Broeckel U, Hengstenberg C, Mayer B et al (2002) A comprehensive linkage analysis for myocardial infarction and its related risk factors. Nat Genet 30:210–214

16. Hauser ER, Crossman DC, Granger C et al (2002) A genome-wide scan in 438 families with early-onset coronary artery disease. Am J Hum Genet 71:459

17. Helgadottir A, Manolescu A, Thorleifsson G et al (2004) The gene encoding 5-lipoxygenase activating protein confers risk of myocardial infarction and stroke. Nat Genet 36:233–239

18. Wang Q, Rao S, Shen GQ et al (2004) Premature myocardial infarction novel susceptibility locus on chromosome 1P34-36 identified by genomewide linkage analysis. Am J Hum Genet 74:262–271

19. Connelly JJ, Wang T, Cox JE et al (2006) GATA2 is associated with familial early-onset coronary artery disease. PLoS Genet 2:e139

20. Wang L, Hauser ER, Shah SH et al (2006) Identification of kalirin gene as a novel coronary artery disease gene through peak-wide association mapping on chromosome 3q13-21. Circulation 114:887

21. Blangero J, Williams JT, Almasy L (2003) Novel family-based approaches to genetic risk in thrombosis. J Thromb Haemost 1:1391–1397

22. Soria JM, Fontcuberta J (2005) New approaches and future prospects for evaluating genetic risk of thrombosis. Haematologica 90:1212–1222

23. Roeder K, Bacanu SA, Wasserman L et al (2006) Using linkage genome scans to improve power of association in genome scans. Am J Hum Genet 78:243–252

24. Wacholder S, Rothman N, Caporaso N (2000) Population stratification in epidemiologic studies of common genetic variants and cancer: quantification of bias. J Natl Cancer Inst 92:1151–1158

25. Helgadottir A, Thorleifsson G, Manolescu A et al (2007) A common variant on chromosome 9p21 affects the risk of myocardial infarction. Science 316:1491–1493

26. Allaart CF, Poort SR, Rosendaal FR et al (1993) Increased risk of venous thrombosis in carriers of hereditary protein C deficiency defect. Lancet 341:134–138

27. (1997) Inherited thrombophilia: memorandum from a joint WHO/International Society on Thrombosis and Haemostasis meeting. Bull World Health Organ 75:177–189.

28. Makris M, Rosendaal FR, Preston FE (1997) Familial thrombophilia: genetic risk factors and management. J Intern Med Suppl 740:9–15

29. Mateo J, Oliver A, Borrell M et al (1997) Laboratory evaluation and clinical characteristics of 2,132 consecutive unselected patients with venous thromboembolism – results of the Spanish Multicentric Study on Thrombophilia (EMET-Study). Thromb Haemost 77:444–451

30. Ridker PM, Goldhaber SZ, Danielson E et al (2003) Long-term, low-intensity warfarin therapy for the prevention of recurrent venous thromboembolism. N Engl J Med 348:1425–1434

31. Egeberg O (1965) Inherited antithrombin deficiency causing thrombophilia. Thromb Diath Haemorrh 13:516–530

32. Lane DA, Olds RJ, Conard J et al (1992) Pleiotropic effects of antithrombin strand 1C substitution mutations. J Clin Invest 90:2422–2433

33. Lane DA, Olds RJ, Boisclair M et al (1993) Antithrombin III mutation database: first update. For the Thrombin and its Inhibitors Subcommittee of the Scientific and Standardization Committee of the International Society on Thrombosis and Haemostasis. Thromb Haemost 70:361–369

34. Finazzi G, Caccia R, Barbui T (1987) Different prevalence of thromboembolism in the subtypes of congenital antithrombin III deficiency: review of 404 cases. Thromb Haemost 58:1094

35. Lane DA, Mannucci PM, Bauer KA et al (1996) Inherited thrombophilia: Part 1. Thromb Haemost 76:651–662

36. Olds RJ, Lane DA, Caso R et al (1992) Antithrombin III Budapest: a single amino acid substitution (429Pro to Leu) in a region highly conserved in the serpin family. Blood 79:1206–1212

37. Sas G, Blasko G, Banhegyi D et al (1974) Abnormal antithrombin III (antithrombin III "Budapest") as a cause of a familial thrombophilia. Thromb Diath Haemorrh 32:105–115

38. Odegard OR, Abildgaard U (1978) Antithrombin III: critical review of assay methods. Significance of variations in health and disease. Haemostasis 7:127–134

39. Tait RC, Walker ID, Perry DJ et al (1994) Prevalence of antithrombin deficiency in the healthy population. Br J Haematol 87:106–112

40. Cosgriff TM, Bishop DT, Hershgold EJ et al (1983) Familial antithrombin III deficiency: its natural history, genetics, diagnosis and treatment. Medicine (Baltimore) 62:209–220

41. Demers C, Ginsberg JS, Hirsh J et al (1992) Thrombosis in antithrombin-III-deficient persons. Report of a large kindred and literature review. Ann Intern Med 116:754–761

42. Martinelli I, Mannucci PM, De Stefano V et al (1998) Different risks of thrombosis in four coagulation defects associated with inherited thrombophilia: a study of 150 families. Blood 92:2353–2358

43. De Stefano V, Leone G, Mastrangelo S et al (1994) Thrombosis during pregnancy and surgery in patients with congenital deficiency of antithrombin III, protein C, protein S. Thromb Haemost 71:799–800

44. De Stefano V, Mastrangelo S, Paciaroni K et al (1995) Thrombotic risk during pregnancy and puerperium in women with APC-resistance-effective subcutaneous heparin prophylaxis in a pregnant patient. Thromb Haemost 74:793–794

45. Chowdhury V, Lane DA, Mille B et al (1994) Homozygous antithrombin deficiency: report of two new cases (99 Leu to Phe) associated with arterial and venous thrombosis. Thromb Haemost 72:198–202

46. Candrina R, Goppini A, Salvi A et al (1986) Arterial thrombosis in antithrombin III deficiency. Clin Lab Haematol 8:267–268

47. Michiels JJ, Hamulyak K (1998) Laboratory diagnosis of hereditary thrombophilia. Semin Thromb Hemost 24:309–320

48. Ranucci M, Isgro G, Cazzaniga A et al (1999) Predictors for heparin resistance in patients undergoing coronary artery bypass grafting. Perfusion 14:437–442

49. Ranucci M, Isgro G, Cazzaniga A et al (2002) Different patterns of heparin resistance: therapeutic implications. Perfusion 17:199–204

50. Menache D, O'malley JP, Schorr JB et al (1990) Evaluation of the safety, recovery, half-life, and clinical efficacy of antithrombin III (human) in patients with hereditary antithrombin III deficiency. Cooperative Study Group. Blood 75:33–39

51. Schwartz RS, Bauer KA, Rosenberg RD et al (1989) Clinical experience with antithrombin III concentrate in treatment of congenital and acquired deficiency of antithrombin. The Antithrombin III Study Group. Am J Med 87:53S–60S

52. Bucur SZ, Levy JH, Despotis GJ et al (1998) Uses of antithrombin III concentrate in congenital and acquired deficiency states. Transfusion 38:481–498

53. Comp PC, Nixon RR, Cooper MR et al (1984) Familial protein S deficiency is associated with recurrent thrombosis. J Clin Invest 74:2082–2088

54. Griffin JH, Evatt B, Zimmerman TS et al (1981) Deficiency of protein C in congenital thrombotic disease. J Clin Invest 68:1370–1373

55. Walker FJ (1984) Regulation of vitamin K-dependent protein S. Inactivation by thrombin. J Biol Chem 259:10335–10339

56. Rezende SM, Simmonds RE, Lane DA (2004) Coagulation, inflammation, and apoptosis: different roles for protein S and the protein S-C4b binding protein complex. Blood 103:1192–1201

57. Grandone E, Margaglione M, Colaizzo D et al (2002) Lower birth-weight in neonates of mothers carrying factor V G1691A and factor II A(20210) mutations. Haematologica 87:177–181

58. Borgel D, Duchemin J, Alhenc-Gelas M et al (1996) Molecular basis for protein S hereditary deficiency: genetic defects observed in 118 patients with type I and type IIa deficiencies. The French Network on Molecular Abnormalities Responsible for Protein C and Protein S Deficiencies. J Lab Clin Med 128:218–227

59. Gomez E, Poort SR, Bertina RM et al (1995) Identification of eight point mutations in protein S deficiency type I – analysis of 15 pedigrees. Thromb Haemost 73:750–755

60. Gandrille S, Borgel D, Eschwege-Gufflet V et al (1995) Identification of 15 different candidate causal point mutations and three polymorphisms in 19 patients with protein S deficiency using a scanning method for the analysis of the protein S active gene. Blood 85:130–138

61. Hayashi T, Nishioka J, Shigekiyo T et al (1994) Protein S Tokushima: abnormal molecule with a substitution of Glu for Lys-155 in the second epidermal growth factor-like domain of protein S. Blood 83:683–690

62. Simmonds RE, Zoller B, Ireland H et al (1997) Genetic and phenotypic analysis of a large (122-member) protein S-deficient kindred provides an explanation for the familial coexistence of type I and type III plasma phenotypes. Blood 89:4364–4370

63. Zoller B, Garcia dF, Dahlback B (1995) Evaluation of the relationship between protein S and C4b-binding protein isoforms in hereditary protein S deficiency demonstrating type I and type III deficiencies to be phenotypic variants of the same genetic disease. Blood 85:3524–3531

64. Bertina RM, Ploos van Amstel HK, van Wijngaarden A et al (1990) Heerlen polymorphism of protein S, an immunologic polymorphism due to dimorphism of residue 460. Blood 76:538–548

65. Dykes AC, Walker ID, McMahon AD et al (2001) A study of Protein S antigen levels in 3788 healthy volunteers: influence of age, sex and hormone use, and estimate for prevalence of deficiency state. Br J Haematol 113:636–641

66. Mahasandana C, Suvatte V, Marlar RA et al (1990) Neonatal purpura fulminans associated with homozygous protein S deficiency. Lancet 335:61–62

67. Coller BS, Owen J, Jesty J et al (1987) Deficiency of plasma protein S, protein C, or antithrombin III and arterial thrombosis. Arteriosclerosis 7:456–462

68. Allaart CF, Aronson DC, Ruys T et al (1990) Hereditary protein S deficiency in young adults with arterial occlusive disease. Thromb Haemost 64:206–210

69. Mosnier LO, Zlokovic BV, Griffin JH (2007) The cytoprotective protein C pathway. Blood 109:3161–3172

70. Aiach M, Gandrille S, Emmerich J (1995) A review of mutations causing deficiencies of antithrombin, protein C and protein S. Thromb Haemost 74:81–89

71. Foster DC, Yoshitake S, Davie EW (1985) The nucleotide sequence of the gene for human protein C. Proc Natl Acad Sci U S A 82:4673–4677

72. Reitsma PH (1997) Protein C deficiency: from gene defects to disease. Thromb Haemost 78:344–350

73. Reitsma PH, te Lintel HW, Koenhen E et al (1990) Application of two neutral MspI DNA polymorphisms in the analysis of hereditary protein C deficiency. Thromb Haemost 64:239–244

74. Tait RC, Walker ID, Reitsma PH et al (1995) Prevalence of protein C deficiency in the healthy population. Thromb Haemost 73:87–93

75. Preston FE, Rosendaal FR, Walker ID et al (1996) Increased fetal loss in women with heritable thrombophilia. Lancet 348:913–916

76. Grewal RP, Goldberg MA (1990) Stroke in protein C deficiency. Am J Med 89:538–539

77. Tripodi A, Franchi F, Krachmalnicoff A et al (1990) Asymptomatic homozygous protein C deficiency. Acta Haematol 83:152–155

78. Lensen RP, Rosendaal FR, Koster T et al (1996) Apparent different thrombotic tendency in patients with factor V Leiden and protein C deficiency due to selection of patients. Blood 88:4205–4208

79. Koster T, Rosendaal FR, Briet E et al (1995) Protein C deficiency in a controlled series of unselected outpatients: an infrequent but clear risk factor for venous thrombosis (Leiden Thrombophilia Study). Blood 85:2756–2761

80. Mustafa S, Mannhalter C, Rintelen C et al (1998) Clinical features of thrombophilia in families with gene defects in protein C or protein S combined with factor V Leiden. Blood Coagul Fibrinolysis 9:85–89

81. Miletich J, Sherman L, Broze G Jr (1987) Absence of thrombosis in subjects with heterozygous protein C deficiency. N Engl J Med 317:991–996

82. De Stefano V, Mastrangelo S, Schwarz HP et al (1993) Replacement therapy with a purified protein C concentrate during initiation of oral anticoagulation in severe protein C congenital deficiency. Thromb Haemost 70:247–249

83. Dahlback B, Carlsson M, Svensson PJ (1993) Familial thrombophilia due to a previously unrecognized mechanism characterized by poor anticoagulant response to activated protein C: prediction of a cofactor to activated protein C. Proc Natl Acad Sci U S A 90:1004–1008

84. Bertina RM, Koeleman BP, Koster T et al (1994) Mutation in blood coagulation factor V associated with resistance to activated protein C. Nature 369:64–67

85. Castoldi E, Brugge JM, Nicolaes GA et al (2004) Impaired APC cofactor activity of factor V plays a major role in the APC resistance associated with the factor V Leiden (R506Q) and R2 (H1299R) mutations. Blood 103:4173–4179

86. Williamson D, Brown K, Luddington R et al (1998) Factor V Cambridge: a new mutation (Arg306→Thr) associated with resistance to activated protein C. Blood 91:1140–1144

87. Chan WP, Lee CK, Kwong YL et al (1998) A novel mutation of Arg306 of factor V gene in Hong Kong Chinese. Blood 91:1135–1139

88. Norstrom E, Thorelli E, Dahlback B (2002) Functional characterization of recombinant FV Hong Kong and FV Cambridge. Blood 100:524–530

89. Steen M, Norstrom EA, Tholander AL et al (2004) Functional characterization of factor V-Ile359Thr: a novel mutation associated with thrombosis. Blood 103:3381–3387

90. Rees DC, Cox M, Clegg JB (1995) World distribution of factor V Leiden. Lancet 346:1133–1134

91. Ridker PM, Miletich JP, Hennekens CH et al (1997) Ethnic distribution of factor V Leiden in 4047 men and women. Implications for venous thromboembolism screening. JAMA 277:1305–1307

92. Zivelin A, Griffin JH, Xu X et al (1997) A single genetic origin for a common Caucasian risk factor for venous thrombosis. Blood 89:397–402

93. Rosendaal FR, Koster T, Vandenbroucke JP et al (1995) High risk of thrombosis in patients homozygous for factor V Leiden (activated protein C resistance). Blood 85:1504–1508

94. Voorberg J, Roelse J, Koopman R et al (1994) Association of idiopathic venous thromboembolism with single point-mutation at Arg506 of factor V. Lancet 343:1535–1536

95. Lindqvist PG, Svensson PJ, Dahlback B et al (1998) Factor V Q506 mutation (activated protein C resistance) associated with reduced intrapartum blood loss – a possible evolutionary selection mechanism. Thromb Haemost 79:69–73

96. Corral J, Iniesta JA, Gonzalez-Conejero R et al (2001) Polymorphisms of clotting factors modify the risk for primary intracranial hemorrhage. Blood 97:2979–2982

97. Donahue BS, Gailani D, Higgins MS et al (2003) Factor V Leiden protects against blood loss and transfusion after cardiac surgery. Circulation 107:1003–1008

98. Faioni EM, Franchi F, Bucciarelli P et al (1999) Coinheritance of the HR2 haplotype in the factor V gene confers an increased risk of venous thromboembolism to carriers of factor V R506Q (factor V Leiden). Blood 94:3062–3066

99. Folsom AR, Cushman M, Tsai MY et al (2002) A prospective study of venous thromboembolism in relation to factor V Leiden and related factors. Blood 99:2720–2725

100. Liang R, Lee CK, Wat MS et al (1998) Clinical significance of Arg306 mutations of factor V gene. Blood 92: 2599–2600

101. de Moerloose P, Reber G, Perrier A et al (2000) Prevalence of factor V Leiden and prothrombin G20210A mutations in unselected patients with venous thromboembolism. Br J Haematol 110:125–129

102. Zuber M, Toulon P, Marnet L et al (1996) Factor V Leiden mutation in cerebral venous thrombosis. Stroke 27:1721–1723

103. Ridker PM, Miletich JP, Buring JE et al (1998) Factor V Leiden mutation as a risk factor for recurrent pregnancy loss. Ann Intern Med 128:1000–1003

104. Kupferminc MJ, Eldor A, Steinman N et al (1999) Increased frequency of genetic thrombophilia in women with complications of pregnancy. N Engl J Med 340:9–13

105. Ho WK, Hankey GJ, Quinlan DJ et al (2006) Risk of recurrent venous thromboembolism in patients with common thrombophilia: a systematic review. Arch Intern Med 166:729–736

106. Juul K, Tybjaerg-Hansen A, Steffensen R et al (2002) Factor V Leiden: The Copenhagen City Heart Study and 2 meta-analyses. Blood 100:3–10

107. Ridker PM, Hennekens CH, Lindpaintner K et al (1995) Mutation in the gene coding for coagulation factor V and the risk of myocardial infarction, stroke, and venous thrombosis in apparently healthy men. N Engl J Med 332:912–917

108. Lalouschek W, Schillinger M, Hsieh K et al (2005) Matched case-control study on factor V Leiden and the prothrombin G20210A mutation in patients with ischemic stroke/transient ischemic attack up to the age of 60 years. Stroke 36: 1405–1409

109. Rosendaal FR, Siscovick DS, Schwartz SM et al (1997) Factor V Leiden (resistance to activated protein C) increases the risk of myocardial infarction in young women. Blood 89:2817–2821

110. Koeleman BP, van Rumpt D, Hamulyak K et al (1995) Factor V Leiden: an additional risk factor for thrombosis in protein S deficient families? Thromb Haemost 74:580–583

111. Zöller B, Berntsdotter A, Garcia de Frutos P et al (1995) Resistance to activated protein C as an additional genetic risk factor in hereditary deficiency of protein S. Blood 85:3518–3523

112. Emmerich J, Rosendaal FR, Cattaneo M et al (2001) Combined effect of factor V Leiden and prothrombin 20210A on the risk of venous thromboembolism – pooled analysis of 8 case-control studies including 2310 cases and 3204 controls. Study Group for Pooled-Analysis in Venous Thromboembolism. Thromb Haemost 86:809–816

113. Lensen R, Bertina RM, Vandenbroucke JP et al (2001) High factor VIII levels contribute to the thrombotic risk in families with factor V Leiden. Br J Haematol 114:380–386

114. Simioni P, Castoldi E, Lunghi B et al (2005) An underestimated combination of opposites resulting in enhanced thrombotic tendency. Blood 106:2363–2365

115. Procare-GEHT Group (2006) ABO blood group but not haemostasis genetic polymorphisms significantly influence thrombotic risk: a study of 180 homozygotes for the Factor V Leiden mutation. Br J Haematol 135:697–702

116. Ridker PM, Hennekens CH, Selhub J et al (1997) Interrelation of hyperhomocyst(e)inemia, factor V Leiden, and risk of future venous thromboembolism. Circulation 95:1777–1782

117. Hirsch DR, Mikkola KM, Marks PW et al (1996) Pulmonary embolism and deep venous thrombosis during pregnancy or oral contraceptive use: prevalence of factor V Leiden. Am Heart J 131:1145–1148

118. Rosendaal FR, Vessey M, Rumley A et al (2002) Hormonal replacement therapy, prothrombotic mutations and the risk of venous thrombosis. Br J Haematol 116:851–854

119. Juul K, Tybjaerg-Hansen A, Schnohr P et al (2004) Factor V Leiden and the risk for venous thromboembolism in the adult Danish population. Ann Intern Med 140:330–337

120. Haim N, Lanir N, Hoffman R et al (2001) Acquired activated protein C resistance is common in cancer patients and is associated with venous thromboembolism. Am J Med 110:91–96

121. Post MS, Rosing J, Van Der Mooren MJ et al (2002) Increased resistance to activated protein C after short-term oral hormone replacement therapy in healthy post-menopausal women. Br J Haematol 119:1017–1023

122. Laszik Z, Mitro A, Taylor FB Jr et al (1997) Human protein C receptor is present primarily on endothelium of large blood vessels: implications for the control of the protein C pathway. Circulation 96:3633–3640

123. Stearns-Kurosawa DJ, Kurosawa S, Mollica JS et al (1996) The endothelial cell protein C receptor augments protein C activation by the thrombin-thrombomodulin complex. Proc Natl Acad Sci U S A 93:10212–10216

124. Medina P, Navarro S, Estelles A et al (2007) Polymorphisms in the endothelial protein C receptor gene and thrombophilia. Thromb Haemost 98:564–569

125. Saposnik B, Reny JL, Gaussem P et al (2004) A haplotype of the EPCR gene is associated with increased plasma levels of sEPCR and is a candidate risk factor for thrombosis. Blood 103:1311–1318

126. Medina P, Navarro S, Estelles A et al (2004) Contribution of polymorphisms in the endothelial protein C receptor gene to soluble endothelial protein C receptor and circulating activated protein C levels, and thrombotic risk. Thromb Haemost 91:905–911

127. Uitte de Willige S, Van Marion V, Rosendaal FR et al (2004) Haplotypes of the EPCR gene, plasma sEPCR levels and the risk of deep venous thrombosis. J Thromb Haemost 2:1305–1310

128. Medina P, Navarro S, Estelles A et al (2005) Influence of the 4600A/G and 4678G/C polymorphisms in the endothelial protein C receptor (EPCR) gene on the risk of venous thromboembolism in carriers of factor V Leiden. Thromb Haemost 94:389–394

129. Grossmann R, Schwender S, Geisen U et al (2002) CBS 844ins68, MTHFR TT677 and EPCR 4031ins23 genotypes in patients with deep-vein thrombosis. Thromb Res 107:13–15

130. Van de Water NS, French JK, McDowell J et al (2001) The endothelial protein C receptor (EPCR) 23bp insert in patients with myocardial infarction. Thromb Haemost 85:749–751

131. Poort SR, Rosendaal FR, Reitsma PH et al (1996) A common genetic variation in the 3′-untranslated region of the prothrombin gene is associated with elevated plasma prothrombin levels and an increase in venous thrombosis. Blood 88:3698–3703

132. Soria JM, Almasy L, Souto JC et al (2000) Linkage analysis demonstrates that the prothrombin G20210A mutation jointly influences plasma prothrombin levels and risk of thrombosis. Blood 95:2780–2785

133. Leroyer C, Mercier B, Oger E et al (1998) Prevalence of 20210 A allele of the prothrombin gene in venous thromboembolism patients. Thromb Haemost 80:49–51

134. Rosendaal FR, Doggen CJ, Zivelin A et al (1998) Geographic distribution of the 20210 G to A prothrombin variant. Thromb Haemost 79:706–708

135. Souto JC, Coll I, Llobet D et al (1998) The prothrombin 20210A allele is the most prevalent genetic risk factor for venous thromboembolism in the Spanish population. Thromb Haemost 80:366–369

136. Brown K, Luddington R, Williamson D et al (1997) Risk of venous thromboembolism associated with a G to A transition at position 20210 in the 3′-untranslated region of the prothrombin gene. Br J Haematol 98:907–909

137. Corral J, Gonzalez-Conejero R, Lozano ML et al (1997) The venous thrombosis risk factor 20210 A allele of the prothrombin gene is not a major risk factor for arterial thrombotic disease. Br J Haematol 99:304–307

138. Cumming AM, Keeney S, Salden A et al (1997) The prothrombin gene G20210A variant: prevalence in a U.K. anticoagulant clinic population. Br J Haematol 98:353–355

139. Hessner MJ, Luhm RA, Pearson SL et al (1999) Prevalence of prothrombin G20210A, factor V G1691A (Leiden), and methylenetetrahydrofolate reductase (MTHFR) C677T in seven different populations determined by multiplex allele-specific PCR. Thromb Haemost 81:733–738

140. Hillarp A, Zoller B, Svensson PJ et al (1997) The 20210 A allele of the prothrombin gene is a common risk factor among Swedish outpatients with verified deep venous thrombosis. Thromb Haemost 78:990–992

141. Lindmarker P, Schulman S, Sten-Linder M et al (1999) The risk of recurrent venous thromboembolism in carriers and non-carriers of the G1691A allele in the coagulation factor V gene and the G20210A allele in the prothrombin gene. DURAC Trial Study Group. Duration of Anticoagulation. Thromb Haemost 81:684–689

142. Grandone E, Margaglione M, Colaizzo D et al (1998) Genetic susceptibility to pregnancy-related venous thromboembolism: roles of factor V Leiden, prothrombin G20210A, and methylenetetrahydrofolate reductase C677T mutations. Am J Obstet Gynecol 179:1324–1328

143. Martinelli I, Sacchi E, Landi G et al (1998) High risk of cerebral-vein thrombosis in carriers of a prothrombin-gene mutation and in users of oral contraceptives. N Engl J Med 338:1793–1797

144. Makris M, Preston FE, Beauchamp NJ et al (1997) Co-inheritance of the 20210A allele of the prothrombin gene increases the risk of thrombosis in subjects with familial thrombophilia. Thromb Haemost 78:1426–1429

145. Atasay B, Arsan S, Gunlemez A et al (2003) Factor V Leiden and prothrombin gene 20210A variant in neonatal thromboembolism and in healthy neonates and adults: a study in a single center. Pediatr Hematol Oncol 20:627–634

146. De Stefano V, Martinelli I, Mannucci PM et al (1999) The risk of recurrent deep venous thrombosis among heterozygous carriers of both factor V Leiden and the G20210A prothrombin mutation. N Engl J Med 341:801–806

147. Margaglione M, Brancaccio V, Giuliani N et al (1998) Increased risk for venous thrombosis in carriers of the prothrombin G→A20210 gene variant. Ann Intern Med 129:89–93

148. Arruda VR, Annichino-Bizzacchi JM, Goncalves MS et al (1997) Prevalence of the prothrombin gene variant (nt20210A) in venous thrombosis and arterial disease. Thromb Haemost 78:1430–1433

149. Croft SA, Daly ME, Steeds RP et al (1999) The prothrombin 20210A allele and its association with myocardial infarction. Thromb Haemost 81:861–864

150. Doggen CJ, Cats VM, Bertina RM et al (1998) Interaction of coagulation defects and cardiovascular risk factors: increased risk of myocardial infarction associated with factor V Leiden or prothrombin 20210A. Circulation 97:1037–1041

151. Eikelboom JW, Baker RI, Parsons R et al (1998) No association between the 20210 G/A prothrombin gene mutation and premature coronary artery disease. Thromb Haemost 80:878–880

152. Ferraresi P, Marchetti G, Legnani C et al (1997) The heterozygous 20210 G/A prothrombin genotype is associated with early venous thrombosis in inherited thrombophilias and is not increased in frequency in artery disease. Arterioscler Thromb Vasc Biol 17:2418–2422

153. Franco RF, Trip MD, Ten Cate H et al (1999) The 20210 G→A mutation in the 3′-untranslated region of the prothrombin gene and the risk for arterial thrombotic disease. Br J Haematol 104:50–54

154. Ridker PM, Hennekens CH, Miletich JP (1999) G20210A mutation in prothrombin gene and risk of myocardial infarction, stroke, and venous thrombosis in a large cohort of US men. Circulation 99:999–1004

155. Rosendaal FR, Siscovick DS, Schwartz SM et al (1997) A common prothrombin variant (20210 G to A) increases the risk of myocardial infarction in young women. Blood 90:1747–1750

156. Martinelli I, Franchi F, Akwan S et al (1997) The transition G to A at position 20210 in the 3′-untranslated region of the prothrombin gene is not associated with cerebral ischemia. Blood 90:3806

157. De Stefano V, Chiusolo P, Paciaroni K et al (1998) Prothrombin G20210A mutant genotype is a risk factor for cerebrovascular ischemic disease in young patients. Blood 91:3562–3565

158. Morange PE, Barthet MC, Henry M et al (1998) A three-generation family presenting five cases of homozygosity for the 20210 G to A prothrombin variant. Thromb Haemost 80:859–860

159. Hooper WC, Roberts S, Dowling N et al (2006) The prevalence of the prothrombin gene variant C20209T in African-Americans and Caucasians and lack of association with venous thromboembolism. Thromb Res 118:767–768

160. Martinelli I, Battaglioli T, Tosetto A et al (2006) Prothrombin A19911G polymorphism and the risk of venous thromboembolism. J Thromb Haemost 4:2582–2586

161. Seligsohn U, Lubetsky A (2001) Genetic susceptibility to venous thrombosis. N Engl J Med 344:1222–1231

162. McCully KS (1996) Homocysteine and vascular disease. Nat Med 2:386–389

163. den Heijer M, Blom HJ, Gerrits WB et al (1995) Is hyperhomocysteinaemia a risk factor for recurrent venous thrombosis? Lancet 345:882–885

164. Wilson KM, McCaw RB, Leo L et al (2007) Prothrombotic effects of hyperhomocysteinemia and hypercholesterolemia in ApoE-deficient mice. Arterioscler Thromb Vasc Biol 27:233–240

165. Dayal S, Wilson KM, Leo L et al (2006) Enhanced susceptibility to arterial thrombosis in a murine model of hyperhomocysteinemia. Blood 108:2237–2243

166. Desouza C, Keebler M, McNamara DB et al (2002) Drugs affecting homocysteine metabolism: impact on cardiovascular risk. Drugs 62:605–616

167. Bazzano LA, He J, Muntner P et al (2003) Relationship between cigarette smoking and novel risk factors for cardio-vascular disease in the United States. Ann Intern Med 138:891–897

168. de Bree A, Verschuren WM, Bjorke-Monsen AL et al (2003) Effect of the methylenetetrahydrofolate reductase 677C→T mutation on the relations among folate intake and plasma folate and homocysteine concentrations in a general population sample. Am J Clin Nutr 77:687–693

169. Gallagher PM, Meleady R, Shields DC et al (1996) Homocysteine and risk of premature coronary heart disease. Evidence for a common gene mutation. Circulation 94:2154–2158

170. Eichinger S, Stumpflen A, Hirschl M et al (1998) Hyperhomocysteinemia is a risk factor of recurrent venous throm-boembolism. Thromb Haemost 80:566–569

171. Ray JG, Shmorgun D, Chan WS (2002) Common C677T polymorphism of the methylenetetrahydrofolate reductase gene and the risk of venous thromboembolism: meta-analysis of 31 studies. Pathophysiol Haemost Thromb 32:51–58

172. Klerk M, Verhoef P, Clarke R et al (2002) MTHFR 677C→T polymorphism and risk of coronary heart disease: a meta-analysis. JAMA 288:2023–2031

173. Lewis SJ, Ebrahim S, Davey SG (2005) Meta-analysis of MTHFR 677C→T polymorphism and coronary heart disease: does totality of evidence support causal role for homocysteine and preventive potential of folate? BMJ 331:1053

174. Love PE, Santoro SA (1990) Antiphospholipid antibodies: anticardiolipin and the lupus anticoagulant in systemic lupus erythematosus (SLE) and in non-SLE disorders. Prevalence and clinical significance. Ann Intern Med 112:682–698

175. Goldberg SN, Conti-Kelly AM, Greco TP (1995) A family study of anticardiolipin antibodies and associated clinical conditions. Am J Med 99:473–479

176. Schur PH (1995) Genetics of systemic lupus erythematosus. Lupus 4:425–437

177. Bugert P, Pabinger I, Stamer K et al (2007) The risk for thromboembolic disease in lupus anticoagulant patients due to pathways involving P-selectin and CD154. Thromb Haemost 97:573–580

178. Brouwer JL, Bijl M, Veeger NJ et al (2004) The contribution of inherited and acquired thrombophilic defects, alone or combined with antiphospholipid antibodies, to venous and arterial thromboembolism in patients with systemic lupus erythematosus. Blood 104:143–148

179. Nojima J, Kuratsune H, Suehisa E et al (2002) Acquired activated protein C resistance is associated with the co-existence of anti-prothrombin antibodies and lupus anticoagulant activity in patients with systemic lupus erythematosus. Br J Haematol 118:577–583

180. Broze GJ Jr (1995) Tissue factor pathway inhibitor and the current concept of blood coagulation. Blood Coagul Fibrinolysis 6(Suppl 1):S7–S13

181. Kleesiek K, Schmidt M, Gotting C et al (1999) The 536C→T transition in the human tissue factor pathway inhibitor (TFPI) gene is statistically associated with a higher risk for venous thrombosis. Thromb Haemost 82:1–5

182. Gonzalez-Conejero R, Lozano ML, Corral J et al (2000) The TFPI 536C→T mutation is not associated with increased risk for venous or arterial thrombosis. Thromb Haemost 83:787–788

183. Le Flem L, Picard V, Emmerich J et al (1999) Mutations in promoter region of thrombomodulin and venous throm-boembolic disease. Arterioscler Thromb Vasc Biol 19:1098–1104

184. Le Flem L, Mennen L, Aubry ML et al (2001) Thrombomodulin promoter mutations, venous thrombosis, and varicose veins. Arterioscler Thromb Vasc Biol 21:445–451

185. Norlund L, Zoller B, Ohlin AK (1997) A novel thrombomodulin gene mutation in a patient suffering from sagittal sinus thrombosis. Thromb Haemost 78:1164–1166

186. Ohlin AK, Norlund L, Marlar RA (1997) Thrombomodulin gene variations and thromboembolic disease. Thromb Haemost 78:396–400

187. Doggen CJ, Kunz G, Rosendaal FR et al (1998) A mutation in the thrombomodulin gene, 127G to A coding for Ala25Thr, and the risk of myocardial infarction in men. Thromb Haemost 80:743–748

188. Ireland H, Kunz G, Kyriakoulis K et al (1997) Thrombomodulin gene mutations associated with myocardial infarction. Circulation 96:15–18

189. Kunz G, Ireland HA, Stubbs PJ et al (2000) Identification and characterization of a thrombomodulin gene mutation coding for an elongated protein with reduced expression in a kindred with myocardial infarction. Blood 95:569–576

190. Li YH, Chen JH, Wu HL et al (2000) G-33A mutation in the promoter region of thrombomodulin gene and its associa-tion with coronary artery disease and plasma soluble thrombomodulin levels. Am J Cardiol 85:8–12

191. Li YH, Chen CH, Yeh PS et al (2001) Functional mutation in the promoter region of thrombomodulin gene in relation to carotid atherosclerosis. Atherosclerosis 154:713–719

192. Norlund L, Holm J, Zoller B et al (1997) A common thrombomodulin amino acid dimorphism is associated with myocardial infarction. Thromb Haemost 77:248–251

193. Norlund L, Holm J, Zoller B et al (1999) The Ala25-Thr mutation in the thrombomodulin gene is not frequent in Swedish patients suffering from ischemic heart disease. Thromb Haemost 82:1367–1368

194. Warner D, Catto A, Kunz G et al (2000) The thrombomodulin gene mutation G(127)→A (Ala25Thr) and cerebrovascular disease. Cerebrovasc Dis 10:359–363

195. Wu KK, Aleksic N, Ahn C et al (2001) Thrombomodulin Ala455Val polymorphism and risk of coronary heart disease. Circulation 103:1386–1389

196. Bezemer ID, Bare LA, Doggen CJ et al (2008) Gene variants associated with deep vein thrombosis. JAMA 299:1306–1314

197. Zehnder JL, Benson RC (1996) Sensitivity and specificity of the APC resistance assay in detection of individuals with factor V Leiden. Am J Clin Pathol 106:107–111

198. Zoller B, He X, Dahlback B (1995) Homozygous APC-resistance combined with inherited type I protein S deficiency in a young boy with severe thrombotic disease. Thromb Haemost 73:743–745

199. Kang SS, Wong PW, Malinow MR (1992) Hyperhomocyst(e)inemia as a risk factor for occlusive vascular disease. Annu Rev Nutr 12:279–298

200. Ross R (1999) Atherosclerosis – an inflammatory disease. N Engl J Med 340:115–126

201. Kullo IJ, Gau GT, Tajik AJ (2000) Novel risk factors for atherosclerosis. Mayo Clin Proc 75:369–380

202. Voetsch B, Loscalzo J (2004) Genetic determinants of arterial thrombosis. Arterioscler Thromb Vasc Biol 24: 216–229

203. Heinrich J, Balleisen L, Schulte H et al (1994) Fibrinogen and factor VII in the prediction of coronary risk. Results from the PROCAM study in healthy men. Arterioscler Thromb 14:54–59

204. Meade TW, Mellows S, Brozovic M et al (1986) Haemostatic function and ischaemic heart disease: principal results of the Northwick Park Heart Study. Lancet 2:533–537

205. Maresca G, Di Blasio A, Marchioli R et al (1999) Measuring plasma fibrinogen to predict stroke and myocardial infarction: an update. Arterioscler Thromb Vasc Biol 19:1368–1377

206. Brown ET, Fuller GM (1998) Detection of a complex that associates with the Bbeta fibrinogen G-455-A polymorphism. Blood 92:3286–3293

207. Carter AM, Mansfield MW, Stickland MH et al (1996) Beta-fibrinogen gene-455 G/A polymorphism and fibrinogen levels. Risk factors for coronary artery disease in subjects with NIDDM. Diabetes Care 19:1265–1268

208. de Maat MP, Kastelein JJ, Jukema JW et al (1998) 455G/A polymorphism of the beta-fibrinogen gene is associated with the progression of coronary atherosclerosis in symptomatic men: proposed role for an acute-phase reaction pattern of fibrinogen. REGRESS group. Arterioscler Thromb Vasc Biol 18:265–271

209. Folsom AR, Aleksic N, Ahn C et al (2001) Beta-fibrinogen gene -455G/A polymorphism and coronary heart disease incidence: the Atherosclerosis Risk in Communities (ARIC) Study. Ann Epidemiol 11:166–170

210. Gardemann A, Schwartz O, Haberbosch W et al (1997) Positive association of the beta fibrinogen H1/H2 gene variation to basal fibrinogen levels and to the increase in fibrinogen concentration during acute phase reaction but not to coronary artery disease and myocardial infarction. Thromb Haemost 77:1120–1126

211. Wang XL, Wang J, McCredie RM et al (1997) Polymorphisms of factor V, factor VII, and fibrinogen genes. Relevance to severity of coronary artery disease. Arterioscler Thromb Vasc Biol 17:246–251

212. Zito F, Di Castelnuovo A, Amore C et al (1997) Bcl I polymorphism in the fibrinogen beta-chain gene is associated with the risk of familial myocardial infarction by increasing plasma fibrinogen levels. A case-control study in a sample of GISSI-2 patients. Arterioscler Thromb Vasc Biol 17:3489–3494

213. Endler G, Mannhalter C (2003) Polymorphisms in coagulation factor genes and their impact on arterial and venous thrombosis. Clin Chim Acta 330:31–55

214. Boekholdt SM, Bijsterveld NR, Moons AH et al (2001) Genetic variation in coagulation and fibrinolytic proteins and their relation with acute myocardial infarction: a systematic review. Circulation 104:3063–3068

215. Martiskainen M, Pohjasvaara T, Mikkelsson J et al (2003) Fibrinogen gene promoter -455 A allele as a risk factor for lacunar stroke. Stroke 34:886–891

216. Standeven KF, Grant PJ, Carter AM et al (2003) Functional analysis of the fibrinogen Aalpha Thr312Ala polymorphism: effects on fibrin structure and function. Circulation 107:2326–2330

217. Carter AM, Catto AJ, Grant PJ (1999) Association of the alpha-fibrinogen Thr312Ala polymorphism with poststroke mortality in subjects with atrial fibrillation. Circulation 99:2423–2426

218. Carter AM, Catto AJ, Kohler HP et al (2000) alpha-fibrinogen Thr312Ala polymorphism and venous thromboembolism. Blood 96:1177–1179

219. Curran JM, Evans A, Arveiler D et al (1998) The alpha fibrinogen T/A312 polymorphism in the ECTIM study. Thromb Haemost 79:1057–1058

220. Kim RJ, Becker RC (2003) Association between factor V Leiden, prothrombin G20210A, and methylenetetrahydrofolate reductase C677T mutations and events of the arterial circulatory system: a meta-analysis of published studies. Am Heart J 146:948–957

221. Reiner AP, Siscovick DS, Rosendaal FR (2001) Hemostatic risk factors and arterial thrombotic disease. Thromb Haemost 85:584–595

222. Margaglione M, D'Andrea G, Giuliani N et al (1999) Inherited prothrombotic conditions and premature ischemic stroke: sex difference in the association with factor V Leiden. Arterioscler Thromb Vasc Biol 19:1751–1756

223. Nowak-Gottl U, Strater R, Heinecke A et al (1999) Lipoprotein (a) and genetic polymorphisms of clotting factor V, prothrombin, and methylenetetrahydrofolate reductase are risk factors of spontaneous ischemic stroke in childhood. Blood 94:3678–3682

224. Inbal A, Freimark D, Modan B et al (1999) Synergistic effects of prothrombotic polymorphisms and atherogenic factors on the risk of myocardial infarction in young males. Blood 93:2186–2190

225. Thomas DP (1988) Overview of venous thrombogenesis. Semin Thromb Hemost 14:1–8

226. Mustard JF, Packham MA, Kinlough-Rathbone RL (1990) Platelets, blood flow, and the vessel wall. Circulation 81:I24–I27

227. Lane DA, Grant PJ (2000) Role of hemostatic gene polymorphisms in venous and arterial thrombotic disease. Blood 95:1517–1532

228. Iacoviello L, Di Castelnuovo A, de Knijff P et al (1998) Polymorphisms in the coagulation factor VII gene and the risk of myocardial infarction. N Engl J Med 338:79–85

229. Doggen CJ, Manger CV, Bertina RM et al (1998) A genetic propensity to high factor VII is not associated with the risk of myocardial infarction in men. Thromb Haemost 80:281–285

230. Folsom AR, Wu KK, Rosamond WD et al (1997) Prospective study of hemostatic factors and incidence of coronary heart disease: the Atherosclerosis Risk in Communities (ARIC) Study. Circulation 96:1102–1108

231. Smith FB, Lee AJ, Fowkes FG et al (1997) Hemostatic factors as predictors of ischemic heart disease and stroke in the Edinburgh Artery Study. Arterioscler Thromb Vasc Biol 17:3321–3325

232. Ariens RA, Philippou H, Nagaswami C et al (2000) The factor XIII V34L polymorphism accelerates thrombin activation of factor XIII and affects cross-linked fibrin structure. Blood 96:988–995

233. Kangsadalampai S, Board PG (1998) The Val34Leu polymorphism in the A subunit of coagulation factor XIII contributes to the large normal range in activity and demonstrates that the activation peptide plays a role in catalytic activity. Blood 92:2766–2770

234. Salomaa V, Matei C, Aleksic N et al (1999) Soluble thrombomodulin as a predictor of incident coronary heart disease and symptomless carotid artery atherosclerosis in the Atherosclerosis Risk in Communities (ARIC) Study: a case-cohort study. Lancet 353:1729–1734

235. Arnaud E, Barbalat V, Nicaud V et al (2000) Polymorphisms in the 5′ regulatory region of the tissue factor gene and the risk of myocardial infarction and venous thromboembolism: the ECTIM and PATHROS studies. Etude Cas-Temoins de l'Infarctus du Myocarde. Paris Thrombosis case-control Study. Arterioscler Thromb Vasc Biol 20:892–898

236. Vijayan KV, Bray PF (2006) Molecular mechanisms of prothrombotic risk due to genetic variations in platelet genes: Enhanced outside-in signaling through the Pro33 variant of integrin beta3. Exp Biol Med (Maywood) 231:505–513

237. Weiss EJ, Bray PF, Tayback M et al (1996) A polymorphism of a platelet glycoprotein receptor as an inherited risk factor for coronary thrombosis. N Engl J Med 334:1090–1094

238. Carter AM, Ossei-Gerning N, Wilson IJ et al (1997) Association of the platelet Pl(A) polymorphism of glycoprotein IIb/IIIa and the fibrinogen Bbeta 448 polymorphism with myocardial infarction and extent of coronary artery disease. Circulation 96:1424–1431

239. Wagner KR, Giles WH, Johnson CJ et al (1998) Platelet glycoprotein receptor IIIa polymorphism P1A2 and ischemic stroke risk: the Stroke Prevention in Young Women Study. Stroke 29:581–585

240. Herrmann SM, Poirier O, Marques-Vidal P et al (1997) The Leu33/Pro polymorphism (PlA1/PlA2) of the glycoprotein IIIa (GPIIIa) receptor is not related to myocardial infarction in the ECTIM Study. Etude Cas-Temoins de l'Infarctus du Myocarde. Thromb Haemost 77:1179–1181

241. Ridker PM, Hennekens CH, Schmitz C et al (1997) PIA1/A2 polymorphism of platelet glycoprotein IIIa and risks of myocardial infarction, stroke, and venous thrombosis. Lancet 349:385–388

242. Ardissino D, Mannucci PM, Merlini PA et al (1999) Prothrombotic genetic risk factors in young survivors of myocardial infarction. Blood 94:46–51

243. Michelson AD, Furman MI, Goldschmidt-Clermont P et al (2000) Platelet GP IIIa Pl(A) polymorphisms display different sensitivities to agonists. Circulation 101:1013–1018

244. Szczeklik A, Undas A, Sanak M et al (2000) Relationship between bleeding time, aspirin and the PlA1/A2 polymorphism of platelet glycoprotein IIIa. Br J Haematol 110:965–967

245. Undas A, Brummel K, Musial J et al (2001) Pl(A2) polymorphism of beta(3) integrins is associated with enhanced thrombin generation and impaired antithrombotic action of aspirin at the site of microvascular injury. Circulation 104:2666–2672

246. Feng D, Lindpaintner K, Larson MG et al (1999) Increased platelet aggregability associated with platelet GPIIIa PlA2 polymorphism: the Framingham Offspring Study. Arterioscler Thromb Vasc Biol 19:1142–1147

247. Reiner AP, Schwartz SM, Kumar PN et al (2001) Platelet glycoprotein IIb polymorphism, traditional risk factors and non-fatal myocardial infarction in young women. Br J Haematol 112:632–636

248. Bottiger C, Kastrati A, Koch W et al (2000) HPA-1 and HPA-3 polymorphisms of the platelet fibrinogen receptor and coronary artery disease and myocardial infarction. Thromb Haemost 83:559–562

249. Hato T, Minamoto Y, Fukuyama T et al (1997) Polymorphisms of HPA-1 through 6 on platelet membrane glycoprotein receptors are not a genetic risk factor for myocardial infarction in the Japanese population. Am J Cardiol 80: 1222–1224

250. Franco RF, Rcitsma PH (2001) Gene polymorphisms of the haemostatic system and the risk of arterial thrombotic disease. Br J Haematol 115:491–506

251. Carlsson LE, Greinacher A, Spitzer C et al (1997) Polymorphisms of the human platelet antigens HPA-1, HPA-2, HPA-3, and HPA-5 on the platelet receptors for fibrinogen (GPIIb/IIIa), von Willebrand factor (GPIb/IX), and collagen (GPIa/IIa) are not correlated with an increased risk for stroke. Stroke 28:1392–1395

252. Carter AM, Catto AJ, Bamford JM et al (1998) Platelet GP IIIa PlA and GP Ib variable number tandem repeat polymorphisms and markers of platelet activation in acute stroke. Arterioscler Thromb Vasc Biol 18:1124–1131

253. Gonzalez-Conejero R, Lozano ML, Rivera J et al (1998) Polymorphisms of platelet membrane glycoprotein Ib associated with arterial thrombotic disease. Blood 92:2771–2776

254. Mercier B, Munier S, Bertault V et al (2000) Myocardial infarction: absence of association with VNTR polymorphism of GP Ibalpha. Thromb Haemost 84:921–922

255. Murata M, Matsubara Y, Kawano K et al (1997) Coronary artery disease and polymorphisms in a receptor mediating shear stress-dependent platelet activation. Circulation 96:3281–3286

256. Sonoda A, Murata M, Ito D et al (2000) Association between platelet glycoprotein Ibalpha genotype and ischemic cerebrovascular disease. Stroke 31:493–497

257. Afshar-Kharghan V, Li CQ, Khoshnevis-Asl M et al (1999) Kozak sequence polymorphism of the glycoprotein (GP) Ibalpha gene is a major determinant of the plasma membrane levels of the platelet GP Ib-IX-V complex. Blood 94:186–191

258. Frank MB, Reiner AP, Schwartz SM et al (2001) The Kozak sequence polymorphism of platelet glycoprotein Ibalpha and risk of nonfatal myocardial infarction and nonfatal stroke in young women. Blood 97:875–879

259. Kunicki TJ, Kritzik M, Annis DS et al (1997) Hereditary variation in platelet integrin alpha 2 beta 1 density is associated with two silent polymorphisms in the alpha 2 gene coding sequence. Blood 89:1939–1943

260. Kritzik M, Savage B, Nugent DJ et al (1998) Nucleotide polymorphisms in the alpha2 gene define multiple alleles that are associated with differences in platelet alpha2 beta1 density. Blood 92:2382–2388

261. Angiolillo DJ, Fernandez-Ortiz A, Bernardo E et al (2004) 807 C/T Polymorphism of the glycoprotein Ia gene and pharmacogenetic modulation of platelet response to dual antiplatelet treatment. Blood Coagul Fibrinolysis 15:427–433

262. Santoso S, Kunicki TJ, Kroll H et al (1999) Association of the platelet glycoprotein Ia C807T gene polymorphism with nonfatal myocardial infarction in younger patients. Blood 93:2449–2453

263. Carlsson LE, Santoso S, Spitzer C et al (1999) The alpha2 gene coding sequence T807/A873 of the platelet collagen receptor integrin alpha2beta1 might be a genetic risk factor for the development of stroke in younger patients. Blood 93:3583–3586

264. Moshfegh K, Wuillemin WA, Redondo M et al (1999) Association of two silent polymorphisms of platelet glycoprotein Ia/IIa receptor with risk of myocardial infarction: a case-control study. Lancet 353:351–354

265. Reiner AP, Kumar PN, Schwartz SM et al (2000) Genetic variants of platelet glycoprotein receptors and risk of stroke in young women. Stroke 31:1628–1633

266. Corral J, Gonzalez-Conejero R, Rivera J et al (1999) Role of the 807 C/T polymorphism of the alpha2 gene in platelet GP Ia collagen receptor expression and function – effect in thromboembolic diseases. Thromb Haemost 81:951–956

267. Croft SA, Hampton KK, Sorrell JA et al (1999) The GPIa C807T dimorphism associated with platelet collagen receptor density is not a risk factor for myocardial infarction. Br J Haematol 106:771–776

268. Burzotta F, Di Castelnuovo A, Amore C et al (1998) 4G/5G promoter PAI-1 gene polymorphism is associated with plasmatic PAI-1 activity in Italians: a model of gene-environment interaction. Thromb Haemost 79:354–358

269. Dawson SJ, Wiman B, Hamsten A et al (1993) The two allele sequences of a common polymorphism in the promoter of the plasminogen activator inhibitor-1 (PAI-1) gene respond differently to interleukin-1 in HepG2 cells. J Biol Chem 268:10739–10745

270. Eriksson P, Kallin B, van 't Hooft FM et al (1995) Allele-specific increase in basal transcription of the plasminogen-activator inhibitor 1 gene is associated with myocardial infarction. Proc Natl Acad Sci U S A 92:1851–1855

271. Gardemann A, Lohre J, Katz N et al (1999) The 4G4G genotype of the plasminogen activator inhibitor 4G/5G gene polymorphism is associated with coronary atherosclerosis in patients at high risk for this disease. Thromb Haemost 82:1121–1126

272. Iwai N, Shimoike H, Nakamura Y et al (1998) The 4G/5G polymorphism of the plasminogen activator inhibitor gene is associated with the time course of progression to acute coronary syndromes. Atherosclerosis 136:109–114

273. Mansfield MW, Stickland MH, Grant PJ (1995) Plasminogen activator inhibitor-1 (PAI-1) promoter polymorphism and coronary artery disease in non-insulin-dependent diabetes. Thromb Haemost 74:1032–1034

274. Margaglione M, Cappucci G, Colaizzo D et al (1998) The PAI-1 gene locus 4G/5G polymorphism is associated with a family history of coronary artery disease. Arterioscler Thromb Vasc Biol 18:152–156

275. Catto AJ, Carter AM, Stickland M et al (1997) Plasminogen activator inhibitor-1 (PAI-1) 4G/5G promoter polymorphism and levels in subjects with cerebrovascular disease. Thromb Haemost 77:730–734

276. Ridker PM, Hennekens CH, Lindpaintner K et al (1997) Arterial and venous thrombosis is not associated with the 4G/5G polymorphism in the promoter of the plasminogen activator inhibitor gene in a large cohort of US men. Circulation 95:59–62

277. Ye S, Green FR, Scarabin PY et al (1995) The 4G/5G genetic polymorphism in the promoter of the plasminogen activator inhibitor-1 (PAI-1) gene is associated with differences in plasma PAI-1 activity but not with risk of myocardial infarction in the ECTIM study. Etude CasTemoins de I'nfarctus du Mycocarde. Thromb Haemost 74:837–841

278. Iacoviello L, Burzotta F, Di Castelnuovo A et al (1998) The 4G/5G polymorphism of PAI-1 promoter gene and the risk of myocardial infarction: a meta-analysis. Thromb Haemost 80:1029–1030

279. Jern C, Ladenvall P, Wall U et al (1999) Gene polymorphism of t-PA is associated with forearm vascular release rate of t-PA. Arterioscler Thromb Vasc Biol 19:454–459

280. van der Bom JG, de Knijff P, Haverkate F et al (1997) Tissue plasminogen activator and risk of myocardial infarction. The Rotterdam Study. Circulation 95:2623–2627

281. Ridker PM, Baker MT, Hennekens CH et al (1997) Alu-repeat polymorphism in the gene coding for tissue-type plasminogen activator (t-PA) and risks of myocardial infarction among middle-aged men. Arterioscler Thromb Vasc Biol 17:1687–1690

282. Steeds R, Adams M, Smith P et al (1998) Distribution of tissue plasminogen activator insertion/deletion polymorphism in myocardial infarction and control subjects. Thromb Haemost 79:980–984

283. Ladenvall P, Wall U, Jern S et al (2000) Identification of eight novel single-nucleotide polymorphisms at human tissue-type plasminogen activator (t-PA) locus: association with vascular t-PA release in vivo. Thromb Haemost 84:150–155

284. Kathiresan S, Yang Q, Larson MG et al (2006) Common genetic variation in five thrombosis genes and relations to plasma hemostatic protein level and cardiovascular disease risk. Arterioscler Thromb Vasc Biol 26:1405–1412

285. Ladenvall P, Johansson L, Jansson JH et al (2002) Tissue-type plasminogen activator -7, 351C/T enhancer polymorphism is associated with a first myocardial infarction. Thromb Haemost 87:105–109

286. Jannes J, Hamilton-Bruce MA, Pilotto L et al (2004) Tissue plasminogen activator -7351C/T enhancer polymorphism is a risk factor for lacunar stroke. Stroke 35:1090–1094

287. Sakharov DV, Plow EF, Rijken DC (1997) On the mechanism of the antifibrinolytic activity of plasma carboxypeptidase B. J Biol Chem 272:14477–14482

288. van Tilburg NH, Rosendaal FR, Bertina RM (2000) Thrombin activatable fibrinolysis inhibitor and the risk for deep vein thrombosis. Blood 95:2855–2859

289. Morange PE, Juhan-Vague I, Scarabin PY et al (2003) Association between TAFI antigen and Ala147Thr polymorphism of the TAFI gene and the angina pectoris incidence. The PRIME Study (Prospective Epidemiological Study of MI). Thromb Haemost 89:554–560

290. Juhan-Vague I, Morange PE, Aubert H et al (2002) Plasma thrombin-activatable fibrinolysis inhibitor antigen concentration and genotype in relation to myocardial infarction in the north and south of Europe. Arterioscler Thromb Vasc Biol 22:867–873

291. Homocysteine Studies Collaboration (2002) Homocysteine and risk of ischemic heart disease and stroke: a meta-analysis. JAMA 288:2015–2022

292. Fletcher O, Kessling AM (1998) MTHFR association with arteriosclerotic vascular disease? Hum Genet 103:11–21

293. Brattstrom L, Wilcken DE, Ohrvik J et al (1998) Common methylenetetrahydrofolate reductase gene mutation leads to hyperhomocysteinemia but not to vascular disease: the result of a meta-analysis. Circulation 98:2520–2526

294. Jacques PF, Bostom AG, Williams RR et al (1996) Relation between folate status, a common mutation in methylenetetrahydrofolate reductase, and plasma homocysteine concentrations. Circulation 93:7–9

295. Cooke JP, Dzau VJ (1997) Nitric oxide synthase: role in the genesis of vascular disease. Annu Rev Med 48:489–509

296. Wang XL, Sim AS, Badenhop RF et al (1996) A smoking-dependent risk of coronary artery disease associated with a polymorphism of the endothelial nitric oxide synthase gene. Nat Med 2:41–45

297. Sigusch HH, Surber R, Lehmann MH et al (2000) Lack of association between 27-bp repeat polymorphism in intron 4 of the endothelial nitric oxide synthase gene and the risk of coronary artery disease. Scand J Clin Lab Invest 60:229–235

298. Stangl K, Cascorbi I, Laule M et al (2000) High CA repeat numbers in intron 13 of the endothelial nitric oxide synthase gene and increased risk of coronary artery disease. Pharmacogenetics 10:133–140

299. Nakayama M, Yasue H, Yoshimura M et al (1999) T-786→C mutation in the 5′-flanking region of the endothelial nitric oxide synthase gene is associated with coronary spasm. Circulation 99:2864–2870

300. Rossi GP, Cesari M, Zanchetta M et al (2003) The T-786C endothelial nitric oxide synthase genotype is a novel risk factor for coronary artery disease in Caucasian patients of the GENICA study. J Am Coll Cardiol 41:930–937

301. Rossi GP, Taddei S, Virdis A et al (2003) The T-786C and Glu298Asp polymorphisms of the endothelial nitric oxide gene affect the forearm blood flow responses of Caucasian hypertensive patients. J Am Coll Cardiol 41:938–945

302. Yamada M, Huang Z, Dalkara T et al (2000) Endothelial nitric oxide synthase-dependent cerebral blood flow augmentation by L-arginine after chronic statin treatment. J Cereb Blood Flow Metab 20:709–717

303. Durrington PN, Mackness B, Mackness MI (2001) Paraoxonase and atherosclerosis. Arterioscler Thromb Vasc Biol 21:473–480

304. Humbert R, Adler DA, Disteche CM et al (1993) The molecular basis of the human serum paraoxonase activity polymorphism. Nat Genet 3:73–76

305. Garin MC, James RW, Dussoix P et al (1997) Paraoxonase polymorphism Met-Leu54 is associated with modified serum concentrations of the enzyme. A possible link between the paraoxonase gene and increased risk of cardiovascular disease in diabetes. J Clin Invest 99:62–66

306. Heijmans BT, Westendorp RG, Lagaay AM et al (2000) Common paraoxonase gene variants, mortality risk and fatal cardiovascular events in elderly subjects. Atherosclerosis 149:91–97

307. Ombres D, Pannitteri G, Montali A et al (1998) The gln-Arg192 polymorphism of human paraoxonase gene is not associated with coronary artery disease in italian patients. Arterioscler Thromb Vasc Biol 18:1611–1616

308. Yamada Y, Metoki N, Yoshida H et al (2006) Genetic risk for ischemic and hemorrhagic stroke. Arterioscler Thromb Vasc Biol 26:1920–1925

309. McPherson R, Pertsemlidis A, Kavaslar N et al (2007) A common allele on chromosome 9 associated with coronary heart disease. Science 316:1488–1491

310. Fuster V, Badimon L, Badimon JJ et al (1992) The pathogenesis of coronary artery disease and the acute coronary syndromes (1). N Engl J Med 326:242–250

311. Ageno W, Prandoni P, Romualdi E et al (2006) The metabolic syndrome and the risk of venous thrombosis: a case-control study. J Thromb Haemost 4:1914–1918

312. Tsai AW, Cushman M, Rosamond WD et al (2002) Cardiovascular risk factors and venous thromboembolism incidence: the longitudinal investigation of thromboembolism etiology. Arch Intern Med 162:1182–1189

313. Hansson PO, Eriksson H, Welin L et al (1999) Smoking and abdominal obesity: risk factors for venous thromboembolism among middle-aged men: "the study of men born in 1913". Arch Intern Med 159:1886–1890

314. Squizzato A, Romualdi E, Ageno W (2006) Why should statins prevent venous thromboembolism? A systematic literature search and a call for action. J Thromb Haemost 4:1925–1927

315. Prandoni P, Bilora F, Marchiori A et al (2003) An association between atherosclerosis and venous thrombosis. N Engl J Med 348:1435–1441

316. Hong C, Zhu F, Du D et al (2005) Coronary artery calcification and risk factors for atherosclerosis in patients with venous thromboembolism. Atherosclerosis 183:169–174

317. Reich LM, Folsom AR, Key NS et al (2006) Prospective study of subclinical atherosclerosis as a risk factor for venous thromboembolism. J Thromb Haemost 4:1909–1913

318. van der Hagen PB, Folsom AR, Jenny NS et al (2006) Subclinical atherosclerosis and the risk of future venous thrombosis in the Cardiovascular Health Study. J Thromb Haemost 4:1903–1908

319. Becattini C, Agnelli G, Prandoni P et al (2005) A prospective study on cardiovascular events after acute pulmonary embolism. Eur Heart J 26:77–83

320. Schulman S, Lindmarker P, Holmstrom M et al (2006) Post-thrombotic syndrome, recurrence, and death 10 years after the first episode of venous thromboembolism treated with warfarin for 6 weeks or 6 months. J Thromb Haemost 4:734–742

321. Prandoni P, Ghirarduzzi A, Prins MH et al (2006) Venous thromboembolism and the risk of subsequent symptomatic atherosclerosis. J Thromb Haemost 4:1891–1896

322. Oscarson M (2003) Pharmacogenetics of drug metabolising enzymes: importance for personalised medicine. Clin Chem Lab Med 41:573–580

323. Weinshilboum R (2003) Inheritance and drug response. N Engl J Med 348:529–537
324. Marin F, Roldan V, Gonzalez-Conejero R et al (2005) Pharmacogenetics in cardiovascular antithrombotic therapy. Curr Med Chem Cardiovasc Hematol Agents 3:357–364
325. Gum PA, Kottke-Marchant K, Poggio ED et al (2001) Profile and prevalence of aspirin resistance in patients with cardiovascular disease. Am J Cardiol 88:230–235
326. Patrono C (2003) Aspirin resistance: definition, mechanisms and clinical read-outs. J Thromb Haemost 1:1710–1713
327. Cooke GE, Bray PF, Hamlington JD et al (1998) PlA2 polymorphism and efficacy of aspirin. Lancet 351:1253
328. Macchi L, Christiaens L, Brabant S et al (2003) Resistance in vitro to low-dose aspirin is associated with platelet PlA1 (GP IIIa) polymorphism but not with C807T(GP Ia/IIa) and C-5T Kozak (GP Ibalpha) polymorphisms. J Am Coll Cardiol 42:1115–1119
329. Cambria-Kiely JA, Gandhi PJ (2002) Aspirin resistance and genetic polymorphisms. J Thromb Thrombolysis 14:51–58
330. Kastrati A, Schomig A, Seyfarth M et al (1999) PlA polymorphism of platelet glycoprotein IIIa and risk of restenosis after coronary stent placement. Circulation 99:1005–1010
331. Laule M, Cascorbi I, Stangl V et al (1999) A1/A2 polymorphism of glycoprotein IIIa and association with excess procedural risk for coronary catheter interventions: a case-controlled study. Lancet 353:708–712
332. Walter DH, Schachinger V, Elsner M et al (1997) Platelet glycoprotein IIIa polymorphisms and risk of coronary stent thrombosis. Lancet 350:1217–1219
333. Angiolillo DJ, Fernandez-Ortiz A, Bernardo E et al (2004) PlA polymorphism and platelet reactivity following clopidogrel loading dose in patients undergoing coronary stent implantation. Blood Coagul Fibrinolysis 15:89–93
334. Januzzi JL, Cannon CP, Theroux P et al (2003) Optimizing glycoprotein IIb/IIIa receptor antagonist use for the non-ST-segment elevation acute coronary syndromes: risk stratification and therapeutic intervention. Am Heart J 146:764–774
335. Wheeler GL, Braden GA, Bray PF et al (2002) Reduced inhibition by abciximab in platelets with the PlA2 polymorphism. Am Heart J 143:76–82
336. Stewart JT, French JK, Theroux P et al (1998) Early noninvasive identification of failed reperfusion after intravenous thrombolytic therapy in acute myocardial infarction. J Am Coll Cardiol 31:1499–1505
337. Montaner J, Fernandez-Cadenas I, Molina CA et al (2003) Safety profile of tissue plasminogen activator treatment among stroke patients carrying a common polymorphism (C-1562T) in the promoter region of the matrix metalloproteinase-9 gene. Stroke 34:2851–2855
338. Weber AA, Meila D, Jacobs C et al (2002) Low incidence of paradoxical platelet activation by glycoprotein IIb/IIIa inhibitors. Thromb Res 106:25–29
339. Marin F, Gonzalez-Conejero R, Lee KW et al (2005) A pharmacogenetic effect of factor XIII valine 34 leucine polymorphism on fibrinolytic therapy for acute myocardial infarction. J Am Coll Cardiol 45:25–29
340. Roldan V, Corral J, Marin F et al (2004) Effect of factor VII -323 Del/Ins polymorphism on the daily variability of factor VIIc and INR in steady anticoagulated patients with acenocoumarol. J Thromb Haemost 2:2264–2265
341. James AH, Britt RP, Raskino CL et al (1992) Factors affecting the maintenance dose of warfarin. J Clin Pathol 45:704–706
342. Hirsh J, Fuster V, Ansell J et al (2003) American Heart Association/American College of Cardiology Foundation guide to warfarin therapy. Circulation 107:1692–1711
343. Aithal GP, Day CP, Kesteven PJ et al (1999) Association of polymorphisms in the cytochrome P450 CYP2C9 with warfarin dose requirement and risk of bleeding complications. Lancet 353:717–719
344. Tabrizi AR, Zehnbauer BA, Borecki IB et al (2002) The frequency and effects of cytochrome P450 (CYP) 2C9 polymorphisms in patients receiving warfarin. J Am Coll Surg 194:267–273
345. Taube J, Halsall D, Baglin T (2000) Influence of cytochrome P-450 CYP2C9 polymorphisms on warfarin sensitivity and risk of over-anticoagulation in patients on long-term treatment. Blood 96:1816–1819
346. Yamazaki H, Inoue K, Chiba K et al (1998) Comparative studies on the catalytic roles of cytochrome P450 2C9 and its Cys- and Leu-variants in the oxidation of warfarin, flurbiprofen, and diclofenac by human liver microsomes. Biochem Pharmacol 56:243–251
347. Hermida J, Zarza J, Alberca I et al (2002) Differential effects of 2C9*3 and 2C9*2 variants of cytochrome P-450 CYP2C9 on sensitivity to acenocoumarol. Blood 99:4237–4239
348. Margaglione M, Colaizzo D, D'Andrea G et al (2000) Genetic modulation of oral anticoagulation with warfarin. Thromb Haemost 84:775–778
349. Tassies D, Freire C, Pijoan J et al (2002) Pharmacogenetics of acenocoumarol: cytochrome P450 CYP2C9 polymorphisms influence dose requirements and stability of anticoagulation. Haematologica 87:1185–1191

350. Schwarz UI, Ritchie MD, Bradford Y et al (2008) Genetic determinants of response to warfarin during initial antico-agulation. N Engl J Med 358:999–1008

351. Anderson JL, Horne BD, Stevens SM et al (2007) Randomized trial of genotype-guided versus standard warfarin dosing in patients initiating oral anticoagulation. Circulation 116:2563–2570

352. Gonzalez-Porras JR, Garcia-Sanz R, Alberca I et al (2006) Risk of recurrent venous thrombosis in patients with G20210A mutation in the prothrombin gene or factor V Leiden mutation. Blood Coagul Fibrinolysis 17:23–28

353. Yoon PW, Scheuner MT, Khoury MJ (2003) Research priorities for evaluating family history in the prevention of com-mon chronic diseases. Am J Prev Med 24:128–135

354. Coppens M, van de Poel MH, Bank I et al (2006) A prospective cohort study on the absolute incidence of venous thromboembolism and arterial cardiovascular disease in asymptomatic carriers of the prothrombin 20210A mutation. Blood 108:2604–2607

355. Middeldorp S, Henkens CM, Koopman MM et al (1998) The incidence of venous thromboembolism in family mem-bers of patients with factor V Leiden mutation and venous thrombosis. Ann Intern Med 128:15–20

356. Middeldorp S, Meinardi JR, Koopman MM et al (2001) A prospective study of asymptomatic carriers of the factor V Leiden mutation to determine the incidence of venous thromboembolism. Ann Intern Med 135:322–327

357. Federici C, Gianetti J, Andreassi MG (2006) Genomic medicine and thrombotic risk: who, when, how and why? Int J Cardiol 106:3–9

358. Andreotti F, Becker RC (2005) Atherothrombotic disorders: new insights from hematology. Circulation 111: 1855–1863

359. Sarasin FP, Bounameaux H (1998) Decision analysis model of prolonged oral anticoagulant treatment in factor V Leiden carriers with first episode of deep vein thrombosis. BMJ 316:95–99

360. Eckman MH, Singh SK, Erban JK et al (2002) Testing for factor V Leiden in patients with pulmonary or venous throm-boembolism: a cost-effectiveness analysis. Med Decis Making 22:108–124

361. Marchetti M, Pistorio A, Barosi G (2000) Extended anticoagulation for prevention of recurrent venous thromboembo-lism in carriers of factor V Leiden – cost-effectiveness analysis. Thromb Haemost 84:752–757

362. Marchetti M, Quaglini S, Barosi G (2001) Cost-effectiveness of screening and extended anticoagulation for carriers of both factor V Leiden and prothrombin G20210A. QJM 94:365–372

363. Baglin C, Brown K, Luddington R et al (1998) Risk of recurrent venous thromboembolism in patients with the factor V Leiden (FVR506Q) mutation: effect of warfarin and prediction by precipitating factors. East Anglian Thrombophilia Study Group. Br J Haematol 100:764–768

364. Christiansen SC, Cannegieter SC, Koster T et al (2005) Thrombophilia, clinical factors, and recurrent venous throm-botic events. JAMA 293:2352–2361

365. Bauer KA (2001) The thrombophilias: well-defined risk factors with uncertain therapeutic implications. Ann Intern Med 135:367–373

366. Brenner B, Hoffman R, Blumenfeld Z et al (2000) Gestational outcome in thrombophilic women with recurrent preg-nancy loss treated by enoxaparin. Thromb Haemost 83:693–697

367. Younis JS, Ohel G, Brenner B et al (2000) The effect of thrombophylaxis on pregnancy outcome in patients with recur-rent pregnancy loss associated with factor V Leiden mutation. BJOG 107:415–419

368. Gris JC, Mercier E, Quere I et al (2004) Low-molecular-weight heparin versus low-dose aspirin in women with one fetal loss and a constitutional thrombophilic disorder. Blood 103:3695–3699

369. van Vlijmen EF, Brouwer JL, Veeger NJ et al (2007) Oral contraceptives and the absolute risk of venous thromboem-bolism in women with single or multiple thrombophilic defects: results from a retrospective family cohort study. Arch Intern Med 167:282–289

370. Nichols WC, Seligsohn U, Zivelin A et al (1997) Linkage of combined factors V and VIII deficiency to chromosome 18q by homozygosity mapping. J Clin Invest 99:596–601

371. Nichols WC, Seligsohn U, Zivelin A et al (1998) Mutations in the ER-Golgi intermediate compartment protein ERGIC-53 cause combined deficiency of coagulation factors V and VIII. Cell 93:61–70

372. Levy GG, Nichols WC, Lian EC et al (2001) Mutations in a member of the ADAMTS gene family cause thrombotic thrombocytopenic purpura. Nature 413:488–494

373. Salomon O, Steinberg DM, Zivelin A et al (1999) Single and combined prothrombotic factors in patients with idio-pathic venous thromboembolism: prevalence and risk assessment. Arterioscler Thromb Vasc Biol 19:511–518

374. Psaty BM, Smith NL, Lemaitre RN et al (2001) Hormone replacement therapy, prothrombotic mutations, and the risk of incident nonfatal myocardial infarction in postmenopausal women. JAMA 285:906–913

375. Edelberg JM, Christie PD, Rosenberg RD (2001) Regulation of vascular bed-specific prothrombotic potential. Circ Res 89:117–124

376. Chang YS, Munn LL, Hillsley MV et al (2000) Effect of vascular endothelial growth factor on cultured endothelial cell monolayer transport properties. Microvasc Res 59:265–277
377. Beekhuizen H, van Furth R (1994) Growth characteristics of cultured human macrovascular venous and arterial and microvascular endothelial cells. J Vasc Res 31:230–239
378. Rupnick MA, Carey A, Williams SK (1988) Phenotypic diversity in cultured cerebral microvascular endothelial cells. In Vitro Cell Dev Biol 24:435–444
379. Christie PD, Edelberg JM, Picard MH et al (1999) A murine model of myocardial microvascular thrombosis. J Clin Invest 104:533–539
380. Edelberg JM, Aird WC, Wu W et al (1998) PDGF mediates cardiac microvascular communication. J Clin Invest 102:837–843
381. Guillot PV, Liu L, Kuivenhoven JA et al (2000) Targeting of human eNOS promoter to the Hprt locus of mice leads to tissue-restricted transgene expression. Physiol Genomics 2:77–83
382. Rosenberg RD, Aird WC (1999) Vascular-bed – specific hemostasis and hypercoagulable states. N Engl J Med 340:1555–1564
383. Nishida M, Springhorn JP, Kelly RA et al (1993) Cell-cell signaling between adult rat ventricular myocytes and cardiac microvascular endothelial cells in heterotypic primary culture. J Clin Invest 91:1934–1941
384. Tabrizi P, Wang L, Seeds N et al (1999) Tissue plasminogen activator (tPA) deficiency exacerbates cerebrovascular fibrin deposition and brain injury in a murine stroke model: studies in tPA-deficient mice and wild-type mice on a matched genetic background. Arterioscler Thromb Vasc Biol 19:2801–2806
385. Koeleman BP, Reitsma PH, Bertina RM (1997) Familial thrombophilia: a complex genetic disorder. Semin Hematol 34:256–264
386. van Boven HH, Reitsma PH, Rosendaal FR et al (1996) Factor V Leiden (FV R506Q) in families with inherited antithrombin deficiency. Thromb Haemost 75:417–421
387. Seligsohn U, Zivelin A (1997) Thrombophilia as a multigenic disorder. Thromb Haemost 78:297–301
388. Auro K, Alanne M, Kristiansson K et al (2007) Combined effects of thrombosis pathway gene variants predict cardiovascular events. PLoS Genet 3:e120
389. Roldan V, Gonzalez-Conejero R, Marin F et al (2005) Five prothrombotic polymorphisms and the prevalence of premature myocardial infarction. Haematologica 90:421–423
390. Hudson M, Herr AL, Rauch J et al (2003) The presence of multiple prothrombotic risk factors is associated with a higher risk of thrombosis in individuals with anticardiolipin antibodies. J Rheumatol 30:2385–2391
391. Potti A, Bild A, Dressman HK et al (2006) Gene-expression patterns predict phenotypes of immune-mediated thrombosis. Blood 107:1391–1396
392. Nurden AT (2006) Polymorphisms and platelet genotyping: the shape of things to come. J Thromb Haemost 4:1194–1196
393. Van Hylckama Vlieg A, Callas PW, Cushman M et al (2003) Inter-relation of coagulation factors and d-dimer levels in healthy individuals. J Thromb Haemost 1:516–522
394. Nesheim M (2001) Myocardial infarction and the balance between fibrin deposition and removal. Ital Heart J 2:641–645
395. Vlassara H, Fuh H, Donnelly T et al (1995) Advanced glycation endproducts promote adhesion molecule (VCAM-1, ICAM-1) expression and atheroma formation in normal rabbits. Mol Med 1:447–456
396. De Cristofaro R, Picozzi M, Morosetti R et al (1996) Effect of sodium on the energetics of thrombin-thrombomodulin interaction and its relevance for protein C hydrolysis. J Mol Biol 258:190–200
397. Ginsburg GS, Shah SH, McCarthy JJ (2007) Taking cardiovascular genetic association studies to the next level. J Am Coll Cardiol 50:930–932
398. Soria JM, Almasy L, Souto JC et al (2002) A quantitative-trait locus in the human factor XII gene influences both plasma factor XII levels and susceptibility to thrombotic disease. Am J Hum Genet 70:567–574
399. Soria JM, Almasy L, Souto JC et al (2003) A new locus on chromosome 18 that influences normal variation in activated protein C resistance phenotype and factor VIII activity and its relation to thrombosis susceptibility. Blood 101:163–167
400. Hennis BC, Van Boheemen PA, Koeleman BP et al (1995) A specific allele of the histidine-rich glycoprotein (HRG) locus is linked with elevated plasma levels of HRG in a Dutch family with thrombosis. Br J Haematol 89:845–852
401. Almasy L, Soria JM, Souto JC et al (2003) A quantitative trait locus influencing free plasma protein S levels on human chromosome 1q: results from the Genetic Analysis of Idiopathic Thrombophilia (GAIT) project. Arterioscler Thromb Vasc Biol 23:508–511
402. Hixson JE, Blangero J (2000) Genomic searches for genes that influence atherosclerosis and its risk factors. Ann N Y Acad Sci 902:1–7

403. Souto JC, Almasy L, Soria JM et al (2003) Genome-wide linkage analysis of von Willebrand factor plasma levels: results from the GAIT project. Thromb Haemost 89:468–474

404. Souto JC, Almasy L, Muniz-Diaz E et al (2000) Functional effects of the ABO locus polymorphism on plasma levels of von Willebrand factor, factor VIII, and activated partial thromboplastin time. Arterioscler Thromb Vasc Biol 20:2024–2028

405. Buil A, Soria JM, Souto JC et al (2004) Protein C levels are regulated by a quantitative trait locus on chromosome 16: results from the Genetic Analysis of Idiopathic Thrombophilia (GAIT) Project. Arterioscler Thromb Vasc Biol 24:1321–1325

406. Berger M, Mattheisen M, Kulle B et al (2005) High factor VIII levels in venous thromboembolism show linkage to imprinted loci on chromosomes 5 and 11. Blood 105:638–644

407. Scott BT, Hasstedt SJ, Bovill EG et al (2002) Characterization of the human prostaglandin H synthase 1 gene (PTGS1): exclusion by genetic linkage analysis as a second modifier gene in familial thrombosis. Blood Coagul Fibrinolysis 13:519–531

408. Almasy L, Soria JM, Souto JC et al (2005) A locus on chromosome 2 influences levels of tissue factor pathway inhibitor: results from the GAIT study. Arterioscler Thromb Vasc Biol 25:1489–1492

409. Rey E, Kahn SR, David M et al (2003) Thrombophilic disorders and fetal loss: a meta-analysis. Lancet 361:901–908

410. Balta G, Altay C, Gurgey A (2002) PAI-1 gene 4G/5G genotype: A risk factor for thrombosis in vessels of internal organs. Am J Hematol 71:89–93

411. Alessio AM, Hoehr NF, Siqueira LH et al (2007) Association between estrogen receptor alpha and beta gene polymorphisms and deep vein thrombosis. Thromb Res 120:639–645

412. Colaizzo D, Amitrano L, Tiscia GL et al (2007) A new JAK2 gene mutation in patients with polycythemia vera and splanchnic vein thrombosis. Blood 110:2768–2769

413. McMahon C, Abu-Elmagd K, Bontempo FA et al (2007) JAK2 V617F mutation in patients with catastrophic intra-abdominal thromboses. Am J Clin Pathol 127:736–743

414. Remacha AF, Estivill C, Sarda MP et al (2007) The V617F mutation of JAK2 is very uncommon in patients with thrombosis. Haematologica 92:285–286

415. Elbaz A, Poirier O, Canaple S et al (2000) The association between the Val34Leu polymorphism in the factor XIII gene and brain infarction. Blood 95:586–591

416. Franco RF, Pazin-Filho A, Tavella MH et al (2000) Factor XIII val34leu and the risk of myocardial infarction. Haematologica 85:67–71

417. Palkimas MP Jr, Skinner HM, Gandhi PJ et al (2003) Polymorphism induced sensitivity to warfarin: a review of the literature. J Thromb Thrombolysis 15:205–212

418. Honda S, Honda Y, Bauer B et al (1995) The impact of three-dimensional structure on the expression of PlA alloantigens on human integrin beta 3. Blood 86:234–242

419. Lazo-Langner A, Knoll GA, Wells PS et al (2006) The risk of dialysis access thrombosis is related to the transforming growth factor-beta1 production haplotype and is modified by polymorphisms in the plasminogen activator inhibitor-type 1 gene. Blood 108:4052–4058

420. Saito K, Nakayama T, Sato N et al (2006) Haplotypes of the plasminogen activator gene associated with ischemic stroke. Thromb Haemost 96:331–336

421. Kelly PJ, Rosand J, Kistler JP et al (2002) Homocysteine, MTHFR 677C→T polymorphism, and risk of ischemic stroke: results of a meta-analysis. Neurology 59:529–536

422. Ozben B, Diz-Kucukkaya R, Bilge AK et al (2007) The association of P-selectin glycoprotein ligand-1 VNTR polymorphisms with coronary stent restenosis. J Thromb Thrombolysis 23:181–187

423. Humphries SE, Luong LA, Ogg MS et al (2001) The interleukin-6 – 174 G/C promoter polymorphism is associated with risk of coronary heart disease and systolic blood pressure in healthy men. Eur Heart J 22:2243–2252

424. O'Leary DH, Polak JF, Kronmal RA et al (1999) Carotid-artery intima and media thickness as a risk factor for myocardial infarction and stroke in older adults. Cardiovascular Health Study Collaborative Research Group. N Engl J Med 340:14–22

425. Pola R, Flex A, Gaetani E et al (2003) Synergistic effect of -174 G/C polymorphism of the interleukin-6 gene promoter and 469 E/K polymorphism of the intercellular adhesion molecule-1 gene in Italian patients with history of ischemic stroke. Stroke 34:881–885

426. van der Meer I, Brouwers GJ, Bulk S et al (2004) Genetic variability of von Willebrand factor and risk of coronary heart disease: the Rotterdam Study. Br J Haematol 124:343–347

427. Durante-Mangoni E, Davies GJ, Ahmed N et al (2002) The prothrombin G20210A polymorphism in patients with myocardial infarction. Blood Coagul Fibrinolysis 13:603–608

428. Belvis R, Santamaria A, Marti-Fabregas J et al (2006) Diagnostic yield of prothrombotic state studies in cryptogenic stroke. Acta Neurol Scand 114:250–253

429. Djousse L, Karamohamed S, Herbert AG et al (2007) Fucosyltransferase 3 polymorphism and atherothrombotic disease in the Framingham Offspring Study. Am Heart J 153:636–639

430. Helgadottir A, Manolescu A, Helgason A et al (2006) A variant of the gene encoding leukotriene A4 hydrolase confers ethnicity-specific risk of myocardial infarction 1. Nat Genet 38:68–74

431. Kastrati A, Koch W, Gawaz M et al (2000) PlA polymorphism of glycoprotein IIIa and risk of adverse events after coronary stent placement. J Am Coll Cardiol 36:84–89

432. Bennett JS, Catella-Lawson F, Rut AR et al (2001) Effect of the Pl(A2) alloantigen on the function of beta(3)-integrins in platelets. Blood 97:3093–3099

433. Gorchakova O, Koch W, Mehilli J et al (2004) PlA polymorphism of the glycoprotein IIIa and efficacy of reperfusion therapy in patients with acute myocardial infarction. Thromb Haemost 91:141–145

434. Chew DP, Bhatt DL, Topol EJ (2001) Oral glycoprotein IIb/IIIa inhibitors: why don't they work? Am J Cardiovasc Drugs 1:421–428

435. Gonzalez-Conejero R, Rivera J, Corral J et al (2005) Biological assessment of aspirin efficacy on healthy individuals: heterogeneous response or aspirin failure? Stroke 36:276–280

436. Quinn MJ, Topol EJ (2001) Common variations in platelet glycoproteins: pharmacogenomic implications. Pharmacogenomics 2:341–352

437. Jefferson BK, Foster JH, McCarthy JJ et al (2005) Aspirin resistance and a single gene. Am J Cardiol 95:805–808

438. Arepally G, McKenzie SE, Jiang XM et al (1997) Fc gamma RIIA H/R 131 polymorphism, subclass-specific IgG anti-heparin/platelet factor 4 antibodies and clinical course in patients with heparin-induced thrombocytopenia and thrombosis. Blood 89:370–375

439. Carlsson LE, Santoso S, Baurichter G et al (1998) Heparin-induced thrombocytopenia: new insights into the impact of the FcgammaRIIa-R-H131 polymorphism. Blood 92:1526–1531

440. Sacchi E, Tagliabue L, Scoglio R et al (1996) Plasma factor VII levels are influenced by a polymorphism in the promoter region of the FVII gene. Blood Coagul Fibrinolysis 7:114–117

Part II
Antithrombotic Therapy for Stable Coronary Atherosclerotic Disease

5

Aspirin in Primary and Secondary Prevention of Cardiovascular Disease

Jinesh Kochar and J. Michael Gaziano

CONTENTS

ABSTRACT For over a century, aspirin has been used for different indications, mainly as an antipyretic, analgesic, and anti-inflammatory agent. However, its cardioprotective properties were discovered only a few decades ago. Initially employed for its antiplatelet effect in secondary prophylaxis of cardiovascular (CVD) events, various large-scale trials have established the role of aspirin in primary prevention of CVD in people at high risk. This chapter summarizes the clinical trial data that demonstrated the efficacy of this drug in both secondary and primary prevention of cardiovascular disease events, the leading cause of death in the US. In addition, an account of the historical perspective on aspirin, its mechanism of action, optimal dose, adverse effects, interaction with other nonsteroidal anti-inflammatory agents, aspirin resistance, and current recommendations for its use in primary prophylaxis of CVD are presented.

Key words: Aspirin; Primary prevention; Stable CAD; Efficacy; Atherosclerosis

HISTORY OF ASPIRIN

With more than 35,000 kg of aspirin (ASA) being consumed daily in the US, it is the most commercially successful synthetic drug in the world (*1*). From a historical perspective, as early as about 3000 BC, ASA, in its crude form, was known to the Egyptians, who employed the decoction of salicylate-containing plants like myrtle or willow leaves for joint pain. Hippocrates of Kos, around 500 BC, recommended extract of willow bark for pain during childbirth. The first scientific description of the beneficial effects of willow bark in ague (fever, usually taken to be malaria) was given in 1763 by Reverend Edward Stone

From: *Contemporary Cardiology: Antithrombotic Drug Therapy in Cardiovascular Disease*
Edited by: A.T. Askari and A.M. Lincoff (eds.), DOI 10.1007/978-1-60327-235-3_5
© Humana Press, a part of Springer Science+Business Media, LLC 2010

of Oxfordshire, UK. In 1876, Thomas MacLagan, a Scottish physician, carried out the first known clinical trial of salicin in a patient with acute rheumatism and reported his findings in *The Lancet*.

The search for the active ingredient in willow bark spanned most of the early and middle 1800s, and a purified form of salicin was obtained by Buchner in 1828. A series of modification of this compound, attempted by European scientists, led to the discovery of salicylic acid as an analgesic and antipyretic agent. Sodium salicylate, the then-commercially available form of this compound had lower gastric tolerability. A Friedrich Bayer & Co. chemist, Felix Hoffmann, in an attempt to improve its tolerability, in 1897 is credited for preparing a purified acetylated form of the molecule. The Bayer Company, on March 6, 1899, first registered the product under the trade name of Aspirin ("a" from acetyl, "spir" from *Spirea ulmania*, a plant containing the compound). By circulating the new drug information to about 30,000 physicians, Bayer is said to have introduced the first mass marketing of a drug. Aspirin's acceptance by the laity has been equally impressive; in 1950, aspirin found a place in the *Guinness Book of Records*, as the most popular pain killer in the world. In existence for over 100 years, aspirin has been a subject of constant attention for its potential role in the treatment or prevention of many acute and chronic conditions.

PHARMACOKINETICS

After oral intake, nondissociated acetylsalicylic acid passively diffuses across the gastric and intestinal mucosa. Enteric coating considerably delays absorption time (peak plasma levels in 3–4 h as compared to 30–40 min for the uncoated aspirin). Once aspirin enters the liver, it is hydrolyzed by esterases. Aspirin has a half-life of about 15–20 min in the human circulation. The mean lifespan of human platelets is approximately 10 days; about 10% of circulating platelets are replaced each day, and 5–6 days following aspirin ingestion, approximately 50% of the platelets function normally. Aspirin thus exhibits a dissociation of pharmacokinetics and pharmacodynamics.

Cumulative effect of low-dose aspirin: In a study done on 46 healthy adults, cumulative daily doses of 0.45 mg/kg of aspirin inhibited the $T \times B_2$ (a stable breakdown product of $T \times A_2$) level to less than 5% by day 7 of therapy *(2)*. For a 133-pound person, a daily dose of as little as 27 mg of aspirin reduced $T \times B_2$ by 36% on day 1, 70% on day 2, 87% on day 3, and 90% on day 4. Greater than 95% inhibition of platelet $T \times B_2$ was maintained for the 30-day period of aspirin administration (Fig. 3).

MECHANISM OF ACTION

After rapid absorption from the stomach and upper small intestine, ASA first comes in contact with platelets in the portal circulation, where it leads to irreversible inactivation of the cyclooxygenase activity of prostaglandin H synthase 1 and synthase 2, referred to as COX-1 and COX-2, respectively (Fig. 1). These enzymes catalyze the conversion of arachidonic acid to PGH_2, which is then converted to the prostaglandins, prostacyclin, and thromboxane A_2 by tissue-specific isomerases. After diffusing through the cell membrane, ASA enters the COX channel, ASA first binds to an arginine 120 residue, and then acetylates the serine 529 residue in COX-1 and serine 516 in COX-2. This prevents access of arachidonic acid to the COX catalytic site. As the anuclear platelets cannot synthesize new enzymes, this effect of ASA remains for the rest of their lifespan. In contrast, the inhibition of COX-2-dependent pathophysiologic processes like hyperalgesia and inflammation, mediated by nucleated cells, requires larger doses of aspirin and frequent dosing because higher levels of ASA are required to inhibit COX-2 than to inhibit COX-1. In addition, unlike platelets, nucleated cells can repeatedly synthesize fresh COX-2, explaining the approximate 100-fold variation in daily doses of aspirin when it is used for anti-inflammatory rather than antithrombotic purposes (Fig. 1).

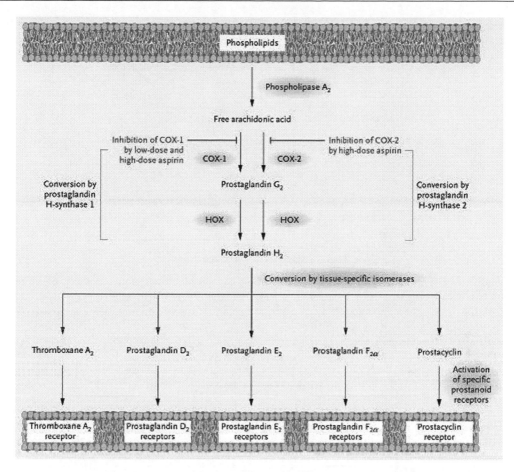

Fig. 1. Mechanism of action of aspirin. Arachidonic acid, a 20-carbon fatty acid containing four double bonds, is liberated from the *sn*2 position of membrane phospholipids by several forms of phospholipase A_2, which are activated by diverse stimuli. Arachidonic acid is converted by cytosolic prostaglandin H synthases, which have both cyclooxygenase and hydroperoxidase (HOX) activity, to the unstable intermediates prostaglandin G_2 and prostaglandin H_2, respectively. The synthases are colloquially termed cyclooxygenases and exist in two forms, cyclooxygenase-1 (COX-1) and cyclooxygenase-2 (COX-2). Low-dose aspirin selectivity inhibits COX-1, whereas high-dose aspirin inhibits both COX-1 and COX-2. Prostaglandin H_2 is converted by tissue-specific isomerases to multiple prostanoids. These bioactive lipids activate specific cell-membrane receptors of the superfamily of G-protein-coupled receptors, such as the thromboxane receptor, the prostaglandin D_2 receptors, the prostaglandin E_2 receptors, the prostaglandin F_2 receptors, and the prostacyclin receptor (*Source*: Patrono et al. *(5)*).

ASPIRIN FOR CARDIOVASCULAR PREVENTION

About 36% of the US adult population, and 80% of those with cardiovascular disease take aspirin for cardiovascular disease prevention, accounting for consumption of 10–20 billion aspirin tablets for cardiovascular disease prevention annually *(3)*.

Secondary Prevention

Over 400 trials have been conducted to evaluate the antiplatelet effects of ASA and other drugs. Aspirin has established benefits in preventing another event in patients with established cardiovascular disease.

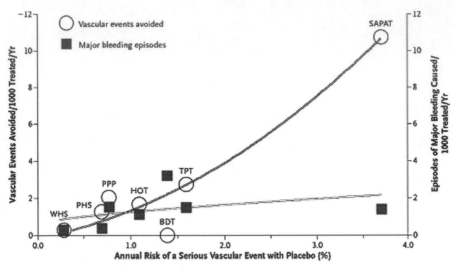

Fig. 2. Benefits and risks of low-dose aspirin in primary-prevention trials. The numbers of vascular events avoided and episodes of major bleeding caused per 1,000 patients treated with aspirin per year plotted from the results of individual placebo-controlled trials of aspirin in different patient populations characterized by various degrees of cardiovascular risk, as noted on the abscissa. *WHS* Women's Health Study, *PHS* Physicians' Health Study, *PPP* Primary Prevention Project, *HOT* Hypertension Optimal Treatment Study, *BDT* British Doctors Trial, *TPT* Thrombosis Prevention Trial, *SAPAT* Swedish Angina Pectoris Aspirin Trial. (*Source*: Patrono et al. *(5)*).

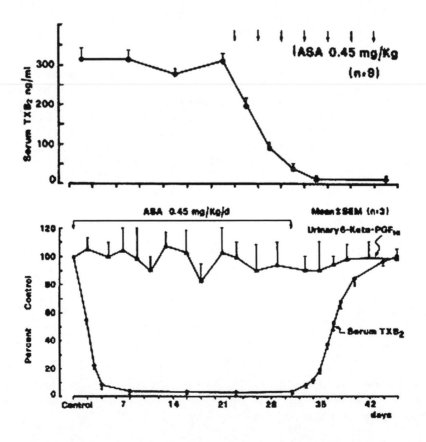

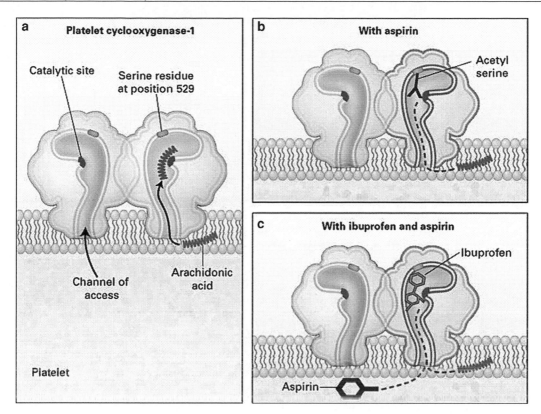

Fig. 4. The effect of aspirin alone and of ibuprofen plus aspirin on platelet cyclooxygenase-1. The platelet prostaglandin G/H synthase-1 (cyclooxygenase-1) is depicted as a dimer. The arachidonic acid substrate gains access to the catalytic site through a hydrophobic channel that leads into the core of the enzyme (**a**). Aspirin blocks the access of arachidonic acid to the catalytic site by irreversibly acetylating a serine residue at position 529 in platelet cyclooxygenase-1, near but not within the catalytic site (**b**). Interpolation of the bulky acetyl residue prevents metabolism of arachidonic acid into the cyclic endoperoxides PGG_2 and PGH_2 for the lifetime of the platelet. Because PGH_2 is metabolized by thromboxane synthase into thromboxane A_2, aspirin prevents the formation of thromboxane A_2 by the platelets until new platelets are generated. Nonsteroidal anti-inflammatory drugs, such as ibuprofen, are reversible, competitive inhibitors of the catalytic site (**c**) whose use results in the reversible inhibition of thromboxane A_2 formation during the dosing interval. Prior occupancy of the catalytic site by ibuprofen prevents aspirin from gaining access to its target serine (*Source*: Catella-Lawson et al (*33*)).

The Antithrombotic Trialists Collaboration conducted a meta-analysis that reviewed 287 studies involving 135,000 patients in comparisons of aspirin versus control and 77,000 patients in comparisons of different antiplatelet regimens (*4*). The main outcome measures included nonfatal myocardial infarction (MI), nonfatal stroke, and vascular death, collectively termed as "serious vascular event."

Fig. 3. (Upper) The effect of low dose (0.45 mg/kg) aspirin on platelet TXB_2. Serum TXB_2 was measured in nine healthy subjects during seven consecutive days without and with (indicated by arrows) aspirin. Each mark on X-axis represents a day. (Lower) The long term effects of low dose (0.45 mg/kg per day) aspirin on platelet TXB_2 and renal PGI_2 synthesis. Serum TXB_2 concentration and urinary excretion of 6-keto-PGF_{1-a} (a prostacycline metabolite) were measured in three healthy subjects before, during and after aspirin therapy. Mean values and standard error of mean are plotted. Arrows indicate duration of aspirin therapy (Source: Patrignani et al. (*2*)).

Overall, aspirin and other antiplatelet drugs led to a 22% risk reduction in serious vascular events in patients with MI, stroke, transient ischemic attack (TIA), coronary artery disease, peripheral vascular disease (PVD), at-risk of pulmonary embolism, or with other high-risk conditions such as diabetes mellitus, hemodialysis, and carotid disease. Exclusion of acute stroke patients increased this figure to 25%. At different doses, aspirin alone reduced the risk of serious vascular events by 23%. At doses of 500–1,500 mg, aspirin reduced the risk of vascular events by 19%. The corresponding risk reduction at doses of 160–325 mg, 75–150 mg, and less than 75 mg were 26%, 32%, and 13%, respectively. It has been suggested that in cardiovascular disease patients with a 4–8% annual risk of a serious vascular event, aspirin prevents 10–20 fatal and nonfatal vascular events in every 1,000 patients treated over a period of 1 year *(5)*. In patients undergoing carotid endarterectomy, risk of stroke, MI, and death within 30 days and 3 months of endarterectomy were lower in patients taking 81 or 325 mg of aspirin daily as compared to those taking 650 or 1,300 mg *(6)*.

Various studies have looked into whether the addition of another antiplatelet agent, with another mechanism of action has additional cardiovascular benefits. The CURE (Clopidogrel in Unstable angina to prevent Recurrent ischemic Events) study randomized 12,562 patients with acute non-ST segment elevation coronary syndrome into two groups: a clopidogrel (a loading dose of 300 mg orally, followed by 75 mg daily) plus aspirin group and a placebo plus aspirin group (75–325 mg) *(7)*. The clopidogrel and aspirin group had a 20% reduced risk of death from cardiovascular causes, nonfatal MI, or ischemic stroke. This effect was more pronounced in patients with high TIMI (Thrombolysis in Myocardial Infarction) risk score (relative risk reduction 45%).

The Clopidogrel for High Atherothrombotic Risk and Ischemic Stabilization, Management and Avoidance (CHARISMA) study randomized people at high cardiovascular risk, defined as either those with pre-existing cardiovascular disease or with cardiovascular risk factors *(8)*. A statistically nonsignificant 8% reduction in nonfatal myocardial infarction, nonfatal ischemic stroke, and mortality from all cardiovascular causes was observed. In a randomized trial comparing the combination of aspirin plus ticlopidine to aspirin alone and aspirin plus warfarin in subjects with coronary stents, the aspirin–ticlopidine combination significantly reduced the incidence of primary endpoints (composite of death from any cause, revascularization of the target lesion without death, evidence of thrombosis of the target vessel on repeated angiography without revascularization, or nonfatal myocardial infarction). The relative risks were 0.15 ($p < 0.001$) and 0.20 ($p = 0.01$), respectively. As compared to aspirin alone, addition of intravenous GP IIb-IIIa antagonist to aspirin was associated with a statistically significant 19% reduction in serious vascular events, translating into preventing 20 vascular events per 1,000 patients in a month. In the Antithrombotic Trialists Collaboration meta-analysis, addition of dipyridamole to aspirin showed a statistically nonsignificant 6% reduction in serious vascular events.

In sum, aspirin reduces the risk of future CVD events, including MI and stroke, in those with CVD. There is no evidence that dose ranges higher than 75–150 mg daily are more effective. The combination of ASA with another antiplatelet agent such as clopidogrel should be reserved for those at the highest risk, including those with acute coronary syndrome and immediately following stent placement.

Primary Prevention

Evaluation of the role of aspirin in primary prevention of cardiovascular events is more complicated, in part because the absolute risk of these events is lower than in secondary prevention. In contrast to the hundreds of trials for secondary prevention, only six large-scale trials have explored the role of aspirin in primary prevention of CVD (Table 1): the British Male Doctors' Trial (BMD) *(9)*, the Hypertension Optimal Treatment Trial (HOT) *(10)*, the Thrombosis Prevention Trial (TPT) *(11)*, the

Table 1

Characteristics of the six major trials of aspirin for primary prevention of cardiovascular disease

Variable	BDT	PHS	TPT	HOT	PPP	WHS
Year	1988	1989	1998	1998	2001	2005
N	5,139	22,071	5,085	18,790	4,495	39,876
% of Women	0	0	0	47	58	100
Aspirin dose	500 mg per day	325 mg every other day	75 mg per day	75 mg per day	100 mg per day	100 mg every other day
Age (years)	<60 (47%) 60–69 (39%) 70–79 (14%)	Mean: 53	Mean: 57.5	Mean: 61.5	<60 (29%) 60–69 (45%) 70–79 (24%)	45–64 (60%) 55–64 (30%) 65 and up (10%)
Additional drug	None	β-carotene	Warfarin	Felodipine ± ACE inhibitor ± β-blocker	Vitamin E	Vitamin E
Study population	Apparently healthy male physicians	Apparently healthy male physicians	Men at high risk of CAD	Men and women with hypertension	Men and women with ≥1 major CVD risk factor	Apparently healthy female health professionals
Mean follow up (years)	6	5	6.4	4	3.6	10.1

Primary Prevention Project (PPP) *(12)*, the U.S. Physicians' Health Study (PHS) *(13)*, and the Women's Health Study (WHS) *(14)* (Fig. 2).

The BMD was one of the first large-scale trials to examine the role of aspirin in the primary prevention of CVD. No significant difference was noted in risk of nonfatal MI in the aspirin or placebo groups. The PHS was a randomized, double-blind, placebo-controlled trial to determine if 325 mg of aspirin every other day decreased cardiovascular mortality and whether beta carotene decreased the incidence of cancer in 22,071 healthy US male physicians. With a statistically significant 44% decrease in the risk of first MI, it was the first of the primary prevention trials reporting the benefits of aspirin in primary prevention of MI. An 18% risk reduction in the composite outcome of MI, stroke, and CVD death was observed (RR: 0.82, 95% CI: 0.70–0.96). However, the small number of strokes and total cardiovascular deaths yielded inconclusive results for aspirin's effect on these outcomes.

The TPT assessed the effects of aspirin and placebo warfarin, placebo aspirin and warfarin, aspirin and warfarin, and placebo aspirin and placebo warfarin. Aspirin was associated with a statistically significant reduction in the incidence of nonfatal stroke, total ischemic heart disease, and nonfatal ischemic heart disease. The HOT study revealed a 36% reduction in fatal and nonfatal MI in hypertensive patients taking aspirin. In people with hypertension, hypercholesterolemia, diabetes, obesity, family history of MI and in the elderly, the PPP demonstrated that 100 mg per day of aspirin reduced the risk of total cardiovascular deaths by 23%, and of cardiovascular mortality by 44%. To date, the largest study of primary prevention of CVD by aspirin is the WHS. This trial, comprising about 40,000 women, did not show a significant difference in the risk of fatal or nonfatal MI and CVD mortality between the aspirin and placebo groups. However, a 24% reduction in the risk of ischemic stroke and a 22% reduction in the risk of TIA were observed. In women 65 and older, aspirin had beneficial effects on major CVD (nonfatal MI, nonfatal stroke and CVD death, MI and ischemic stroke). Age modified the effect of aspirin on major CVD and MI; in women 65 and older, aspirin showed a significant 26% reduction in the risk of major CVD and 30% in the risk of ischemic stroke. Additionally, this was the only age group in which aspirin significantly reduced the risk of MI.

Various meta-analyses have analyzed the primary prevention trials to summarize the overall effectiveness of primary prophylaxis with aspirin *(15–19)*. A recent meta-analysis of data from all six primary prevention trials has shown that aspirin reduces the risk of nonfatal MI by 25%, total coronary heart disease by 23%, and total cardiovascular events by 15%. No statistically significant decrease in stroke, fatal coronary heart disease, and all-cause mortality was noted with aspirin *(15)*. Similar results have been reported by other meta-analyses *(16–18)*. It is interesting to note that although statistically not significant, the addition of WHS data to the other five trials in the meta-analysis by Bartolucci et al. showed that aspirin was better than placebo for decreasing the risk of stroke and all-cause mortality *(15)*. More studies are required to clarify the exact role of aspirin for these outcomes.

Thus, aspirin reduces the risk of first nonfatal MI and CHD. Overall, aspirin has clear benefits in preventing CVD events in men and women.

ADVERSE EFFECTS OF LOW-DOSE ASPIRIN

In a sex-specific meta-analysis of the six primary prevention trials, aspirin use was associated with a 70% increased risk of major bleeding events in men and women; this translated into causing one major bleeding event per 400 women and per 303 men over 6.4 years of aspirin use *(19)*. Gastrointestinal tract perforation, ulceration, and bleeding are expected adverse effects in that they are, at least in part, explained by inhibition of prostaglandin synthesis produced by aspirin. Gastrointestinal bleeding risk is dose dependent; higher doses are associated with higher rates of bleeding *(20,21)*. A case-control study has suggested that proton pump inhibitors are more effective than H_2 receptor antagonists in preventing upper GI bleeds associated with aspirin use *(22)*. At least five randomized controlled trials of healthy volunteers have suggested that enteric-coated aspirin is associated with endoscopically documented decreased risk of gastric mucosal injury *(23)*. Aspirin hypersensitivity is an uncommon adverse effect, and desensitization therapy may be helpful in permitting the continued use of aspirin.

ASPIRIN MAY NOT ALWAYS WORK

While aspirin can reduce the risk of primary or secondary events, some patients may not get the maximal benefit. Many factors may underlie such a reduction in the effect of aspirin (Table 2), including but not limited to noncompliance, cigarette smoking, drug–drug interactions, drug–disease interactions, and biochemical aspirin resistance. Noncompliance with aspirin can be related to habitual noncompliance to medications, or its adverse effects, chiefly gastric. Cigarette smoking has been shown to interfere with the antiplatelet activity of aspirin. The WHS has demonstrated a reduction in risk of CVD events among nonsmokers but not among smokers. Smoking may interfere with aspirin's effect on platelets by increasing F_2 isoprostanes, which have prothrombotic and vasoconstrictor effects *(24)*.

Certain NSAIDs, including ibuprofen and indomethacin, have been shown to antagonize the antiplatelet effects of aspirin. These drugs may interfere with access of aspirin to the COX-1 binding site (Fig. 4). Whether or not this interaction translates into clinically important events remains to be

Table 2
**Possible causes of recurrent ischemic vascular events among patients taking aspirin
(Adapted from Hankey et al. *(34)*)**

Nonatherothrombotic causes
- Embolism from the heart (red, fibrin thrombi; vegetations; calcium; tumor; prostheses)
- Arteritis

Poor aspirin bioavailability
- Poor compliance
- Inadequate dose
- Concurrent intake of certain nonsteroidal anti-inflammatory drugs (for example ibuprofen, indomethacin), possibly preventing the access of aspirin to cyclooxygenase-1 binding site

Alternative mechanisms of platelet activation
- Platelet activation by pathways that are not blocked by aspirin (for example, red cell-induced platelet activation: stimulation of collagen, adenosine diphosphate, epinephrine, and thrombin receptors on platelets)
- Increased platelet sensitivity to collagen and adenosine diphosphate
- Biosynthesis of thromboxane by pathways that are not blocked by aspirin (for example, by cyclooxygenase-2 in monocytes and macrophages, and vascular endothelial cells)

High platelet turnover
- Increased production of platelets by the bone marrow in response to stress (for example, after coronary artery bypass surgery), introducing into blood stream newly formed platelets unexposed to aspirin during the 24-h dose interval (aspirin is given once daily and has only a 20 min half-life)

Genetic polymorphisms
- Polymorphisms involving platelet glycoprotein Ia/IIa, Ib/V/IX, and IIb/IIIa receptors, and collagen and von Willebrand factor receptors
- Polymorphisms of cyclooxygenase-1, cyclooxygenase-2, thromboxane A_2-synthase, or other arachidonate metabolism enzymes
- Factor XIII Val34Leu polymorphism, leading to variable inhibition of factor XIII activation by low-dose aspirin

more clearly defined with few, observational studies available. In one study of 7,107 patients discharged on low-dose aspirin (<325 mg/day) after their first hospital admission for CV disease, patients taking aspirin plus ibuprofen had an increased risk of all-cause mortality (adjusted hazard ratio: 1.93, 95% CI: 1.30–2.87, $p=0.0011$) and cardiovascular mortality (1.73, 1.05–2.84, $p=0.0305$) compared with those taking aspirin alone (25). More recent data lend some doubt to the adverse interaction between ibuprofen and aspirin (26,27). Among 70,316 patients discharged after admission for an MI a similar risk of death was seen in patients discharged on aspirin alone, aspirin and ibuprofen, or on aspirin and another NSAID (26). A recent nested case-control study further supports the lack of an adverse interaction between ibuprofen, other NSAIDs, and aspirin (27). Due to over-the-counter availability of these drugs and frequent coexistence of painful conditions such as arthritis in those who may use aspirin, it is important to look for such interactions.

The term "aspirin resistance" suffers from a lack of consensus definition and validity. It has been varyingly defined as recurrence of coronary heart disease, stroke, and peripheral vascular disease despite prescription of a regular therapeutic dose of aspirin ("clinical aspirin resistance"), or persistent ex vivo platelet activation, measured by platelet function tests, despite aspirin use ("biochemical" or "laboratory aspirin resistance"). A recent meta-analysis showed that patients with laboratory aspirin resistance have higher risk of clinical aspirin resistance (28). Laboratory tests to investigate platelet function include optical platelet aggregation tests, PFA-100, P-selectin flow cytometry, urinary thromboxane excretion analysis, etc. No study has shown a clear benefit from routine screening for aspirin resistance. There is some indication that genetic factors like polymorphism PLA1/A2 of the gene encoding for glycoprotein IIIa might be associated with altered platelet function and increased risk of cardiovascular events. Although unclear from current research, clopidogrel or ticlopidine might be effective alternatives for clinical failure of aspirin.

Overall, aspirin remains the most cost-effective drug for secondary prevention of atherothrombotic disease; factors like cigarette smoking, compliance, and interactions with NSAIDs should be identified and addressed.

RECOMMENDATIONS

Aspirin decreases the incidence of a first CVD event in adults at an increased risk of heart disease. The absolute risk reduction is lower than that seen in secondary prevention; however, the incidence of gastric side effects is comparable. There are various guidelines for decision making in prescribing aspirin for primary prevention of CVD.

Aspirin is clearly indicated for secondary prevention among those with any form of cardiovascular disease. In this setting, it is safe and highly cost effective. For primary prevention, the use of aspirin requires a risk assessment. The U.S. Preventive Services Task Force (USPSTF) recommends that overall risk assessment be done before initiating primary prophylaxis with aspirin. These risk factors are age, sex, diabetes, elevated total cholesterol, low HDL cholesterol, elevated blood pressure, family history of CAD, and smoking (29). Men older than 40 years of age, postmenopausal women, and younger adults at high risk of CAD might benefit from aspirin therapy; the estimated 5-year magnitude of which is shown in Table 3. It is recommended that the risks and benefits of aspirin therapy be discussed with the patient at least every 5 years in middle age and older people or when other cardiovascular risk factors are detected. According to the USPSTF 2009 guidelines, there is a grade A recommendation for use of aspirin to prevent MI in men age 45–79, and ischemic stroke in women age 55–79. There is insufficient evidence to recommend aspirin in other age groups.

Table 3

The USPSTF estimates of benefits and harms of aspirin for primary prophylaxis
(5 years of therapy to 1,000 individuals) (Adapted from Hayden et al. (*18*))

Benefits and harms	Baseline risk of coronary heart disease over 5 years		
	1%	*3%*	*5%*
Total mortality	No effect	No effect	No effect
CHD events avoided	1–4	4–12	6–20
Hemorrhagic strokes caused	0–2	0–2	0–2
Major GI bleeding events caused	2–4	2–4	2–4

To estimate the 10-year risks, double the baseline risks; i.e., 5-year risk of 1% = 10-year risk of 2%, and so on
These estimates are based on a 28% risk reduction in coronary heart disease events in aspirin-treated subjects
Major GI bleeding events may be 2–3 times higher in people older than 70 years

The American Heart Association (AHA) guidelines for Primary Prevention of Cardiovascular Diseases and Stroke suggest low-dose aspirin (75–160 mg/day) for persons with a 10-year CAD risk of more than or equal to 10% (instead of >6% 10-year risk of CAD suggested by USPSTF) *(30)*. The underlying rationale for this difference is to improve the risk-benefit ratio. It is also recommended that persons with diabetes or with a 10-year CAD risk >20% be considered equivalent to persons with established CAD.

Similar recommendations have been made by the American Diabetes Association. Low-dose aspirin (75–162 mg) has been recommended to men and women with type 1 or type 2 diabetes at increased cardiovascular risk, including those over 40 years of age or who have additional risk factors (family history of CVD, hypertension, smoking, dyslipidemia, albuminuria) *(31)*. Aspirin therapy is not associated with an increased risk for retinal or vitreous hemorrhage.

The European Society of Cardiology recommends aspirin prophylaxis in high-risk individuals, such as treated hypertensive patients whose blood pressure is well controlled and men at "particularly high" CHD risk *(32)*. The Society does not recommend such therapy in all high-risk individuals. The definition of "particularly high" risk is not clearly described.

To sum up, we recommend aspirin for primary prophylaxis of CAD in high-risk individuals, as defined by USPSTF, after individual evaluation of the patient.

ACKNOWLEDGMENTS

Dr. Gaziano has received a research grant from McNeil Consumer Products and honoraria from Bayer. He is a consultant for Bayer and for McNeil Consumer Products.

REFERENCES

1. Jack DB (1997) One hundred years of aspirin. Lancet 350(9075):437–439
2. Patrignani P, Filabozzi P, Patrono C (1982) Selective cumulative inhibition of platelet thromboxane production by low-dose aspirin in healthy subjects. J Clin Invest 69(6):1366–1372
3. Ajani UA, Ford ES, Greenland KJ, Giles WH, Mokdad AH (2006) Aspirin use among U.S. adults: Behavioral Risk Factor Surveillance System. Am J Prev Med 30(1):74–77
4. Antithrombotic Trialists' Collaboration (2002) Collaborative meta-analysis of randomised trials of antiplatelet therapy for prevention of death, myocardial infarction, and stroke in high risk patients. BMJ 324(7329):71–86
5. Patrono C, Garcia Rodriguez LA, Landolfi R, Baigent C (2005) Low-dose aspirin for the prevention of atherothrombosis. N Engl J Med 353(22):2373–2383

6. Taylor DW, Barnett HJ, Haynes RB et al (1999) Low-dose and high-dose acetylsalicylic acid for patients undergoing carotid endarterectomy: a randomised controlled trial. ASA and Carotid Endarterectomy (ACE) Trial Collaborators. Lancet 353(9171):2179–2184

7. Yusuf S, Zhao F, Mehta SR, Chrolavicius S, Tognoni G, Fox KK (2001) Effects of clopidogrel in addition to aspirin in patients with acute coronary syndromes without ST-segment elevation. N Engl J Med 345(7):494–502

8. Bhatt DL, Fox KA, Hacke W et al (2006) Clopidogrel and aspirin versus aspirin alone for the prevention of atherothrombotic events. N Engl J Med 354(16):1706–1717

9. Peto R, Gray R, Collins R et al (1988) Randomised trial of prophylactic daily aspirin in British male doctors. Br Med J (Clin Res Ed) 296(6618):313–316

10. Hansson L, Zanchetti A, Carruthers SG et al (1998) Effects of intensive blood-pressure lowering and low-dose aspirin in patients with hypertension: principal results of the Hypertension Optimal Treatment (HOT) randomised trial. HOT Study Group. Lancet 351(9118):1755–1762

11. (1998) Thrombosis prevention trial: randomised trial of low-intensity oral anticoagulation with warfarin and low-dose aspirin in the primary prevention of ischaemic heart disease in men at increased risk. The Medical Research Council's General Practice Research Framework. Lancet 351(9098):233–241.

12. de Gaetano G, Collaborative Group of the Primary Prevention Project (2001) Low-dose aspirin and vitamin E in people at cardiovascular risk: a randomised trial in general practice. Collaborative Group of the Primary Prevention Project. Lancet 357(9250):89–95

13. (1989) Final report on the aspirin component of the ongoing Physicians' Health Study. Steering Committee of the Physicians' Health Study Research Group. N Engl J Med 321(3):129–135.

14. Ridker PM, Cook NR, Lee IM et al (2005) A randomized trial of low-dose aspirin in the primary prevention of cardiovascular disease in women. N Engl J Med 352(13):1293–1304

15. Bartolucci AA, Howard G (2006) Meta-analysis of data from the six primary prevention trials of cardiovascular events using aspirin. Am J Cardiol 98(6):746–750

16. Eidelman RS, Hebert PR, Weisman SM, Hennekens CH (2003) An update on aspirin in the primary prevention of cardiovascular disease. Arch Intern Med 163(17):2006–2010

17. Sanmuganathan PS, Ghahramani P, Jackson PR, Wallis EJ, Ramsay LE (2001) Aspirin for primary prevention of coronary heart disease: safety and absolute benefit related to coronary risk derived from meta-analysis of randomised trials. Heart 85(3):265–271

18. Hayden M, Pignone M, Phillips C, Mulrow C (2002) Aspirin for the primary prevention of cardiovascular events: a summary of the evidence for the U.S. Preventive Services Task Force. Ann Intern Med 136(2):161–172

19. Berger JS, Roncaglioni MC, Avanzini F, Pangrazzi I, Tognoni G, Brown DL (2006) Aspirin for the primary prevention of cardiovascular events in women and men: a sex-specific meta-analysis of randomized controlled trials. JAMA 295(3):306–313

20. Farrell B, Godwin J, Richards S, Warlow C (1991) The United Kingdom transient ischaemic attack (UK-TIA) aspirin trial: final results. J Neurol Neurosurg Psychiatry 54(12):1044–1054

21. The Dutch TIA Trial Study Group (1991) A comparison of two doses of aspirin (30 mg vs. 283 mg a day) in patients after a transient ischemic attack or minor ischemic stroke. The Dutch TIA Trial Study Group. N Engl J Med 325(18):1261–1266

22. Lanas A, Garcia-Rodriguez LA, Arroyo MT et al (2007) Effect of antisecretory drugs and nitrates on the risk of ulcer bleeding associated with nonsteroidal anti-inflammatory drugs, antiplatelet agents, and anticoagulants. Am J Gastroenterol 102(3):507–515

23. Walker J, Robinson J, Stewart J, Jacob S (2007) Does enteric-coated aspirin result in a lower incidence of gastrointestinal complications compared to normal aspirin? Interact Cardiovasc Thorac Surg 6(4):519–522

24. Morrow JD, Frei B, Longmire AW et al (1995) Increase in circulating products of lipid peroxidation (F2-isoprostanes) in smokers. Smoking as a cause of oxidative damage. N Engl J Med 332(18):1198–1203

25. MacDonald TM, Wei L (2003) Effect of ibuprofen on cardioprotective effect of aspirin. Lancet 361(9357):573–574

26. Curtis JP, Wang Y, Portnay EL, Masoudi FA, Havranek EP, Krumholz HM (2003) Aspirin, ibuprofen, and mortality after myocardial infarction: retrospective cohort study. BMJ 327(7427):1322–1323

27. Garcia Rodriguez LA, Varas-Lorenzo C, Maguire A, Gonzalez-Perez A (2004) Nonsteroidal antiinflammatory drugs and the risk of myocardial infarction in the general population. Circulation 109(24):3000–3006

28. Snoep JD, Hovens MM, Eikenboom JC, van der Bom JG, Huisman MV (2007) Association of laboratory-defined aspirin resistance with a higher risk of recurrent cardiovascular events: a systematic review and meta-analysis. Arch Intern Med 167(15):1593–1599

29. Aspirin for the primary prevention of cardiovascular events (2002) recommendation and rationale. Ann Intern Med 136(2):157–160

30. Pearson TA, Blair SN, Daniels SR et al (2002) AHA Guidelines for Primary Prevention of Cardiovascular Disease and Stroke: 2002 Update: Consensus Panel Guide to Comprehensive Risk Reduction for Adult Patients Without Coronary or Other Atherosclerotic Vascular Diseases. American Heart Association Science Advisory and Coordinating Committee. Circulation 106(3):388–391
31. Colwell JA (2004) Aspirin therapy in diabetes. Diabetes Care 27(Suppl 1):S72–S73
32. Prevention of coronary heart disease in clinical practice (1998) Recommendations of the Second Joint Task Force of European and other Societies on coronary prevention. Eur Heart J 19(10):1434–1503
33. Catella-Lawson F, Reilly MP, Kapoor SC et al (2001) Cyclooxygenase inhibitors and the antiplatelet effects of aspirin. N Engl J Med 345(25):1809–1817
34. Hankey GJ, Eikelboom JW (2004) Aspirin resistance. BMJ 328(7438):477–479

6 Thienopyridines in Stable Coronary Disease

Marcus D. Flather and Dipak Kotecha

Contents

ABSTRACT Antiplatelet agents including aspirin and clopidogrel have an established role in reducing the risk of death, stroke and myocardial infarction, and other complications of cardiovascular disease. Aspirin is the standard acute and long-term antiplatelet agent, although clopidogrel alone is slightly more effective than aspirin alone. Several randomized trials have tested the effects of clopidogrel added to aspirin compared to aspirin alone and beneficial effects in the region of 10–20% proportional reductions in risk have been observed in acute coronary syndromes (ST-elevation and non-ST-elevation) and percutaneous coronary intervention. In the chronic setting, where there are far more patients who could potentially benefit, there has been no proven effect of adding clopidogrel to aspirin compared to aspirin alone. In the CHARISMA trial there were trends to benefit in subgroups with pre-existing vascular disease or a prior vascular event. The combination of clopidogrel plus aspirin compared to aspirin alone increases the risk of major bleeding by about 30%. A simple pooling of published data suggests that the overall benefit of adding clopidogrel to aspirin in patients with acute or chronic vascular disease decreases the risk of cardiovascular death, myocardial infarction, and stroke by a proportional 10% and an absolute 1% (with greater effects in higher-risk patients) which is clinically worthwhile. Further work is needed to test the effects of clopidogrel when added to aspirin in patients with a prior stroke, myocardial infarction, or peripheral arterial disease as there may be worthwhile benefits that were not apparent in the CHARISMA trial.

Key words: Clopidogrel; Ticlopidine; CHARISMA trial; Stable CAD; Atherosclerosis

From: *Contemporary Cardiology: Antithrombotic Drug Therapy in Cardiovascular Disease*
Edited by: A.T. Askari and A.M. Lincoff (eds.), DOI 10.1007/978-1-60327-235-3_6
© Humana Press, a part of Springer Science+Business Media, LLC 2010

INTRODUCTION

Prevention of vascular events such as death, myocardial infarction (MI), and stroke is a key part of the management of cardiovascular disease both among patients with a prior history of vascular disease, and apparently healthy individuals with cardiovascular risk factors. Emphasis on a healthy lifestyle including appropriate eating habits, regular exercise, and avoidance of cigarette smoking is a standard approach to prevention of cardiovascular disease, but this approach is time consuming and proving efficacy has been difficult *(1,2)*. Thus for patients with established vascular disease there is an emphasis on pharmacological therapies with proven benefits including statins, antiplatelet agents, angiotensin-converting enzyme inhibitors, and beta blockers *(3)*. In addition the careful management of important risk factors such as hypertension, diabetes, and hyperlipidemia through pharmacological and nonpharmacological methods is essential *(4)*.

Aspirin has clinically useful antiplatelet effects by inhibiting the enzyme cyclooxygenase and reducing thromboxane A2 which is involved in platelet activity. Numerous studies have established aspirin as a key long-term antithrombotic agent that is well tolerated and effective. In high-risk patients it reduces the risk of nonfatal myocardial infarction by 30%, nonfatal stroke by 25% and overall vascular death by around 15% *(5)*. Unfortunately, a considerable number of patients suffer a further event despite aspirin treatment *(6)*.

The search for new antithrombotic therapies that augment the protective effects of aspirin (or substitute in patients with intolerance) has identified several promising agents. These include oral anticoagulants (warfarin and the direct thrombin inhibitors), oral glycoprotein IIb/IIIa receptor antagonists (which were found to have an adverse effect in spite of good biological rationale) *(7)*, and more recently the oral thienopyridine clopidogrel. The latter is slightly more effective than aspirin alone, and in combination with aspirin has additional benefits in patients with acute coronary syndromes (ACS).

In this chapter we review data from the larger clinical trials about the potential benefits and risks of longer-term thienopyridine treatment in patients with coronary, cerebral, and peripheral vascular disease.

THIENOPYRIDINES

The two main thienopyridines are clopidogrel and prasugrel, but newer agents including short-acting intravenous compounds are under investigation *(8,9)*. Prasugrel is relatively new and has been investigated in patients with ACS with evidence of efficacy and will be discussed in other chapters. Both act on the P2Y12 (ADP) receptor on the platelet, decrease platelet reactivity, and provide irreversible platelet inhibition. Clopidogrel is a prodrug which is converted to an active metabolite with a short half-life in the liver before exerting its antiplatelet effect, whereas prasugrel is immediately effective resulting in a quicker onset of action. Clopidogrel is one of the most carefully studied antithrombotic agents, and it is estimated that more than 100,000 patients have been enrolled in randomized trials involving clopidogrel.

BRIEF REVIEW OF THIENOPYRIDINE TRIALS

Thienopyridines, mainly clopidogrel, have been studied in several disease areas including chronic vascular disease (CAD, cerebrovascular, and PAD either separately or in combination), ACS, percutaneous coronary intervention (PCI), and atrial fibrillation (Table 1). The first study to show the safety and efficacy of clopidogrel was the CAPRIE trial which randomized 19,185 patients with a history of prior stroke, prior MI, or PAD to either clopidogrel 75 mg or aspirin

Table 1

Results from the major randomized trials of clopidogrel plus aspirin

Trial name	Patients studied	Treatment group	Control group	Composite vascular outcome	Months of follow up	Treatment N (%)	Control N (%)	HR (95%CI) P-value	Major bleeds HR (95% CI) P-value
Acute coronary syndromes									
CURE	Non-ST elevation ACS	Clopidogrel 300mg loading then 75mg daily Aspirin 75–325mg	Placebo clopidogrel+aspirin	CV death, stroke, MI	9	582/6,259 (9.3%)	719/6,303 (11.4%)	0.80 (0.72–0.90) P<0.001	1.38 (1.13–1.67) P=0.001
CLARITY	ST elevation ACS (fibrinolysis)	Clopidogrel 300mg load followed by 75mg+aspirin 150–325mg load then 75–162mg daily	Placebo clopidogrel+aspirin	CV death, MI	30 days (treatment up to 8 days)	89/1,752a (5.1%)	100/1,739a (5.8%)	0.89 P=NS	1.26 P=0.24 (TIMI major or minor)
COMMIT	ST elevation or bundle branch block ACS (50% fibrinolysis)	Clopidogrel 75mg Aspirin 162mg	Placebo clopidogrel plus aspirin	Death, MI, stroke	Up to 1 month Mean 16 days	2,125/22,958 (9.3%)	2311/22,891 (10.1%)	0.91 (0.86–0.97) P=0.002	1.1
PCI, stable vascular disease and risk factors									
CREDO	PCI	Clopidogrel 300mg loading then 75mg daily Aspirin 325mg	Placebo loading, active clopidogrel for 28 days post PCI, then placebo+aspirin throughout	Death, stroke, MI	12	89/1,053 (8.5%)	122/1,063 (11.5%)	0.73 (0.56–0.96) P=0.02	1.31 P=0.07
CHARISMA	CAD, CVD, PAD or combination of risk factors	Clopidogrel 75mg Aspirin 75–162mg	Placebo clopidogrel plus aspirin	CV death, MI, stroke	Median 28 months	534/7,802 (6.8%)	573/7,801 (7.3%)	0.93 (0.83–1.05) P=0.22	1.25 (0.97–1.61) P=0.09
Cerebrovascular disease									
MATCH	Prior stroke or TIA	Clopidogrel 75mg Aspirin 75mg	Clopidogrel 75mg Placebo aspirin	Vascular death, ischemic stroke, MI	18	445/3,797 (11.7%)	473/3,802 (12.4%)	0.94 (0.83–1.07) P=0.36	1.36 (0.86–1.86) P<0.001
Atrial fibrillation									
ACTIVE-W	Atrial fibrillation with high-risk features	Clopidogrel 75mg Aspirin 75–100mg	Warfarin or other oral anticoagulant (OAC)	CV death, MI, stroke	15 months	234/3,335 (7.0%)	OAC 165/3,371 (4.9%)	1.44 (1.18–1.76) P=0.0003	1.10 (0.83–1.45) P=0.53
ACTIVE-A	Atrial fibrillation with high-risk features	Clopidogrel 75mg Aspirin 75–100mg	Placebo clopidogrel plus aspirin	CV death, MI, stroke	36 months				

aEstimated from published data where information is not exactly as required for the table. *ACS* Acute coronary syndrome, *CAD* Coronary artery disease, *CVD* Cerebrovascular disease, *HR* Hazard ratio, *95% CI* 95% Confidence intervals, *OAC* Oral anticoagulation, *PAD* Peripheral arterial disease, *PCI* Percutaneous coronary intervention, *TIA* Transient ischemic attack

325 mg *(10)*. The annual rates of death, stroke, or MI over the average 2 years of follow-up were 5.3% and 5.8%, respectively (HR: 0.91; 95%: 0.83–0.97; *P*=0.04). Although there was a slight benefit of clopidogrel over aspirin, there was no change in clinical practice because the cost of clopidogrel was much higher than aspirin and the effects size considered small. Importantly CAPRIE established the efficacy and safety of clopidogrel as a useful antiplatelet agent and an alternative treatment if patients could not tolerate aspirin. The next major trial was the CURE trial, discussed in detail in other chapters, which enrolled 12,562 patients with ACS without ST elevation on the presenting ECG and randomized patients to a combination of clopidogrel plus aspirin (C+A; loading dose of clopidogrel 300 mg followed by 75 mg) or aspirin alone (75–300 mg) for up to 1 year (mean duration of treatment about 9 months) on top of other standard treatments (Table 1) *(11)*. The risk of cardiovascular death, stroke, or MI was 9.3% in the C+A group and 11.4% in the aspirin alone group (HR: 0.80; 95%CI: 0.72–0.90; *P*<0.001) establishing this as a standard approach for the management of ACS without persistent ST elevation. Following the success of the CURE trial clopidogrel was investigated for the management of cerebrovascular disease and atrial fibrillation as well as ACS with ST elevation.

The CLARITY-TIMI 28 trial *(12)* and COMMIT CCS-2 *(13)* studies were complementary trials evaluating clopidogrel plus aspirin for the management of ST elevation ACS. CLARITY was an angiographic study in patients treated with fibrinolysis as the method of reperfusion and enrolled 3,491 patients randomized to C+A or aspirin alone. Rates of occluded arteries (TIMI flow grade 0 or 1) were 11.7% in the C+A group and 18.4% in the aspirin alone group (HR: 0.59; 95% CI: 0.48–0.72; *P*<0.001, Table 6.1) which was the main driver of the primary outcome composite assessed at angiography of an occluded infarct related artery, death, or MI. COMMIT was a large pragmatic study of 45,852 patients with mainly ST elevation myocardial infarction enrolled in China randomized to either C+A (75 mg clopidogrel + 162 mg aspirin) or aspirin alone and treated for 4 weeks. The rate of death, stroke, or MI occurred in 9.2% in the C+A group and 10.1% in aspirin alone (HR: 0.91; 95% CI: 0.86–0.97; *P*=0.002), and there was a significant reduction in all cause mortality (HR: 0.93; 95% CI: 0.83–0.99; *P*=0.03). These two trials have established clopidogrel as a standard approach for patients with ST elevation ACS treated with fibrinolysis. Previous smaller trials had shown benefits of clopidogrel in patients undergoing PCI with stenting, and therefore the use of clopidogrel is standard practice for patients with ST elevation MI undergoing primary PCI *(14)*.

The MATCH trial investigated the effects of clopidogrel in patients with established cerebrovascular disease by comparing clopidogrel alone with C+A in 7,599 patients followed for a mean of 18 months *(15)*. This study design was different from CURE, CLARITY, and COMMIT as the control group was treated with clopidogrel alone, rather than aspirin alone as in the other trials. The primary outcome of death, stroke, MI, or cardiovascular hospitalization occurred in 15.7% patients in the C+A group compared to 16.7% in the clopidogrel alone group (HR: 0.93; 95%CI: 0.84–1.05). This trial did not support the routine use of C+A in patients with prior stroke or transient ischemic attack, but this combination could be superior to aspirin alone which was not tested in MATCH. The ACTIVE-W trial investigated the role of C+A for the management of atrial fibrillation (AF) treated with warfarin *(16)*. 6,706 patients with AF and additional risk factors for stroke, MI, or death were randomized in an open label design to warfarin or C+A and followed for a mean of 18 months. The annual risk of stroke, death, or MI was 5·6 in the C+A group compared to 3·9% on warfarin (HR: 1·44; 95% CI: 1·18–1.76; *P*=0.0003) driven mainly by the excess of nonfatal strokes. Overall mortality and major bleeding rates were similar between the two groups. Thus ACTIVE W did not support the use of C+A as a replacement treatment for oral anticoagulation for AF, especially in those already stabilized on warfarin (most of the ACTIVE-W patients). The ACTIVE trial is also investigating the role of C+A compared to aspirin alone in patients who cannot tolerate warfarin (ACTIVE A), and also the role of irbesartan, an angiotensin-II antagonist for vascular protection in patients with AF (ACTIVE I) *(17)*.

Other studies have evaluated the longer-term role of clopidogrel in patients undergoing PCI in the nonacute setting in particular the CREDO trial which enrolled 2,116 patients who underwent PCI with stent placement randomized to C+A (loading dose of 300 mg followed by 75 mg) or aspirin alone (with all patients receiving 28 days of open label clopidogrel following the procedure) *(18)*. At 1 year, the hazard ratio for the primary outcome of death, stroke, or MI for C+A compared to aspirin alone was 0.73 (95% CI: 0.65–0.0.96; $P=0.02$) providing support for a loading dose of clopidogrel prior to PCI and continuing for up to a year. There is much discussion about the exact role of clopidogrel in the context of PCI and stenting *(19)*. There is general agreement that a loading dose of 300 mg is a standard approach and higher doses are being investigated in the large CURRENT trial *(20)*. Clinical guidelines suggest continuation of clopidogrel therapy (in addition to aspirin) for a minimum of 1 month (ideally 12) following bare-metal stent insertion and for at least 12 months after drug-cluting stent PCI *(21)*. Longer-term use of thienopyridines has been associated with improved outcomes in bare metal stents with a relative risk reduction of 65% for the composite of death, MI, and stroke comparing 180-day with 30-day treatment *(22)*. Early stopping of dual antiplatelet therapy following implantation of drug eluting stents is associated with early and late stent-thrombosis *(23,24)*. The main trial that evaluated the role of clopidogrel for longer-term vascular protection in patients at risk of vascular events (either with established vascular disease, or with risk factors) was CHARISMA which is discussed in more detail as follows *(25)*.

THE CHARISMA TRIAL

The CHARISMA trial set out to answer the question "could a combination of clopidogrel and aspirin provide greater vascular protection than aspirin alone in a wide range of stable patients in at risk of vascular events" *(25)*. Eligibility criteria for entry were broad — patients could qualify if they had a clear diagnosis of coronary, cerebrovascular, or peripheral arterial disease (without a definite prior stroke or MI), or if they had a combination of risk factors such as diabetes, hyperc-holesterolemia, hypertension, or smoking (without a clear prior history of vascular disease). The trial enrolled 15,603 patients randomized to C+A or aspirin alone and followed for a median of 28 months. The primary outcome of cardiovascular death, stroke, or MI occurred in 6.8% of the C+A group and 7.3% of the aspirin alone group (relative risk: 0.93; 95%CI: 0.83–1.05; $P=0.22$) suggesting a trend in favor of C+A in this broad population (Table 2). A secondary outcome that included rates of cardiovascular hospitalization was marginally significant in favor of C+A. Patients with no clear history of vascular disease made up about 20% of the total, and in this subgroup there was a trend to an adverse effect of C+A on the primary outcome and a higher rate of cardiovascular death (3.9% C+A vs. 2.2% on aspirin alone). In contrast, in those patients with clear evidence of prior vascular disease rates of the primary outcome were 6.9% vs. 7.9% ($P=0.046$) with no apparent difference in rates of death in this subgroup (Table 2, Fig. 2). Overall rates of major bleeding in the C+A group were 1.7% compared to 1.3% in the aspirin group ($P=0.09$), and there was a significant excess of moderate bleeding.

The results of CHARISMA appear disappointing because there is no clear indication for the use of clopidogrel in this large population of community-based patients that are at moderate to high risk of vascular events. Recent data from the American Heart Association estimate that there may be 15 million people in the United States with prior stroke, MI, or symptomatic PAD *(26)*. If their annual risk of death, stroke, or MI was 3% there would be about 450,000 events each year and just a 1%

Table 2
Major subgroups of the CHARISMA trial

Subgroup of interest	N (%) of total CHARISMA population (total N = 15,603)	CV death, MI, stroke (Clopidogrel plus aspirin)	CV Death, MI, stroke (Placebo clopidogrel plus aspirin)	HR	95%CI	P
Symptomatic vascular disease	12,153 (78%)	6.9%	7.9%	0.88	0.77–1.0	0.05
Prior MI, prior stroke, PAD	9,478 (61%)	7.3%	8.8%	0.83	0.72–0.96	0.01
PAD	3,096 (19.8%)	7.6%	8.9%	0.85	0.66–1.08	0.18
Asymptomatic	3,284 (21%)	6.6%	5.5%	1.2	0.91–1.59	0.20
Primary prevention	2,289 (14.7%)	5.7%	4.7%	1.2		0.30

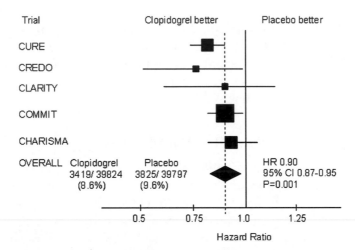

Fig. 1. Horizontal box and whiskers plot of the results of the randomized trials of clopidogrel versus placebo on a background of aspirin. *Squares* represent point estimates of the hazard ratio for each trial, and the *horizontal lines* represent the 95% confidence intervals around these estimates. The *size of the squares* represents the relative amount of statistical information in the trial which is influenced by the number of patients and number of events. The overall pooled hazard ratio, confidence intervals, and *P*-value were estimated using a simple proportional formula. Refer to Table 1 for details of the trials.

reduction would avoid 4,500 events. These estimates reinforce the need for trials like CHARISMA which can have profound public health benefits even if they show moderate treatment benefits of the order of 10–20% proportional reductions.

POOLED ANALYSIS OF LARGE TRIALS OF CLOPIDOGREL PLUS ASPIRIN

Table 1 and Fig. 1 summarize the available published evidence from the large trials of C+A and show that about 80,000 patients have been randomized into these studies. The overall hazard ratio for death, stroke, and MI is about 0.90 (*P*<0.001) with an absolute reduction of 1% in favor of C+A compared to aspirin alone. The average increase in the risk of major bleeds requiring hospitalization and/or transfusion is about 30%.

ADDITIONAL ANALYSES FROM CHARISMA

A number of additional analyses have been undertaken by the CHARISMA investigators and probably the most important issue is to try and understand if the effects in patients with and without prior vascular disease are due to play of chance (i.e., there is no real difference in effect of C+A compared to aspirin) or whether there may be a genuine qualitative interaction. In the context of assessing therapeutic effects in subgroups of clinical trials, a *quantitative* interaction is a difference of effect in amount or quantity, but still in the same direction (this would be an *expected* interaction), and a *qualitative* interaction is a difference in direction of effect (evidence of apparent harm one group and apparent benefit in another which is usually *unexpected*) *(27)*.

The CAPRIE trial had already established the benefit and safety of clopidogrel compared to aspirin, and therefore it was logical to undertake an analysis of the "CAPRIE like" patients in the CHARISMA trial, i.e., those with a prior MI, prior stroke, or symptomatic PAD. There were 9,478 patients who met these criteria (61% of the total CHARISMA population and 78% of those with any prior vascular disease), and the primary outcome of CV death, stroke, or MI occurred in 7.3% in the C+A group versus 8.8% in the aspirin alone group (HR: 0.83; 95% CI: 0.72–0.96; $P=0.01$) suggesting that there were potentially greater benefits of C+A in these patients than in the CHARISMA group overall (Table 2, Fig. 2) *(28)*. The trend for benefit in the CAPRIE-like cohort was also greater than the broader group of patients who had evidence of prior vascular disease but not necessarily a prior stroke or MI. Additionally, hospitalizations for ischemia were significantly decreased, 11.4% versus 13.2%, respectively (HR: 0.86; 95% CI: 0.76–0.96; $P=0.008$). There was no significant difference in the rate of severe bleeding: 1.7% versus 1.5% (HR: 1.12; 95% CI: 0.81–1.53; $P=0.50$) but moderate bleeding was significantly increased: 2.0% versus 1.3% (HR: 1.60; 95% CI: 1.16–2.20; $P=0.004$). A similar trend was found in the PAD subgroup (Table 2, Fig. 2) *(29)*. A more detailed analysis of the asymptomatic or primary prevention cohort confirmed the original findings in the main report of CHARISMA, but it has been difficult to elucidate the mechanism of potential harm in this group (Table 2) *(30)*. One hypothesis was that the excess risk is caused by increased bleeding, but rates of fatal bleeds were similar to the overall group, and also similar whether patients were on C+A or aspirin alone. About 80% of patients in the asymptomatic populations of CHARISMA were diabetic, and there is a possibility that these patients may be more prone to plaque hemorrhage and therefore a worse outcome, as a result of intensive antiplatelet treatment with C+A, but this remains speculation at present.

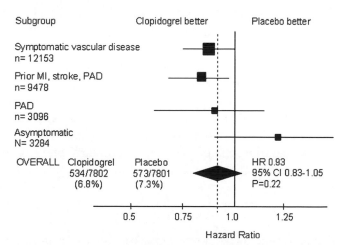

Fig. 2. Major subgroups are shown from the CHARISMA trial. Details of the *squares* and *horizontal lines* are the same as for Fig. 1. The interaction test for heterogeneity between the symptomatic and asymptomatic group was about 0.045. Refer to Table 2 for more details of these subgroups. *MI* myocardial infarction; *PAD* peripheral arterial disease.

Of greater importance is the potential benefit of C+A in apparently stable patients at high risk of vascular events, a clear hypothesis generated by the CHARISMA trial. This hypothesis has a sound basis both in the previous CAPRIE results and the subgroup analyses from CHARISMA itself. A clinical trial randomizing patients to a combination of a thienopyridine (clopidogrel or prasugrel) in combination with aspirin compared to aspirin alone in patients with prior MI, prior stroke, or symptomatic PAD would be important, but it seems unlikely that this will be carried by industry as the patent life of clopidogrel is running out and the focus for prasugrel at present is still in ACS.

THIENOPYRIDINES IN STABLE CORONARY ARTERY DISEASE

Data on the effects of C+A in the subgroup of patients with CAD have not been published from the CHARISMA trial, but presentations of these data and interpretation from the available publications suggest that an expected proportional reduction of about 15% for CAD patients is consistent with the CAPRIE like cohort subgroup. In the main publication of CHARISMA, subgroup analyses suggest that patients with prior MI had a trend to benefit from C+A whereas those without prior MI who appeared to have little benefit *(25)*.

SHOULD DUAL ANTIPLATELET TREATMENT
BE STARTED IN STABLE PATIENTS?

There is little clear evidence to routinely add a thienopyridine to aspirin in patients with stable coronary, cerebrovascular, or symptomatic PAD, and no evidence to start this regimen for primary prevention in patients without evidence of vascular disease. Clearly clopidogrel is indicated in patients who need vascular protection and cannot tolerate aspirin which is supported by the CAPRIE data.

The REACH registry which ran concurrently with the CHARISMA trial with similar eligibility criteria in an observational study design, documented characteristics, treatments, and outcomes in 68,000 patients *(31)*. One important finding of the REACH registry is that patients with vascular disease in more than one territory (coronary, cerebrovascular, or peripheral) have a greater risk of adverse outcomes than patients with either no documented vascular disease or disease in a single territory. Annual average risk of death, stroke, or MI in the REACH registry was between 4% and 5% compared to the overall risk in CHARISMA which was 3%. This suggests that future studies of dual antiplatelet therapy for the protection of vascular events in an outpatient setting should focus on patients with a prior vascular event, symptomatic peripheral arterial disease, or patients with evidence of disease in more than one vascular territory.

It is also important to review the findings of giving clopidogrel to patients with stable cerebrovascular disease and peripheral arterial disease (PAD). In both situations there is no clear evidence for adding clopidogrel to aspirin in spite of a good rationale for more intensive antiplatelet therapy than aspirin alone (although in the case of patients with prior stroke, dipyridamole is often added to aspirin). There have not been any specific trials in PAD to evaluate the long-term protective effects of a thienopyridine added to aspirin and the MATCH trial, one of the largest secondary prevention stroke trials, did not confirm the benefits of dual antiplatelet therapy compared to clopidogrel alone *(15)*.

DISCUSSION

Inferences about the potential benefits of adding a thienopyridine to aspirin for secondary prevention of vascular events can be drawn from the ACS studies such as CURE and TRITON-TIMI 38 *(11,32)*. The pattern of underlying risk and benefit is very similar in these trials indicating the main absolute and proportional benefits are achieved early on (within about a month of the acute event), but careful review of later effects (e.g., >1 month after the acute event) also indicates evidence of benefit *(32,33)*. This raises the question about the duration of treatment after an acute event in patients, and what level of underlying risk do patients need to have to expect benefit from a thienopyridine added to aspirin. This in turn leads to the issue of the mechanism of action of antiplatelet therapy, the balance of benefit and risk, and the issue of variability of response or "resistance." A recent position paper from the Working Group on Thrombosis of the European Society of Cardiology *(1)* identifies pharmacody-namic resistance to clopidogrel (for example potential gene polymorphism in the P2Y12 receptor) and pharmacokinetic resistance. The latter includes issues with absorption, inadequate dosage, and impaired liver metabolism. Due to the scarcity of prospective trials linking platelet measurements with outcome, assessment of platelet function is not currently recommended *(34)* For research centers encountering patients with recurrent vascular events, suggested tests include functional assessment of clopidogrel resistance using adenosine diphosphate-induced aggregation and biochemical assessment using vasodilator-stimulated phosphoprotein (VASP) assays.

Noncompliance with clopidogrel treatment is also a major concern *(35)*. In a study of 2,360 patients successfully revascularized with drug-eluting stents, 32.4% had some degree of bleeding, predominantly nuisance bleeds (85.7%) but also including internal (13.6%; epistaxis, gastrointestinal, hematuria, etc.) and more substantial bleeds (0.7%; intracranial, life-threatening or requiring transfusion) *(36)*. In the nuisance bleeding group, 11.1% ceased clopidogrel therapy and 5% stopped aspirin.

Antiplatelet agents reduce the activity of platelets (with variable effects on the traditional model of adhesion, activation, and aggregation) imparting a benefit in patients at relatively high risk of arterial thrombotic complications, a situation that is particularly evident during ACS or PCI (in the latter case there is arterial injury which increases thrombotic risk). Where patients have recovered from the acute event (e.g., >6 months later) the evidence for routinely adding a thienopyridine to aspirin is limited. However this is where an assessment of ongoing risk is important and the methods to do this either rely on traditional scoring systems such as Framingham or SCORE (the latter is a validated European risk prediction model) *(37,38)*, or to use simple clinical surrogates as a history of prior MI, stroke, or symptomatic vascular disease, or disease in more than one vascular territory. Even with an assessment of risk of future vascular events at >5% per annum, the addition of a thienopyridine to aspirin is specu-lative at present and is not based on solid evidence, especially as there is an ongoing bleeding hazard in the region of 1.3 times that of aspirin alone. Further trials to clarify this important question are urgently needed.

REFERENCES

1. Böhm M, Werner C, Jakobsen A, Heroys J, Ralph A, Rees T, Shaw M (2008) Treating to protect: current cardiovascular treatment approaches and remaining needs. Medscape J Med 10(Suppl):S3
2. Ebrahim S, Beswick A, Burke M, Davey Smith G. (2006) Multiple risk factor interventions for primary prevention of coronary heart disease. Cochrane Database Syst Rev (4):CD001561. Review.
3. Sanz G, Fuster V (2009) Fixed-dose combination therapy and secondary cardiovascular prevention: rationale, selection of drugs and target population. Nat Clin Pract Cardiovasc Med 6(2):101–110 Epub 2008 Dec 23
4. Yusuf S, Hawken S, Ounpuu S, Dans T, Avezum A, Lanas F, McQueen M, Budaj A, Pais P, Varigos J, Lisheng L, INTER-HEART Study Investigators (2004) Effect of potentially modifiable risk factors associated with myocardial infarction in 52 countries (the INTERHEART study): case-control study. Lancet 364(9438):937–952
5. Antithrombotic Trialists' Collaboration (2002) Collaborative meta-analysis of randomised trials of antiplatelet therapy for prevention of death, myocardial infarction, and stroke in high risk patients. BMJ 324:71–86
6. Van de Werf F (2007) Dual antiplatelet therapy in high-risk patients. Eur Heart J 9(Supplement D):D3–D9
7. Steinhubl SR, Schneider DJ, Berger PB, Becker RC (2008) Determining the efficacy of antiplatelet therapies for the individual: lessons from clinical trials. J Thromb Thrombolysis 26(1):8–13 Epub 2007 Nov 1

8. Toth PP (2009) The potential role of prasugrel in secondary prevention of ischemic events in patients with acute coronary syndromes. Postgrad Med 121(1):59–72

9. Norgard NB (2008) Abu-Fadel M Future prospects in anti-platelet therapy: a review of potential P2Y12 and thrombin receptor antagonists. Recent Pat Cardiovasc Drug Discov 3(3):194–200

10. Gent M, CAPRIE Steering Committee (1996) A randomised, blinded, trial of clopidogrel versus aspirin in patients at risk of ischaemic events(CAPRIE). Lancet 348:1329–1339

11. Yusuf S, Zhao F, Mehta SR, Chrolavicius S, Tognoni G, Fox KK, Clopidogrel in Unstable Angina to Prevent Recurrent Events Trial Investigators (2001) Effects of clopidogrel in addition to aspirin in patients with acute coronary syndromes without ST-segment elevation. N Engl J Med 345(7):494–502

12. Sabatine MS, Cannon CP, Gibson CM, López-Sendón JL, Montalescot G, Theroux P, Claeys MJ, Cools F, Hill KA, Skene AM, McCabe CH, Braunwald E, CLARITY-TIMI 28 Investigators (2005) Addition of clopidogrel to aspirin and fibrinolytic therapy for myocardial infarction with ST-segment elevation. N Engl J Med 352(12):1179–1189 Epub 2005 Mar 9

13. Chen ZM, Jiang LX, Chen YP, Xie JX, Pan HC, Peto R, Collins R, Liu LS (2005) Addition of clopidogrel to aspirin in 45,852 patients with acute myocardial infarction: randomised placebo-controlled trial. COMMIT (ClOpidogrel and Metoprolol in Myocardial Infarction Trial) collaborative group. Lancet 366(9497):1607–1621

14. Vlaar PJ, Svilaas T, Damman K, de Smet BJ, Tijssen JG, Hillege HL, Zijlstra F (2008) Impact of pretreatment with clopidogrel on initial patency and outcome in patients treated with primary percutaneous coronary intervention for ST-segment elevation myocardial infarction: a systematic review. Circulation 118(18):1828–1836 Epub 2008 Oct 13. Review

15. Diener HC, Bogousslavsky J, Brass LM, Cimminiello C, Csiba L, Kaste M, Leys D, Matias-Guiu J, Rupprecht HJ, MATCH investigators (2004) Aspirin and clopidogrel compared with clopidogrel alone after recent ischaemic stroke or transient ischaemic attack in high-risk patients (MATCH): randomised, double-blind, placebo-controlled trial. Lancet 364(9431):331–337

16. Connolly S, Pogue J, Hart R, Pfeffer M, Hohnloser S, Chrolavicius S, Yusuf S (2006) ACTIVE Investigators Clopidogrel plus aspirin versus oral anticoagulation for atrial fibrillation in the Atrial fibrillation Clopidogrel Trial with Irbesartan for prevention of Vascular Events (ACTIVE W): a randomised controlled trial. Lancet 367(9526):1903–1912

17. Connolly S, Yusuf S, Budaj A, Camm J, Chrolavicius S, Commerford PJ, Flather M, Fox KA, Hart R, Hohnloser S, Joyner C, Pfeffer M, Anand I, Arthur H, Avezum A, Bethala-Sithya M, Blumenthal M, Ceremuzynski L, De Caterina R, Diaz R, Flaker G, Frangin G, Franzosi MG, Gaudin C, Golitsyn S, Goldhaber S, Granger C, Halon D, Hermosillo A, Hunt D, Jansky P, Karatzas N, Keltai M, Lanas F, Lau CP, Le Heuzey JY, Lewis BS, Morais J, Morillo C, Oto A, Paolasso E, Peters RJ, Pfisterer M, Piegas L, Pipillis T, Proste C, Sitkei E, Swedberg K, Synhorst D, Talajic M, Trégou V, Valentin V, van Mieghem W, Weintraub W, Varigos J (2006) The Active Steering Committee; ACTIVE Investigators, Rationale and design of ACTIVE: the atrial fibrillation clopidogrel trial with irbesartan for prevention of vascular events. Am Heart J 151(6):1187–1193

18. Steinhubl SR, Berger PB, Mann JT III, Fry ET, DeLago A, Wilmer C, Topol EJ, CREDO Investigators (2002) Early and sustained dual oral antiplatelet therapy following percutaneous coronary intervention: a randomized controlled trial. Clopidogrel for the Reduction of Events During Observation. JAMA 288(19):2411–2420 Erratum in: JAMA. 2003 Feb 26;289(8):987

19. Buonamici P, Marcucci R, Migliorini A, Gensini GF, Santini A, Paniccia R, Moschi G, Gori AM, Abbate R, Antoniucci D (2007) Impact of platelet reactivity after clopidogrel administration on drug-eluting stent thrombosis. J Am Coll Cardiol 49(24):2312–2317

20. Mehta SR, Bassand JP, Chrolavicius S, Diaz R, Fox KA, Granger CB, Jolly S, Rupprecht HJ, Widimsky P, Yusuf S, CURRENT-OASIS 7 Steering Committee (2008) Design and rationale of CURRENT-OASIS 7: a randomized, 2 x 2 factorial trial evaluating optimal dosing strategies for clopidogrel and aspirin in patients with ST and non-ST-elevation acute coronary syndromes managed with an early invasive s. Am Heart J 156(6):1080.e1–1088.e1 Epub 2008 Nov 1

21. King SB III, Smith SC Jr, Hirshfeld JW Jr, Jacobs AK, Morrison DA, Williams DO, Feldman TE, Kern MJ, O'Neill WW, Schaff HV, Whitlow PL, ACC/AHA/SCAI, Adams CD, Anderson JL, Buller CE, Creager MA, Ettinger SM, Halperin JL, Hunt SA, Krumholz HM, Kushner FG, Lytle BW, Nishimura R, Page RL, Riegel B, Tarkington LG, Yancy CW (2008) 2007 focused update of the ACC/AHA/SCAI 2005 guideline update for percutaneous coronary intervention: a report of the American College of Cardiology/American Heart Association Task Force on Practice guidelines. J Am Coll Cardiol 51(2):172–209

22. Bernardi V, Szarfer J, Summay G, Mendiz O, Sarmiento R, Alemparte MR, Gabay J, Berger PB (2007) Long-term versus short-term clopidogrel therapy in patients undergoing coronary stenting (from the Randomized Argentine Clopidogrel Stent [RACS] trial). Am J Cardiol 99(3):349–352

23. Iakovou I, Schmidt T, Bonizzoni E, Ge L, Sangiorgi GM, Stankovic G, Airoldi F, Chieffo A, Montorfano M, Carlino M, Michev I, Corvaja N, Briguori C, Gerckens U, Grube E, Colombo A (2005) Incidence, predictors, and outcome of thrombosis after successful implantation of drug-eluting stents. JAMA 293(17):2126–2130

24. Pfisterer M, Brunner-La Rocca HP, Rickenbacher P, Hunziker P, Mueller C, Nietlispach F, Leibundgut G, Bader F, Kaiser C, BASKET Investigators (2009) Long-term benefit-risk balance of drug-eluting vs. bare-metal stents in daily practice: does stent diameter matter? Three-year follow-up of BASKET. Eur Heart J 30(1):16–24

25. Bhatt DL, Fox KA, Hacke W, Berger PB, Black HR, Boden WE, Cacoub P, Cohen EA, Creager MA, Easton JD, Flather MD, Haffner SM, Hamm CW, Hankey GJ, Johnston SC, Mak KH, Mas JL, Montalescot G, Pearson TA, Steg PG, Steinhubl SR, Weber MA, Brennan DM, Fabry-Ribaudo L, Booth J, Topol EJ, CHARISMA Investigators (2006) Clopidogrel and aspirin versus aspirin alone for the prevention of atherothrombotic events. N Engl J Med 354(16):1706–1717 Epub 2006 Mar 12

26. American Heart Association. Heart and Stroke Statistics 2008. http://www.americanheart.org/downloadable/heart/1200078608862HS_Stats%202008.final.pdf

27. Yusuf S, Wittes J, Probstfield J, Tyroler HA (1991) Analysis and interpretation of treatment effects in subgroups of patients in randomized clinical trials. JAMA 266(1):93–98

28. Bhatt DL, Flather MD, Hacke W, Berger PB, Black HR, Boden WE, Cacoub P, Cohen EA, Creager MA, Easton JD, Hamm CW, Hankey GJ, Johnston SC, Mak KH, Mas JL, Montalescot G, Pearson TA, Steg PG, Steinhubl SR, Weber MA, Fabry-Ribaudo L, Hu T, Topol EJ, Fox KA, CHARISMA Investigators (2007) Patients with prior myocardial infarction, stroke, or symptomatic peripheral arterial disease in the CHARISMA trial. J Am Coll Cardiol 49(19):1982–1988 Epub 2007 Apr 11

29. Cacoub PP, Bhatt DL, Steg PG, Topol EJ, Creager MA, CHARISMA Investigators (2009) Patients with peripheral arterial disease in the CHARISMA trial. Eur Heart J 30(2):192–201 Epub 2009 Jan 9

30. Wang TH, Bhatt DL, Fox KA, Steinhubl SR, Brennan DM, Hacke W, Mak KH, Pearson TA, Boden WE, Steg PG, Flather MD, Montalescot G, Topol EJ, CHARISMA Investigators (2007) An analysis of mortality rates with dual-antiplatelet therapy in the primary prevention population of the CHARISMA trial. Eur Heart J 28(18):2200–2207

31. Steg PG, Bhatt DL, Wilson PW, D'Agostino R Sr, Ohman EM, Röther J, Liau CS, Hirsch AT, Mas JL, Ikeda Y, Pencina MJ, Goto S, REACH Registry Investigators (2007) One-year cardiovascular event rates in outpatients with atherothrombosis. JAMA 297(11):1197–1206

32. Wiviott SD, Braunwald E, McCabe CH, Montalescot G, Ruzyllo W, Gottlieb S, Neumann FJ, Ardissino D, De Servi S, Murphy SA, Riesmeyer J, Weerakkody G, Gibson CM, Antman EM, TRITON-TIMI 38 Investigators (2007) Prasugrel versus clopidogrel in patients with acute coronary syndromes. N Engl J Med 357(20):2001–2015

33. Yusuf S, Mehta SR, Zhao F, Gersh BJ, Commerford PJ, Blumenthal M, Budaj A, Wittlinger T, Fox KA, Clopidogrel in Unstable angina to prevent Recurrent Events Trial Investigators (2003) Early and late effects of clopidogrel in patients with acute coronary syndromes. Circulation 107(7):966–972

34. Kuliczkowski W, Witkowski A, Polonski L, Watala C, Filipiak K, Budaj A, Golanski J, Sitkiewicz D, Pregowski J, Gorski J, Zembala M, Opolski G, Huber K, Arnesen H, Kristensen SD, De Caterina R (2009) Interindividual variability in the response to oral antiplatelet drugs: a position paper of the Working Group on antiplatelet drugs resistance appointed by the Section of Cardiovascular Interventions of the Polish Cardiac Society, endorsed by the Working Group on Thrombosis of the European Society of Cardiology. Eur Heart J 30(4):426–435

35. Kuchulakanti PK, Chu WW, Torguson R, Ohlmann P, Rha S-W, Clavijo LC, Kim S-W, Bui A, Gevorkian N, Xue Z, Smith K, Fournadjieva J, Suddath WO, Satler LF, Pichard AD, Kent KM, Waksman R (2006) Correlates and Long-Term Outcomes of Angiographically Proven Stent Thrombosis With Sirolimus- and Paclitaxel-Eluting Stents. Circulation 113(8):1108–1113

36. Roy P, Bonello L, Torguson R, de Labriolle A, Lemesle G, Slottow TLP, Steinberg DH, Kaneshige K, Xue Z, Satler LF, Kent KM, Suddath WO, Pichard AD, Lindsay J, Waksman R (2008) Impact of "Nuisance" Bleeding on Clopidogrel Compliance in Patients Undergoing Intracoronary Drug-Eluting Stent Implantation. Am J Cardiol 102(12):1614–1617

37. Scheltens T, Verschuren WM, Boshuizen HC, Hoes AW, Zuithoff NP, Bots ML, Grobbee DE (2008) Estimation of cardiovascular risk: a comparison between the Framingham and the SCORE model in people under 60 years of age. Eur J Cardiovasc Prev Rehabil 15(5):562–566

38. de Ruijter W, Westendorp RG, Assendelft WJ, den Elzen WP, de Craen AJ, le Cessie S, Gussekloo J (2009) Use of Framingham risk score and new biomarkers to predict cardiovascular mortality in older people: population-based observational cohort study. BMJ 338:a3083. doi:10.1136/bmj.a3083

Part III
Antithrombotic Therapy for NSTE ACS

7

Antiplatelet Therapies in Unstable Angina and Non-ST Segment Elevation Myocardial Infarction

Saif Anwaruddin and Deepak L. Bhatt

CONTENTS

ABSTRACT The central role of the platelet in the pathophysiology of acute coronary syndromes (ACS) has been well established. The significant morbidity and mortality associated with ACS has fostered great interest and effort in identifying various antiplatelet and antithrombotic regimens as well as developing novel agents in order to abrogate the platelet and its associated prothrombotic effects. Aspirin remains the integral component of all therapeutic strategies for ACS. When used in combination with thienopyridines (i.e., clopidogrel), GP IIb/IIIa inhibitors (abciximab, eptifibatide, tirofiban), or both, patients have experienced improved outcomes in this setting. However, with more potent antiplatelet regimens comes an increased risk of bleeding. Thus, the search for more potent antiplatelet agents with a decreased risk of bleeding continues for this patient population.

Key words: Acute coronary syndromes; Aspirin; Clopidogrel; Glycoprotein IIb/IIIa inhibitors; Non-T-segment-elevation myocardial infarction; Percutaneous coronary intervention; ST segment-elevation myocardial infarction; Thienopyridines

INTRODUCTION

Improved understanding of the relationship between inflammation, thrombosis, and acute coronary syndromes (ACS) has fostered advances in management which have dramatically altered the approach and outcomes related to this disease *(1)*. Although advances in percutaneous coronary intervention

From: *Contemporary Cardiology: Antithrombotic Drug Therapy in Cardiovascular Disease*
Edited by: A.T. Askari and A.M. Lincoff (eds.), DOI 10.1007/978-1-60327-235-3_7
© Humana Press, a part of Springer Science+Business Media, LLC 2010

(PCI) have improved the ability to restore flow in an infarct related artery, the majority of benefits can be attributed to enhanced adjunctive pharmacotherapies.

The inciting events of a non-ST-segment-elevation myocardial infarction (NSTEMI) are, most often, erosion and rupture of atherosclerotic plaque(s) within the coronary tree *(1)*. With the rupture of the atherosclerotic plaque, the sub-endothelial matrix and lipid core of the plaque are exposed to circulating pro-thrombotic factors including tissue factor and von Willebrand Factor (vWF). vWF, a key component to the initiation of thrombosis, binds to the subendothelial collagen matrix and is then able to bind platelets via the combination of shear stress and the glycoprotein (GP) 1b receptor *(2,3)*. The binding of vWF to the GP 1b receptor has been shown to be important in platelet activation via the $P2Y_{12}$ ADP receptor *(4)*. Once the initial defect in the endothelium has been covered by platelets, the process of further platelet recruitment, activation, and cross-linking with fibrinogen begins. This sequence of events forms the basis for understanding the importance of antiplatelet and antithrombotic therapies in NSTEMI.

In the minority of cases, NSTEMI is caused by a fixed stenosis leading to a secondary reduction in epicardial coronary blood flow such that the oxygen supply cannot meet an increased demand (i.e., tachycardia, sepsis, etc). This chapter will expound upon the importance of platelet biology and will discuss the present and future of antiplatelet pharmacotherapy for NSTEMI.

PLATELETS: CONNECTING INFLAMMATION AND THROMBOSIS

Despite their size, platelets are complex and display a wide functionality. In the setting of plaque rupture, after initial platelet response, activated platelets are then able to attract other platelets to the site of injury in a paracrine fashion. This is mediated through platelet-derived factors such as adenosine diphosphate (ADP) and thromboxane A2 (TXA-2). Platelet activation results in a conformational change that includes the externalization of glycoprotein IIb/IIIa (GP IIb/IIIa) receptors, essential receptors that facilitate the cross-binding of platelets to fibrinogen and the formation of a stable thrombus. Since there are several pathways that facilitate platelet activation, different antiplatelet therapies are often used in combination to optimize outcomes.

In addition to their prothrombotic properties, platelets can exert potent inflammatory effects through a variety of platelet-derived receptors, adhesion molecules, and mediators including CD40L and P-selectin. Interactions between these molecules and receptors on the surface of other cell types ultimately leads to the recruitment of leukocytes, further release of inflammatory mediators, and the perpetuation of a prothrombotic state *(5,6)*.

Clinically, sCD40L has been related to adverse outcomes in patients presenting with ACS *(7)* and following presentation for ACS *(8)*. The use of glycoprotein IIb/IIIa inhibitors, such as abciximab, has been shown to be of benefit in those with ACS, especially with elevated levels of sCD40L *(7)*. P-selectin has also been shown to predict adverse cardiovascular events in otherwise healthy patients *(9)*.

CURRENT ANTIPLATELET THERAPIES IN NON-ST-SEGMENT MYOCARDIAL INFARCTION

Aspirin

The intra-platelet metabolism of arachadonic acid into TXA2 facilitates activation of other platelets. These steps are driven by the action of the enzyme, cyclo-oxygenase-1 (COX-1). Aspirin is a well-known irreversible inhibitor of the COX-1 enzyme and, subsequently, of TXA2 production and platelet activation. Because of its potent antithrombotic properties, aspirin use in coronary atherosclerosis has been studied extensively.

The beneficial effects of aspirin in unstable angina/NSTEMI have been demonstrated across broad populations of patients, with either short or long-term administration, and in comparison to other antithrombotic therapies. A few landmark trials, conducted prior to the widespread use of clopidogrel, glycoprotein IIb/IIIa inhibitors, and an early invasive approach, established aspirin as the backbone of therapy for patients with an ACS. The Veterans Administration (VA) Cooperative Study was one of the first multicenter, double-blinded, randomized trials examining the use of 324 mg of aspirin vs. placebo for 12 weeks in 1,266 men with unstable angina *(10)*. The use of aspirin was associated with a significant reduction in the rate of death or myocardial infarction ($p=0.0005$). The beneficial effects of aspirin were shown to be durable, despite cessation of aspirin therapy at 12 weeks, with a significantly lower mortality at 1 year in those treated with aspirin ($p=0.008$). One caveat of this study was the introduction of beta-blocker therapy during the study period and the fact that it was not accounted for in the study protocol.

Cairns et al. reported the results of the Canadian Multicenter Trial in 1985 *(11)*. Five hundred fifty five patients with unstable angina were enrolled in this randomized, double-blinded, prospective study and received 325 mg of aspirin (4×/day), sulfinpyrazone 200 mg, a combination of both therapies, or placebo *(11)*. While enrollment was not limited to men and follow up was over a longer period, the results were equally dramatic with a significant reduction in the composite of death and nonfatal myocardial infarction over a mean of 18 months ($p=0.008$). There was no apparent benefit with sulfinpyrazone.

Aspirin has also been examined in comparison to heparin in patients with NSTEMI. The Research Group on Instability in Coronary Artery Disease (RISC) study examined 796 Swedish men with unstable angina and compared the effects of intravenous heparin therapy for 5 days after presentation, lower dose aspirin (75 mg/day oral) for 1 year, both the above, or neither *(12)*. Over a follow-up period of 3 months, there was a clear reduction in the rate of death or non-fatal myocardial infarction in those patients who received aspirin. The use of IV heparin alone did not confer any obvious benefit; however, during the first 5 days of the study, the combination of heparin and aspirin together resulted in a significant reduction of the primary combined endpoint as compared to heparin or placebo. The benefit of heparin in ACS was, however, observed in a study by Theroux et al., examining the benefit of intravenous heparin, aspirin (325 mg oral 2×/daily), the combination, or placebo in patients with ACS *(13)*.

Despite the obvious benefit of aspirin in these patients, many patients do not receive appropriate antiplatelet therapy. The Reduction of Atherothrombosis for Continued Health (REACH) Registry reported that among 40,450 patients with established CAD, between 10 and 15% of those previously revascularized were not on any antiplatelet therapy. Furthermore, of those only on medical therapy for atherosclerotic disease, more than 20% did not receive any antiplatelet therapy *(14)*.

ASPIRIN DOSING

Aspirin is likely to be one of the most widely used drugs in the world. There are many indications for its use in cardiovascular disease – it has been shown to be of benefit in the setting of ACS, in chronic stable coronary disease, and in high-risk primary prevention. However , the optimal dosing strategy for each of these situations is unknown. The studies described above vary in the dosing of aspirin used in ACS. The benefit, however, appears to be similar and lasting despite the wide variation in dosing. The benefit of aspirin in preventing myocardial infarction and ischemic stroke may be countered by an increased risk of bleeding (primarily gastrointestinal) and hemorrhagic stroke *(15,16)*. In gastric mucosa, the inhibition of cyclo-oxygenase-1 (COX-1) results in a reduction in prostaglandin production. Subsequent studies have documented that long term aspirin use has been associated with increased risk of gastric and duodenal ulceration *(17)*. Data from healthy adult volunteers suggest that very high doses of aspirin (2,600 mg/day) can lead to gastric mucosal injury independent of a prostaglandin-mediated mechanism *(18)*. It has been previously demonstrated that inhibition of platelet-derived thromboxane occurs at considerably lower doses of aspirin (19,20). To optimize the dose of aspirin would involve selecting a dose low enough to ensure proper and complete platelet inhibition without significantly increasing the risk of bleeding.

The optimal dosing of aspirin in the setting of primary prevention of coronary atherosclerosis has been examined. A systematic review examining aspirin use in the prevention of cardiovascular disease has concluded that the optimal daily dose of aspirin should be between 75 and 81 mg daily to optimize antiplatelet activity without substantially increasing the risk of bleeding complications (21).

In the setting of higher risk patients, aspirin dosing becomes a more critical issue. Often, in these patients, antiplatelet agents or antiplatelet and antithrombotic agents in combination are used. The risk of bleeding increases substantially with the combination of these agents (22). Furthermore, elderly patients appear to be at significantly higher risk of bleeding complications, primarily gastrointestinal bleeding, with a combination of agents vs. aspirin alone (23). Data from this same observational cohort identified age, renal failure, peptic ulcer disease, diabetes, and bleeding during hospitalization for acute MI as risk factors for bleeding in elderly patients.

The Antithrombotic Trialists' Collaboration (ATC) examined the question of aspirin dosing in patients at higher risk of arterial or venous thrombosis, or in those with an acute thrombotic event. A meta-analysis of 287 studies examining 135,000 patients was conducted to examine the benefit of various types of antiplatelet and antithrombotic therapies in reducing non-fatal myocardial infarction, non-fatal stroke, or vascular death. In terms of efficacy, there appeared to be no difference in the proportional reduction in serious vascular events when comparing doses of 75–150 mg (32%±6%) to higher daily doses such as 160–325 mg (26%±3%) or 500–1,500 mg (19%±3%). Daily doses less than 75 mg/day appeared to have a slightly smaller benefit (24).

In a substudy of the Clopidogrel in Unstable angina to prevent Recurrent Events (CURE) trial, investigators examined the question of aspirin dosing (≤100 mg, 101–199 mg, and ≥199 mg) in the setting of clopidogrel vs. placebo ACS (25). In 12,562 patients with ACS, an increasing dose of aspirin resulted in a higher risk of major bleeding, without an increase in efficacy and authors conclude that dosing between 75 and 100 mg/day may be optimal, irrespective of clopidogrel use.

The DUTCH TIA Trial Study Group reported that 30 mg of aspirin per day was as effective in reducing recurrent events as 283 mg of aspirin per day. In 3,131 patients with a prior TIA, 30 mg of aspirin was also associated with fewer side effects, including a significant reduction in minor bleeding complications (26).

Despite the data from these studies, it appears that practice trends are quite different. The Can Rapid Risk Stratification of Unstable Angina Patients Suppress Adverse Outcomes with Early Implementation of the American College of Cardiology/American Heart Association Guidelines (CRUSADE) initiative suggested that up to 24.1% of patients hospitalized for ACS did not receive aspirin at discharge and of those who did, the majority of patients received 325 mg/day dosing (27).

For post elective PCI or PCI for ACS, the ACC/AHA/ESC guidelines recommend 325 mg of aspirin once daily for those patients with evidence of aspirin resistance. In addition, it is recommended that the aspirin be dosed at the 325 mg level for 1 month following bare metal stent implantation, for 3 months following sirolimus-eluting stent implantation and for 6 months following paclitaxel-eluting stent implantation prior to decreasing the dose to 81 mg indefinitely.

ADP Receptor Blockade (Thienopyridines)

Clopidogrel and ticlopidine are the two currently available drugs, which act to inhibit the function of the ADP receptor, $P2Y_{12}$. Both of these drugs are present as pro-drugs and require metabolism into an active form by the liver. ADP mediated activation of the $P2Y_{12}$ receptor results in further platelet activation in the form of platelet aggregation and response to other platelet stimuli resulting in a heightened prothrombotic state. Ticlopidine use has been limited given the association with serious side effects including neutropenia and thrombotic thrombocytopenic purpura *(28)*.

Ticlopidine

Ticlodipine has been examined in the context of acute coronary syndromes and in the setting of elective percutaneous coronary intervention (PCI). A randomized, multicenter trial examined patients with unstable angina randomized to conventional therapy alone ($n=338$) vs. conventional therapy plus ticlopidine 250 mg b.i.d. ($n=314$). The investigators followed patients for 6 months and found that those treated with a combination of conventional therapy and ticlopidine had a relative risk reduction of 46.8% in vascular death whereas a relative risk reduction in non fatal myocardial infarction of 46.1% was noted in the group treated with combination therapy *(29)*.

Ticlopidine was also examined in the context of acute myocardial infarction following thrombolysis in 1,470 patients randomized to either aspirin (160 mg/day) or ticlopidine (500 mg/day). There was a similar rate of death, recurrent myocardial infarction, angina or stroke in both of these groups (8.0%, $p=0.966$). Furthermore there was no significant difference in the rate of adverse reactions between the two groups *(30)*.

In the setting of PCI, the use of ticlopidine has been examined (Table 1). A meta-analysis examined 13,955 patients enrolled in these trials and found that clopidogrel provided an advantage with regard to major adverse cardiac events and notably all cause mortality at 30 days ($p=0.001$), suggesting improved efficacy of clopidogrel over ticlopidine in the setting of PCI *(31)*.

Clopidogrel

The use of clopidogrel in both secondary prevention and ACS been extensively examined. In the Clopidogrel vs. Aspirin in Patients at Risk of Ischemic Events (CAPRIE) trial, clopidogrel was compared to aspirin for purposes of secondary prevention. In 19,185 patients, the use of clopidgrel was associated with an 8.7% reduction in the risk of ischemic stroke, vascular death, or myocardial infarction without an increase in adverse events *(32)*.

Given the potential complimentary role of ADP receptor inhibitors to aspirin in platelet inhibition, it is no surprise that the combination serves as a potent antithrombotic entity *(33)*. In the setting of PCI, the Clopidogrel for Reduction of Events During Observation (CREDO) study examined the combination of clopidogrel and aspirin in 2,116 patients undergoing PCI with patients randomized to either a 300 mg-loading dose of clopidogrel followed by 75 mg/day for 1 year vs. 75 mg/day for 28 days *(34)*. At 28 days, the group receiving the loading dose of clopidogrel had an 18.5% relative risk reduction in a combined endpoint of death, myocardial infarction, or urgent target vessel revascularization ($p=0.23$). At 1 year, there was an observed 26.9% relative risk reduction in the same combined endpoint ($p=0.02$) and the curves started to separate quite early from randomzation. Interestingly, a post-hoc analysis suggested that patients randomized to a loading dose of 300 mg of clopidogrel greater than 6 h before PCI experienced a 38.6% relative risk reduction in the combined endpoint vs. no benefit in those receiving the loading dose <6 h to PCI.

In the setting of ACS, clopidogrel has been examined in many trials. In acute ST elevation myocardial infarction (STEMI), the use of clopidogrel has been examined in two large trials. The Clopidogrel and Metoprolol in Myocardial Infarction Trial (COMMIT) assessed the effect of either aspirin or aspirin and clopidogrel in 45,852 patients with AMI. In those receiving both aspirin and

Table 1
Trials of ticlopidine in the setting of percutaneous coronary intervention

Trial	# of Pts	Treatment groups	Primary endpoint	Results	Comments
CLASSICS (66)	n = 1,020	Randomized to:300 mg Clopidogrel loading then 75 mg/day/325 mg ASA vs. 75 mg Clopidogrel and ASA 325 vs. 250 mg bid Ticlopidine/325 mg ASA	Combined: major bleeding complications, neutropenia, thrombocytopenia, or discontinuation due to noncardiac adverse event	Primary endpoint occurred in 9.1% of ticlopidine group vs. 4.6% of clopidogrel ($p = 0.005$)	No difference in major adverse cardiac events between the groups noted
FANSTASTIC Study (67)	n = 485	Randomized to ASA (100–325 mg/day) and:Ticlopidine 250 mg bid × 6 weeks vs. oral anticoagulants for 6 weeks	Combined: bleeding, or peripheral vascular complications, secondary include cardiac events and duration of hospitalization	Primary endpoint: 13.5% of ticlopidine vs. 21% of oral anticoagulation ($p = 0.03$). MACE and hospital duration were shorter in the ticlopidine group ($p = 0.01$ and $p = 0.0001$)	
Muller et al. (68)	n = 700	Randomized to 4 weeks of 500 mg/day of ticlopidine or 75 mg/day of clopidogrel after elective/urgent PCI (ASA as standard of care)	Combined primary cardiac: of death, urgent TVR, stent thrombosis, or non fatal MI within 30 days	No difference in the primary cardiac endpoint which occurred in 1.7% on ticlopidine and 3.1% on clopidogrel ($p = 0.24$)	Noncardiac events were higher in the ticlopidine population ($p = 0.01$)
Taniuchi et al. (69)	n = 1,016 (522 to clopidogrel and 494 to ticlopidine)	Randomized to either clopidogrel or ticlopidine after PCI. Patients on 325 mg/day of ASA and GP IIb/IIIa inhibitor at discretion of operator	Primary: Failure to complete thienopyridine therapy in addition to ASA. Secondary combined endpoints were thrombocytopenia, bleeding, cardiac death, NSTEMI, stent thrombosis or TVR	The primary endpoint occurred in more patients on ticlopidine ($p = 0.04$). There were no differences in the other outcomes between groups	No significant differences in rates of thrombocytopenia between groups using GPIIb/IIIa inhibitors

	n				
Dangas et al. (70)	n=827	Retrospective, examining those having undergone PCI and then received either clopidogrel or ticlopidine in addition to ASA. Ticlopidine was loaded at 500 mg pre PCI and then 250 mg bid for 2–4 weeks	30-day follow up to examine the incidence of stent thrombosis	While not statistically significant, there was a slightly higher rate of subacute stent thrombosis with ASA and clopidogrel	A total of only 6 episodes of subacute stent thrombosis occurred in the study at 30 days
Berger et al. (71)	n=500 consecutive patients with clopidogrel and 827 consecutive patients receiving ticlopidine	Comparison of consecutive patients having received clopidogrel after PCI vs. those having received ticlopidine (non randomized)	30-day incidence of adverse cardiac events including death, non-fatal MI, repeat PCI or bypass surgery	There was no significant difference in outcomes between the two groups with regards to adverse cardiac outcomes	Patients treated with clopidogrel were older, had more severe angina and more frequent MI within preceding 24 h

CLASSICS Clopidogrel Aspirin Stent International Cooperative Study; *FANTASTIC* full anticoagulation vs. aspirin and ticlopidine after intracoronary stenting; *MACE* Major adverse cardiac events; *TVR* target vessel revascularization; *MI* myocardial infarction; *ASA* aspirin; *GP IIb/IIIa* glycoprotein IIb/IIIa inhibitor; *PCI* percutaneous coronary intervention; *NSTEMI* non-ST segment elevation myocardial infarction clopidogrel, there was a significant reduction in mortality ($p=0.03$) and in the risk of death, reinfarction, and stroke ($p=0.002$) *(35)*.

The other large study examining the efficacy of clopidogrel in AMI was the Clopidogrel as Adjunctive Reperfusion Therapy Thrombolysis in Myocardial Infarction 28 (CLARITY-TIMI 28) Trial, which randomized 3,491 patients with AMI to clopidogrel vs. placebo following fibrinolysis for AMI. In those receiving clopidogrel in addition to fibrinolysis and aspirin, there was a 20% risk reduction of a combined endpoint of 30 day death from cardiovascular causes, myocardial infarction, or need for urgent revascularization *(36)*.

In the setting of unstable angina/NSTEMI, the CURE trial examined the question of whether the addition of clopidogrel to aspirin in the setting of unstable angina or NSTEMI led to a reduction in the first primary outcome, a combination of death from cardiovascular causes, non fatal myocardial infarction, or stroke. A second primary endpoint consisting of the first primary endpoint or recurrent ischemia was also examined. In total 12,562 patients were randomized to either aspirin and placebo or aspirin and clopidogrel (300 mg loading dose and then 75 mg/day). Patients were eligible if they presented within 24 h of onset of symptoms *(37)*. Patients randomized to clopidogrel and aspirin were noted to have a 20% relative risk reduction in the first primary outcome ($p<0.001$). Within this first primary outcome, patients receiving clopidogrel and aspirin had a 40% reduction in ST elevation myocardial infarctions. Furthermore, the same group had a 14% relative risk reduction in the second primary endpoint. This benefit came at the expense of a significant increase in major bleeding in the treatment group ($p=0.001$), although not in life threatening bleeding ($p=0.13$) *(37)*.

The benefit of clopidogrel therapy in ACS was noticeable in the first 24 h following treatment. At this time point there was a statistically significant reduction in the combined second primary endpoint. Withholding clopidogrel treatment by even 1 day resulted in a significant loss in the benefit observed during the first day of treatment. It is unclear if part of the short term benefit is due to the possibility of prevention of rebound hypercoagulability following heparin cessation *(38)*. Incremental benefit of clopidogrel therapy was noted between 30 days and 12 months from randomization with an 18% relative risk reduction in the combined primary endpoint *(39)*.

PCI-CURE was a planned prospective substudy of the original CURE trial. This intention to treat analysis examined 2,658 patients with UA or NSTEMI who underwent PCI. Patients were pretreated with a combination of aspirin and placebo or clopidogrel for a median of 6 days prior to PCI. Following PCI, >80% of patients were placed on an "open-label" thienopyridine for 4 weeks, after which the original study drug (placebo or clopidogrel) was resumed. The primary combined endpoint of cardiovascular death, myocardial infarction, or urgent target-vessel revascularization was seen in 6.4% of the placebo group vs. 4.5% for the treatment group ($p=0.03$) *(40)*. This benefit was observed at both 30 days post-PCI and up to 8 months post-PCI for cardiovascular death and myocardial infarction. Interestingly, the group randomized to clopidogrel showed less utilization of a glycoprotein IIb/IIIa inhibitor. Furthermore, the benefit of clopidogrel was realized regardless of the timing of PCI following presentation *(41)*.

In summary, the current data on thienopyridine, primarily clopidogrel, use suggests that their efficacy is about equivalent to that of aspirin. Furthermore, the combination of dual antiplatelet therapy (aspirin and thienopyridine) provides an incremental benefit beyond either of them alone in elective PCI and across the spectrum of ACS (NSTEMI and STEMI). In the setting of elective PCI, early pretreatment with a thienopyridine may provide more benefit than starting at or after the time of PCI. It is also important to realize that the effects of this therapy begin early after initiation and last up to 1 year.

Drug Eluting Stent Thrombosis and Clopidogrel Therapy

Recent enthusiasm for the use of drug eluting stents (DES) in reducing clinical and angiographic restenosis seen with bare metal stents has been dampened by the very real and catastrophic risk of stent thrombosis. Stent thrombosis, both subacute and late, in DES has been observed following PCI. McFadden et al. reported four cases of angiographically confirmed late stent thrombosis following PCI with DES *(42)*. Nasser et al. also reported two cases of stent thrombosis occurring in the setting of non-cardiac surgery following cessation of all antiplatelet therapy *(43)*.

The Basel Stent Kosten Effektiviats Trial – Late Thrombotic Events (BASKET-LATE) study examined this question in patients randomized to either bare metal stents or drug eluting stents. Following PCI, patients were treated with dual antiplatelet therapy for 6 months and after this time clopidogrel was discontinued. The rates of nonfatal myocardial infarction and cardiac death or nonfatal myocardial infarction were significantly higher in the group receiving DES after dual antiplatelet therapy was stopped. Furthermore, cardiac death or the combination of cardiac death and nonfatal MI were more frequently related to thrombosis *(44)*.

However, the issue regarding the true incidence of stent thrombosis remains controversial. This was partly driven by the lack of a consistent definition of stent thrombosis, be it angiographic or clinical. There have been several studies, including many meta-anlayses of larger clinical trials of drug eluting stents, attempting to quantify the risk associated with DES use vs. bare metal stents and they are described in Table 2. The rate of DES stent thrombosis after 1 year remains low overall. In some of these studies, the rate remains even lower than others. This may, in part, be due to "off label" vs. "on label" usage of these coronary devices. "Real world" or increased off-label usage of DES appears to confer a higher risk of stent thrombosis as noted in the Swedish Coronary Angioplasty and Angiography Registry (SCAAR) study, which used propensity analysis to compare 19,771 patients, who had undergone PCI with either BMS or DES *(45)*. They concluded that over a 3-year period the risk of death was significantly higher with DES use. Although the specifics relating to duration of clopidogrel therapy were not reported, the excess mortality as compared to the large-scale clinical trials raises concern. Iakovou and colleagues examined this question of predictors of stent thrombosis in a "real world" population and at 9 months follow up found that there was a higher rate of stent thrombosis than noted in the clinical trial data and that premature discontinuation of antiplatelet therapy, the presence of diabetes, left ventricular dysfunction, renal failure, and bifurcation lesions were predictive of stent thrombosis *(46)*.

The role of dual antiplatelet therapy following PCI with DES appears to have meaningful significance in reducing clinical events associated with DES. In an observational study of 4,666 patients undergoing PCI with either DES ($n=1,501$) or BMS ($n=3,165$), the ongoing use of clopidogrel therapy was associated with lower rates of death up to 1 year and death or MI up to 2 years *(47)*. Similar findings were seen in a prospective analysis of 500 patients having received DES for acute MI where cessation of thienopyridine therapy by 30 days post PCI was associated with higher mortality rates *(48)*. These findings are in contrast to clinical trial data, which tested the duration of dual antiplatelet therapy for either 3 or 6 months. Currently, the optimal duration of dual antiplatelet therapy following PCI with DES is not known. Although recommendations currently call for dual antiplatelet therapy for at least 1 year following PCI with DES, the optimal duration of therapy, in terms of risks and benefits, is not known.

Table 2

Studies examining the risk of stent thrombosis associated with drug eluting stent vs. bare metal stent use with at least 1 year of follow up

Study	# of patients	Design	Follow up	Results	Comments
Stone et al. (72)	1,748 for sirolimus vs. placebo and 3,513 for paclitaxel vs. placebo	Pooled analysis of 4 trials of sirolimus stents vs. BMS and 5 trials of paclitaxel stents vs. BMS	4 years	After 1 year, rates of ST were higher vs. BMS in both types of DES, however, no increase in death or MI at 4 years	While rates of TVR were lower in either DES group, after 1 year, there was significantly higher rates of ST in both the DES groups
Bavry et al. (73)	6,675	Meta-analysis on 14 clinical trials of either paclitaxel or sirolimus eluting stents	>1 year follow up	Rates of ST were significantly higher in both DES types vs. BMS, although overall rates remained low	The true risk of ST with DES increased >6–12 months after procedure
Kastrati et al. (74)	4,958	Meta-analyis of 14 clinical trials of sirolimus vs. BMS with primary endpoint of all cause mortality, but also examining ST	12.1–58.9 months mean follow up interval	Rates of death, myocardial infarction, and need for revasc were all lower with sirolimus eluting stents	While the overall risk of ST was no different, after 1 year, the risk of ST with SES was slightly higher
Mauri et al. (75)	878 with SES 1,400 with PES 2,267 with BMS	Pooled analysis of 8 trials of both PES and SES vs. BMS. Readjudicated outcomes according to the ARC definition of ST	4 years	Rates of ST by ARC definition did not differ significantly between either DES group and BMS group	Authors suggest that differences in mortality rates between DES and BMS are not all attributable to ST
Airoldi et al. (76)	3,021 with DES vs. BMS at 4 institutions	Prospective observational cohort, examining the incidence of ST	18 months	Within 6 months, discontinuation of thienopyridine therapy was strongest predictor of ST. At 18 months, 1.9% had ST	Discontinuation of thienopyridine therapy did not predict ST beyond 6 months

Ong et al. (77)	2,006 patients with SES or PES	Prospective observational cohort examining angiographically proven ST	Mean of 1.5 years	Angiographically proven late ST occurred with an incidence of 0.35%	ST occurred in this population in patients on only antiplatelet mono-therapy
Lagerqvist et al. (45)	6,033 with DES, 13,738 with BMS	Retrospective, propensity matched study comparing outcomes between DES and BMS usage	3 years	After 6 months, there was a significantly higher mortality rate with DES use	Reflects "off label" use, however, unclear if the early gain observed with DES is due to clopidogrel use at this time, not accurately quantified

BMS Bare metal stent; ST stent thrombosis; TVR target vessel revascularization; DES drug eluting stent; SES sirolimus eluting stent; PES paclitaxel eluting stent; ARC academic research consortium

Table 3

Select major trials of GP IIb/IIIa inhibitors in acute coronary syndromes and elective PCI

Trial	GP IIb/IIIa inibitor	Design	# of patients	Results	Comments
EPIC (78)	Abciximab	Prospective, double blind, high risk pts (ACS, or high risk anatomy) on ASA and heparin randomized to abciximab vs. placebo	2,099	At 30 days, 35% reduction in primary endpoint of death, nonfatal MI, unplanned surg. revasc, or refractory ischemia req. IABP or unplanned percutaneous procedure	The benefits of treatment were noted out to 6 months and 3 years with regards to the primary composite endpoint
EPILOG (79)	Abciximab	Prospective double blind trial of elective or urgent PCI of abciximab vs. placebo	2,792	At 30 days, significant reduction in primary endpoint noted in abciximab group	The benefit comes at no increased risk of bleeding. Furthermore, the benefits of treatment noted out to 1 year (80)
CAPTURE (81)	Abciximab	Prospective double blind randomized to abciximab vs. placebo after angiography and prior to PCI for ACS not responsive to medications	1,265	At 30 days, composite endpoint of death, MI, or urgent intervention was lower in the treatment group (p=0.012)	Major bleeding was more frequent in the treatment group
ADMIRAL (82)	Abciximab	Prospective, double blind, randomized to abciximab vs. placebo at time of PCI for STEMI	400	At 30 days and 6 months, primary endpoint (death, MI, urgent TVR) was lower in the treatment group	Angiographic analysis at 30 days and 6 months revealed more TIMI 3 flow in the treatment group vs. placebo
RAPPORT (83)	Abciximab	Prospective double blind, randomized to placebo vs. abciximab prior to PCI for STEMI (<12 h)	483	At 6 months, no difference in primary efficacy endpoint (death, MI or any TVR) between the two groups	At 7 days and at 30 days, early death, any TVR or re-infarction were significantly reduced. At 6 months, treatment group had significant reduction in death, MI or urgent TVR
CADILLAC (84)	Abciximab	Prospective, 2×2 factorial, testing combination of PTCA vs. stenting and abciximab vs. placebo	2,082	At 6 months, the difference in the primary endpoint was noted in those with stents, irrespective of abciximab status	The reduction in the composite endpoint at 6 months was driven by a significant reduction in rates of ischemia driven TVR
EPISTENT (85)	Abciximab	Prospective, examining stenting with placebo, stenting with abciximab, or PTCA with abciximab	2,399	At both 30 days and 6 months, the primary endpoint (death, MI, urgent revasc) was lower in stenting and abciximab group	The benefit was observed at 1 year in the stenting and abciximab group. The benefit was noted regardless of whether the patients had elective PCI or urgent PCI
GUSTO IV ACS (86)	Abciximab	Prospective, ACS pts randomized to placebo vs. abciximab bolus and 24 h infusion or abciximab bolus and 48 h infusion with no planned intervention	7,800	Primary endpoint of death or MI at 30 days was no different between the three groups	No added benefit in patients with positive biomarkers of myonecrosis

Trial	Drug	Design	n	Primary endpoint	Comments
PURSUIT (87)	Eptifibatide	Pts w. UA/NSTEMI randomized to eptifibatide vs. placebo for up to 72 h	10,948	At 30 days, primary composite endpoint of death, non fatal MI was lower in the eptifibatide group	The benefit of eptifibatide was noted in patients treated with only medical management or early revascularization
ESPRIT (88)	Eptifibatide	Prospective, elective PCI, randomized to eptifibatide or placebo in addition to asa, heparin and thienopyridine	2,064	Primary endpoint at 30 days of death, MI, urgent TVR and bailout therapy was significantly lower in the treatment arm	Major bleeding was higher in the treatment arm ($p=0.027$). At 1 year the benefits of eptifibatide treatment were still present
IMPACT II (89)	Eptifibatide	Prospective, prior to PCI, randomized to placebo, eptifibatide bolus +0.5 µg/kg/min infusion, or eptifibatide bolus +0.75 µg/kg/min infusion	4,010	Composite endpoint at 30 days of death, MI or unplanned or repeat revascularization was no different between the groups	By treatment-received analysis, the bolus +0.5 µg/kg/min infusion group had a significant reduction in the composite endpoint ($p=0.04$). There was no increase in the rates of major bleeding noted
PRISM (90)	Tirofiban	Prospective, double blind, ACS pts randomized to IV heparin vs. tirofiban for 48 h	3,232	Primary endpt of death, MI or refractory ischemia at 48 h was significantly lower in the tirofiban group	The benefits of tirofiban at 30 days from randomization were in those high risk patients with positive troponin values (91)
PRISM-PLUS (92)	Tirofiban	Prospective, double blind, ACS pts randomized to either IV heparin, tirofiban or tirofiban and IV heparin prior to PCI	1,915	7 day composite primary endpt of death, MI or refractory ischemia was lower in group with the combination of IV heparin and tirofiban	The benefit of the combination of heparin and tirofiban remained at 30 days and there was no increase in major bleeding in the combination therapy group

EPIC Evaluation of c7E3 to prevent ischemic complications; *EPILOG* platelet glycoprotein IIb/IIIa receptor blockade and low dose heparin during percutaneous coronary revascularization; *CAPTURE* c7E3 fab antiplatelet therapy in unstable refractory angina. *ADMIRAL* abciximab before direct angioplasty and stenting in myocardial infarction regarding acute and long term follow up; *RAPPORT* ReoPro and primary PTCA organization and randomization trial; *CADILLAC* controlled abciximab and device investigation to lower late angioplasty complications trial; *EPISTENT* evaluation of platelet IIb/IIIa inhibitor for stenting trial; *GUSTO IV ACS* global utilization strategies to open occluded coronary arteries trial IV in acute coronary syndromes; *PURSUIT* platelet glycoprotein IIb/IIIa in unstable angina: receptor suppression using integrelin therapy; *ESPRIT* enhanced suppression of the platelet IIb/IIIa receptor with integrellin therapy; *IMPACT II* integrellin to minimize platelet aggregation and coronary thrombosis II; *PRISM* platelet receptor inhibition in ischemic syndrome management; *PRISM-PLUS* platelet receptor inhibition in ischemic syndrome management limited by unstable signs and symptoms; *ACS* acute coronary syndrome; *MI* myocardial infarction; *IABP* intraaortic balloon pump counterpulsation; *PCI* percutaneous coronary intervention; *STEMI* ST elevation myocardial infarction; *TVR* target vessel revascularization; *TIMI* thrombolysis in myocardial infarction; *PTCA* percutaneous transluminal coronary angioplasty; *UA/NSTEMI* unstable angina, non-ST elevation myocardial infarction; *IV* intravenous

GLYCOPROTEIN IIB/IIIA INHIBITORS IN ACUTE CORONARY SYNDROMES

The role of the GP IIb/IIIa receptor in platelet aggregation and thrombus stability has led to the use of glycoprotein IIb/IIIa inhibitors in the setting of PCI and ACS. The rationale in the use of the inhibitors is to prevent the binding of the GP IIb/IIIa receptor to fibrinogen or circulating vWF, thus preventing platelet aggregation and formation and stabilization of the thrombus.

There are three forms of intravenous GP IIb/IIIa inhibitiors available and approved for clinical use. Those are eptifibatide, abciximab, and tirofiban. There has been investigational work done in the area of oral GP IIb/IIIa inhibitors, which have not demonstrated any benefit and will not be expounded upon at this time. The intravenous GP IIb/IIIa inhibitors have been assessed in both the context of ACS and elective PCI. Table 3 discusses the important studies of glycoprotein IIb/IIIa inhibitors for ACS and for elective PCI. It is important to carefully understand the indications and the populations studied in each of these large trials as these may account for the noted differences in results. Meta-analyses of some of these large trials of GP IIb/IIIa inhibitors have reinforced the benefit of these agents in both the UA/NSTEMI (49) and ST STEMI populations (50).

The relative benefits of each of these antiplatelet agents may vary significantly based on the context in which the medication is being administered. In the modern era, with the use of aspirin, heparin (or LMWH), and clopidogrel in the setting of ACS, the concomitant use of a GP IIb/IIIa inhibitor has been questioned. The Intracoronary Stenting and Antithrombotic Regimen: Rapid and Early Action for Coronary Treatment 2 (ISAR-REACT-2) examined this question in the setting of PCI for ACS. In higher risk patients undergoing PCI for NSTEMI, this study examined the utility of adding abciximab to aspirin, IV heparin, and 600 mg of clopidogrel. At total of 2,022 patients were randomized to abciximab or placebo and while there were no significant differences between the groups in terms of bleeding, there was a significant reduction in the primary composite endpoint of death, myocardial infarction, or urgent TVR noted in troponin positive patients in favor of abciximab (51).

GP IIb/IIIa inhibitors have demonstrated utility across the broad spectrum of ACS patients, particularly in the higher risk troponin positive patients, as shown in post-hoc analyses. Furthermore, the benefit of this drug is really observed in the context of undergoing PCI while receiving the drug. Although no data has demonstrated the benefit of the combination of GP IIb/IIIa inhibitors and thienopyridine therapy over either therapy alone in the medical management of ACS patients, the combination of these medications appears to be more potent than a single agent during PCI for ACS.

NOVEL ANTIPLATELET THERAPIES ON THE HORIZON

Many new antiplatelet agents are currently under investigation for use in ACS and elective PCI. The hope is to achieve more rapid and more sustained platelet inhibition with less inconsistency than with currently available agents. There are several new ADP receptor antagonists currently being examined in clinical trials.

Cangrelor is an intravenous ADP P2Y$_{12}$ receptor subtype inhibitor that is direct acting and does not require conversion to an active form. Phase II clinical studies in the setting of elective PCI have shown cangrelor to be efficacious (100% inhibition of platelet aggregation at 4 µg/kg dose) yet safe when compared with standard medical therapies. Furthermore, in addition to achieving rapid and reversible inhibition of platelet function, there is a more rapid return to baseline bleeding times in comparison to abciximab (52). Phase II clinical studies in the setting of ACS have clearly demonstrated the safety of this agent as an adjunct to aspirin and heparin therapy without an increase in serious bleeding events (53). The Clinical Trial Comparing Cangrelor to Clopidogrel in Subjects who Require Percutaneous Coronary Intervention (CHAMPION-PCI) (54) is a mutli-center clinical trial currently enrolling patients to demonstrate either superiority or non-inferiority of cangrelor to clopidogrel in the setting of PCI. The Clinical Trial Comparing Treatment with Cangrelor (In Combination With Usual Care), to Usual Care in Subjects Who Require Percutaneous Coronary Intervention (CHAMPION-PLATFORM) *(55)* will measure the composite of all cause mortality, myocardial ischemia, and ischemia driven revascularization as an assessment of cangrelor vs. usual care in patients undergoing PCI.

Prasugrel is an ADP $P2Y_{12}$ receptor irreversible antagonist, which like the currently available thienopyridines, requires conversion to an active prodrug form. The potential advantage of this ADP receptor antagonist is the potent antiplatelet effect *(56)* and more rapid onset of action demonstrated in comparison to currently available thienoyridines *(57)*. These effects are a result of enzymatic transformation of the prodrug to an active metabolite in the plasma phase – not dependent upon hepatic function. Early phase clinical trials have demonstrated the safety and efficacy of prasugrel *(58–60)*. The Phase III Trial to Assess Improvement in Therapeutic Outcomes by Optimizing Platelet Inhibition with Prasugrel-Thrombolysis in Myocardial Infarction 38 (TRITON-TIMI 38) examined the efficacy of prasugrel in comparison to clopidogrel in patients with ACS undergoing PCI. A total of 13,608 patients with ACS were randomized to loading and maintenance dosing of either prasugrel or clopidogrel. While there was a 19% reduction in the primary efficacy end point of cardiovascular death, non fatal myocardial infarction or nonfatal stroke with prasugrel ($p<0.001$), this was counterbalanced by an increase in the rate of life threatening bleeding ($p=0.01$) *(61)*. Furthermore, among those patients with an initial primary endpoint event, those treated with prasugrel had fewer recurrent events ($p=0.016$) and less cardiovascular mortality ($p=0.008$) when compared to the clopidogrel treatment arm *(62)*. Although the overall clinical efficacy appears to favor prasugrel over clopidogrel in ACS, the increased rates of major bleeding events with prasugrel are cause for concern. The Prasugrel in Comparison to Clopidogrel for Inhibition of Platelet Activation and Aggregation-Thrombolysis in Myocardial Infarction 44 (PRINCIPLE-TIMI 44) examined the question of dosing with regard to both prasugrel and clopidogrel *(63)*.

AZD6140 is a novel, non-thienopyridine ADP $P2Y_{12}$ receptor inhibitor. This oral reversible ADP receptor inhibitor belongs to a class of agents termed cyclopentyltriazolopyrimidines that do not require metabolism to an active state. In a double blind, parallel group study, 200 patients with atherosclerosis were randomized to either 50, 100, or 200 mg twice daily, or 400 mg once daily or clopidogrel 75 mg. Nearly complete platelet inhibition was achieved with AZD6140 doses greater than 100 mg bid. At higher dose ranges of AZD6140, there were slightly higher rates of minor/mild bleeding and one reported major bleeding event at a dose of 400 mg once daily. Furthermore, there was a slight increase in non-heart failure or bronchospasm related symptoms of dyspnea with increasing doses of AZD6140 *(64)*. The Phase III Platelet Inhibition and Patient Outcomes (PLATO) trial will compare the effectiveness of AZD6140 against clopidogrel in patients with acute coronary syndromes *(65)*.

CONCLUSION

The ability to modulate platelet activity effectively and safely has proved to be an advantage in many different types of cardiovascular disease. Platelet inhibition has improved outcomes in both elective PCI and, especially, in ACS. Activated platelets appear to provide a key link between inflammation and thrombosis. As such, inhibiting platelet activation by one of many pathways serves not only to inhibit thrombus formation, but also appears to temper the inflammatory component in ACS and in the setting of PCI. Effective antiplatelet therapy has also been shown to be of primary importance in the prevention of stent thrombosis following PCI with drug eluting stents. The goal of newer agents is to improve efficacy, to reduce time to peak platelet inhibition, and to provide a more uniform response among patients. There are several new agents, which are currently under investigation to answer questions on efficacy and safety. Time will tell whether these agents will significantly alter practice and outcomes. What is certain is that an improved understanding of platelet function will allow for the development of more specific therapies that will likely enhance our ability to safely and effectively control platelets.

REFERENCES

1. Buffon A, Biasucci LM, Liuzzo G, D'Onofrio G, Crea F, Maseri A (2002) Widespread coronary inflammation in unstable angina. N Engl J Med 347:5–12
2. Andre P, Denis CV, Ware J et al (2000) Platelets adhere to and translocate on von Willebrand factor presented by endothelium in stimulated veins. Blood 96:3322–3328
3. Eto K, Isshiki T, Yamamoto H et al (1999) AJvW-2, an anti-vWF monoclonal antibody, inhibits enhanced platelet aggregation induced by high shear stress in platelet-rich plasma from patients with acute coronary syndromes. Arterioscler Thromb Vasc Biol 19:877–882
4. Goto S, Tamura N, Eto K, Ikeda Y, Handa S (2002) Functional significance of adenosine 5'-diphosphate receptor (P2Y(12)) in platelet activation initiated by binding of von Willebrand factor to platelet GP Ibalpha induced by conditions of high shear rate. Circulation 105:2531–2536
5. Wagner AH, Guldenzoph B, Lienenluke B, Hecker M (2004) CD154/CD40-mediated expression of CD154 in endothelial cells: consequences for endothelial cell-monocyte interaction. Arterioscler Thromb Vasc Biol 24:715–720
6. Andre P, Prasad KS, Denis CV et al (2002) CD40L stabilizes arterial thrombi by a beta3 integrin–dependent mechanism. Nat Med 8:247–252
7. Heeschen C, Dimmeler S, Hamm CW et al (2003) Soluble CD40 ligand in acute coronary syndromes. N Engl J Med 348:1104–1111
8. Varo N, de Lemos JA, Libby P et al (2003) Soluble CD40L: risk prediction after acute coronary syndromes. Circulation 108:1049–1052
9. Ridker PM, Buring JE, Rifai N (2001) Soluble P-selectin and the risk of future cardiovascular events. Circulation 103:491–495
10. Lewis HD Jr, Davis JW, Archibald DG et al (1983) Protective effects of aspirin against acute myocardial infarction and death in men with unstable angina. Results of a veterans administration cooperative study. N Engl J Med 309:396–403
11. Cairns JA, Gent M, Singer J et al (1985) Aspirin, sulfinpyrazone, or both in unstable angina. Results of a Canadian multicenter trial. N Engl J Med 313:1369–1375
12. (1990) Risk of myocardial infarction and death during treatment with low dose aspirin and intravenous heparin in men with unstable coronary artery disease. The RISC Group. Lancet 336:827–830
13. Theroux P, Ouimet H, McCans J et al (1988) Aspirin, heparin, or both to treat acute unstable angina. N Engl J Med 319:1105–1111
14. Steinberg BA, Steg PG, Bhatt DL, Fonarow GC, Zeymer U, Cannon CP (2007) Comparisons of guideline-recommended therapies in patients with documented coronary artery disease having percutaneous coronary intervention versus coronary artery bypass grafting versus medical therapy only (from the REACH International Registry). Am J Cardiol 99:1212–1215
15. He J, Whelton PK, Vu B, Klag MJ (1998) Aspirin and risk of hemorrhagic stroke: a meta-analysis of randomized controlled trials. JAMA 280:1930–1935
16. Gorelick PB, Weisman SM (2005) Risk of hemorrhagic stroke with aspirin use: an update. Stroke 36:1801–1807
17. Kurata JH, Abbey DE (1990) The effect of chronic aspirin use on duodenal and gastric ulcer hospitalizations. J Clin Gastroenterol 12:260–266
18. Lee M, Cryer B, Feldman M (1994) Dose effects of aspirin on gastric prostaglandins and stomach mucosal injury. Ann Intern Med 120:184–189
19. FitzGerald GA, Oates JA, Hawiger J et al (1983) Endogenous biosynthesis of prostacyclin and thromboxane and platelet function during chronic administration of aspirin in man. J Clin Invest 71:676–688
20. Kallmann R, Nieuwenhuis HK, de Groot PG, van Gijn J, Sixma JJ (1987) Effects of low doses of aspirin, 10 mg and 30 mg daily, on bleeding time, thromboxane production and 6-keto-PGF1 alpha excretion in healthy subjects. Thromb Res 45:355–361
21. Campbell CL, Smyth S, Montalescot G, Steinhubl SR (2007) Aspirin dose for the prevention of cardiovascular disease: a systematic review. JAMA 297:2018–2024
22. Hallas J, Dall M, Andries A et al (2006) Use of single and combined antithrombotic therapy and risk of serious upper gastrointestinal bleeding: population based case-control study. BMJ 333:726

23. Buresly K, Eisenberg MJ, Zhang X, Pilote L (2005) Bleeding complications associated with combinations of aspirin, thienopy-ridine derivatives, and warfarin in elderly patients following acute myocardial infarction. Arch Intern Med 165:784–789

24. Antithrombotic Trialists' Collaboration (2002) Collaborative meta-analysis of randomised trials of antiplatelet therapy for prevention of death, myocardial infarction, and stroke in high risk patients. BMJ 324:71–86

25. Peters RJ, Mehta SR, Fox KA et al (2003) Effects of aspirin dose when used alone or in combination with clopidogrel in patients with acute coronary syndromes: observations from the clopidogrel in unstable angina to prevent recurrent events (CURE) study. Circulation 108:1682–1687

26. (1991) A comparison of two doses of aspirin (30 mg vs. 283 mg a day) in patients after a transient ischemic attack or minor ischemic stroke. The Dutch TIA Trial Study Group. N Engl J Med 325:1261–1266

27. Tickoo S, Roe MT, Peterson ED et al (2007) Patterns of aspirin dosing in non-ST-elevation acute coronary syndromes in the CRUSADE quality improvement initiative. Am J Cardiol 99:1496–1499

28. Bennett CL, Weinberg PD, Rozenberg-Ben-Dror K, Yarnold PR, Kwaan HC, Green D (1998) Thrombotic thrombocy-topenic purpura associated with ticlopidine. A review of 60 cases. Ann Intern Med 128:541–544

29. Balsano F, Rizzon P, Violi F et al (1990) Antiplatelet treatment with ticlopidine in unstable angina. A controlled multi-center clinical trial. The studio della ticlopidina nell'angina instabile group. Circulation 82:17–26

30. Scrutinio D, Cimminiello C, Marubini E, Pitzalis MV, Di Biase M, Rizzon P (2001) Ticlopidine versus aspirin after myocardial infarction (STAMI) trial. J Am Coll Cardiol 37:1259–1265

31. Bhatt DL, Bertrand ME, Berger PB et al (2002) Meta-analysis of randomized and registry comparisons of ticlopidine with clopidogrel after stenting. J Am Coll Cardiol 39:9–14

32. (1996) A randomised, blinded, trial of clopidogrel versus aspirin in patients at risk of ischaemic events (CAPRIE). CAPRIE Steering Committee. Lancet 348:1329–1339

33. Cadroy Y, Bossavy JP, Thalamas C, Sagnard L, Sakariassen K, Boneu B (2000) Early potent antithrombotic effect with combined aspirin and a loading dose of clopidogrel on experimental arterial thrombogenesis in humans. Circulation 101:2823–2828

34. Steinhubl SR, Berger PB, Mann JT III et al (2002) Early and sustained dual oral antiplatelet therapy following percu-taneous coronary intervention: a randomized controlled trial. JAMA 288:2411–2420

35. Chen ZM, Jiang LX, Chen YP et al (2005) Addition of clopidogrel to aspirin in 45, 852 patients with acute myocardial infarction: randomised placebo-controlled trial. Lancet 366:1607–1621

36. Sabatine MS, Cannon CP, Gibson CM et al (2005) Addition of clopidogrel to aspirin and fibrinolytic therapy for myo-cardial infarction with ST-segment elevation. N Engl J Med 352:1179–1189

37. Yusuf S, Zhao F, Mehta SR, Chrolavicius S, Tognoni G, Fox KK (2001) Effects of clopidogrel in addition to aspirin in patients with acute coronary syndromes without ST-segment elevation. N Engl J Med 345:494–502

38. Di Nisio M, Bijsterveld NR, Meijers JC, Levi M, Buller HR, Peters RJ (2005) Effects of clopidogrel on the rebound hypercoagulable state after heparin discontinuation in patients with acute coronary syndromes. J Am Coll Cardiol 46:1582–1583

39. Yusuf S, Mehta SR, Zhao F et al (2003) Early and late effects of clopidogrel in patients with acute coronary syndromes. Circulation 107:966–972

40. Mehta SR, Yusuf S, Peters RJ et al (2001) Effects of pretreatment with clopidogrel and aspirin followed by long-term therapy in patients undergoing percutaneous coronary intervention: the PCI-CURE study. Lancet 358:527–533

41. Lewis BS, Mehta SR, Fox KA et al (2005) Benefit of clopidogrel according to timing of percutaneous coronary inter-vention in patients with acute coronary syndromes: further results from the clopidogrel in unstable angina to prevent recurrent events (CURE) study. Am Heart J 150:1177–1184

42. McFadden EP, Stabile E, Regar E et al (2004) Late thrombosis in drug-eluting coronary stents after discontinuation of antiplatelet therapy. Lancet 364:1519–1521

43. Nasser M, Kapeliovich M, Markiewicz W (2005) Late thrombosis of sirolimus-eluting stents following noncardiac surgery. Catheter Cardiovasc Interv 65:516–519

44. Pfisterer M, Brunner-La Rocca HP, Buser PT et al (2006) Late clinical events after clopidogrel discontinuation may limit the benefit of drug-eluting stents: an observational study of drug-eluting versus bare-metal stents. J Am Coll Cardiol 48:2584–2591

45. Lagerqvist B, James SK, Stenestrand U, Lindback J, Nilsson T, Wallentin L (2007) Long-term outcomes with drug-eluting stents versus bare-metal stents in Sweden. N Engl J Med 356:1009–1019

46. Iakovou I, Schmidt T, Bonizzoni E et al (2005) Incidence, predictors, and outcome of thrombosis after successful implantation of drug-eluting stents. JAMA 293:2126–2130

47. Eisenstein EL, Anstrom KJ, Kong DF et al (2007) Clopidogrel use and long-term clinical outcomes after drug-eluting stent implantation. JAMA 297:159–168

48. Spertus JA, Kettelkamp R, Vance C et al (2006) Prevalence, predictors, and outcomes of premature discontinuation of thienopyridine therapy after drug-eluting stent placement: results from the PREMIER registry. Circulation 113:2803–2809

49. Boersma E, Harrington RA, Moliterno DJ et al (2002) Platelet glycoprotein IIb/IIIa inhibitors in acute coronary syndromes: a meta-analysis of all major randomised clinical trials. Lancet 359:189–198

50. Montalescot G, Borentain M, Payot L, Collet JP, Thomas D (2004) Early vs late administration of glycoprotein IIb/IIIa inhibitors in primary percutaneous coronary intervention of acute ST-segment elevation myocardial infarction: a meta-analysis. JAMA 292:362–366

51. Kastrati A, Mehilli J, Neumann FJ et al (2006) Abciximab in patients with acute coronary syndromes undergoing percutaneous coronary intervention after clopidogrel pretreatment: the ISAR-REACT 2 randomized trial. JAMA 295:1531–1538

52. Greenbaum AB, Grines CL, Bittl JA et al (2006) Initial experience with an intravenous P2Y12 platelet receptor antagonist in patients undergoing percutaneous coronary intervention: results from a 2-part, phase II, multicenter, randomized, placebo- and active-controlled trial. Am Heart J 151:689 e1–689 e10

53. Jacobsson F, Swahn E, Wallentin L, Ellborg M (2002) Safety profile and tolerability of intravenous AR-C69931MX, a new antiplatelet drug, in unstable angina pectoris and non-Q-wave myocardial infarction. Clin Ther 24:752–765

54. A clinical trial comparing cangrelor to clopidogrel in subjects who require percutaneous coronary intervention (CHAMPION-PCI). Available at http://clinicaltrials-nccs.nlm.nih.gov/ct/show/NCT00305162. Accessed 15 Nov 2007

55. A clinical trial comparing treatment with cangrelor (in combination with usual care), in subjects who require percutaneous coronary intervention. Available at http://clinicaltrials-nccs.nlm.nih.gov/ct/show/NCT00385138. Accessed 15 Nov 2007

56. Niitsu Y, Jakubowski JA, Sugidachi A, Asai F (2005) Pharmacology of CS-747 (prasugrel, LY640315), a novel, potent antiplatelet agent with in vivo P2Y12 receptor antagonist activity. Semin Thromb Hemost 31:184–194

57. Brandt JT, Payne CD, Wiviott SD et al (2007) A comparison of prasugrel and clopidogrel loading doses on platelet function: magnitude of platelet inhibition is related to active metabolite formation. Am Heart J 153:66 e9–66 e16

58. Matsushima N, Jakubowski JA, Asai F et al (2006) Platelet inhibitory activity and pharmacokinetics of prasugrel (CS-747) a novel thienopyridine P2Y12 inhibitor: a multiple-dose study in healthy humans. Platelets 17:218–226

59. Asai F, Jakubowski JA, Naganuma H et al (2006) Platelet inhibitory activity and pharmacokinetics of prasugrel (CS-747) a novel thienopyridine P2Y12 inhibitor: a single ascending dose study in healthy humans. Platelets 17:209–217

60. Wiviott SD, Antman EM, Winters KJ et al (2005) Randomized comparison of prasugrel (CS-747, LY640315), a novel thienopyridine P2Y12 antagonist, with clopidogrel in percutaneous coronary intervention: results of the joint utilization of medications to block platelets optimally (JUMBO)-TIM 26 trial. Circulation 111:3366–3373

61. Wiviott SD, Braunwald E, McCabe CH et al (2007) Prasugrel versus clopidogrel in patients with acute coronary syndromes. N Engl J Med 357:2001–2015

62. Murphy SA, Antman EM, Wiviott SD et al (2008) Reduction in recurrent cardiovascular events with prasugrel compared with clopidogrel in patients with acute coronary syndromes from the TRITON-TIMI 38 trial. Eur Heart J 29(20):2473–2479

63. Protocol H7T-MC-TABL(a) PRasurgrel IN Comparison to Clopidogrel for Inhibition of PLatelet Activation and AggrEgation (PRINCIPLE) – TIMI 44. Available at http://clinicaltrials-nccs.nlm.nih.gov/ct/show/NCT00357968. Accessed 15 Nov 2007

64. Husted S, Emanuelsson H, Heptinstall S, Sandset PM, Wickens M, Peters G (2006) Pharmacodynamics, pharmacokinetics, and safety of the oral reversible P2Y12 antagonist AZD6140 with aspirin in patients with atherosclerosis: a double-blind comparison to clopidogrel with aspirin. Eur Heart J 27:1038–1047

65. A randomised, double-blind, parallel group, phase 3, efficacy and safety study of AZD6140 compared with clopidogrel for prevention of vascular events in patients with non-ST or ST elevation acute coronary syndromes (ACS) [PLATO- a study of PLATelet inhibition and patient outcomes]. Available at http://clinicaltrials-nccs.nlm.nih.gov/ct/show/NCT00391872. Accessed 15 Nov 2007

66. Bertrand ME, Rupprecht HJ, Urban P, Gershlick AH (2000) Double-blind study of the safety of clopidogrel with and without a loading dose in combination with aspirin compared with ticlopidine in combination with aspirin after coronary stenting: the clopidogrel aspirin stent international cooperative study (CLASSICS). Circulation 102:624–629

67. Bertrand ME, Legrand V, Boland J et al (1998) Randomized multicenter comparison of conventional anticoagulation versus antiplatelet therapy in unplanned and elective coronary stenting. The full anticoagulation versus aspirin and ticlopidine (fantastic) study. Circulation 98:1597–1603

68. Muller C, Buttner HJ, Petersen J, Roskamm H (2000) A randomized comparison of clopidogrel and aspirin versus ticlopidine and aspirin after the placement of coronary-artery stents. Circulation 101:590–593

69. Taniuchi M, Kurz HI, Lasala JM (2001) Randomized comparison of ticlopidine and clopidogrel after intracoronary stent implantation in a broad patient population. Circulation 104:539–543

70. Dangas G, Mehran R, Abizaid AS et al (2001) Combination therapy with aspirin plus clopidogrel versus aspirin plus ticlopidine for prevention of subacute thrombosis after successful native coronary stenting. Am J Cardiol 87:470–472 A7

71. Berger PB, Bell MR, Rihal CS et al (1999) Clopidogrel versus ticlopidine after intracoronary stent placement. J Am Coll Cardiol 34:1891–1894

72. Stone GW, Moses JW, Ellis SG et al (2007) Safety and efficacy of sirolimus- and paclitaxel-eluting coronary stents. N Engl J Med 356:998–1008

73. Bavry AA, Kumbhani DJ, Helton TJ, Borek PP, Mood GR, Bhatt DL (2006) Late thrombosis of drug-eluting stents: a meta-analysis of randomized clinical trials. Am J Med 119:1056–1061

74. Kastrati A, Mehilli J, Pache J et al (2007) Analysis of 14 trials comparing sirolimus-eluting stents with bare-metal stents. N Engl J Med 356:1030–1039

75. Mauri L, Hsieh WH, Massaro JM, Ho KK, D'Agostino R, Cutlip DE (2007) Stent thrombosis in randomized clinical trials of drug-eluting stents. N Engl J Med 356:1020–1029

76. Airoldi F, Colombo A, Morici N et al (2007) Incidence and predictors of drug-eluting stent thrombosis during and after discontinuation of thienopyridine treatment. Circulation 116:745–754

77. Ong AT, McFadden EP, Regar E, de Jaegere PP, van Domburg RT, Serruys PW (2005) Late angiographic stent thrombosis (LAST) events with drug-eluting stents. J Am Coll Cardiol 45:2088–2092

78. (1994) Use of a monoclonal antibody directed against the platelet glycoprotein IIb/IIIa receptor in high-risk coronary angioplasty. The EPIC investigation. N Engl J Med 330:956–961

79. (1997) Platelet glycoprotein IIb/IIIa receptor blockade and low-dose heparin during percutaneous coronary revascularization. The EPILOG investigators. N Engl J Med 336:1689–1696

80. Lincoff AM, Tcheng JE, Califf RM et al (1999) Sustained suppression of ischemic complications of coronary intervention by platelet GP IIb/IIIa blockade with abciximab: one-year outcome in the EPILOG trial. Evaluation in PTCA to Improve Long-term Outcome with abciximab GP IIb/IIIa blockade. Circulation 99:1951–1958

81. (1997) Randomised placebo-controlled trial of abciximab before and during coronary intervention in refractory unstable angina: the CAPTURE Study. Lancet 349:1429–1435

82. Montalescot G, Barragan P, Wittenberg O et al (2001) Platelet glycoprotein IIb/IIIa inhibition with coronary stenting for acute myocardial infarction. N Engl J Med 344:1895–1903

83. Brener SJ, Barr LA, Burchenal JE et al (1998) Randomized, placebo-controlled trial of platelet glycoprotein IIb/IIIa blockade with primary angioplasty for acute myocardial infarction. ReoPro and Primary PTCA Organization and Randomized Trial (RAPPORT) Investigators. Circulation 98:734–741

84. Stone GW, Grines CL, Cox DA et al (2002) Comparison of angioplasty with stenting, with or without abciximab, in acute myocardial infarction. N Engl J Med 346:957–966

85. EPISTENT Investigators (1998) Randomised placebo-controlled and balloon-angioplasty-controlled trial to assess safety of coronary stenting with use of platelet glycoprotein-IIb/IIIa blockade. Lancet 352:87–92

86. Simoons ML (2001) Effect of glycoprotein IIb/IIIa receptor blocker abciximab on outcome in patients with acute coronary syndromes without early coronary revascularisation: the GUSTO IV-ACS randomised trial. Lancet 357:1915–1924

87. (1998) Inhibition of platelet glycoprotein IIb/IIIa with eptifibatide in patients with acute coronary syndromes. The PURSUIT trial investigators. Platelet glycoprotein IIb/IIIa in unstable angina: receptor suppression using integrilin therapy. N Engl J Med 339:436–443

88. ESPRIT Investigators (2000) Novel dosing regimen of eptifibatide in planned coronary stent implantation (ESPRIT): a randomised, placebo-controlled trial. Lancet 356:2037–2044

89. Randomised placebo-controlled trial of effect of eptifibatide on complications of percutaneous coronary intervention. IMPACT II. Integrellin to Minimise Platelet Aggregation and Coronary Thrombosis II. Lancet 1997. May 17, 349(9063):1422–1428

90. (1998) A comparison of aspirin plus tirofiban with aspirin plus heparin for unstable angina. Platelet receptor inhibition in ischemic syndrome management (PRISM) study investigators. N Engl J Med 338:1498–1505

91. Heeschen C, Hamm CW, Goldmann B, Deu A, Langenbrink L, White HD (1999) Troponin concentrations for stratification of patients with acute coronary syndromes in relation to therapeutic efficacy of tirofiban. PRISM study investigators. Platelet receptor inhibition in ischemic syndrome management. Lancet 354:1757–1762

92. (1998) Inhibition of the platelet glycoprotein IIb/IIIa receptor with tirofiban in unstable angina and non-Q-wave myocardial infarction. Platelet Receptor Inhibition in Ischemic Syndrome Management in Patients Limited by Unstable Signs and Symptoms (PRISM-PLUS) Study Investigators. N Engl J Med 338:1488–1497

8

Unfractionated Heparin and Enoxaparin for the Management of Non-ST-Segment Elevation Acute Coronary Syndromes

Pierluigi Tricoci and Kenneth W. Mahaffey

CONTENTS

ABSTRACT Unfractionated heparin (UFH) and low-molecular-weight heparin (LMWH) are antithrombin agents used to treat patients with non-ST-segment elevation acute coronary syndromes (NSTE ACS). Among LMWH agents, enoxaparin has the strongest evidence for use in NSTE ACS. While heparins were the only antithrombin drugs recommended for NSTE ACS treatment during the last decade, new developments in antithrombotic drugs – particularly bivalirudin and fondaparinux – have broadened the list of agents from which physicians may choose.

This chapter will focus on pharmacology and clinical data for enoxaparin and UFH in the management of patients with NSTE ACS, while clinical trials comparing heparins with new antithrombin agents will be described in detail in other chapters.

Key words: Acute coronary syndromes; Unfractionated heparin; Enoxaparin; Antithrombin; NSTE ACS

From: *Contemporary Cardiology: Antithrombotic Drug Therapy in Cardiovascular Disease*
Edited by: A.T. Askari and A.M. Lincoff (eds.), DOI 10.1007/978-1-60327-235-3_8
© Humana Press, a part of Springer Science+Business Media, LLC 2010

STRUCTURE AND MECHANISM OF ACTION

Unfractionated heparin (UFH) is a mixture of heparins, which are highly sulfated, negatively charged glycosaminoglycans. The molecules in the mixture are heterogeneous in molecular weight ranging from 3,000 to 30,000 Da *(1)*. Heparins act as indirect inhibitors of coagulation factors, because antithrombin, a natural regulator of the coagulation cascade, is required as a cofactor for the anticoagulant effect. Antithrombin and heparins form a complex that inhibits thrombin (factor IIa), factors Xa, IXa, XIa, and XIIa *(1)*. Among those factors, thrombin and factor Xa are the most sensitive to antithrombin/heparin inhibition *(1)*. UFH has a more potent effect on thrombin than on factor Xa, with an anti-IIa/anti-Xa activity ratio of approximately ten *(1)*. The weight of the heparin molecules determines the capability to inhibit factor IIa and the anti-IIa/anti-Xa ratio. In fact, the inhibitory effect on thrombin requires that a heparin molecule binds antithrombin and thrombin simultaneously. This complex can be formed only by heparin molecules with at least 18 saccharides *(1)*. The inhibition of factor Xa requires a heparin molecule to contain a specific pentasaccharidic sequence *(2)*. The pentasaccharide is a heparin sequence that binds antithrombin, producing a high anti-Xa effect without anti-IIa effect. Therefore, small heparin molecules containing pentasaccharide are highly selective in inhibiting factor Xa *(2)*. Approximately 30% of UFH molecules contain the requisite pentasaccharide *(1)*.

Low-molecular-weight heparins (LMWHs) are derived from depolymerization of UFH resulting in an average molecular weight that is approximately one-third of UFH (2,000–9,000 Da) *(3)*. The various LMWH agents commercially available differ in the method adopted to achieve depolymerization. Enoxaparin is obtained by alkaline depolymerization of heparin benzyl ester. Enoxaparin has an average molecular weight of approximately 4,500 Da *(4)*. Given their smaller size, LMWHs are less capable of inhibiting thrombin and therefore act more specifically as factor Xa inhibitors *(1)*. The anti-IIa/anti-Xa ratio for commercially available LMWH is typically from 1:2 to 1:4, and 1:3 for enoxaparin *(5)*. Selective factor Xa inhibition has been proposed as a potential pharmacological advantage of LMWH over UFH because factor Xa is located upstream in the coagulation cascade. However, no evidence confirms that anti-Xa activity is clinically superior to anti-IIa activity, or that anti-Xa selectivity represents a clinical advantage.

PHARMACOKINETICS

Circulating molecules contained in UFH mixtures bind to several plasma proteins and only 30% bind antithrombin, thus producing an actual anticoagulant effect *(1)*. Heparin molecules also bind endothelial cells and macrophages. These nonspecific protein- and cell-binding properties of heparin render its anticoagulant effect unpredictable *(1)*. The clearance of heparin from plasma occurs in two phases. The first, rapid, saturable phase is the consequence of the cell-binding properties of heparin. The second, slow, nonsaturable mechanism is mediated by renal clearance. As a consequence of this complex elimination, the anticoagulant effect of heparin is not linear at therapeutic doses *(1)*.

The most recognized pharmacologic advantage of LMWH over UFH is the pharmacokinetic profile. In fact, the lower molecular size of LMWH results in limited binding to plasma protein and cells *(4)*. This has two main reported consequences. First, the dose–response relationship is more predictable for LMWH, eliminating the need for monitoring in most clinical situations. Second, because of the lack of a rapid cell-mediated clearance mechanism, LMWH has a longer half-life and therefore can be administered at longer intervals without continuous infusion. Moreover, the higher subcutaneous bioavailability of LMWH obviates the need for intravenous infusion. The main elimination mechanism for LMWH is renal, with potential risk of accumulation in patients with renal insufficiency and need for dose adjustment *(1)*.

HEPARIN MONITORING AND DOSING

UFH

Given the unpredictability of the UFH anticoagulant effect, monitoring is required in clinical practice. The most common method for monitoring UFH therapy is the activated prothrombin time assay (aPTT) *(6)*. The activated clotting time (ACT) is used when a higher level of anticoagulation is needed, such as in percutaneous coronary intervention (PCI) and coronary artery bypass surgery (CABG) *(1)*. The aPTT is sensitive to the inhibitory effects of heparin on thrombin, factor Xa, and factor IXa; however, it is most sensitive to factor IIa activity *(6)*.

Despite the almost universal use of aPTT to monitor UFH therapy, there remains uncertainty about the optimal level of anticoagulation in patients with non-ST-segment elevation acute coronary syndromes (NSTE ACS). Several studies have investigated the relationship between aPTT, recurrent cardiovascular events, and bleeding in patients with ACS treated with UFH. In the Organization to Assess Strategies in Ischemic Syndromes 2 (OASIS 2) trial, values of aPTT<60 s were associated with an increased risk of ischemic complication compared with an aPTT>60 s. At the same time, there was a 7% increase in bleeding for each 10-s increase in aPTT *(7)*. Among patients treated with fibrinolysis in the Global Use of Strategies To Open Occluded Coronary Arteries I (GUSTO I) trial, an aPTT between 50 and 70 s at 12 h was found to be associated with the lowest rate of bleeding and ischemic complication *(8)*. The Thrombolysis in Myocardial Infarction IIIB (TIMI IIIB) trial failed to show differences in either aPTT values or protamine heparin concentrations among NSTE ACS patients with and without ischemic complications. Moreover, anticoagulation with heparin to achieve aPTT>2.0 times control did not appear to offer additional clinical benefit *(9)*. The GUSTO IIB trial, in which the target aPTT was prespecified at 50–70 s, showed a significant relationship between increasing 12-h aPTT and increasing rate of 30-day death or reinfarction; an aPTT between 50 and 60 s was associated with the lowest risk of bleeding *(10)*. Findings were similar in an analysis of the relationship of aPTT with ischemic events and bleeding in the Platelet IIb/IIIa Antagonism for the Reduction of Acute coronary syndrome events in a Global Organization Network (PARAGON), a study, which used blinded, central adjustment of heparin infusion rate based on a standard algorithm and a standard device for measuring aPTT *(11)*. Based on these data, current guidelines recommend an aPTT range between 50 and 70 s or between 1.5 and 2.0 times the laboratory control value for treatment of patients with NSTE ACS *(12)*. However, the significant variability in aPTT reagent sensitivity is a well-known problem *(6)*. In fact, aPTT measures obtained at different laboratories are not directly comparable due to the availability of numerous assays which may differ in thromboplastin reagents and coagulometer instruments *(13,14)*. It has been shown that, for a known heparin anti-Xa units of 0.3 U/ml, the corresponding aPTT varied from 48 to 108 s depending on method of determination used *(13,14)*. In practice, this means that the same patient treated at two different hospitals may require two very different heparin doses to achieve the same aPTT effect, resulting in two very different plasma heparin levels and possibly in vivo anticoagulant effect. To correct this lack of standardization of aPTT measurement, the College of American Pathologists and the American College of Chest Physicians recommended against the use of a fixed aPTT therapeutic range in favor of establishing a local therapeutic range by determining the aPTT range that, with the local assay, corresponds to heparin anti-Xa activity between 0.3 and 0.7 U/L (or protamine titration heparin levels of 0.2 to 0.4 U/ml) for the treatment of venous thromboembolism and 0.3–0.6 U/L for coronary indications such as NSTE ACS. However, the use of such heparin therapeutic levels, particularly in the setting of ACS, has never been validated in large outcome studies so the precise relationship between actual heparin concentration and outcomes remains unknown. Potential problems may also occur in anti-Xa measurement with the lack of standardization across assays. In addition, the relationship between anti-Xa activity and outcomes has not been appropriately examined in large populations.

Appropriate initial dosing of UFH is important to increase the likelihood that a patient achieves therapeutic anticoagulation levels. Because weight is a major determinant of the antithrombotic effect of UFH, weight-adjusted nomograms have been developed and have been shown to produce a more predictable anticoagulant effect and an increased chance of achieving therapeutic anticoagulation *(10,15–17)*. Moreover, a fixed dose of heparin results in marked initial over-anticoagulation in patients with ACS *(15)* and causes a significant increase in the rate of major bleeding *(18,19)*. Thus, American College of Cardiology (ACC)/American Heart Association (AHA) guidelines recommend an initial bolus dose of 60 U/kg (maximum 4,000 U) and an initial infusion of 12 U/kg/h (maximum1,000 U/h) *(12)*. The anticoagulant effect should be measured 6 h after the initiation of the therapy.

Enoxaparin

Enoxaparin, like other LMWHs, does not require monitoring in most clinical situations, and a fixed weight- and renal-adjusted dosing regimen is used to treat patients with NSTE ACS. The recommended dosing regimen of enoxaparin in NSTE ACS is 1 mg/kg every 12 h. A single daily dose of 1 mg/kg is recommended for patients with creatinine clearance <30 ml/min, to avoid drug accumulation and bleeding. A recent study in the setting of ST-segment elevation myocardial infarction treated with fibrinolysis, the Enoxaparin and Thrombolysis Reperfusion for Acute Myocardial Infarction Treatment, Thrombolysis in Myocardial Infarction 25 (ExTRACT-TIMI 25) study used a more conservative dosing regimen of enoxaparin in older patients treated with thrombolysis. Patients aged 75 years or older received a 0.75 mg/kg subcutaneous dose every 12 h (maximum 75 mg total) *(20)*.

Monitoring is not usually clinically required; however, anti-factor Xa assays are available to monitor therapy with LMWH. These anti-Xa assays have been used mostly for research aiming to establish a correlation between measures of LMWH effect and outcomes. Nonetheless, anti-Xa assays are also suggested for clinical monitoring of LMWH therapy in special populations such as patients with obesity and/or renal insufficiency *(1)*. Some studies have shown increased risk of bleeding with elevated anti-Xa levels (>0.8 U/ml) *(21)*, whereas others have failed to confirm this association *(22–24)*. Another analysis in an unselected NSTE ACS population showed that anti-Xa activity <0.5 U/ml with LMWH was associated with an increased risk of recurrent ischemic events at 30 days *(25)*.

An anti-Xa-dependent point-of-care assay (ENOX time) has been developed to monitor enoxaparin therapy. In a study evaluating ENOX times in patients undergoing PCI treated with enoxaparin, the test showed moderate correlation with laboratory-assessed anti-Xa level and no significant association with ischemic complication in the multivariable model, whereas increased ENOX times were associated with increased risk of bleeding *(26)*.

The American College of Chest Physicians guidelines recommend a therapeutic anti-Xa range for enoxaparin to be between 0.6 and 1.0 U/ml peak values for twice-daily regimens *(1)*.

CLINICAL TRIALS OF UFH IN NSTE ACS

Six randomized clinical trials have compared UFH and aspirin versus aspirin alone and provide the foundation of evidence for the use of UFH in patients with NSTE ACS. These trials, however, would be considered small by current standards, as none included more than 400 patients *(27–32)*. Nonetheless, they showed a relative risk reduction of 50–60% in the incidence of myocardial infarction within 1 week. In a systematic overview of these six randomized trials, UFH was associated with a statistically nonsignificant 33% reduction in the risk of death or myocardial infarction (relative risk [RR] 0.67; 95% confidence interval [CI] 0.44–1.02) *(33)*.

CLINICAL TRIALS OF LMWH IN NSTE ACS

Trials of LMWH versus Placebo

LMWH was clinically tested when therapy with UFH was already considered the standard of care, and therefore most trials with LMWH were performed against UFH as the control treatment. Two large trials, however, compared LMWH versus placebo: FRagmin during InStability in Coronary Artery Disease (FRISC) and the subsequent FRISC II trial (34,35). The FRISC trial compared 6-day dalteparin (120 U/kg twice a day) followed by 7,500 U once daily up to 45 days versus placebo in 1,506 patients with NSTE ACS (34). The rate of death or new myocardial infarction at 6 days was lower in the dalteparin group than in the placebo group (1.8% vs. 4.8%; RR 0.37; 95% CI 0.20–0.68). The benefit persisted at 40 days, although an increased risk of reinfarction was observed following dalteparin dose reduction. No differences were observed in the rates of death and myocardial infarction 4–5 months after the end of treatment.

The FRISC II trial further investigated the effect of long-term dalteparin in 2,267 patients with NSTE ACS. After a minimum of 5 days of treatment with open-label dalteparin, patients received subcutaneous dalteparin twice daily or placebo for 3 months. Similar to the FRISC trial, FRISC II showed a significant reduction of death or myocardial infarction in the dalteparin group at 30 days (3.1% vs. 5.9%; RR 0.53; 95% CI 0.35–0.80), which was no longer significant at 3 months (6.7% vs. 8.0%; RR 0.81; 95% CI 0.60–1.10).

Trials with LMWH versus UFH

A total of nine randomized clinical trials have compared LMWH and UFH, including six evaluating enoxaparin (Table 1). These trials have been completed over an extended period of time with changing patient demographics, concomitant medications, and management strategies.

FIRST LARGE RANDOMIZED CLINICAL TRIALS OF ENOXAPARIN VERSUS UFH IN NSTE ACS

The first two large randomized clinical trials comparing enoxaparin versus UFH in the treatment of patients with NSTE ACS were the Efficacy and Safety of Subcutaneous Enoxaparin in Non-Q-wave Coronary Events (ESSENCE) trial and the TIMI 11B trial (36,37). The ESSENCE trial randomized 3,171 patients with NSTE ACS to receive either subcutaneous enoxaparin (1 mg/kg twice daily) or intravenous UFH, for a minimum of 48 h to a maximum of 8 days. The primary end point was the composite of 14-day death, myocardial infarction, or recurrent angina. Patients in the enoxaparin group had a significant reduction in the incidence of the primary end point (16.6% vs. 19.8%; odds ratio [OR] 0.80; 95% CI 0.67–0.96). Also, at 30 days, the incidence of the composite triple end points remained significantly lower in the enoxaparin group (19.8% vs. 23.3%; OR 0.81; 95% CI 0.68–0.96). All bleeding was significantly higher in the enoxaparin group (18.4% vs. 14.2%; $P=0.001$), although major bleeding was not significantly different (6.5% vs. 7.0%; $P=0.57$). The 1-year follow up of the ESSENCE trial showed a sustained benefit of enoxaparin on the triple composite end point (32.0% vs. 35.7%; $P=0.022$) (38).

The TIMI 11B trial included 3,910 patients with NSTE ACS who received either enoxaparin (initial 30 mg intravenous bolus followed by subcutaneous injections of 1.0 mg/kg every 12 h) or 3–8 days of UFH infusion (initial 70 U/kg bolus and initial infusion of 15 U/kg/h; target aPTT 1.5–2.5 times the control) (37). The trial also had an outpatient phase during which patients in the enoxaparin group continued to receive the drug (40 mg subcutaneously every 12 h for patients weighing <65 kg and 60 mg for those weighing ≥65 kg) for an additional 35 days after hospital discharge, and patients in the UFH group received subcutaneous injections of placebo. The primary end point was the composite

Table 1
Randomized clinical trials of enoxaparin versus unfractionated heparin in NSTE ACS

Trial	Sample	Enoxaparin dosing	UFH initial dosing	Ischemic event rates and risk estimates (95% confidence intervals)	Major bleeding
Trials in the setting of an early conservative strategy					
ESSENCE (36)	3,171	Enoxaparin 1 mg/kg SC twice daily	UFH IV bolus (usually 5,000 U) and continued IV infusion	Death, MI, or recurrent angina At 14 days: enoxaparin 16.6%, UFH 19.8% (OR 0.80 [0.67–0.96]) At 30 days: enoxaparin 19.8%, UFH 23.3% (OR 0.81 [0.68–0.96])	At 30 days: enoxaparin 6.5%, UFH 7% (P=0.57)
TIMI 11B (37)	3,910	Inpatient: enoxaparin 30 mg IV bolus followed by 1 mg/kg SC every 12 h Outpatient: enoxaparin 40 mg SC every 12 h (patients <65 kg) or 60 mg SC twice per day (patients ≥65 kg)	Inpatient: UFH 70 U/kg IV bolus and 15 U/h IV infusion Outpatient: placebo SC twice per day	Death, MI, urgent revascularizationAt 48 h: enoxaparin 5.5%, UFH 7.3% (OR 0.75 [0.58–0.97]) At 8 days: enoxaparin 12.4%, UFH 14.5% (OR 0.83 [0.69–1.00]) At 14 days: enoxaparin 14.2%, UFH 16.7% (OR 0.82 [0.69–0.98]) At 43 days: enoxaparin 17.3%, UFH 19.7% (OR 0.85 [0.72–1.00])	At 48 h: enoxaparin 0.8%, UFH 0.7%; (P=0.14) End of index hospitalization: enoxaparin 1.5%, UFH 1% (P=0.143) Between Day 8 and Day 43: enoxaparin 2.9%, placebo 2.9% (P=0.021)

Trials in the setting of concomitant therapy with a GP IIb/IIIa inhibitor

ACUTE II (46)	525	Enoxaparin 1 mg/kg SC every 12 h	UFH 5,000 U IV bolus and maintenance infusion at 1,000 U/h IV adjusted to aPTT	Death at 30 days: enoxaparin 2.5%, UFH 1.9% (RR 1.3 [0.06–3.93]) MI at 30 days: enoxaparin 6.7%, UFH 7.1% (RR 0.94 [0.45–2.56])	Within 24 h of drug discontinuation: Enoxaparin 0.3%, UFH 1% (P=0.57)
INTERACT (47)	746	Enoxaparin 1 mg/kg SC every 12 h	UFH 70 U/kg IV bolus followed by 15 U/kg/h IV infusion	Death or MI at 30 days: enoxaparin 5.0%, UFH 9.0% (RR 0.55 [0.30–0.96])	At 96 h: enoxaparin 1.8%, UFH 4.6% (P=0.03)
A to Z (48)	3,987	Enoxaparin 1 mg/kg SC every 12 h	UFH 60 U/kg (maximum 4,000 U) IV bolus followed by 12 U/kg/h IV infusion (maximum 900 U/h)	Death, MI, or refractory ischemia within 7 days of tirofiban initiation: enoxaparin 8.4%, UFH 9.4% (HR 0.88 [0.71–1.08])	Within 24 h of tirofiban: enoxaparin 0.9%, UFH 0.4% (P=0.05)

Trial in the setting of an early invasive strategy

SYNERGY (52)	10,027	Enoxaparin 1 mg/kg SC every 12 h	UFH 60 U/kg IV bolus (maximum 5,000 U) followed by 12 U/kg/h (maximum 1,000 U/h)	Death or MI at 30 days: enoxaparin 14.0%, UFH 14.5% (HR 0.96 [0.86–1.06])	In-hospital TIMI major: enoxaparin 9.1%, UFH 7.6% (P=0.008) In-hospital GUSTO severe: enoxaparin 2.7%, UFH 2.2% (P=0.08)

GP glycoprotein; *GUSTO* global use of strategies to open occluded coronary arteries; *HR* hazard ratio; *MI* myocardial infarction; *NSTE ACS* non-ST-segment elevation acute coronary syndromes; *OR* odds ratio; *RR* relative risk; *SC* subcutaneous; *TIMI* Thrombolysis in Myocardial Infarction; *UFH* unfractionated heparin of death, myocardial infarction, or urgent revascularization. At 8 days, the primary end point occurred in 12.4% of patients in the enoxaparin group and 14.5% of patients in the UFH group (OR 0.83; 95% CI 0.69–1.00). This benefit was sustained in the outpatient phase of the study (17.3% vs. 19.7%; OR 0.85; 95% CI 0.72–1.00), but there was no further additional benefit of enoxaparin. The rate of major bleeding during the inpatient phase was not significantly different between the two groups (1.5% enoxaparin vs. 1.0 UFH; $P=0.143$), whereas the rate of minor bleeding was higher in the enoxaparin group, mostly due to ecchymosis reported at the injection site (9.5% vs. 2.5%; $P<0.001$). In the outpatient phase, patients treated with enoxaparin had a significantly higher rate of major (2.9% vs. 1.5%; $P=0.021$) and minor (19.3% vs. 5.2%; $P<0.001$) bleeding compared with placebo.

The results of the ESSENCE and TIMI 11B trials were analyzed as part of a prespecified systematic overview (39). The meta-analysis estimated that, overall, enoxaparin provided a 20% benefit over UFH in reduction of death and serious cardiac ischemic events. Moreover, pooled data demonstrated an 18–23% relative risk reduction of the composite of death or myocardial infarction, whereas the two trials individually did not show a significant reduction in this combined end point (36,37). The reduction of events occurred only in the first days of treatment, although it was sustained through 43 days. The drawback was the increase in the rate of minor bleeding associated with enoxaparin treatment (OR 2.38; 95% CI 1.98–2.85).

Results of trials with other LMWHs (dalteparin and nadroparin) have not been consistent with those of ESSENCE and TIMI 11B in showing superiority compared with UFH, thus negating a "class effect" of LMWHs. The FRIC trial failed to show a significant benefit of subcutaneous dalteparin compared with intravenous UFH during the acute phase of hospitalization in reducing the risk of death, myocardial infarction, or recurrent angina (9.3% dalteparin vs. 7.6% UFH; RR 1.18; 95% CI 0.84–1.66), with no benefit of dalteparin over placebo during prolonged treatment (up to 45 days) (40). Similarly, the FRAXiparine in Ischemic Syndrome (FRAXIS) trial showed that treatment with nadroparin for 6 days was not superior to UFH and that a more prolonged regimen (14 days) of nadroparin did not provide any additional benefit (41). The reason for the heterogeneity of results between trials with enoxaparin and those with dalteparin and nadroparin is not clear. Differences in LMWH preparations, anti-Xa/anti-IIa factor ratios, dose regimens, populations studied, and trial design have been proposed as possible explanations.

Despite the favorable results achieved by enoxaparin in the ESSENCE and TIMI 11B trials, there were scientific and practical barriers that limited widespread adoption of enoxaparin in clinical practice during the subsequent years. First, the ACC/AHA guidelines gave only a class IIa recommendation on the preference of enoxaparin over UFH (42). Second, management of patients with NSTE ACS continued to evolve with more common use of coronary catheterization and an early invasive strategy, and physicians struggled with integration of new pharmacotherapy and invasive approaches. Third, glycoprotein (GP) IIb/IIIa inhibitors and clopidogrel were also introduced, and the impact of these agents on bleeding and efficacy outcomes with enoxaparin had not been studied (42). In the pooled ESSENCE/TIMI 11B populations, only approximately 13% of patients underwent PCI during initial hospitalization, and use of clopidogrel and GP IIb/IIIa inhibitors was rare (39). Moreover, the trials of GP IIb/IIIa receptor antagonists – in both the setting of PCI and medically managed NSTE ACS patients – were conducted using concomitant antithrombin therapy with UFH (43,44), and ESSENCE and TIMI 11b mandated that patients received open-label UFH during coronary procedures to achieve ACT greater than 350 s (36,37). As a consequence, UFH remained the preferred antithrombotic drug among patients undergoing an early invasive strategy as did the practice of switching to UFH during PCI for those patients treated with enoxaparin.

A number of subsequent studies have reevaluated enoxaparin in a more contemporary NSTE ACS treatment setting, including concomitant GP IIb/IIIa receptor inhibition and an early invasive strategy.

TRIALS OF LMWH VERSUS UFH IN ADDITION TO A GP IIb/IIIa INHIBITOR

The Antithrombotic Combination Using Tirofiban and Enoxaparin (ACUTE) II trial, which followed the pilot ACUTE trial, evaluated the safety of adding enoxaparin to tirofiban in patients with NSTE ACS *(45,46)*. A total of 525 patients treated with tirofiban were randomized to receive enoxaparin (1 mg/kg every 12 h) or UFH (5,000 U initial bolus, 1,000 U/h initial infusion) for 24–96 h *(46)*. The total TIMI major or minor bleeding rate was not different between the two groups (3.5% vs. 4.8% for enoxaparin and UFH, respectively; OR 1.4; 95% CI 0.6–3.4). Although the trial was not powered to evaluate efficacy, no differences in the rate of death or myocardial infarction were observed, but recurrent ischemia was less frequent in the enoxaparin group.

The Integrilin and Enoxaparin Randomised Assessment of Acute Coronary Syndrome Treatment (INTERACT) trial randomized 746 patients with NSTE ACS treated with eptifibatide to receive open-label enoxaparin (1 mg/kg subcutaneously twice daily) or UFH (70 U/kg initial bolus, 15 kg/h infusion) for 48 h *(47)*. The primary safety outcome (96-h major non-CABG-related bleeding) was significantly lower in the enoxaparin group than in the UFH group (1.8% vs. 4.6%; $P=0.03$), but the rate of minor bleeding was higher in the enoxaparin group (30.3% vs. 20.8%; $P=0.003$). The trial also found lower rates of ischemic episodes detected by continuous electrocardiogram evaluation (primary efficacy outcome) and of 30-day death or myocardial infarction in the enoxaparin group.

The largest trial conducted to compare enoxaparin and UFH on a background therapy with GP IIb/IIIa inhibition was the prospective, international, open-label, randomized A to Z trial *(48)*. The objective of the study was to assess the noninferiority of enoxaparin (1 mg/kg every 12 h) compared with weight-adjusted intravenous UFH in patients with NSTE ACS treated with tirofiban. The treatment strategy (early invasive vs. conservative) was left to the discretion of the treating physician. The primary end point of the trial was the composite of death, myocardial infarction, or refractory ischemia at 7 days. Among the 3,987 patients randomized in the study, 8.4% experienced a primary end point event in the enoxaparin group and 9.4% in the UFH group (hazard ratio [HR] 0.88; 95% CI 0.71–1.08), meeting the prespecified criterion for noninferiority but not the criterion for superiority. Interestingly, the trial indicated a trend on the primary end point in favor of enoxaparin among patients who did not receive antithrombotic treatment prior to randomization (HR 0.77; 95% CI 0.53–1.11). The rate of any TIMI bleeding was 3.0% in the enoxaparin group and 2.2% in the UFH group ($P=0.13$).

TRIALS OF LMWH VERSUS UFH IN PATIENTS UNDERGOING AN EARLY INVASIVE STRATEGY

The Superior Yield of the New Strategy of Enoxaparin, Revascularization, and Glycoprotein IIb/IIIa Inhibitors (SYNERGY) trial was designed to compare enoxaparin with UFH in patients planned to undergo an early invasive strategy *(49)*. There were several reasons why such a trial was needed. First, patients undergoing an early invasive strategy are different from those treated conservatively with regards to demographic characteristics and risk profiles *(50)*. Second, the use of an early invasive strategy had been shown to reduce ischemic events in NSTE ACS, and therefore it was not clear whether therapy with enoxaparin would reproduce the benefit observed in the setting of a conservative strategy *(51)*. Third, patients undergoing PCI more often receive triple antiplatelet therapy, including aspirin, clopidogrel, and a GP IIb/IIIa inhibitor. Fourth, interventional cardiologists have been reluctant to use enoxaparin during PCI because of a lack of anticoagulant monitoring and also because of concerns regarding sheath management. Finally, the SYNERGY trial evaluated enoxaparin and UFH in a high-risk population, whereas previous trials included a broader NSTE ACS population, mostly at low to moderate risk.

SYNERGY was a randomized, open-label trial including 10,027 high-risk NSTE ACS patients *(52)*. Patients received either subcutaneous enoxaparin or weight-adjusted aPTT-titrated intravenous UFH. The primary efficacy outcome was the composite of death or nonfatal myocardial infarction during the first 30 days after randomization. The goal of the trial was primarily to demonstrate the superiority of enoxaparin over UFH, and subsequently to test for noninferiority if superiority was not demonstrated. The primary end point occurred in 14.0% of patients in the enoxaparin group and 14.5% of patients in the UFH group (OR 0.96; 95% CI 0.86–1.06). Thus, enoxaparin failed to demonstrate superiority but met the criterion for noninferiority. Overall, enoxaparin was associated with a significant increase in the risk of TIMI major bleeding (9.1% vs. 7.6%; $P=0.008$) and a nonsignificant trend toward increase in the rate of GUSTO severe bleeding (2.7% vs. 2.2%; $P=0.08$) and transfusions (17.0% vs. 16.0%; $P=0.16$). The SYNERGY trial allowed patients to be randomized even if an antithrombin had been started prior to randomization, and a total of 75% of patients had actually received either UFH or LMWH. The analysis of patients who did not receive any prerandomization therapy or who received consistent pre- and postrandomization therapy showed a reduced risk of 30-day death or myocardial infarction among those randomized to receive enoxaparin (13.9% vs. 15.9%; HR 0.82; 95% CI 0.72–0.94) and no differences in blood transfusion (16.9% vs. 17.0%). In subgroup analyses specifically addressing the impact of prerandomization treatment, after adjustment for differences in baseline characteristics, consistent therapy with enoxaparin was associated with a reduced risk of 30-day death or myocardial infarction, with a trend toward increased risk of bleeding *(53)*.

OVERVIEW OF TRIALS COMPARING LMWH AND UFH IN NSTE ACS

Trials comparing UFH and enoxaparin in NSTE ACS conducted at different times and with different concomitant medication and treatment strategies have produced different results. Enoxaparin was shown to be superior to UFH in trials where patients were mostly treated with a conservative approach and with no use of dual or triple antiplatelet therapy *(36,37)*. Trials performed with a background therapy of GP IIb/IIIa inhibition and a trial performed in the setting of an early invasive strategy with high rates of PCI, clopidogrel, and GP IIb/IIIa inhibitor use have shown substantial equivalence of the two treatments on the efficacy side, and some advantage of UFH in terms of bleeding risk *(48,52)*.

Petersen et al. performed a systematic overview of all six randomized clinical trials comparing enoxaparin and UFH in NSTE ACS (including >22,000 patients) to investigate whether differences in the relative efficacy and safety exist between the two drugs across time and evolution of NSTE ACS treatment *(54)*. At 30 days, the rate of death was similar for enoxaparin and UFH (3.0% vs. 3.0%; OR 1.00; 95% CI 0.85–1.17), but there was a mild, yet significant, benefit in the composite of death or myocardial infarction at 30 days in patients treated with enoxaparin (10.1% vs. 11.0%; OR 0.91; 95% CI 0.83–0.99) (Fig. 1). The size of effect of enoxaparin on 30-day death or MI was greater among patients who did not receive prerandomization antithrombin therapy (8.0% vs. 9.4%; OR 0.81; 95% CI 0.70–0.94). No significant difference was found in odds of blood transfusion (OR 1.01; 95% CI 0.89–1.14) or major bleeding (OR 1.04; 95% CI 0.83–1.30) at 7 days after randomization. Similar results were found in patients who did not receive prerandomization therapy. The data from this meta-analysis seem to support the concept that enoxaparin, when used consistently during the course of hospitalization, may be superior to UFH, without a significant toll in terms of bleeding.

MANAGEMENT OF ANTITHROMBIN THERAPY DURING PCI IN NSTE ACS PATIENTS

UFH historically has been the antithrombin agent of choice during PCI, even after the introduction of LMWH. The main reasons for this preference likely derive from the familiarity of interventional cardiologists with the drug and the ability to monitor the anticoagulant effect prior to the procedure and to sheath removal. Moreover, because of limited experience with LMWH use, the first trials on

Death or Myocardial Infarction at 30 Days

| Trial | Events, No./Total (%) | | OR (95% CI) |
	Enoxaparin	UFH	
ESSENCE[7]	94/1607 (5.8)	118/1564 (7.5)	0.76 (0.58-1.01)
TIMI 11B[8]	145/1953 (7.4)	163/1957 (8.3)	0.88 (0.70-1.11)
ACUTE II[18]	25/315 (7.9)	17/210 (8.1)	0.97 (0.51-1.83)
INTERACT[17]	19/380 (5.0)	33/366 (9.0)	0.54 (0.30-0.96)
A to Z[15]	137/1852 (7.4)	139/1768 (7.9)	0.94 (0.73-1.20)
SYNERGY[16]	696/4992 (14.0)	722/4982 (14.5)	0.96 (0.86-1.07)
Overall	1116/11099 (10.1)	1192/10847 (11.0)	0.91 (0.83-0.99)

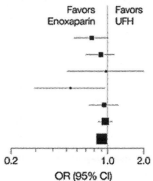

Death or Myocardial Infarction at 30 Days

| Trial | Events, No./Total (%) | | OR (95% CI) |
	Enoxaparin	UFH	
ESSENCE[7]	94/1607 (5.8)	118/1564 (7.5)	0.76 (0.58-1.01)
TIMI 11B[8]	81/1257 (6.4)	97/1242 (7.8)	0.81 (0.60-1.10)
INTERACT[17]	14/304 (4.6)	24/295 (8.1)	0.55 (0.28-1.08)
A to Z[15]	43/589 (7.3)	37/537 (6.9)	1.06 (0.68-1.67)
SYNERGY[16]	165/1212 (12.6)	44/1228 (14.8)	0.84 (0.68-1.05)
Overall	397/4969 (8.0)	458/4866 (9.4)	0.81 (0.70-0.94)

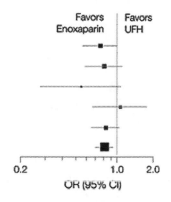

Fig. 1. Meta-analysis of six randomized clinical trials comparing enoxaparin and UFH in NSTE ACS. *Top panel* shows the odds ratios for 30-day death or myocardial infarction in all patients included in the meta-analysis. *Bottom panel* shows the odds ratios for 30-day death or myocardial infarction among patients who did not receive an antithrombin agent prior to randomization. From Ref. *(54)* (permission request pending).

enoxaparin mandated the use of open-label UFH even during PCI *(36,37)*. Consequently, a widely adopted strategy in clinical practice for patients treated with enoxaparin and undergoing PCI was to "hold" the morning injection of enoxaparin and administer additional UFH bolus prior to the PCI. The practice of "holding then switching" has been also endorsed by previous ACC/AHA guidelines *(42)*.

However, clinical studies published over the years have consistently shown that PCI can be safely performed in patients who are receiving standard doses of enoxaparin. In a cohort of 451 consecutive NSTE ACS patients treated with standard enoxaparin dose for 48 h, Collet et al. showed that, when PCI was performed within 8 h of the last dose of enoxaparin, no in-hospital abrupt closures or urgent revascularizations occurred after PCI *(55)*. In the National Investigators Collaborating on Enoxaparin (NICE) 1 study groups, registry patients undergoing PCI received enoxaparin 1.0 mg/kg intravenously (without abciximab), whereas those enrolled in the NICE 4 registry received 0.75 mg/kg of enoxaparin intravenously in addition to abciximab. Bleeding events and ischemic outcomes assessed in-hospital and at 30 days post-PCI were infrequent and not superior to historical control *(56)*.

In the SYNERGY trial, in patients assigned to enoxaparin and undergoing PCI within 8 h of the last subcutaneous injection, no additional anticoagulant (neither enoxaparin nor UFH) was to be given *(52)*. For those who received the last enoxaparin dose 8 or more hours before the PCI, an additional intravenous bolus of 0.3 mg/kg of enoxaparin was to be given before the procedure. The trial found no differences in ischemic complication during PCI between patients treated with enoxaparin and those treated with UFH – including abrupt closures, threatened abrupt closures, or emergency CABG – and no differences in the rate of 30-day death or myocardial infarction *(57)*. The possibility of safely performing PCI under anticoagulation with enoxaparin was specifically investigated and confirmed in the Safety and Efficacy of Enoxaparin in Percutaneous Coronary Intervention Patients, an International Randomized Evaluation (STEEPLE) trial *(58)*. The trial randomized 3,528 patients undergoing elective PCI to receive enoxaparin (0.5 mg/kg or 0.75 mg/kg) or ACT-adjusted UFH dose. The primary end point was the incidence of non-CABG-related major or minor bleeding. Patients in the enoxaparin 0.5 mg/kg group had a significant reduction in the rate of non-CABG-related bleeding compared with UFH (5.9% vs. 8.5%; absolute difference –2.6; 95% CI [–4.7, –0.6]), whereas, among patients in the enoxaparin 0.75 mg/kg group, the difference was nonsignificant (6.5% vs. 8.5%; absolute difference –2.0; 95% CI –4.0–0.0). The rate of major bleeding was significantly lower in both enoxaparin groups compared with UFH.

Overall, these results have important implications for the management of patients with NSTE ACS undergoing PCI. In fact, they indicate that UFH and enoxaparin are both adequate choices for use in the performance of PCI in patients with NSTE ACS.

CLINICAL PERSPECTIVE AND CURRENT GUIDELINE RECOMMENDATIONS

Despite decades of use in clinical practice, several key issues regarding heparin remain unresolved. The first is related to the unpredictability of the pharmacologic effect of UFH and the need to monitor its antithrombotic effect to calculate the dosing. Infusion doses of UFH are based on complex protocols which are poorly standardized across hospitals, and, as a consequence, the clinical trial results may not be observed in routine clinical practice *(59)*. There is also uncertainty about the appropriate tool for measuring the anticoagulant effect and the optimal therapeutic range. In fact, the widely used aPTT measurement is poorly standardized, making it almost impossible to directly compare the reference ranges across laboratories *(1)*. The therapeutic aPTT range itself is not well established. Recent heparin guidelines recommend using heparin anti-Xa assay to establish the local aPTT, but the therapeutic heparin anti-Xa range with UFH in NSTE ACS has never been studied *(1)*. Enoxaparin overcomes some of these limitations of UFH because of its more predictable pharmacology, the better standardization of dosing regimens, and the lack of need for monitoring in most clinical situations.

One clinically important issue with enoxaparin is the need for decreased dose in patients with chronic kidney disease. Current dosing guidelines include an increase of the dosing interval from 12 to 24 h in patients with creatinine clearance <30 ml/min. It is unclear, however, whether a more conservative dosing regimen may be warranted in patients with more modest degrees of renal dysfunction *(60)* or with other characteristics such as advanced age.

Clinical experiences suggest that routine switching from enoxaparin to UFH is common, despite data to support continued therapy and the protective effect of enoxaparin on thrombotic complication during PCI. For example, SYNERGY, in which no periprocedural monitoring of enoxaparin therapy was used, demonstrated no procedural differences in ischemic events compared with UFH. Although potential confounders complicate the interpretation of the risk of events occurring in postrandomization groups, these data, along with the demonstrated comparable efficacy of enoxaparin and UFH during PCI, should discourage the adoption of switching between heparins *(49,58)*.

Currently, physicians may choose from among four different agents for antithrombin therapy in NSTE ACS: UFH, enoxaparin, fondaparinux, and bivalirudin. The recently revised ACC/AHA and European Society of Cardiology guidelines have incorporated the results of clinical trials of bivalirudin and fondaparinux and consequently have expanded the list of recommended drugs *(12,61–63)*.

Table 2
Class of recommendation and level of evidence regarding NSTE ACS antithrombin therapies in 2007 ACC/AHA and ESC guidelines

Class of recommendation, level of evidence	Urgent/early invasive strategy		Conservative/non-urgent invasive strategy	
	ESC	ACC/AHA	ESC	ACC/AHA
I, A		Enoxaparin, UFH	Fondaparinux	Enoxaparin, UFH
I, B	Bivalirudin	Bivalirudin, fondaparinux		Fondaparinux[a]
I, C	UFH			
IIa, B	Enoxaparin		Enoxaparin[b], LMWH, UFH	Enoxaparin, fondaparinux[c]

[a]Fondaparinux preferred if there is an increased risk of bleeding
[b]Enoxaparin recommended only if the risk of bleeding is low
[c]Enoxaparin or fondaparinux preferred over UFH unless CABG is planned <24 h
ACC American College of Cardiology; AHA American Heart Association; ESC European Society of Cardiology; NSTE ACS nNon-ST-segment elevation acute coronary syndromes; UFH unfractionated heparin

The ACC/AHA and ESC guidelines interpreted these results differently, however, thereby highlighting the complexities and pitfalls in the design of such trials and in inferences from subgroup analyses (Table 2). The ACC/AHA guidelines have given a class I recommendation to each of the four agents. Given the larger number of available randomized clinical trial data, UFH and enoxaparin have a level of evidence A, whereas bivalirudin and fondaparinux – which are supported by only one trial in the NSTE ACS population – have a level of evidence B. Nonetheless, current guidelines do not indicate any preference as to which agent should be chosen in patients undergoing an early invasive strategy. In patients undergoing conservative treatment, the guidelines express a preference for enoxaparin or fondaparinux (class IIb), with fondaparinux being the agent of choice for patients at risk of bleeding (class I).

The ESC guidelines indicated a preference for bivalirudin use among patients undergoing an urgent early invasive strategy (IB), with UFH as a possible alternative (IC). Enoxaparin has only been attributed a class IIa, and fondaparinux has not been included as a possible choice in the setting of rapid cardiac catheterization. In patients who receive a conservative approach or a delayed catheterization, the ESC guidelines clearly indicate fondaparinux as the preferred choice (IA), as opposed to enoxaparin and UFH (IIa and B, respectively).

In our view, there are several factors to be taken into account when deciding which antithrombin agent should be used. These include the treatment strategy (invasive vs. conservative), the institutional standard practice of time to cardiac catheterization (same day vs. next day vs. other), the use of upstream GP IIb/IIIa inhibitors, the use of clopidogrel as initial medical therapy, the presence of renal disease, and the overall risk of bleeding. However, none of these factors has been clearly proven to be critical to predict the benefit/risk of each currently available antithrombotic drug relative to another, and they mostly derive from informal evaluation of the populations included in trials, the concomitant medication used, and the treatment strategies adopted.

For high-risk patients requiring a GP IIb/IIIa inhibitor who do not undergo cardiac catheterization in the first few hours, enoxaparin or UFH may still represent the first choice, particularly if enoxaparin is used consistently. In patients with renal disease, those at higher risk of bleeding, and those who are treated conservatively, fondaparinux may be the treatment of choice. Finally, bivalirudin may represent the optimal choice for those patients undergoing expedited PCI with no planned use of GP IIb/IIIa inhibitors, in patients not at high risk, or in those pretreated with clopidogrel prior to PCI. As stated above, those recommendations should be seen more as general criteria from which to choose, rather than as guidelines supported by scientific evidence from specific randomized clinical investigations. However, rather than deciding on a case-by-case basis, it is recommended that each hospital adopt a protocol indicating the antithrombin of choice to be used locally. The protocol should indicate specific instructions relative to dosing, timing of administration, monitoring (as needed), and management of the therapy in case of catheterization, PCI, or CABG. The protocol should also specify special situations in which another agent may be preferable.

A protocol-based approach has several potential advantages. First, it ensures that patients admitted to the hospital receive consistent treatment, thereby avoiding changes in therapy within the same hospital. For the same reason, patients who come from another hospital and have already received an antithrombin drug should continue the treatment started at the first hospital rather than switching to accommodate local or personal preferences. Second, the adoption of a protocol with a "first-choice" drug increases the familiarity of physicians and other health care professionals with the chosen agent. Increased familiarity and specific dosing guidelines may decrease the risk of dosing errors and is even more critical for those therapies with more complex dosing regimens (64).

In conclusion, despite the developments in new antithrombotic drugs, UFH and enoxaparin still represent valuable choices for the treatment of patients with NSTE ACS and retain an ACC/AHA guideline recommendation of class I, level of evidence A. Appropriate dosing, consistency of therapy, and adequate management of therapy during invasive procedures are critical to optimize the balance of efficacy and safety when these drugs are used.

REFERENCES

1. Hirsh J, Raschke R (2004) Heparin and low-molecular-weight heparin: the Seventh ACCP Conference on Antithrombotic and Thrombolytic Therapy. Chest 126(3 suppl):188S–203S
2. Walenga JM, Jeske WP, Bara L et al (1997) Biochemical and pharmacologic rationale for the development of synthetic heparin pentasaccharide. Thromb Res 86(1):1–36
3. Fareed J, Jeske W, Hoppensteadt D et al (1998) Low-molecular-weight heparins: pharmacologic profile and product differentiation. Am J Cardiol 82(5B):3L–10L
4. Fareed J, Hoppensteadt D, Walenga J et al (2003) Pharmacodynamic and pharmacokinetic properties of enoxaparin: implications for clinical practice. Clin Pharmacokinet 42(12):1043–1057
5. Antman EM, Handin R (1998) Low-molecular-weight heparins: an intriguing new twist with profound implications. Circulation 98(4):287–289
6. Bates SM, Weitz JI (2005) Coagulation assays. Circulation 112(4):e53–e60
7. Anand SS, Yusuf S, Pogue J et al (2003) Relationship of activated partial thromboplastin time to coronary events and bleeding in patients with acute coronary syndromes who receive heparin. Circulation 107(23):2884–2888
8. Granger CB, Hirsh J, Califf RM et al (1996) Activated partial thromboplastin time and outcome after thrombolytic therapy for acute myocardial infarction: results from the GUSTO-I trial. Circulation 93(5):870–878
9. Becker RC, Cannon CP, Tracy RP et al (1996) Relation between systemic anticoagulation as determined by activated partial thromboplastin time and heparin measurements and in-hospital clinical events in unstable angina and non-Q wave myocardial infarction. Thrombolysis in Myocardial Ischemia III B Investigators. Am Heart J 131(3):421–433
10. Lee MS, Wali AU, Menon V et al (2002) The determinants of activated partial thromboplastin time, relation of activated partial thromboplastin time to clinical outcomes, and optimal dosing regimens for heparin treated patients with acute coronary syndromes: a review of GUSTO-IIb. J Thromb Thrombolysis 14(2):91–101
11. Newby LK, Harrington RA, Bhapkar MV et al (2002) An automated strategy for bedside aPTT determination and unfractionated heparin infusion adjustment in acute coronary syndromes: insights from PARAGON A. J Thromb Thrombolysis 14(1):33–42
12. Anderson JL, Adams CD, Antman EM et al (2007) ACC/AHA 2007 guidelines for the, management of patients with unstable angina/non-ST-elevation myocardial infarction: a report of the American College of Cardiology/American

Heart Association Task Force on Practice Guidelines (Writing Committee to Revise the 2002 Guidelines for the Management of Patients With Unstable Angina/Non-ST-Elevation Myocardial Infarction) developed in collaboration with the American College of Emergency Physicians, the Society for Cardiovascular Angiography and Interventions, and the Society of Thoracic Surgeons endorsed by the American Association of Cardiovascular and Pulmonary Rehabilitation and the Society for Academic Emergency Medicine. J Am Coll Cardiol 50(7):e1–e157

13. Bates SM, Weitz JI, Johnston M et al (2001) Use of a fixed activated partial thromboplastin time ratio to establish a therapeutic range for unfractionated heparin. Arch Intern Med 161(3):385–391

14. Brill-Edwards P, Ginsberg JS, Johnston M et al (1993) Establishing a therapeutic range for heparin therapy. Ann Intern Med 119(2):104–109

15. Hochman JS, Wali AU, Gavrila D et al (1999) A new regimen for heparin use in acute coronary syndromes. Am Heart J 138(2 Pt 1):313–318

16. Hassan WM, Flaker GC, Feutz C et al (1995) Improved anticoagulation with a weight-adjusted heparin nomogram in patients with acute coronary syndromes: a randomized trial. J Thromb Thrombolysis 2(3):245–249

17. Becker RC, Ball SP, Eisenberg P et al (1999) A randomized, multicenter trial of weight-adjusted intravenous heparin dose titration and point-of-care coagulation monitoring in hospitalized patients with active thromboembolic disease. Antithrombotic Therapy Consortium Investigators. Am Heart J 137(1):59–71

18. (1994) Use of a monoclonal antibody directed against the platelet glycoprotein IIb/IIIa receptor in high-risk coronary angioplasty. The EPIC Investigation. N Engl J Med 330(14):956–961

19. (1997) Platelet glycoprotein IIb/IIIa receptor blockade and low-dose heparin during percutaneous coronary revascularization. The EPILOG Investigators. N Engl J Med 336(24):1689–1696

20. Antman EM, Morrow DA, McCabe CH et al (2006) Enoxaparin versus unfractionated heparin with fibrinolysis for ST-elevation myocardial infarction. N Engl J Med 354(14):1477–1488

21. Nieuwenhuis HK, Albada J, Banga JD et al (1991) Identification of risk factors for bleeding during treatment of acute venous thromboembolism with heparin or low-molecular-weight heparin. Blood 78(9):2337–2343

22. Bara L, Leizorovicz A, Picolet H et al (1992) Correlation between anti-Xa and occurrence of thrombosis and haemorrhage in post-surgical patients treated with either Logiparin (LMWH) or unfractionated heparin. Post-surgery Logiparin Study Group. Thromb Res 65(4–5):641–650

23. Walenga JM, Hoppensteadt D, Fareed J (1991) Laboratory monitoring of the clinical effects of low-molecular-weight heparins. Thromb Res Suppl 14:49–62

24. Prandoni P, Lensing AW, Buller HR et al (1992) Comparison of subcutaneous low-molecular-weight heparin with intravenous standard heparin in proximal deep-vein thrombosis. Lancet 339(8791):441–445

25. Montalescot G, Collet JP, Tanguy ML et al (2004) Anti-Xa activity relates to survival and efficacy in unselected acute coronary syndrome patients treated with enoxaparin. Circulation 110(4):392–398

26. Moliterno DJ, Hermiller JB, Kereiakes DJ et al (2003) A novel point-of-care enoxaparin monitor for use during percutaneous coronary intervention: Results of the Evaluating Enoxaparin Clotting Times (ELECT) Study. J Am Coll Cardiol 42(6):1132–1139

27. Telford AM, Wilson C (1981) Trial of heparin versus atenolol in prevention of myocardial infarction in intermediate coronary syndrome. Lancet 1(8232):1225–1228

28. Williams DO, Kirby MG, McPherson K et al (1986) Anticoagulant treatment of unstable angina. Br J Clin Pract 40(3):114–116

29. Neri Serneri GG, Gensini GF, Poggesi L et al (1990) Effect of heparin, aspirin, or alteplase in reduction of myocardial ischaemia in refractory unstable angina. Lancet 335(8690):615–618

30. Holdright D, Patel D, Cunningham D et al (1994) Comparison of the effect of heparin and aspirin versus aspirin alone on transient myocardial ischemia and in-hospital prognosis in patients with unstable angina. J Am Coll Cardiol 24(1):39–45

31. Theroux P, Waters D, Qiu S et al (1993) Aspirin versus heparin to prevent myocardial infarction during the acute phase of unstable angina. Circulation 88(5 Pt 1):2045–2048

32. Cohen M, Adams PC, Hawkins L et al (1990) Usefulness of antithrombotic therapy in resting angina pectoris or non-Q-wave myocardial infarction in preventing death and myocardial infarction (a pilot study from the Antithrombotic Therapy in Acute Coronary Syndromes Study Group). Am J Cardiol 66(19):1287–1292

33. Oler A, Whooley MA, Oler J et al (1996) Adding heparin to aspirin reduces the incidence of myocardial infarction and death in patients with unstable angina. A meta-analysis. JAMA 276(10):811–815

34. Low-molecular-weight heparin during instability in coronary artery disease (1996) Fragmin during Instability in Coronary Artery Disease (FRISC) study group. Lancet 347(9001):561–568

35. (1999) Long-term low-molecular-mass heparin in unstable coronary artery disease: FRISC II prospective randomised multicentre study. FRagmin and Fast Revascularisation during InStability in Coronary artery disease Investigators. Lancet 354(9180):701–707.

36. Cohen M, Demers C, Gurfinkel EP et al (1997) A comparison of low-molecular-weight heparin with unfractionated heparin for unstable coronary artery disease. Efficacy and Safety of Subcutaneous Enoxaparin in Non-Q-Wave Coronary Events Study Group. N Engl J Med 337(7):447–452

37. Antman EM, McCabe CH, Gurfinkel EP et al (1999) Enoxaparin prevents death and cardiac ischemic events in unstable angina/non-Q-wave myocardial infarction: results of the Thrombolysis In Myocardial Infarction (TIMI) 11B trial. Circulation 100(15):1593–1601

38. Goodman SG, Cohen M, Bigonzi F et al (2000) Randomized trial of low-molecular-weight heparin (enoxaparin) versus unfractionated heparin for unstable coronary artery disease: one-year results of the ESSENCE study Efficacy and Safety of Subcutaneous Enoxaparin in Non-Q-Wave Coronary Events. J Am Coll Cardiol 36(3):693–698

39. Antman EM, Cohen M, Radley D et al (1999) Assessment of the treatment effect of enoxaparin for unstable angina/non-Q-wave myocardial infarction TIMI 11B-ESSENCE meta-analysis. Circulation 100(15):1602–1608

40. Klein W, Buchwald A, Hillis SE et al (1997) Comparison of low-molecular-weight heparin with unfractionated heparin acutely and with placebo for 6 weeks in the management of unstable coronary artery disease Fragmin in unstable coronary artery disease study (FRIC). Circulation 96(1):61–68

41. (1999) Comparison of two treatment durations (6 days and 14 days) of a low-molecular-weight heparin with a 6-day treatment of unfractionated heparin in the initial management of unstable angina or non-Q-wave myocardial infarction: FRAX.I.S. (FRAxiparine in Ischaemic Syndrome). Eur Heart J 20(21):1553–1562.

42. Braunwald E, Antman EM, Beasley JW et al (2002) ACC/AHA 2002 guideline update for the management of patients with unstable angina and non-ST-segment elevation myocardial infarction–summary article: a report of the American College of Cardiology/American Heart Association Task Force on Practice Guidelines (Committee on the Management of Patients With Unstable Angina). J Am Coll Cardiol 40(7):1366–1374

43. Boersma E, Harrington RA, Moliterno DJ et al (2002) Platelet glycoprotein IIb/IIIa inhibitors in acute coronary syndromes: a meta-analysis of all major randomised clinical trials. Lancet 359(9302):189–198

44. Karvouni E, Katritsis DG, Ioannidis JP (2003) Intravenous glycoprotein IIb/IIIa receptor antagonists reduce mortality after percutaneous coronary interventions. J Am Coll Cardiol 41(1):26–32

45. Cohen M, Theroux P, Weber S et al (1999) Combination therapy with tirofiban and enoxaparin in acute coronary syndromes. Int J Cardiol 71(3):273–281

46. Cohen M, Theroux P, Borzak S et al (2002) Randomized double-blind safety study of enoxaparin versus unfractionated heparin in patients with non-ST-segment elevation acute coronary syndromes treated with tirofiban and aspirin: the ACUTE II study. The Antithrombotic Combination Using Tirofiban and Enoxaparin study. Am Heart J 144(3):470–477

47. Goodman SG, Fitchett D, Armstrong PW et al (2003) Randomized evaluation of the safety and efficacy of enoxaparin versus unfractionated heparin in high-risk patients with non-ST-segment elevation acute coronary syndromes receiving the glycoprotein IIb/IIIa inhibitor eptifibatide. Circulation 107(2):238–244

48. Blazing MA, de Lemos JA, White HD et al (2004) Safety and efficacy of enoxaparin vs unfractionated heparin in patients with non-ST-segment elevation acute coronary syndromes who receive tirofiban and aspirin: a randomized controlled trial. JAMA 292(1):55–64

49. Torbicki A, Perrier A, Konstantinides SV et al. Guidelines on the diagnosis and management of acute pulmonary embolims: The Task Force for the Diagnosis and Management of Acute Pulmonary Embolism of the European Society of Cardiology (ESC). Eur Heart J 2008: 29:2276–2315

50. Kearon C, Kahn SR, Agnelli G, Goldhaber S, Raskob GE, Comerota AJ. Antithrombotic therapy for venous thromboembolic disease: American College of Chest Physicians Evidence-Based Clinical Practice Guidelines (8th Edition). Chest 2008; 133(6 Suppl):454S–545S.

51. Mehta SR, Steg PG, Granger CB et al (2005) Randomized, blinded trial comparing fondaparinux with unfractionated heparin in patients undergoing contemporary percutaneous coronary intervention: Arixtra Study in Percutaneous Coronary Intervention: a randomized evaluation (ASPIRE) pilot. Circulation 111(11):1390–1397

52. Ferguson JJ, Califf RM, Antman EM et al (2004) Enoxaparin vs unfractionated heparin in high-risk patients with non-ST-segment elevation acute coronary syndromes managed with an intended early invasive strategy: primary results of the SYNERGY randomized trial. JAMA 292(1):45–54

53. Cohen M, Mahaffey KW, Pieper K et al (2006) A subgroup analysis of the impact of prerandomization antithrombin therapy on outcomes in the SYNERGY trial: enoxaparin versus unfractionated heparin in non-ST-segment elevation acute coronary syndromes. J Am Coll Cardiol 48(7):1346–1354

54. Petersen JL, Mahaffey KW, Hasselblad V et al (2004) Efficacy and bleeding complications among patients randomized to enoxaparin or unfractionated heparin for antithrombin therapy in non-ST-segment elevation acute coronary syndromes: a systematic overview. JAMA 292(1):89–96

55. Collet JP, Montalescot G, Lison L et al (2001) Percutaneous coronary intervention after subcutaneous enoxaparin pretreatment in patients with unstable angina pectoris. Circulation 103(5):658–663

56. Kereiakes DJ, Grines C, Fry E et al (2001) Enoxaparin and abciximab adjunctive pharmacotherapy during percutaneous coronary intervention. J Invasive Cardiol 13(4):272–278

57. White HD, Kleiman NS, Mahaffey KW et al (2006) Efficacy and safety of enoxaparin compared with unfractionated heparin in high-risk patients with non-ST-segment elevation acute coronary syndrome undergoing percutaneous coronary intervention in the Superior Yield of the New Strategy of Enoxaparin, Revascularization and Glycoprotein IIb/IIIa Inhibitors (SYNERGY) trial. Am Heart J 152(6):1042–1050

58. Montalescot G, White HD, Gallo R et al (2006) Enoxaparin versus unfractionated heparin in elective percutaneous coronary intervention. N Engl J Med 355(10):1006–1017

59. Favaloro EJ, Bonar R, Sioufi J et al (2005) An international survey of current practice in the laboratory assessment of anticoagulant therapy with heparin. Pathology 37(3):234–238

60. Mahaffey KW, Levine G, Gallo R et al (2005) Relationships between renal function, age, and obesity and outcomes in high-risk patients with acute coronary syndromes: results from SYNERGY. J Am Coll Cardiol 45(Suppl A):214A Abstract 812–4

61. Stone GW, McLaurin BT, Cox DA et al (2006) Bivalirudin for patients with acute coronary syndromes. N Engl J Med 355(21):2203–2216

62. Klok FA, Mos IC, Huisman MV. Brain-type natriuretic peptide levels in the prediction of adverse outcome in patients with pulmonary embolism: a systematic review and meta-analysis. Am J Respir Crit Care Med 2008; 178(4):425–430

63. Task Force for Diagnosis and Treatment of Non-ST-Segment Elevation Acute Coronary Syndromes of European Society of Cardiology (2007) Guidelines for the diagnosis and treatment of non-ST-segment elevation acute coronary syndromes. The Task Force for the Diagnosis and Treatment of Non-ST-Segment Elevation Acute Coronary Syndromes of the European Society of Cardiology. Eur Heart J 28(13):1598–1660

64. Alexander KP, Chen AY, Roe MT et al (2005) Excess dosing of antiplatelet and antithrombin agents in the treatment of non-ST-segment elevation acute coronary syndromes. JAMA 294(24):3108–3116

9 Direct Thrombin Inhibitors in Acute Coronary Syndromes

Tyler L. Taigen, James E. Harvey, and A. Michael Lincoff

Contents

Abstract The acute coronary syndromes (ACS) represent a continuum of athereothrombotic diseases that result from near instantaneous platelet activation and the initiation of the coagulation cascade most often following plaque erosion/rupture. Due to the central role of thrombin in clot formation, many therapies have aimed at inhibiting the action of thrombin to slow or reverse the coagulation cascade and to minimize the morbidity of ACS. While unfractionated heparin has been the stalwart agent for the management of ACS, several unfavorable characteristics such as the inability to inhibit clot-bound thrombin and a vulnerability to circulating inhibitors have prompted the search for alternative agents. Direct thrombin inhibitors (DTIs) were developed in an effort to effectively block the prothrombotic effects of thrombin without the associated increase in hemorrhagic events seen with the use of heparin. Early trials evaluating the DTI hirudin for management of unstable angina (UA) and non-ST-elevation myocardial infarction (NSTEMI) were largely disappointing. More recent data has demonstrated significantly lower bleeding rates with a similar effect on ischemic endpoints with the use of the DTI, bivalirudin, across the spectrum of ACS. As a result, the use of bivalirudin for most patients presenting with UA, NSTEMI, or STEMI is increasing. In this chapter, the data regarding the use of DTI in ACS will be presented and suggestions for their use in specific clinical scenarios will be given.

Key words: Direct thrombin inhibitors; bivalirudin; antithrombin; Acute coronary syndromes; intervention

From: *Contemporary Cardiology: Antithrombotic Drug Therapy in Cardiovascular Disease*
Edited by: A.T. Askari and A.M. Lincoff (eds.), DOI 10.1007/978-1-60327-235-3_9
© Humana Press, a part of Springer Science+Business Media, LLC 2010

INTRODUCTION

Acute coronary syndromes (ACS) represent a continuum of atherothrombotic disease and include unstable angina (UA), non-ST segment elevation myocardial infarction (NSTEMI), and ST-segment-elevation myocardial infarction (STEMI). Central to the development of an acute coronary syndrome is atherosclerotic plaque erosion and/or rupture, the mechanism of which remains poorly understood but involves factors that induce plaque vulnerability. With plaque rupture, subendothelial collagen is exposed and tissue factor is released resulting in near instantaneous platelet activation and the initiation of the coagulation cascade, respectively.

Once initiated, the coagulation cascade rapidly facilitates the generation of thrombin which in turn serves a number of essential functions (Table 1). Thrombin formation induces platelet activation, activation of factors V, VIII and XI, and the generation of more thrombin. Thrombin triggers platelet activation by protease-activated receptors (PARs) which leads to the production of thromboxane, serotonin and ADP. Clot formation is further amplified by thrombin-induced activation of the glycoprotein IIb/IIIa integrin receptor to bind fibrinogen and the von-Willebrand factor resulting in platelet aggregation. The intrinsic and extrinsic coagulation cascades unite in the conversion of fibrinogen to fibrin and cross-linking fibrin, leading to a stable thrombus. In addition, thrombin also plays a role in endothelial vasoconstriction, smooth muscle cell proliferation, and cytokine release (1). The final product is a fibrin-platelet clot which limits or obstructs blood flow through a coronary artery and results in an acute coronary syndrome.

The central role that thrombin plays in clot formation provides a unique opportunity for therapeutic intervention. There are two classes of anticoagulants aimed at inhibiting thrombin, the heparins (unfractionated heparin, low molecular weight heparin (LMWH), and fondaparinux, a synthetic heparin pentasaccharide) and the direct thrombin inhibitors (DTIs).

Heparins are indirect thrombin inhibitors and require a cofactor, antithrombin (formerly antithrombin III). Upon binding to antithrombin, a conformational change occurs which converts the enzyme from a slow to a rapid inhibitor of thrombin. The heparin–antithrombin complex inactivates thrombin, as well as factor VII, IX, and X. This in turn inhibits the activation of factor V and VIII, and decreases platelet activation and aggregation (Fig. 1).

Notwithstanding the strong anticoagulation properties, there are important intrinsic limitations associated with the use of heparin (Table 2) (2–4). Perhaps most significant is that the large heparin–antithrombin complex cannot inactivate thrombin bound within a clot (2). The thrombin molecule has three receptors which regulate its enzymatic activity: the catalytic site and two exosites. Exosite-1 is the substrate binding domain for alignment of the peptide bonds to the catalytic site. Exosite 2 is the heparin binding site (Fig. 1). Following the attachment of thrombin to fibrin within a clot, exosite 2 is protected from the heparin–antithrombin complex. Thus, clot bound thrombin continues to exert thrombogenic effects despite the use of heparin. Secondly, heparin is vulnerable to suppression by circulating inhibitors including platelet factor 4 and heparinase (4). Heparin also exhibits variable

Table 1
Effects of thrombin on coagulation

Effect	Mechanism of action
Increased platelet activation	Activates platelet protease-activated receptor
	Activates platelet Gp IIb/IIIa integrin receptor
Increased generation of thrombin	Activates autocatalytic feedback loop
Propagates and stabilizes clot formation	Catalyzes cross-link of fibrin clot

Table 2
Comparison of heparin and direct thrombin inhibitors

Unfractionated heparin	Direct thrombin inhibitors
Unable to inhibit thrombin bound to fibrin clot due to steric hindrance	Inhibits thrombin bound to fibrin clot
Indirectly inhibits thrombin through antithrombin cofactor	Directly inhibits thrombin without cofactor
Reduced potency with antithrombin cofactor deficiency	No dependence upon cofactor
Unpredictable bioavailability due to non-specific binding to circulating or vascular proteins	Little or no non-specific binding
Variable potency depending upon distribution of molecular size in natural mixture	Consistent potency
Inhibited by platelet factor 4 and other circulating inhibitors	No circulating inhibitors
Activates platelets	No platelet activation. Inhibits thrombin-mediated pathway of platelet activation
Antibody-mediated heparin-induced thrombocytopenia syndrome (HITS)	No heparin-induced thrombocytopenia or cross-reaction with HITS antibodies

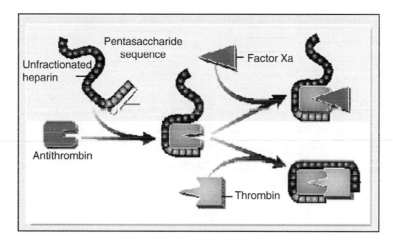

Fig. 1. Schematic representation of the interaction between antithrombin and heparin and its effect on the binding of antithrombin with factor Xa and thrombin. Heparin binds with antithrombin via a specific pentasaccharide binding site.

bioavailability and non-linear pharmacokinetics. The animal source and manufacturing process results in non-uniform sized molecules, approximately only a third of which have the unique pentasaccharide sequence required to effectively activate antithrombin. Heparin binds numerous tissues and plasma proteins leading to unpredictable active plasma levels and variable dosing from patient to patient. Heparin also appears to have an inherent platelet activating effect (5). In addition, extended heparin use may result in heparin-induced thrombocytopenia (HIT) in 2.5–3% of the patients (6). HIT is particularly a matter of concern in patients with acute coronary syndrome, as it is results in a prothrombotic state. Lastly, observations from several trials have suggested a potential reactivation of thrombin leading to coronary ischemia in the hours following heparin discontinuation. (7,8) Another theoretical limitation is that heparin should have limited effectiveness in patients with antithrombin deficiency, however, clinically this appears to be irrelevant (9).

In an effort to overcome some of the unfavorable pharmacokinetic and pharmacodynamic characteristics of UFH, LMWH was developed. LMWHs are approximately 5,000 dalton heparin fragments produced through the enzymatic or chemical depolymerization of UFH *(10)*. Whether injected IV or SC, LMWHs have a more predictable onset of action than does UFH and LMWHs have a decreased propensity to bind to plasma proteins and platelets *(11,12)*. This is believed to explain the greater bioavailability and diminished platelet activation and incidence of HIT observed with the use of LMWHs as compared to UFH. Like UFH, LMWH binds with AT through a unique pentasaccharide segment resulting in the accelerated AT-mediated inactivation of factor Xa, thus inhibiting the coagulation cascade. LMWH also inactivates thrombin, however, it does so to a lesser degree than does UFH. Different LMWH preparations have varying ratios of polysaccharide chain lengths, the majority of which are less than 18 units in length. Because the inactivation of thrombin requires the heparin molecule to have at least 18 saccharide units, the anticoagulant effects LMWH are predominantly due to its inhibition of factor X and less so to its inhibition of thrombin *(13)*. The overall result is a longer and a more predictable anticoagulation effect that does not require frequent monitoring or dose adjustment and is feasible for SC delivery *(14)*. Early trials comparing the LMWH enoxaparin to UFH among patients with UA/NSTEMI treated with aspirin and conservative management revealed a decrease in ischemic events with no difference in hemorrhagic complications *(15–17)*. While these data were promising, they had significant limitations. Most importantly, these trials did not employ an early invasive strategy or the adjunctive use of Gp IIbIIIa inhibitors in the treatment of ACS and thus, it was not possible to extrapolate these trials to include contemporary practice patterns *(18)*. To resolve this, the SYNERGY trial randomized 10,000 high-risk patients with ACS to receive either enoxaparin or UFH with concomitant Gp IIbIIIa inhibitor as per the physician's discretion and an early invasive strategy of catheterization and revascularization *(19,20)*. There was no statistically-significant difference between the two groups in the primary endpoint of death or MI (14.5% vs. 14.0% in the UFH and enoxaparin arms, respectively, $p = 0.4$); however, major bleeding occurred more frequently among patients in the enoxaparin arm (7.6% vs. 9.1% respectively, $p = 0.008$). Similarly, multiple studies comparing the use of enoxaparin vs. UFH in patients presenting with STEMI and undergoing fibrinolytic therapy were performed *(21–23)*. While each of these trials showed enoxaparin to have similar or improved efficacy in reducing death and MI when compared to UFH, they also revealed significantly increased risk of hemorrhagic complications. The use of enoxaparin compared to UFH in patients with STEMI and primary PCI has not been well evaluated.

OVERVIEW OF DIRECT THROMBIN INHIBITORS

The inherent limitations of heparins led to the investigation of alternative strategies to inhibit thrombin. DTIs bind directly to the catalytic and/or substrate recognition (exosite 1) sites of thrombin, in contrast to heparin which binds antithrombin *(1)*. Hirudin, the prototype DTI, and other recently developed synthetic analogues are potent anticoagulants with different pharmacokinetic and pharmacodynamic properties. Bivalent DTIs bind the catalytic site and the substrate binding site (exosite 1) whereas univalent DTIs only bind the catalytic site (Fig. 2). DTIs have several important advantages over heparin (Table 2). In contrast to heparin, DTIs are not subject to steric hindrance and are able to inactivate thrombin bound within a clot. DTIs do not require a cofactor and there are no circulating inhibitors. DTIs have more reliable therapeutic responses as in general they do not bind plasma proteins. They do not cause the immune-mediated syndrome of HIT. Finally, whereas heparin has been shown to intrinsically activate platelets *(3)*, DTIs do not share this effect and actually inhibit the thrombin-mediated pathway of platelet aggregation (Table 2).

Initial studies using animal models to compare DTIs to heparin in suppression of arterial and venous thrombosis suggested a possible benefit with DTIs. Enthusiasm for their use however was tempered by the results of several large trials in the 1990s. It appeared that DTIs, primarily hirudin, provided only minimal benefit beyond that of heparin in protection against ischemic events, and yet increased hemorrhagic events. More recent evidence has suggested the therapeutic benefit of synthetic analogues, in particular bivalirudin, initially in the attenuation of peri-procedural ischemic complications of percutaneous intervention and later in the treatment of ACS.

SPECIFIC DIRECT THROMBIN INHIBITORS

Hirudin

Hirudin is a naturally occurring molecule originally isolated from the saliva of the medicinal leech (*Hirudo medicinalis*) over 30 years ago (Table 3). It is a 65-amino-acid polypeptide which bivalently and irreversibly binds thrombin with high affinity *(24)*. Hirudin can be administered intravenously or subcutaneously and is almost exclusively excreted by the kidneys. The half-life of hirudin is approximately 60 min; however this can be significantly prolonged in the presence of renal dysfunction. Hirudin is contraindicated for patients with a creatinine clearance <15 ml/min. Formation of antibodies directed against hirudin may occur in up to 40% of patients, and anaphylactic reactions have been reported *(25,26)*. Moreover, anti-hirudin antibodies may lead to an increased half-life and subsequent drug accumulation *(27)*. Plasma levels of partial thromboplastin times (PTT) increase proportionally with dosing over a range of 0.1–0.4 mg/kg. Dosing adjustments should be made until a steady state aPTT of 1.5–2.5 times the initial baseline value is achieved. Hirudin is FDA-approved for treatment of HIT. Lepirudin is a recombinant form of hirudin derived from yeast cells with virtually the same pharmacokinetic and pharmacodynamic properties.

Table 3

Properties and FDA indications for use of parenteral DTIs : Hirudin, Bivalirudin, and Argatroban

	Hirudin	*Bivalirudin*	*Argatroban*
Type of molecule	65 amino acid polypeptide	20 amino acid peptide	Synthetic arginine derivative
Mass (daltons)	7,000	1,980	527
Thrombin binding sites	Catalytic, exosite I	Catalytic, exosite I	Catalytic
Thrombin binding kinetics	Irreversible	Reversible on proteolytic cleavage	Reversible, competitive
Clearance	Renal	Predominantly endogenous circulating peptidases, minor renal	Hepatic
Elimination half-life	60 min	25 min	54 min
Produces antibodies?	Yes	No	No
FDA indication(s)	Treatment of HIT	1. AC in patients undergoing PCI. 2. ACS (with ASA) undergoing PTCA	1. Treatment of HIT 2. During PCI in patients who have or are at risk for HIT

Bivalirudin

Bivalirudin is a 20-amino acid synthetic analogue of hirudin. Like hirudin, it bivalently binds with high affinity to both the catalytic and exosite-1 recognition sites of thrombin (Fig. 2). Unlike hirudin, thrombin inhibition by bivalirudin is reversible *(1,28)*. Upon binding to thrombin, bivalirudin is quickly cleaved into two fragments which only weakly interact with thrombin. The half-life of biva-lirudin is approximately 25 min, a factor which may contribute to the lower rate of bleeding compli-cations compared with hirudin. Bivalirudin is administered intravenously and plasma levels are directly proportional to dosing. For percutaneous coronary intervention, an initial bolus of 0.75 mg/kg is followed by a continuous infusion of 1.75 mg/kg/h for the duration of the procedure. For man-agement of ACS outside of percutaneous interventional procedures, the initial dose is 0.1 mg/kg, followed by a continuous infusion of 0.25 mg/kg/h. Therapeutic steady state is achieved when the PTT is 1.5–2.5 times the baseline value. Bivalirudin fragments are degraded by endogenous pepti-dases in the blood, and are primarily excreted by the kidneys. Although clearance is only modestly effected by decreased renal insufficiency, dose adjustments and careful monitoring is suggested in patients with creatinine clearance <30 ml/min (decrease infusion rate to 1 mg/kg/h) and dialysis dependent patients (decrease infusion to 0.25 mg/kg/h). Bivalirudin is approved for use as an anti-coagulant in patients undergoing percutaneous coronary intervention electively or during an acute coronary syndrome.

Argatroban

Argatroban is a small synthetic molecule derived from L-arginine, which acts as a reversible uni-valent thrombin inhibitor. In contrast to bivalirudin or hirudin, argatroban is hepatically metabolized through the cytokine P450 pathway, and approximately half of a given intravenous dose is bound by plasma proteins. Dosing precautions are advised in patients with hepatic dysfunction, but are not required in patients with renal insufficiency *(29)*. Plasma levels are linearly related to intravenous dosing, and the half-life of argatroban is approximately 54 min. In percutaneous coronary interven-tion, an initial bolus dose of 350 mcg/kg is followed by infusion of 25 mcg/kg/min, with additional boluses of 150 mcg/kg and increase in infusion as necessary to achieve an activated clotting time (ACT) of 300–450 s. When given for treatment of HIT, dose adjustment should be made until a steady state aPTT of 1.5–3.0 times the initial baseline value is achieved. Argatroban has not been linked to immune-mediated responses. Argatroban is approved for use in the treatment of HIT, and during percutaneous coronary intervention in patients who have or are at risk for HIT.

Orally Active Direct Thrombin Inhibitors

Ximelagatran was the first orally-active DTI (Fig. 2). It is a small molecule which requires metabo-lization after ingestion to melagatran, a univalent inhibitor of the catalytic site on thrombin. Melagatran has a half-life of 5 h, and is excreted in the urine. Use of this agent has been limited by an alarming number of unpredictable incidents of severe hepatotoxicity. In 2004 the FDA Advisory Committee rec-ommended against its approval, and the sponsoring company terminated its development 2 years later.

Dabigatran etexilate is another orally active DTI under investigation to determine its safety and efficacy in the treatment of venous and arterial thromboembolic disorders *(30)*.

CLINICAL USE OF DIRECT THROMBIN INHIBITORS IN UNSTABLE ANGINA AND NSTEMI

Thrombus formation at the site of plaque disruption leading to partial or subtotal occlusion of a coronary artery is the key step in the pathogenesis of UA and non-transmural myocardial infarction.

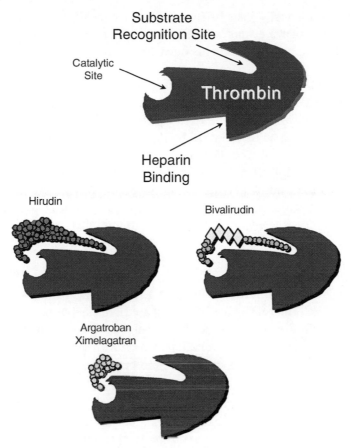

Fig. 2. Schematic representation of thrombin with substrate recognition sites (exosites 1 and 2) and the active catalytic site. Binding patterns of bivalent (hirudin and bivalirudin) and univalent (argatroban and Ximelagatran) are shown.

Coronary artery plaque disruption results in exposure of subendothelial collagen and tissue factor to circulating clotting factors. The activation of thrombin is a critical early step in the activation of the clotting cascade, platelet activation and ultimately in the formation of a platelet-fibrin clot. Based on the limitations of heparins and the advantages of DTIs discussed above, recent investigation has focused on using DTI as primary anticoagulant agents in the treatment of ACS.

The use of DTIs in the treatment of ACS has been evaluated by a number of clinical trials. Two large trials the Global Utilization of Strategies to Open Occluded Coronary Arteries (GUSTO-II) *(31)*, and the Organization to Assess Strategies for Ischemic Syndromes (OASIS-2) trial *(32)* focused on the use of recombinant hirudin in the treatment of ACS. GUSTO IIb was a multicenter international trial that compared heparin to low dose hirudin (0.1 mg/kg bolus followed by 0.1 mg/kg/h infusion; goal aPTT 60–85 s) in 12,142 patients enrolled in 1994 and 1995 with either ST elevation (4,131 patients) or non-ST elevation (8,011 patients) myocardial infarctions *(33)*. At 24 h, hirudin therapy was associated with a statistically-significant reduction in the incidence of death or recurrent myocardial infarction (1.3% vs. 2.1% with heparin, $p=0.001$). By 30 days, however, this difference was only marginally significant with 8.9% and 9.8% of patients in the hirudin and heparin arms respectively reaching the study's primary endpoint of death or non-fatal myocardial infarction ($p=0.06$). Of those patients who presented without ST elevation, the difference in incidence of death or recurrent ischemia was less impressive and statistically insignificant (8.3% for hirudin vs. 9.1% for heparin, $p = 0.22$). The trend toward reduced ischemic events was offset by an increase in the incidence of moderate and severe bleeding defined as the need for transfusion with hirudin (9.7%) compared to heparin (8.6%, $p = 0.04$).

A subsequent trial, OASIS II, evaluated a similar hypothesis that hirudin would be a superior anti-coagulant to heparin in patients with UA or non-ST elevation myocardial infarction (32). In this trial, 10,141 patients were enrolled from August 1996 to April 1998 and randomized to standard dose UFH vs. high dose hirudin (0.4 mg/kg bolus followed by 0.15 mg/kg/h infusion; goal aPTT 60–100 s). At 7 days, patients treated with hirudin were less likely to develop the primary endpoints of cardiovascular death or new myocardial infarction (3.6% vs. 4.2% with heparin, $p = 0.077$). Moreover, hirudin therapy was associated with a statistically significant reduction in the secondary composite endpoint of cardiovascular death, myocardial infarction or refractory angina at 7 days (5.6% vs. 6.7% with heparin, $p = 0.0125$). Differences were particularly apparent in higher risk patients for whom an intervention was eventually required. Similar to GUSTO II, the risk of major bleed was higher in the hirudin group than in the heparin treated group (1.2% vs. 0.7%, $p = 0.01$).

A meta-analysis performed by the Direct Thrombin Inhibitor Trialists' Collaborative Group compared safety and efficacy of four different DTIs from 11 randomized trials and 35,970 patients who presented with UA, NSTEMI, and STEMI (34). Compared with heparin, patients treated with DTIs had a significant reduction in the primary efficacy endpoint of death or myocardial infarction (4.3% vs. 5.1%) at 30 days. Notably the treatment benefit was seen with bivalent DTIs, hirudin and bivalirudin, but not with the univalent DTIs, inogatran or argatroban. This finding held true in the subset of patients who presented without ST elevation with primary endpoint occurring in 3.7% with DTIs versus 4.6% with heparin (Odds Ratio 0.80 (0.70–0.92)). Perhaps most significant given the results of the OASIS II and GUSTO II trials, there was an increase in major bleeding with hirudin but an actual reduction in bleeding with bivalirudin.

The finding that improved antithrombotic efficacy may be obtained without an associated increase in major bleeding was first demonstrated in the Bivalirudin Angioplasty Trial (BAT). The BAT trial enrolled 4,098 patients with either UA or postinfarction angina between March 1993 and July 1994 (35). Patients were randomly assigned to receive either heparin or bivalirudin prior to angiography. Although there was no difference in the primary endpoint of death in the hospital, myocardial infarction, abrupt vessel closure or cardiac derived clinical decline between bivalirudin and heparin (11.4% vs. 12.2%, $p = 0.44$), there was a significant reduction in incidence of major hemorrhage seen in patients treated with bivalirudin compared with heparin (3.8% vs. 9.8%, $p < 0.001$). Although the mechanism is unclear, it has been suggested that the reduction in bleeding seen with bivalirudin is due to its reversible binding of thrombin and shorter half-life (35). The results of the BAT trial suggested bivalirudin could provide at least equal reduction in ischemic complications without resulting in an increased risk of bleeding.

Taken together, the results of the individual trials and the meta-analysis comparing DTIs to heparin in the setting of ACS suggest a modest superiority of DTIs over heparin in reducing ischemic events, which in the case of hirudin is achieved at the cost of increased bleeding. The meta-analysis demonstrated heterogeneity of DTIs both in terms of clinical benefit and incidence of major bleeding. The greatest benefit in the meta analysis appeared to be derived from patients treated with bivalirudin who later underwent percutaneous coronary intervention (34), in whom the BAT trial revealed bivalirudin could actually reduce bleeding rates.

The relevance of the results from early studies to current clinical practice is limited. Overall management strategies during the majority of these trials were conservative in contrast to current strategies of early angiography and aggressive percutaneous coronary intervention. Additionally, when the effectiveness of DTIs could be evaluated in the setting of percutaneous intervention, it was in an era prior to the widespread use of coronary stents. Another limitation is that newer anti-coagulants such as thienopyridines and glycoprotein IIb/IIIa inhibitors which have been shown to be clearly beneficial were not yet part of the treatment strategy for ACS at the time of the early trials. Moreover, despite the notable benefit of reduced bleeding with bivalirudin noted in the BAT trial and the DTI meta-analysis, the majority of the initial investigations were focused on huridin.

Based on its favorable safety profile compared with other DTIs and the results of the BAT trial, bivalirudin received approval for use as an anticoagulation strategy in percutaneous intervention. However, widespread use of bivalirudin in this setting did not occur until The Randomized Evaluation in PCI Linking Angiomax to Reduced Clinical Events (REPLACE-2) trial suggested bivalirudin could be used as an alternative anticoagulation strategy instead of heparin and GPIIa/IIIb inhibition (36). The REPLACE-2 trial demonstrated bivalirudin to be non-inferior to heparin plus glycoprotein IIb/IIIa blockade in reducing ischemic complications associated with PCI, while significantly reducing rate of major in-hospital bleeding (4.1% in heparin plus GPIIa/IIIb vs. 2.4% in bivalirudin alone, $p=0.001$).

The intent of the REPLACE-2 trial was to evaluate the use of bivalirudin during elective or urgent PCI, and the study did not include patients with acute myocardial infarctions or who were given antithrombotic therapy prior to PCI for high-risk acute coronary syndrome (36). Therefore, to assess the role of bivalirudin across the spectrum of care from contemporary medical pretreatment through early angiography and PCI in the setting of moderate- or high-risk ACS, the Acute Catheterization and Urgent Intervention Triage Strategy (ACUITY) trial was performed (37). This trial enrolled 13,819 patients, all of whom were to receive immediate aspirin and undergo angiography within 72 h of presentation; the administration of clopidogrel was at the discretion of the local investigator. Patients were assigned to one of three arms for anticoagulation: unfractionated or low molecular weight heparin plus a glycoprotein IIb/IIIa inhibitor (heparin plus GpIIb/IIIa inhibitor), bivalirudin plus a glycoprotein IIb/IIIa inhibitor (bivalirudin plus GpIIb/IIIa inhibitor), or bivalrudin plus provi-sional use of a glycoprotein IIb/IIIa inhibitor (per the discretion of the investigator; bivalirudin alone). Both bivalirudin alone and with GpIIb/IIIa inhibition, compared to heparin plus a GpIIb/IIIa inhibitor, were associated with non-inferior 30 day rates of the primary endpoint of death, myocar-dial infarction, or unplanned revascularization (Fig. 3). Rates of major hemorrhage were similar for the bivalirudin plus GpIIb/IIIa inhibitor arm and the heparin plus GpIIb/IIIa inhibitor arm (5.3% vs. 5.7%, respectively, $p=0.38$), while bivalirudin alone was associated with significantly less major bleeding (3.0%, $p<0.001$). In a subgroup analysis, it is worth noting that treatment with bivalirudin alone without pretreatment with clopidogrel prior to angiography showed a marginally significant increase in ischemic events (9.1% vs. 7.1% with heparin plus GpIIb/IIIa inhibition, $p=0.054$) Subsequent more detailed post hoc analysis suggested that outcomes in the bivalirudin monotherapy arm were similar to those in the heparin plus GP IIb/IIIa inhibitor group as long as clopidogrel was administered before or within 30 min of completing the PCI procedure (38). Thus, while the data from ACUITY were by no means conclusive that bivalirudin monotherapy without clopidogrel pre-treatment is inferior to treatment with heparin plus a GpIIb/IIIa inhibitor, the apparent relationship was noted and led to the recommendation in the ACC/AHA 2007 Guidelines for the Management of Unstable Angina/Non-ST Elevation Myocardial Infarction that bivalirudin monotherapy be used with clopidogrel loading (39). The results from ACUITY support those from REPLACE-2 in dem-onstrating that the use of bivalirudin is associated with a similar incidence of ischemic events, yet significantly less major bleeding complications when compared to treatment with heparin and a

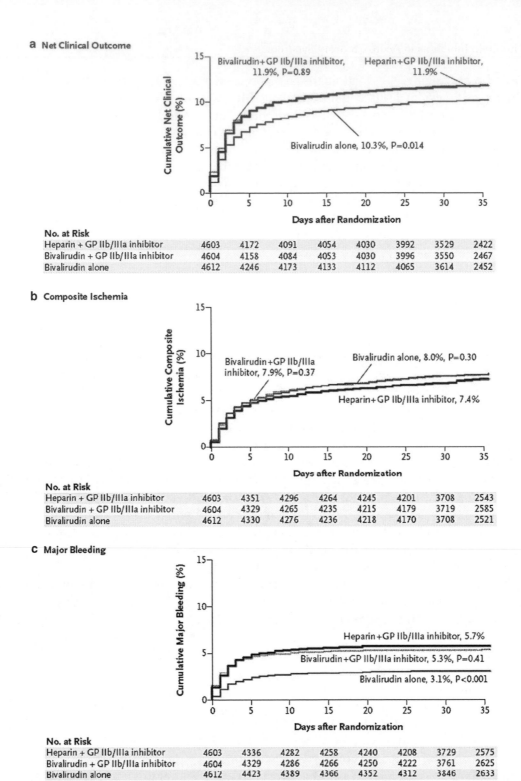

Fig. 3. Kaplan–Meier Time-to-Event Curves for the end points of net clinical outcome (**a**), composite ischemia (**b**), and major bleeding (**c**). Outcomes at 30 days in the ACUITY trial comparing bivalirudin with and without glycoprotein IIb/IIIa to heparin and glycoprotein IIb/IIIa blockade in the treatment of acute coronary syndromes. The primary end points were measured at 30+5 days; thus, follow-up is reported to 35 days. The event rate for each curve refers to the cumulative rate at 35 days. *P* values are for comparisons with the control group (unfractionated heparin or enoxaparin plus glycoprotein IIb/IIIa inhibitors). GP denotes glycoprotein. The thick solid line represents heparin plus GP IIb/IIIa inhibitor; the dotted line, bivalirudin plus GP IIb/IIIa inhibitor; and the thin solid line, bivalirudin alone.

glycoprotein IIb/IIIa inhibitor, and thus is an acceptable alternative for the management of UA, NSTEMI and during elective or urgent PCI (36,37).

CLINICAL USE OF DIRECT THROMBIN INHIBITORS IN STEMI

In contrast to UA or NSTEMI, the majority of patients with STEMIs have occlusive coronary thrombi with little or no blood flow to the effected area of myocardium (40). Therapy for this condition is therefore focused on immediate reperfusion with either fibrinolysis or percutaneous intervention. Early trials focused on the usefulness of DTIs in conjunction with fibrinolytics in the treatment of STEMIs. GUSTO-IIa (31,33) and TIMI-9a (41) assessed hirudin in this setting, but both studies were terminated early after initial analysis revealed higher bleeding rates within the hirudin treatment arms. Although, the trials were restarted with lower doses of hirudin, treatment with hirudin was associated with similar rates of ischemic events compared with heparin (31,33)(42). Moreover, primary endpoints of death or myocardial re-infarction at 30 days were not significantly different between the hirudin and heparin groups in GUSTO-IIb (hirudin 9.9% vs. heparin 11.3%) or TIMI 9b (hirudin 9.7% vs. heparin 9.5%). As was the case for patients with UA and NSTEMIs, hirudin treatment was associated with a higher rate of bleeding in patients with STEMI. The Hirulog and Early Reperfusion or Occlusion (HERO-2) trial compared the use of bivalirudin to heparin in patients with ST elevation myocardial infarctions undergoing fibinolysis with streptokinase (43). The results were similarly disappointing with no difference in the primary endpoint of 30 day mortality in patients treated with bivalirudin (10.8%) compared to heparin (10.9%), and there were higher rates of bleeding in the bivalirudin arm. Taken together, these studies demonstrate that the use of DTIs appear to offer no benefit over heparin in the setting of fibrinolysis for treatment of acute STEMI.

The results of these trials evaluating the use of DTIs in the treatment of ST-segment elevation myocardial infarctions thus suggested that DTI's do not provide a net benefit over heparin among patients undergoing fibrinolysis. The Harmonizing Outcomes with Revascularization and Stents in Acute Myocardial Infarction (HORIZONS-AMI) study was designed to test whether direct thrombin inhibition could provide a benefit in patients with ST elevation myocardial infarctions who underwent early percutaneous intervention (44). A total of 3,602 patients presenting with STEMI were randomly assigned to receive heparin plus glycoprotein IIb/IIIa blockade or bivalirudin alone and then underwent emergent percutaneous coronary intervention (Fig. 4) (44). All patients were treated with optimal platelet inhibition including aspirin and clopidogrel. At 30 days, those treated with bivalirudin monotherapy showed similar rates of major cardiovascular events when compared to heparin plus a GpIIa/IIIb inhibitor. However, bivalirudin monotherapy resulted in significantly lower 30 day rates of death from cardiovascular causes (1.8% vs. 2.9% with heparin plus GpIIb/IIIa inhibition, $p = 0.03$) and death from all causes (2.1% vs. 3.1% with heparin plus GIIb/IIIa inhibition, $p = 0.047$). Equally notable was that bivalirudin monotherapy was associated with significantly less major hemorrhage (5.0% vs. 8.4% with heparin plus GpIIb/IIIa inhibition, $p < 0.001$, Fig. 4). As shown in Fig. 4, there was an apparent initial increase in ischemic cardiovascular endpoints (death, reinfarction, target vessel revascularization for ischemia, and stroke) in the bivalirudin arm, however, this difference was no longer evident at 30 days when overall rates were similar (5.4% vs. 5.5% with heparin and GpIIb/IIIa inhibition, respectively, $p = 0.95$). In addition, the authors note that in the 3,124 patients in whom stents were implanted, stent thrombosis occurred in 17 more patients within the first 24 h in the bivalirudin arm. However, that trend was later reversed with seven fewer incidents of stent thrombosis in the bivalirudin arm during the period from the 24 h to 30 days. At 30 days, there was no significant difference in stent thrombosis between the bivalirudin group (2.5%) and the heparin and glycoprotein group (1.9%, $p = 0.30$).

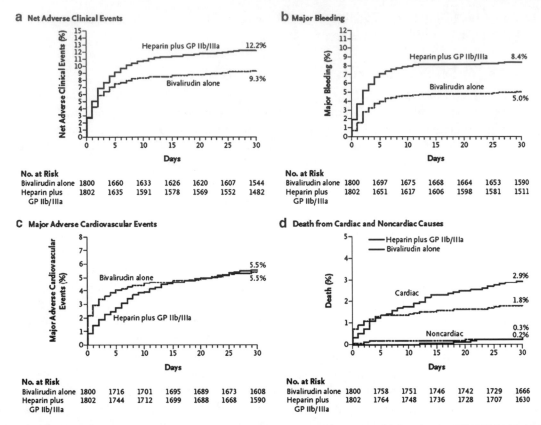

Fig. 4. HORIZONS-AMI: Time to event curves through 30 days. Outcomes at 30days in the HORIZONS-AMI trial comparing bivalirudin to heparin and glycoprotein IIb/IIIa in the treatment of STEMI.

SAFETY AND EFFICACY OF SWITCHING ANTICOAGULANT THERAPY

Most patients presenting with ACS are currently treated with UFH or LMWH initiated in the ambulance, the emergency department, or in a transferring hospital before PCI. In such patients, it has been suggested that switching from UFH to LMWH or vice versa may be associated with an increased rate of death or myocardial infarction at 30 days and an increase in the need for blood transfusion *(19)*. Thus, the safety of changing antithrombin therapy from a heparin to a DTI once therapy has been initiated has been called into question. The small randomized SWITCH trial among 91 patients with non-ST elevation ACS treated with enoxaparin demonstrated that subsequent switching to bivalirudin for PCI was not associated with increased risk of major bleeding when compared to those who did not have a change in antithrombin therapy *(45)*. This finding was independent of the duration of time between the last administration of enoxaparin and PCI.

A subsequent analysis of the REPLACE-2 study evaluated the incidence of hemorrhage among patients who were pretreated with UFH or LWMH during the 48 h prior to PCI *(46)*. When compared to those who did not receive pretreatment, there was no difference in the rates of major or minor bleeding nor non-CABG related blood transfusion in patients who received bivalirudin during PCI (Table 6). Interestingly, those who received heparin pretreatment and then received heparin and additional glycoprotein IIb/IIIa inhibition did have a significant increase in bleeding complications when compared to

Table 4

Major trials of DTIs in ST-elevation acute myocardial infarction

		TIMI 9B	GUSTO IIb	HERO-2	HORIZONS-AMI
Number of patients		3,002	4,131	17,073	3,602
Direct thrombin inhibitor		Hirudin	Hirudin	Bivalirudin	Bivalirudin
Dose	DTI	0.1 mg/kg bolus 0.1 mg/kg-h×4 days	0.25 mg/kg bolus 0.5 mg/kg-h×12 h, then 0.25 mg/kg-h×36 h	0.1 mg/kg bolus 0.1 mg/kg-h×3–5 days	0.75 mg/kg bolus 1.75 mg/kg/h until completion of PCI
	UH	5000 U bolus 1000 U/h×4 days, aPTT=55–85 s	5000 U bolus 1000 U/h×48 h, aPTT=50–75 s	5000 U bolus 1000 U/h×3–5 days, aPTT=60–85 s	60 IU/kg bolus rebolused as necessary for goal ACT 200–250 s.
Fibrinolytic agent		TPA – 64% SK – 36%	TPA – 69% SK – 31%	SK – 100%	N/A (Primary PCI used)
Endpoint follow-up		30 days	30 days	96h	30 days
Death (%)	DTI	6.1	10.8	5.9	2.1
	UH	5.0	10.9	6.2	3.1
Reinfarction (%)	DTI	4.3	1.6*	5.0	1.8
	UH	5.0	2.3*	6.0	1.8
Death or reinfarction (%)	DTI	9.7	12.6	9.9	5.4
	UH	9.3	13.6	11.3	5.5
Intracranial hemorrhage (%, in-hospital)	DTI	0.4	0.6	0.5	Not reported
	UH	0.7	0.4	0.4	Not reported
Major bleeding (%, in-hospital)	DTI	3.4	0.7	1.1	3.1**
	UH	3.8	0.5	1.5	5.0**

All p=N.S. except *p=0.001, **p=0.002

DTI direct thrombin inhibitor, SK streptokinase, TPA tissue plasminogen activator, UFH unfractionated heparin. GUSTO Global Use of Strategies to Open Occluded Coronary Arteries (21), HERO Hirulog and Early Reperfusion or Occlusion (23), TIMI Thrombolysis and Thrombin Inhibition in Myocardial Infarction (22), HORIZONS-AMI Harmonizing Outcomes with Revascularization and Stents in Acute Myocardial Infarction Trial

Table 5
Major trials of DTIs in non-ST-elevation acute coronary syndromes

		Gusto IIb	Oasis-2	Acuity
Number of patients		8,011	10,141	13,819
Direct thrombin inhibitor (DTI)		Hirudin	Hirudin	Bivalirudin
Dose	DTI	0.1 mg/kg bolus	0.4 mg/kg bolus	0.1 mg/kg bolus
		0.1 mg/kg-h×3–5 days	0.15 mg/kg-h×3 days	0.25 mg/kg/h until PCI[¶]
	UFH	5,000 U bolus	5,000 U bolus	60 U/kg bolus
		1000 U/h×3–5 days, aPTT=60–85 s	15 U/kg-h×3 days, aPTT=60–105 s	12 U/kg-h until PCI[b], aPTT=50–75 s
	LMWH	N/A	N/A	1 mg/kg q12 h[a]
Endpoint follow-up		30 days	7 days	30 days
Death (%)	DTI	3.7	NR	1.6
	UFH	3.9	NR	1.3[c]
Reinfarction (%)	DTI	5.6	NR	5.4
	UFH	6.4	NR	4.9[c]
Death or reinfarction (%)	DTI	8.3	3.6**	7.8
	UFH	9.1	4.2**	7.3[c]
Intracranial hemorrhage (%, in-hospital)	DTI	0.2*	0	<0.1
	UFH	0.02*	0	<0.1[c]
Major bleeding (%, in-hospital)	DTI	1.3*	1.2***	0.9[‡]
	UFH	0.9*	0.7***	1.9[c,‡]

[a]Additional 0.3 mg/kg LMWH given if last dose given >8 h. before PCI
[b]Anticoagulation could be continued past completion of PCI at the discretion of the physician
[c]Number represents percentage of patients in whom endpoint occurred while receiving either UFH or LMWH and a GpIIbIIa inhibitor in the ACUITY trial
All p=N.S. except *p=0.06,**p=0.066, ***p=0.01, ‡ $p \le 0.001$
DTI direct thrombin inhibitor, NR not reported, UFH unfractionated heparin

those who received no pretreatment (Table 6). It is worth noting that patients in this study could not receive bivalirudin within 8 h of administration of LMWH or 6 h of administration of UFH unless the ACT was less than 175 s. Nevertheless, there was no association between time of discontinuation of heparin therapy to the time of PCI and incidence of major or minor bleeding (Fig. 5).

More recently, an analysis of patients who received heparin prior to randomization in the ACUITY trial assessed the safety of switching from prerandomization UFH or enoxaparin to bivalirudin as compared with continuation of their heparin therapy in the setting of non-ST elevation ACS managed with an invasive strategy (47). Here the authors found that patients switching to bivalirudin had similar rates of ischemia (6.9% vs. 7.4%, p=0.52), less major bleeding (2.8% vs. 5.8%, p<0.01), and improved net clinical outcomes (9.2% vs. 11.9%, p<0.01) compared with those who had been randomized to continue their prerandomization heparin.

To date, there are no published studies that evaluate the safety and efficacy of switching from heparin therapy to a DTI in the setting of STEMI. However, in HORIZONS-AMI, approximately two-thirds of patients randomized to treatment with bivalirudin received UFH prior to PCI. There was no significant difference in bleeding between those who received preprocedural heparin and those who did not (4.8% with preprocedural heparin vs. 5.2% without, p=0.47).

Table 6

Bleeding rates associated with different antithrombin transitions (Adapted with permission)

Variable	Naïve→bivalirudin* (n = 2,345)	UFH→bivalirudin (n = 287)	LMWH→bivalirudin (n = 258)	Naïve→GP IIb/IIIa/UFH (n = 2,325)	UFH→GP IIb/IIIa/UFH (n = 349)	LMWH→GP IIb/IIIa/UFH (n = 313)
Protocol major bleeding	2.3%*	1.7%	2.7%	3.6%	4.9%	5.8%
Protocol minor bleeding	13.4%*	13.6%	14.0%	25.0%	28.9%	29.1%
Protocol major/minor bleeding	15.6%*	15.3%	16.7%	28.6%†	33.8%	34.8%
TIMI major/minor bleeding	1.9%*	1.4%	1.9%	3.5%	4.3%	5.4%
≥2 Non-CABG transfusions	0.8%*	1.1%	1.2%	1.0%†	2.3%	2.9%

*p=NS for all three-way comparisons versus bivalirudin alone

†p<0.05 for two-way comparison versus GP IIb/IIIa, UFH-naïve as well as two-way comparisons of UFH- naïve versus either preceding UFH or preceding LMWH

CABG coronary artery bypass grafting; GP glycoprotein; LMWH low molecular weight heparin; UFH unfractionated heparin

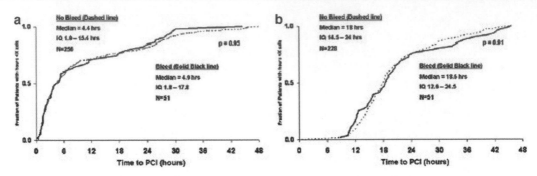

Fig. 5. Time from last dose of antithrombin until PCI in patients who received bivalirudin by incidence of major or minor bleeding (**a**) unfractionated heparin (**b**) low-molecular-weight heparin.

Interestingly, preprocedural administration of heparin was also associated with a weak trend toward reduced major adverse cardiovascular events at 30 days in the bivalirudin group (4.6% vs. 7.2% without preprocedure heparin, $p=0.08$)

While these data are not conclusive, they strongly suggest that in patients presenting with both non-ST elevation and ST elevation ACS in whom an invasive strategy is planned, it is safe to switch from heparin to bivalirudin prior to PCI. Randomized trials designed to better evaluate this are currently underway.

RECOMMENDATIONS FOR USE OF DIRECT THROMBIN INHIBITORS IN ACS

There are many possible anticoagulation and antiplatelet regimens available. Our recommendations for choice of agents are as follows:

UA/NSTEMI

In patients presenting with UA or NSTEMI, we recommend initiation of anticoagulation in addition to antiplatelet therapy as soon as possible. The anticoagulant chosen reflects the clinical scenario.

- For patients in whom an urgent or emergent invasive strategy is planned (patient to be immediately taken to the catheterization laboratory), we recommend the use of bivalirudin. UFH is an acceptable alternative.
- For patients in whom an early invasive strategy is selected, we recommend the use of bivalirudin. Enoxaparin, UFH, and Fondaparinux are acceptable alternatives.
- For patients who are at a high risk of bleeding in whom an early invasive strategy is selected, we recommend the use of bivalirudin. Fondaparinux which is the preferred alternative over UFH or enoxaparin.
- For patients in whom an early conservative strategy is planned, we recommend the use of enoxaparin. UFH and fondaparinux are acceptable alternatives.
- For patients who are at a high risk of bleeding in whom an early conservative strategy is selected, we recommend the use of fondaparinux.

STEMI

For patients presenting with STEMI, the choice of agent depends upon whether the planned treatment strategy is primary PCI, thrombolytic therapy, or no reperfusion.

- For patients with STEMI referred for primary PCI, we recommend the use of bivalirudin (with provisional use of a Gp IIb/IIIa inhibitor) in addition to an oral antiplatelet agent as soon as possible. UFH (plus planned use of a GpIIb/IIIa inhibitor) in addition to an oral antiplatelet agent is an acceptable alternative.
- For patients presenting with STEMI who are at low risk for bleeding and are undergoing reperfusion therapy with fibrinolytic therapy, we recommend the use of enoxaparin. UFH is an acceptable alternative.

- For patients presenting with STEMI who are at high risk for bleeding and are undergoing reperfusion therapy with fibrinolytic therapy, we recommend the use of fondaparinux.
- For patients presenting with STEMI in whom no reperfusion therapy is planned, we recommend the use of enoxaparin or fondaparinux; the latter particularly if the patient is at increased risk of bleeding.

SUMMARY

Millions of people are admitted to hospitals in the united states every year with ACS. The underlying pathophyiology involves a complex cascade of clotting factor activation and platelet activation and aggregation leading to thrombus formation. Thus, thrombus formation results in impaired coronary blood flow and subsequent manifestations of the acute coronary syndrome. Thrombus causing partial occlusion of the lumen results in UA or non-STEMI, and complete occlusion typically results in STEMI. Thrombin plays a central role in the activation of clotting factor and platelets leading to the formation of intracoronary clots and the acute coronary syndrome. While heparin is a beneficial therapy in this disease state, patients with ACS continue to have high rates of ischemic and hemorrhagic complications *(34)*. DTIs have several important advantages over heparin which may lead to reduced ischemic events and hemorrhagic complications.

Early trials involving DTIs focused on the treatment of ACS with the prototypical DTI, hirudin. While a modest reduction in ischemic events was reported, the benefits were offset by an increase in bleeding complications. Hirudin was found to have a surprisingly narrow therapeutic window, and its use has since been limited to treatment of patients with HIT. The synthetic analogue, bivalirudin, has a shorter half life and, in contrast to hirudin, binds reversibly to thrombin. Subsequent trials have demonstrated bivalirudin as an alternative to heparin with comparable ischemic events and reduced bleeding complications. The REPLACE-2 trial showed that the use of bivalirudin during percutaneous intervention was associated with significantly less bleeding *(36)*. Later the ACUITY trial *(37)* and HORIZONS-AMI trial *(44)* demonstrated that bivalirudin as compared to heparin and glycoprotein IIb/IIIa blockade was associated with similar rates of recurrent ischemic events and significantly lower rates of bleeding in moderate to high risk patients with ACS and STEMIs, respectively. As a whole, the evidence over the last 15 years suggests that DTIs are superior anticoagulants in the treatment of all forms of the acute coronary syndrome.

REFERENCES

1. Weitz JI, Bates ER (2003) Direct thrombin inhibitors in cardiac disease. Cardiovasc Toxicol 3:13–25
2. Weitz JI, Hudoba M, Massel D, Maraganore J, Hirsh J (1990) Clot-bound thrombin is protected from inhibition by heparin-antithrombin III but is susceptible to inactivation by antithrombin III-independent inhibitors. J Clin Invest 86:385–391
3. Hirsh J (1991) Heparin. N Engl J Med 324:1565–1574
4. Eitzman DT, Chi L, Saggin L, Schwartz RS, Lucchesi BR, Fay WP (1994) Heparin neutralization by platelet-rich thrombi. Role of platelet factor 4. Circulation 89:1523–1529
5. Sobel M, Fish WR, Toma N et al (2001) Heparin modulates integrin function in human platelets. J Vasc Surg 33:587–594
6. Martel N, Lee J, Wells PS (2005) Risk for heparin-induced thrombocytopenia with unfractionated and low-molecular-weight heparin thromboprophylaxis: a meta-analysis. Blood 106:2710–2715
7. Bijsterveld NR, Peters RJ, Murphy SA, Bernink PJ, Tijssen JG, Cohen M (2003) Recurrent cardiac ischemic events early after discontinuation of short-term heparin treatment in acute coronary syndromes: results from the Thrombolysis in Myocardial Infarction (TIMI) 11B and Efficacy and Safety of Subcutaneous Enoxaparin in Non-Q-Wave Coronary Events (ESSENCE) studies. J Am Coll Cardiol 42:2083–2089
8. Theroux P, Waters D, Lam J, Juneau M, McCans J (1992) Reactivation of unstable angina after the discontinuation of heparin. N Engl J Med 327:141–145

9. Marciniak E, Gockerman JP (1977) Heparin-induced decrease in circulating antithrombin-III. Lancet 2:581–584
10. Weitz JI (1997) Low-molecular-weight heparins. N Engl J Med 337:688–698
11. Bara L, Billaud E, Gramond G, Kher A, Samama M (1985) Comparative pharmacokinetics of a low molecular weight heparin (PK 10 169) and unfractionated heparin after intravenous and subcutaneous administration. Thromb Res 39:631–636
12. Young E, Wells P, Holloway S, Weitz J, Hirsh J (1994) Ex-vivo and in-vitro evidence that low molecular weight heparins exhibit less binding to plasma proteins than unfractionated heparin. Thromb Haemost 71:300–304
13. Hirsh J, Warkentin TE, Raschke R, Granger C, Ohman EM, Dalen JE (1998) Heparin and low-molecular-weight heparin: mechanisms of action, pharmacokinetics, dosing considerations, monitoring, efficacy, and safety. Chest 114:489S–510S
14. Cosmi B, Fredenburgh JC, Rischke J, Hirsh J, Young E, Weitz JI (1997) Effect of nonspecific binding to plasma proteins on the antithrombin activities of unfractionated heparin, low-molecular-weight heparin, and dermatan sulfate. Circulation 95:118–124
15. Cohen M, Demers C, Gurfinkel EP et al (1997) A comparison of low-molecular-weight heparin with unfractionated heparin for unstable coronary artery disease. Efficacy and Safety of Subcutaneous Enoxaparin in Non-Q-Wave Coronary Events Study Group. N Engl J Med 337:447–452
16. Antman EM, McCabe CH, Gurfinkel EP et al (1999) Enoxaparin prevents death and cardiac ischemic events in unstable angina/non-Q-wave myocardial infarction. Results of the thrombolysis in myocardial infarction (TIMI) 11B trial. Circulation 100:1593–1601
17. Bozovich GE, Gurfinkel EP, Antman EM, McCabe CH, Mautner B (2000) Superiority of enoxaparin versus unfractionated heparin for unstable angina/non-Q-wave myocardial infarction regardless of activated partial thromboplastin time. Am Heart J 140:637–642
18. Cannon CP, Weintraub WS, Demopoulos LA et al (2001) Comparison of early invasive and conservative strategies in patients with unstable coronary syndromes treated with the glycoprotein IIb/IIIa inhibitor tirofiban. N Engl J Med 344:1879–1887
19. Ferguson JJ, Califf RM, Antman EM et al (2004) Enoxaparin vs unfractionated heparin in high-risk patients with non-ST-segment elevation acute coronary syndromes managed with an intended early invasive strategy: primary results of the SYNERGY randomized trial. Jama 292:45–54
20. Mahaffey KW, Cohen M, Garg J et al (2005) High-risk patients with acute coronary syndromes treated with low-molecular-weight or unfractionated heparin: outcomes at 6 months and 1 year in the SYNERGY trial. Jama 294:2594–2600
21. Assessment of the Safety and Efficacy of a New Thrombolytic Regimen (ASSENT)-3 Investigators (2001) Efficacy and safety of tenecteplase in combination with enoxaparin, abciximab, or unfractionated heparin: the ASSENT-3 randomised trial in acute myocardial infarction. Lancet 358:605–613
22. Wallentin L, Goldstein P, Armstrong PW et al (2003) Efficacy and safety of tenecteplase in combination with the low-molecular-weight heparin enoxaparin or unfractionated heparin in the prehospital setting: the Assessment of the Safety and Efficacy of a New Thrombolytic Regimen (ASSENT)-3 PLUS randomized trial in acute myocardial infarction. Circulation 108:135–142
23. Antman EM, Morrow DA, McCabe CH et al (2006) Enoxaparin versus unfractionated heparin with fibrinolysis for ST-elevation myocardial infarction. N Engl J Med 354:1477–1488
24. Tsuda Y, Szewczuk Z, Wang J, Yue SY, Purisima E, Konishi Y (1995) Interactions of hirudin-based inhibitor with thrombin: critical role of the IleH59 side chain of the inhibitor. Biochemistry 34:8708–8714
25. Eichler P, Friesen HJ, Lubenow N, Jaeger B, Greinacher A (2000) Antihirudin antibodies in patients with heparin-induced thrombocytopenia treated with lepirudin: incidence, effects on aPTT, and clinical relevance. Blood 96:2373–2378
26. Huhle G, Hoffmann U, Song X, Wang LC, Heene DL, Harenberg J (1999) Immunologic response to recombinant hirudin in HIT type II patients during long-term treatment. Br J Haematol 106:195–201
27. Jang IK, Brown DF, Giugliano RP et al (1999) A multicenter, randomized study of argatroban versus heparin as adjunct to tissue plasminogen activator (TPA) in acute myocardial infarction: myocardial infarction with novastan and TPA (MINT) study. J Am Coll Cardiol 33:1879–1885
28. Maraganore JM, Chao B, Joseph ML, Jablonski J, Ramachandran KL (1989) Anticoagulant activity of synthetic hirudin peptides. J Biol Chem 264:8692–8698
29. Swan SK, Hursting MJ (2000) The pharmacokinetics and pharmacodynamics of argatroban: effects of age, gender, and hepatic or renal dysfunction. Pharmacotherapy 20:318–329
30. Hauel NH, Nar H, Priepke H, Ries U, Stassen JM, Wienen W (2002) Structure-based design of novel potent nonpeptide thrombin inhibitors. J Med Chem 45:1757–1766

31. (1994) Randomized trial of intravenous heparin versus recombinant hirudin for acute coronary syndromes. The Global Use of Strategies to Open Occluded Coronary Arteries (GUSTO) IIa Investigators. Circulation 90:1631–1637.

32. (1999) Effects of recombinant hirudin (lepirudin) compared with heparin on death, myocardial infarction, refractory angina, and revascularisation procedures in patients with acute myocardial ischaemia without ST elevation: a randomised trial. Organisation to Assess Strategies for Ischemic Syndromes (OASIS-2) Investigators. Lancet 353:429–438

33. (1996) A comparison of recombinant hirudin with heparin for the treatment of acute coronary syndromes. The Global Use of Strategies to Open Occluded Coronary Arteries (GUSTO) IIb investigators. N Engl J Med 335:775–782.

34. Direct Thrombin Inhibitor Trialists' Collaborative Group (2002) Direct thrombin inhibitors in acute coronary syndromes: principal results of a meta-analysis based on individual patients' data. Lancet 359:294–302

35. Bittl JA, Strony J, Brinker JA et al (1995) Treatment with bivalirudin (Hirulog) as compared with heparin during coronary angioplasty for unstable or postinfarction angina. Hirulog Angioplasty Study Investigators. N Engl J Med 333:764–769

36. Lincoff AM, Bittl JA, Harrington RA et al (2003) Bivalirudin and provisional glycoprotein IIb/IIIa blockade compared with heparin and planned glycoprotein IIb/IIIa blockade during percutaneous coronary intervention: REPLACE-2 randomized trial. Jama 289:853–863

37. Stone GW, McLaurin BT, Cox DA et al (2006) Bivalirudin for patients with acute coronary syndromes. N Engl J Med 355:2203–2216

38. Lincoff AM, Steinhubl SR, Manoukian SV et al (2008) Influence oftiming of clopidogrel treatment on theefficacy and safety of bivalirudin in patients with non-st-segment elevation acute coronary syndromes undergoing percutaneous coronary intervention: an analysis of the ACUITY (Acute Catheterization and Urgent Intervention Triage strategY) trial. J Am Coll Intv 1:639–648

39. Anderson JL, Adams CD, Antman EM et al (2007) ACC/AHA 2007 guidelines for the management of patients with unstable angina/non-ST-Elevation myocardial infarction: a report of the American College of Cardiology/American Heart Association Task Force on Practice Guidelines (Writing Committee to Revise the 2002 Guidelines for the Management of Patients With Unstable Angina/Non-ST-Elevation Myocardial Infarction) developed in collaboration with the American College of Emergency Physicians, the Society for Cardiovascular Angiography and Interventions, and the Society of Thoracic Surgeons endorsed by the American Association of Cardiovascular and Pulmonary Rehabilitation and the Society for Academic Emergency Medicine. J Am Coll Cardiol 50:e1–e157

40. DeWood MA, Spores J, Notske R et al (1980) Prevalence of total coronary occlusion during the early hours of transmural myocardial infarction. N Engl J Med 303:897–902

41. Antman EM (1994) Hirudin in acute myocardial infarction. Safety report from the Thrombolysis and Thrombin Inhibition in Myocardial Infarction (TIMI) 9A Trial. Circulation 90:1624–1630

42. Antman EM (1996) Hirudin in acute myocardial infarction. Thrombolysis and Thrombin Inhibition in Myocardial Infarction (TIMI) 9B trial. Circulation 94:911–921

43. White H (2001) Thrombin-specific anticoagulation with bivalirudin versus heparin in patients receiving fibrinolytic therapy for acute myocardial infarction: the HERO-2 randomised trial. Lancet 358:1855–1863

44. Stone GW, Witzenbichler B, Guagliumi G et al (2008) Bivalirudin during primary PCI in acute myocardial infarction. N Engl J Med 358:2218–2230

45. Waksman R, Wolfram RM, Torguson RL et al (2006) Switching from Enoxaparin to Bivalirudin in Patients with Acute Coronary Syndromes without ST-segment Elevation who Undergo Percutaneous Coronary Intervention. Results from SWITCH – a multicenter clinical trial. J Invasive Cardiol 18:370–375

46. Gibson CM, Ten Y, Murphy SA et al (2007) Association of prerandomization anticoagulant switching with bleeding in the setting of percutaneous coronary intervention (A REPLACE-2 analysis). Am J Cardiol 99:1687–1690

47. White HD, Chew DP, Hoekstra JW et al (2008) Safety and efficacy of switching from either unfractionated heparin or enoxaparin to bivalirudin in patients with non-ST-segment elevation acute coronary syndromes managed with an invasive strategy: results from the ACUITY (Acute Catheterization and Urgent Intervention Triage strategY) trial. J Am Coll Cardiol 51:1734–1741

10

Synthetic Factor Xa Inhibition in Acute Coronary Syndromes

Michael S. Kim, Robert L. Page, and Ivan P. Casserly

CONTENTS

ABSTRACT Over the last decade, several advances in the management of patients with acute coronary syndrome have been made. Despite these therapeutic advances, the risk of major adverse cardiovascular events related to acute coronary syndrome remains significant. These findings have led to continued efforts to find more efficacious antiplatelet agents and anticoagulants to help reduce the risk of recurrent ischemic events. This chapter reviews the clinical data pertaining to the novel anticoagulant fondaparinux for the treatment of acute coronary syndrome.

Key words: Fondaparinux; Acute coronary syndrome; Anticoagulant

INTRODUCTION

Over the last decade, several advances in the management of patients with acute coronary syndromes (ACS) have been made. Specifically, the use of various antiplatelet agents *(1–7)*, anticoagulants *(8–12)*, lipid-lowering agents *(13–15)*, and an invasive strategy in both appropriate clinical settings and specific patient subsets *(16–18)* have been shown to reduce morbidity and mortality from ACS. Despite these therapeutic advances, the risk of major adverse cardiovascular events (MACE) related to an ACS remains significant: patients presenting with unstable angina (UA) or non-ST elevation myocardial infarction (NSEMI) and ST-elevation MI (STEMI) have a 1-month MACE rate of 10–15% and 4–6%, respectively (Fig. 1). These findings have led to continued efforts to find more efficacious antiplatelet agents and anticoagulants to help reduce the risk of recurrent ischemic events. However, recent data demonstrating a relationship between major bleeding events

From: *Contemporary Cardiology: Antithrombotic Drug Therapy in Cardiovascular Disease*
Edited by: A.T. Askari and A.M. Lincoff (eds.), DOI 10.1007/978-1-60327-235-3_10
© Humana Press, a part of Springer Science+Business Media, LLC 2010

at the time of an ACS and subsequent morbidity and mortality *(19–22)* (Fig. 2) underscore the importance of improved safety for newer antiplatelet agents and anticoagulants in achieving maximal net clinical benefit.

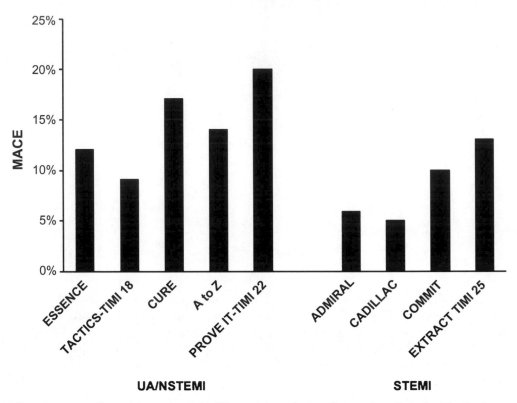

Fig. 1. Major adverse cardiovascular event (MACE) rates in major cardiovascular clinical trials. In the represented trials, MACE was defined as cardiovascular death, myocardial infarction, target vessel revascularization, refractory ischemia, and/or stroke.

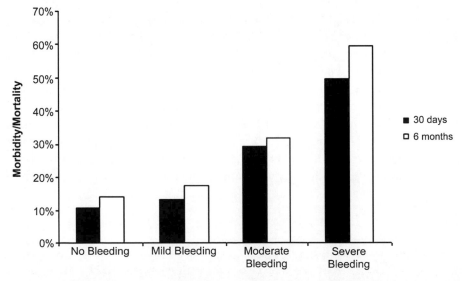

Fig. 2. Thirty-day and six-month death or myocardial infarction rates by worsening Global Strategies for Opening Occluded Coronary Arteries (GUSTO) bleeding severity. Adapted from Rao SV et al. (2005) Am J Cardiol 96(9):1200–6.

In this chapter, we review the clinical data pertaining to the novel anticoagulant Fondaparinux (Arixtra – GlaxoSmithKline, Middlesex, UK) for the treatment of ACS.

FONDAPARINUX SODIUM – SELECTIVE FACTOR XA INHIBITOR

Fondaparinux sodium is a synthetic pentasaccharide and represents the first commercially available selective factor Xa inhibitor *(23)*. Fondaparinux is composed of three D-glucosamine units separated by one D-glucuronic acid unit and one L-iduronic acid unit, each with several sulfonate groups in key positions (Fig. 3). X-ray crystallography studies have shown that it selectively binds to the heparin binding site on antithrombin *(24)* which induces a permanent conformational change in the antithrombin molecule. This conformational change results in antithrombin having an enhanced affinity for factor Xa, resulting in an approximate 300-fold increase in the inhibition of factor Xa. Once factor Xa is bound, fondaparinux is released from antithrombin, allowing it to consecutively bind several antithrombin molecules (Fig. 4). Unlike both unfractionated heparin (UFH) and low-molecular weight heparin (LMWH), fondaparinux does not interact with other plasma proteins (including factor IIa). It is this selectivity for factor Xa which results in the predictable pharmacologic profile described below.

While fondaparinux contains critical structural features that allow it to tightly bind to antithrombin *(25,26)*, a lone methyl group on the end of the molecule prevents it from nonspecifically binding to other plasma proteins *(27)*. Because it does not interact with plasma proteins (e.g., thrombin) other than antithrombin, fondaparinux exhibits a very predictable dose-response. Pharmacodynamic studies in young healthy volunteers reveal that subcutaneously administered fondaparinux has a bioavailability of 100%, displays a rapid onset of action (reaching half maximum plasma concentration within 25 min, and a maximum plasma concentration within 2 h), and has a dose-independent half-life of approximately 15 h, making it well suited for a once-daily dosing regimen *(28)*. Intravenous adminis-

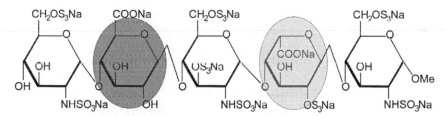

Fig. 3. Molecular structure of fondaparinux sodium. Three D-glucosamine units are separated by one D-glucuronic acid unit (*red*) and one L-iduronic acid unit (*yellow*).

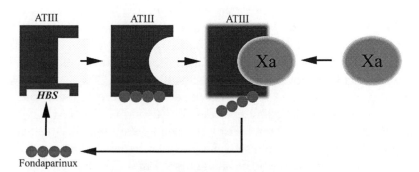

Fig. 4. Mechanism of action of fondaparinux (see associated text for detailed description). *ATIII* antithrombin III; *HBS* heparin binding site.

tration of fondaparinux demonstrates a similar pharmacokinetic profile, with peak plasma levels and activity area under the curve being linearly related to the dose administered.

When fondaparinux is administered in repeated subcutaneous doses, steady-state plasma concentrations are achieved after 3 or 4 days. In addition, the fraction of administered fondaparinux recovered in the urine ranges between 64% and 77% (29). Given that the kidneys are the primary route of its elimination (there is no evidence thus far in pharmacologic studies that fondaparinux undergoes any significant hepatic metabolism) (30), the drug should be used with caution in patients with altered renal function and is contraindicated in patients with severe renal impairment (i.e., creatinine clearance <30 ml/min).

Multiple dose ranging studies with fondaparinux have been performed. The PENTUA (Pentasaccharide in Unstable Angina) (31), PENTALYSE (synthetic PENTasaccharide as an Adjunct to fibrinoLYsis in ST-Elevation acute myocardial infarction) (32), and ASPIRE (Arixtra Study in Percutaneous coronary intervention: a Randomized Evaluation) (33) studies examined various fondaparinux doses in patients with ACS, STEMI, and patients undergoing PCI, respectively. Across all these studies, there did not appear to be a clear dose response with respect to clinical efficacy, with lower dosages (2.5–4 mg) achieving similar efficacy to the highest dosages (5–12 mg) (31).

FONDAPARINUX IN ACS – CLINICAL TRIALS

With several pilot studies suggesting that fondaparinux may be as effective as LMWH and UFH in the treatment of patients with ACS (31,32), two large, randomized clinical trials were performed to formally evaluate the safety and efficacy of fondaparinux in the setting of ACS. Prior to these studies, the ASPIRE trial was performed to evaluate the optimal dosing of fondaparinux for patients in these trials who required PCI.

Percutaneous Coronary Intervention

The Arixtra Study in Percutaneous Coronary Intervention: a Randomized Evaluation (ASPIRE) trial (33) was a randomized, blinded, phase II trial comparing two doses of intravenous fondaparinux (2.5 and 5 mg) with UFH (100 units/kg without concomitant glycoprotein IIb/IIIa antagonist; 65 units/kg with concomitant glycoprotein IIb/IIIa antagonist) in 350 patients undergoing PCI. The major indications for PCI were acute coronary syndrome (79%) or stable angina (20%). This study was a necessary prerequisite for the subsequent large OASIS-5 and -6 trials to help determine the optimal dosing of fondaparinux for patients in those trials who would require PCI.

The ASPIRE trial was a safety study, with the primary outcome consisting of the composite of major and minor bleeding events 48 h after PCI. Efficacy of fondaparinux was also investigated as a secondary outcome consisting of a composite of death, MI, urgent revascularization, and bailout use of glycoprotein IIb/IIIa antagonist over the same 48-h study period.

When compared to patients receiving UFH, patients receiving fondaparinux experienced a nonsignificant trend toward fewer bleeding episodes (7.6% vs. 6%, $P=0.61$) (Fig. 5a). In addition, there was a nonsignificant trend toward lower rates of bleeding with the lower (2.5 mg) dose of fondaparinux (3.4% vs. 9.6%, $P=0.06$). These results were similar in patients who received either planned or unplanned intravenous glycoprotein IIb/IIIa antagonists. Finally, with regard to efficacy, composite efficacy outcomes were equal between the fondaparinux and UFH groups, with no obvious dose response noted between the 2.5 and 5 mg fondaparinux dosing groups (Fig. 5b).

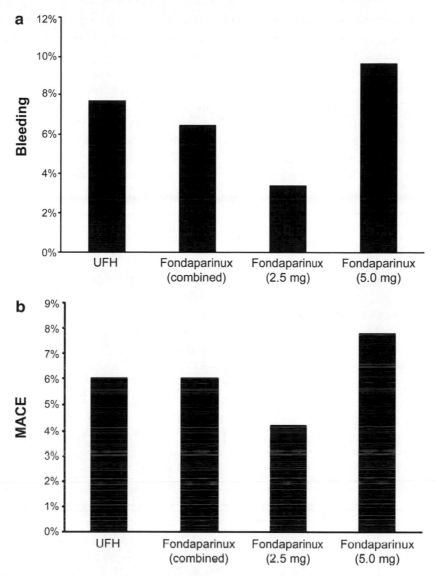

Fig. 5. (**a**) Total bleeding and (**b**) major adverse cardiovascular event (MACE) rates with UFH and varying doses of fondaparinux in ASPIRE. MACE was defined as death, myocardial infarction, urgent revascularization, and/or bailout glycoprotein IIb/IIIa inhibitor use; *UFH* unfractionated heparin.

The similar clinical efficacy and trend toward improved safety with the 2.5 mg dosing of fondaparinux formed the basis for that dosing recommendation during PCI in the subsequent OASIS-5 and OASIS-6 trials. To date, there are no larger studies supporting the use of fondaparinux in elective PCI.

OASIS-5 – UA/NSTEMI

The Fifth Organization to Assess Strategies for Ischemic Syndromes (OASIS-5) trial was a randomized, double-blinded, noninferiority trial comparing low-dose fondaparinux (2.5 mg once daily by subcutaneous injection) with enoxaparin (1 mg/kg twice daily by subcutaneous injection) in 20,078 patients with UA or NSTEMI *(34)*. The study's primary objective was to determine whether therapy with fondaparinux was noninferior to enoxaparin with respect to the occurrence of death, myocardial infarction (MI), or refractory ischemia at 9 days. In addition, the study's main safety outcome was the occurrence of bleeding at 9 days. Secondary outcomes included evaluating these same endpoints at predetermined follow-up periods of 30 days and study end (maximum of 180 days).

The results of OASIS-5 are shown in Table 1. There was no difference in the primary endpoint of death, MI, or refractory ischemia at 9 days between the two study groups (5.8% in the fondaparinux arm vs. 5.7% in the enoxaparin arm, $P=0.007$ for noninferiority). At 30 and 180-days follow-up, however, there was a trend toward a lower combined incidence of death, MI, and refractory ischemia with fondaparinux compared to enoxaparin. This difference was driven largely by a reduction in mortality in the fondaparinux arm, which reached statistical significance at the 30 day time point, and was of borderline statistical significance at 180 days. Analysis of the primary safety outcome revealed that the rate of major bleeding at 9 days was significantly lower in the fondaparinux group compared to the enoxaparin group (2.2% vs. 4.1%; $P<0.0001$). Specifically, treatment of patients with fondaparinux resulted in substantial reductions in both fatal and severe bleeding, with significant reductions in retroperitoneal hematoma and major bleeding requiring surgical intervention or transfusions. Major bleeding in this study was associated with significantly higher rates of death, recurrent infarction and stroke, which may explain the delayed benefit in mortality observed in the fondaparinux arm of this study, and underscores the importance of preventing major bleeding episodes during the treatment of ACS. A sub-analysis of bleeding outcomes based on baseline renal function demonstrated that the largest reduction in major bleeding events occurred in those with the most significant baseline renal dysfunction (i.e., GFRs<71 ml/min per 1.73 cm^2) (35).

The results of a prospectively specified analysis of the PCI cohort of the OASIS-5 study were recently published (36). Of the initial cohort of over 20,000 patients, 6,238 patients underwent PCI. The algorithm used to determine the dosing of anticoagulant used at the time of PCI is shown in Fig. 6. At 9 days, there was a similar incidence of ischemic events (death, MI, or stroke) in the fondaparinux and enoxaparin groups (6.3% vs. 6.2%, $P=0.79$), and a significant reduction in the incidence of major bleeding (2.4% vs. 5.1%, $P<0.00001$). These findings were maintained at the 30-day and 6-month follow-up time points. Despite the overall net clinical benefit in the fondaparinux arm of this substudy, the major issue of concern that was raised by this analysis involved an increased rate of guide catheter thrombosis in

Table 1
Clinic al outcomes in OASIS-5

Time (days)	Clinical endpoint	Fondaparinux (%)	Enoxaparin (%)	P-value (Noninferiority)	P-value (Superiority)
9	Death, MI, refractory ischemia	5.8	5.7	0.007	–
	Major bleeding	2.2	4.1	–	<0.001
	Death	1.8	1.9	0.005	–
30	Death, MI, refractory ischemia	8.0	8.6	–	0.13
	Major bleeding	3.1	5.0	–	<0.001
	Death	2.9	3.5	–	0.02
180	Death, MI, refractory ischemia	12.3	13.2	–	0.06
	Major bleeding	4.3	5.8	–	<0.001
	Death	5.8	6.5	–	0.05

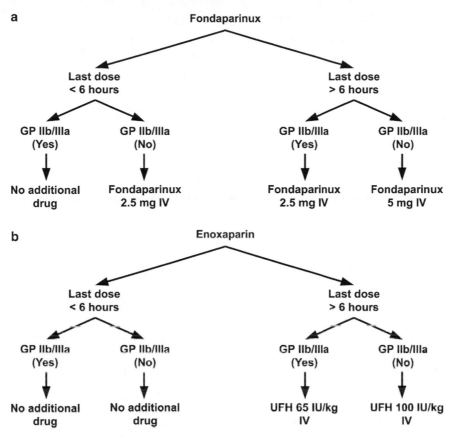

Fig. 6. Drug dosing in the PCI cohort of OASIS-5. (**a**) Fondaparinux arm; (**b**) Enoxaparin arm. *GP IIb/IIIa* Glycoprotein IIb/IIIa inhibitor; *UFH* Unfractionated heparin.

the fondaparinux arm (0.9% vs. 0.4%). The occurrence of catheter-related thrombus was associated with a very high rate of MI and stroke (27% and 5.4%, respectively) underscoring the significant morbidity of such an event. An amendment to the OASIS-5 protocol was made following an interim analysis of these events allowing the use of open label UFH at the discretion of the investigator. In the remainder of the study, nine of the ten events of catheter-related thrombus in the fondaparinux arm occurred in patients who did not receive adjunctive UFH. Despite the fact that overall outcomes in the PCI subset with fondaparinux were reassuring in this study, interventional cardiologists will likely be concerned by the potential for an uncommon but serious event such as guide catheter thrombosis. This may hamper the widespread application of fondaparinux in patients with ACS. The ability to provide a point-of-care assay to assess the anticoagulant effect of selective Xa inhibitors, and to correlate this measurement with clinical outcomes might be a first step in addressing this important issue. In addition, the efficacy and safety of the strategy of upstream fondaparinux with the use of standard UFH at the time of PCI as recommended by the study authors needs to be tested in prospective clinical studies.

In summary, OASIS-5 demonstrated that low-dose fondaparinux was equivalent to enoxaparin in its short-term efficacy in preventing ischemic events among high-risk patients with UA or NSTEMI and resulted in a substantial reduction in major bleeding, a finding that was associated with a reduction in long-term morbidity and mortality. Although there was an overall net clinical benefit in the PCI cohort, the issue of guide catheter thrombosis needs to be addressed and effective strategies for its prevention in patients receiving fondaparinux therapy are required.

OASIS-6 – STEMI

The Sixth Organization for the Assessment of Strategies for Ischemic Syndromes (OASIS-6) trial was a randomized, double-blinded trial comparing fondaparinux to "usual care" in 12,092 patients with STEMI *(37)*. The trial design was complex in that patients were allocated to two separate strata based on the need for antithrombotic therapy, as determined by the enrolling physician (Fig. 7). The first stratum included patients lacking a strict indication for antithrombotic therapy. Patients in this stratum were randomized to fondaparinux or placebo. The second stratum included patients in whom antithrombotic therapy was indicated, such as those who received fibin-specific lytic therapy, were undergoing PCI, or were managed conservatively with no reperfusion therapy. All patients in this stratum were randomized to fondaparinux or UFH. Patients in stratum 2 who underwent PCI were prerandomized to one of four possible drug regimens (UFH alone, GpIIb/IIIa inhibitor alone, UFH and Gp IIb/IIIa inhibitor, or neither medication). Subsequent dosing of the randomized agent (i.e., fondaparinux or UFH) was based on the prerandomized regimen.

The study's primary endpoint was death or recurrent MI at 30 days. Secondary outcomes included evaluation of these same clinical endpoints at 9 days and at study's end (3–6 months). The primary safety outcome was the incidence of bleeding complications at 9 days.

In the pooled analysis of patients from both strata, treatment with fondaparinux resulted in a significant reduction in the composite endpoint of death or MI at 9 and 30 days (primary endpoint), and at 3–6 months (Table 2). Somewhat surprisingly, treatment with fondaparinux resulted in a significant reduction in overall mortality at all three time points. In terms of bleeding complications, there was a trend toward fewer severe and major bleeding episodes with fondaparinux at 9 days. Overall, the results were consistent for patients in stratum 1 and 2.

The sub-analysis of outcomes in patients from stratum 2, however, revealed some important findings that suggested a distinct dichotomy of clinical response to fondaparinux based on the performance of primary PCI. At study end, patients who received fondaparinux and did not undergo primary PCI had a significantly lower incidence of death or reinfarction (14.9% vs. 19%, $P = 0.008$) and demonstrated a trend toward less major bleeding events at 9 days (Fig. 8). In contrast, patients who received fondaparinux

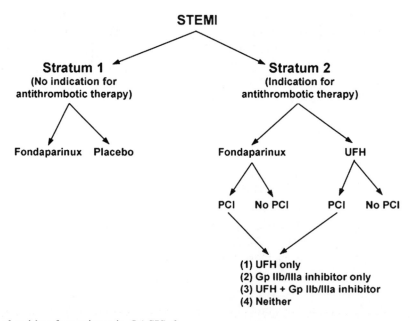

Fig. 7. Treatment algorithm for patients in OASIS-6.

Table 2
Clinical outcomes in OASIS-6

Time (days)	Clinical endpoint	Fondaparinux (%)	Placebo or UFH (%)
9	Death or reinfarction	7.4	8.9
	Severe bleeding	1.0	1.3
	Major bleeding	1.8	2.1
	Death	6.1	7.0
30	Death or reinfarction	9.7	11.2
	Death	7.8	8.9
Study end	Death or reinfarction	13.4	14.8
	Death	10.5	11.6

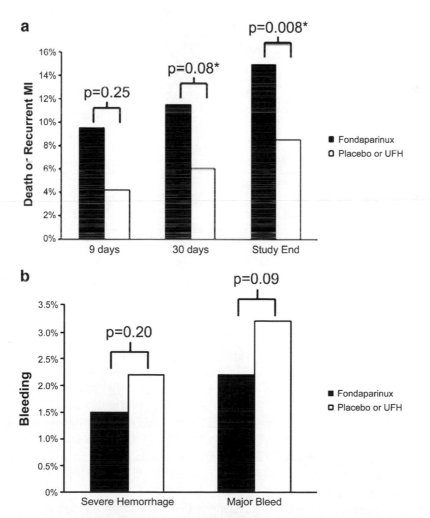

Fig. 8. Clinical and safety outcomes in patients not undergoing PCI in OASIS-6. (**a**) Incidence of death or recurrent myocardial infarction (MI); (**b**) Incidence of bleeding.

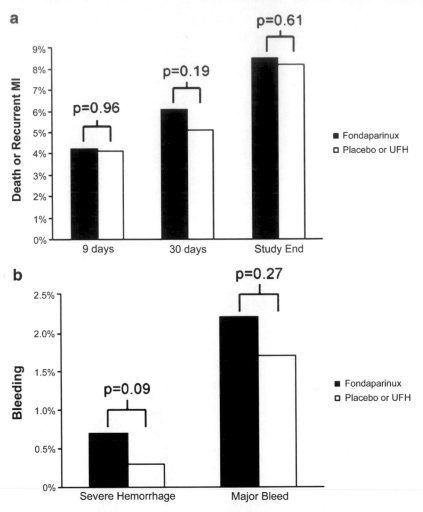

Fig. 9. Clinical and safety outcomes of patients undergoing PCI in OASIS-6. (**a**) Incidence of death or recurrent myocardial infarction (MI); (**b**) Incidence of bleeding.

and underwent PCI, derived no mortality benefit at 3–6 months (6.1% vs. 5.9%), and had a trend toward an increased incidence of major bleeding episodes at 9 days (Fig. 9). The explanation for this dichotomy is not entirely clear. Patients undergoing PCI in stratum 2 were at lower predicted risk and received a shorter duration of antithrombotic therapy compared to patients who received thrombolytic therapy or no reperfusion therapy. In addition, the specter of guide catheter thrombosis was again observed in the fondaparinux arm of this trial, with 22 events in patients treated with fondaparinux and no events in the UFH arm. The adverse consequence(s) of guide catheter thrombosis may have contributed to the overall lack of benefit observed in the PCI cohort. These data underscore how rare catheter thrombosis occurs in patients receiving standard treatment with UFH, and will certainly create reluctance on the part of interventional cardiologists to abandon the gold standard of anticoagulation in favor of more novel anticoagulants which have not proven the same degree of procedural safety. In a post hoc analysis, the investigators did report that among patients who were randomized to the fondaparinux arm and who received adjunctive UFH at the time of PCI, clinical event rates were similar to controls. This suggests that the addition of UFH at the time of PCI in patients who have received upstream fondaparinux for the treatment of STEMI may largely prevent adverse complications and may ultimately prove to be the best treatment strategy for this subset of patients.

ACC UA/NSTEMI GUIDELINES – UPDATE 2007

The use of fondaparinux is now specifically addressed in the most recent American College of Cardiology/American Heart Association (ACC/AHA) guidelines for the management of an unstable angina and NSTEMI *(38)*.

Fondaparinux receives a Class I indication for use in patients with UA/NSTEMI in whom a conservative strategy is selected. Furthermore, fondaparinux is recommended as the anticoagulant agent of choice in patients who have an increased risk of bleeding and in whom a noninvasive strategy is selected. In all cases, treatment with fondaparinux should be initiated at a subcutaneous dose of 2.5 mg administered daily once a conservative strategy has been planned and continued for the duration of hospitalization or up to 8 days. Given the concern of guide catheter thrombosis raised in the OASIS-5 and OASIS-6 trials, the task force also recommends the administration of adjunctive UFH (50–60 units/kg) at the time of PCI in patients who receive upstream fondaparinux.

COST-ANALYSIS OF FONDAPARINUX IN ACS

Economic data on the use of fondaparinux are limited to its use in the prevention and treatment of venous thromboembolism where it has clearly demonstrated overall cost-efficacy *(39,40)*. Although health economic studies on the use of fondaparinux in ACS have yet to be carried out, interpolation of existing data suggests that fondaparinux usage may result in an overall health care cost savings for several reasons, including lower and uncomplicated administration doses and decreased rates of bleeding when compared to traditional antithrombotic therapies in specific patient subsets. Further studies formally investigating the cost-effectiveness of this novel antithrombotic agent, however, are required.

CONCLUSION

Fondaparinux is a unique antithrombotic agent that selectively inhibits factor Xa. Until recently, the role of fondaparinux in ACS remained undefined. The OASIS-5 and OASIS-6 trials, however, have demonstrated the overall safety and efficacy of fondaparinux in the treatment of patients presenting with UA, NSTEMI, and STEMI. The major challenge for the more widespread application of this agent in these clinical settings is the management of the subset of ACS patients who ultimately require PCI. Prospective randomized studies documenting the efficacy and safety of using adjunctive UFH at the time of PCI in patients receiving fondaparinux would aid significantly in this regard.

REFERENCES

1. (2002) Collaborative meta-analysis of randomised trials of antiplatelet therapy for prevention of death, myocardial infarction, and stroke in high risk patients. BMJ 324(7329):71–86.
2. Boersma E, Harrington RA, Moliterno DJ, White H, Simoons ML (2002) Platelet glycoprotein IIb/IIIa inhibitors in acute coronary syndromes. Lancet 360(9329):342–343
3. Chen ZM, Jiang LX, Chen YP et al (2005) Addition of clopidogrel to aspirin in 45,852 patients with acute myocardial infarction: randomised placebo-controlled trial. Lancet 366(9497):1607–1621
4. Montalescot G, Barragan P, Wittenberg O et al (2001) Platelet glycoprotein IIb/IIIa inhibition with coronary stenting for acute myocardial infarction. N Engl J Med 344(25):1895–1903

5. Peters RJ, Mehta SR, Fox KA et al (2003) Effects of aspirin dose when used alone or in combination with clopidogrel in patients with acute coronary syndromes: observations from the Clopidogrel in Unstable angina to prevent Recurrent Events (CURE) study. Circulation 108(14):1682–1687

6. Stone GW, Grines CL, Cox DA et al (2002) Comparison of angioplasty with stenting, with or without abciximab, in acute myocardial infarction. N Engl J Med 346(13):957–966

7. Yusuf S, Zhao F, Mehta SR, Chrolavicius S, Tognoni G, Fox KK (2001) Effects of clopidogrel in addition to aspirin in patients with acute coronary syndromes without ST-segment elevation. N Engl J Med 345(7):494–502

8. (1988) Randomized trial of intravenous streptokinase, oral aspirin, both, or neither among 17,187 cases of suspected acute myocardial infarction: ISIS-2. ISIS-2 (Second International Study of Infarct Survival) Collaborative Group. J Am Coll Cardiol 12(6 Suppl A):3A–13A.

9. Antman EM, Morrow DA, McCabe CH et al (2006) Enoxaparin versus unfractionated heparin with fibrinolysis for ST-elevation myocardial infarction. N Engl J Med 354(14):1477–1488

10. Cohen M, Demers C, Gurfinkel EP et al (1998) Low-molecular-weight heparins in non-ST-segment elevation ischemia: the ESSENCE trial. Efficacy and Safety of Subcutaneous Enoxaparin versus intravenous unfractionated heparin, in non-Q-wave Coronary Events. Am J Cardiol 82(5B):19L–24L

11. Eikelboom JW, Quinlan DJ, Mehta SR, Turpie AG, Menown IB, Yusuf S (2005) Unfractionated and low-molecular-weight heparin as adjuncts to thrombolysis in aspirin-treated patients with ST-elevation acute myocardial infarction: a meta-analysis of the randomized trials. Circulation 112(25):3855–3867

12. Mahaffey KW, Granger CB, Collins R et al (1996) Overview of randomized trials of intravenous heparin in patients with acute myocardial infarction treated with thrombolytic therapy. Am J Cardiol 77(8):551–556

13. Cannon CP, Braunwald E, McCabe CH et al (2004) Intensive versus moderate lipid lowering with statins after acute coronary syndromes. N Engl J Med 350(15):1495–1504

14. Cannon CP, Steinberg BA, Murphy SA, Mega JL, Braunwald E (2006) Meta-analysis of cardiovascular outcomes trials comparing intensive versus moderate statin therapy. J Am Coll Cardiol 48(3):438–445

15. de Lemos JA, Blazing MA, Wiviott SD et al (2004) Early intensive vs a delayed conservative simvastatin strategy in patients with acute coronary syndromes: phase Z of the A to Z trial. JAMA 292(11):1307–1316

16. Antman EM, Anbe DT, Armstrong PW et al (2004) ACC/AHA guidelines for the management of patients with ST-elevation myocardial infarction; A report of the American College of Cardiology/American Heart Association Task Force on Practice Guidelines (Committee to Revise the 1999 Guidelines for the Management of patients with acute myocardial infarction). J Am Coll Cardiol 44(3):E1–E211

17. Mehta SR, Cannon CP, Fox KA et al (2005) Routine vs selective invasive strategies in patients with acute coronary syndromes: a collaborative meta-analysis of randomized trials. JAMA 293(23):2908–2917

18. Smith SC Jr, Feldman TE, Hirshfeld JW Jr et al (2006) ACC/AHA/SCAI 2005 Guideline Update for Percutaneous Coronary Intervention-Summary Article: A Report of the American College of Cardiology/American Heart Association Task Force on Practice Guidelines (ACC/AHA/SCAI Writing Committee to Update the 2001 Guidelines for Percutaneous Coronary Intervention). J Am Coll Cardiol 47(1):216–235

19. Eikelboom JW, Mehta SR, Anand SS, Xie C, Fox KA, Yusuf S (2006) Adverse impact of bleeding on prognosis in patients with acute coronary syndromes. Circulation 114(8):774–782

20. Moscucci M, Fox KA, Cannon CP et al (2003) Predictors of major bleeding in acute coronary syndromes: the Global Registry of Acute Coronary Events (GRACE). Eur Heart J 24(20):1815–1823

21. Rao SV, O'Grady K, Pieper KS et al (2006) A comparison of the clinical impact of bleeding measured by two different classifications among patients with acute coronary syndromes. J Am Coll Cardiol 47(4):809–816

22. Rao SV, O'Grady K, Pieper KS et al (2005) Impact of bleeding severity on clinical outcomes among patients with acute coronary syndromes. Am J Cardiol 96(9):1200–1206

23. Choay J, Petitou M, Lormeau JC, Sinay P, Casu B, Gatti G (1983) Structure-activity relationship in heparin: a synthetic pentasaccharide with high affinity for antithrombin III and eliciting high anti-factor Xa activity. Biochem Biophys Res Commun 116(2):492–499

24. Jin L, Abrahams JP, Skinner R, Petitou M, Pike RN, Carrell RW (1997) The anticoagulant activation of antithrombin by heparin. Proc Natl Acad Sci U S A 94(26):14683–14688

25. Petitou M, Duchaussoy P, Lederman I, Choay J, Sinay P (1988) Binding of heparin to antithrombin III: a chemical proof of the critical role played by a 3-sulfated 2-amino-2-deoxy-D-glucose residue. Carbohydr Res 179:163–172

26. Petitou M, Lormeau JC, Choay J (1988) Interaction of heparin and antithrombin III. The role of O-sulfate groups. Eur J Biochem 176(3):637–640

27. Petitou M, Duchaussoy P, Lederman I et al (1987) Synthesis of heparin fragments: a methyl alpha-pentaoside with high affinity for antithrombin III. Carbohydr Res 167:67–75

28. Petitou M, Duchaussoy P, Herbert JM et al (2002) The synthetic pentasaccharide fondaparinux: first in the class of antithrombotic agents that selectively inhibit coagulation factor Xa. Semin Thromb Hemost 28(4):393–402
29. Donat F, Duret JP, Santoni A et al (2002) The pharmacokinetics of fondaparinux sodium in healthy volunteers. Clin Pharmacokinet 41(Suppl 2):1–9
30. Lieu C, Shi J, Donat F et al (2002) Fondaparinux sodium is not metabolised in mammalian liver fractions and does not inhibit cytochrome P450-mediated metabolism of concomitant drugs. Clin Pharmacokinet 41(Suppl 2):19–26
31. Simoons ML, Bobbink IW, Boland J et al (2004) A dose-finding study of fondaparinux in patients with non-ST-segment elevation acute coronary syndromes: the Pentasaccharide in Unstable Angina (PENTUA) Study. J Am Coll Cardiol 43(12):2183–2190
32. Coussement PK, Bassand JP, Convens C et al (2001) A synthetic factor-Xa inhibitor (ORG31540/SR9017A) as an adjunct to fibrinolysis in acute myocardial infarction. The PENTALYSE study. Eur Heart J 22(18):1716–1724
33. Mehta SR, Steg PG, Granger CB et al (2005) Randomized, blinded trial comparing fondaparinux with unfractionated heparin in patients undergoing contemporary percutaneous coronary intervention: Arixtra Study in Percutaneous Coronary Intervention: a Randomized Evaluation (ASPIRE) Pilot. Circulation 111(11):1390–1397
34. Yusuf S, Mehta SR, Chrolavicius S et al (2006) Comparison of fondaparinux and enoxaparin in acute coronary syndromes. N Engl J Med 354(14):1464–1476
35. Fox KA, Bassand JP, Mehta SR et al (2007) Influence of renal function on the efficacy and safety of fondaparinux relative to enoxaparin in non ST-segment elevation acute coronary syndromes. Ann Intern Med 147(5):304–310
36. Mehta SR, Granger CB, Eikelboom JW et al (2007) Efficacy and safety of fondaparinux versus enoxaparin in patients with acute coronary syndromes undergoing percutaneous coronary intervention: results from the OASIS-5 trial. J Am Coll Cardiol 50(18):1742–1751
37. Yusuf S, Mehta SR, Chrolavicius S et al (2006) Effects of fondaparinux on mortality and reinfarction in patients with acute ST-segment elevation myocardial infarction: the OASIS-6 randomized trial. JAMA 295(13):1519–1530
38. Anderson JL, Adams CD, Antman EM et al (2007) ACC/AHA 2007 guidelines for the management of patients with unstable angina/non ST-elevation myocardial infarction: a report of the American College of Cardiology/American Heart Association Task Force on Practice Guidelines (Writing Committee to Revise the 2002 Guidelines for the Management of Patients With Unstable Angina/Non ST-Elevation Myocardial Infarction): developed in collaboration with the American College of Emergency Physicians, the Society for Cardiovascular Angiography and Interventions, and the Society of Thoracic Surgeons: endorsed by the American Association of Cardiovascular and Pulmonary Rehabilitation and the Society for Academic Emergency Medicine. Circulation 116(7):e148–e304
39. Sullivan SD, Davidson BL, Kahn SR, Muntz JE, Oster G, Raskob G (2004) A cost-effectiveness analysis of fondaparinux sodium compared with enoxaparin sodium as prophylaxis against venous thromboembolism: use in patients undergoing major orthopaedic surgery. Pharmacoeconomics 22(9):605–620
40. Sullivan SD, Kwong L, Nutescu E (2006) Cost-effectiveness of fondaparinux compared with enoxaparin as prophylaxis against venous thromboembolism in patients undergoing hip fracture surgery. Value Health 9(2):68–76

11

Antiplatelet Therapies: Aspirin, Clopidogrel and Thienopyridines, and Glycoprotein IIb/IIIa Inhibitors for the Management of ST-Segment Elevation Myocardial Infarction

Rory B. Weiner and Marc S. Sabatine

CONTENTS

ABSTRACT Platelet adhesion, aggregation, and activation play a key role in initiating and propagating coronary thrombosis. This provides opportunities to pharmacologically interfere with platelet function and antiplatelet therapies are a central component in the treatment of acute coronary syndromes. Whether the reperfusion strategy for ST-segment elevation myocardial infarction (STEMI) is pharmacologic or catheter-based, the use of adjunctive antiplatelet therapy can reduce the rate of death and ischemic complications. Aspirin, an irreversible inhibitor of platelet cyclooxygenase 1, provides mortality benefit to STEMI patients and is a cornerstone of therapy. Thienopyridines inhibit platelet activation and aggregation by targeting the $P2Y_{12}$ adenosine diphosphate (ADP) receptor and have been shown to provide mortality benefit in STEMI patients. Clopidogrel is preferred over ticlopidine due to a more favorable side effect profile. The Clopidogrel as Adjunctive Reperfusion Therapy – Thrombolysis in Myocardial Infarction 28 trial (CLARITY – TIMI 28) and the Clopidogrel and Metoprolol Infarction Trial/the Second Chinese Cardiac Study (COMMIT/CCS – 2) are two recent landmark trials demonstrating mortality benefit with clopidogrel in patients receiving pharmacologic reperfusion for STEMI. The glycoprotein (GP) IIb/IIIa receptor mediates platelet aggregation induced by all physiologic agonists and blockade of the receptor, either by monoclonal antibodies (abciximab) or by small molecules (eptifibatide and tirofiban), can be used in adjunctive treatment of STEMI, particularly in patients receiving primary percutaneous intervention (PCI). Novel antiplatelet agents, which may address issues relating to variability in response and irreversibility of inhibitor effects, are under active investigation and will better refine the role of antiplatelet therapy in this clinical setting and lead to further improvement in patient outcomes.

From: *Contemporary Cardiology: Antithrombotic Drug Therapy in Cardiovascular Disease*
Edited by: A.T. Askari and A.M. Lincoff (eds.), DOI 10.1007/978-1-60327-235-3_11
© Humana Press, a part of Springer Science+Business Media, LLC 2010

Key words: Platelet; ST-segment elevation myocardial infarction (STEMI); Aspirin; Clopidogrel; Glycoprotein (GP) IIb/IIIa inhibitor

BACKGROUND

Platelet adhesion, aggregation, and activation play a key role in initiating and propagating coronary thrombosis. In response to vascular injury, platelets interact with components of the subendothelial matrix, notably collagen and von Willebrand factor *(1)*. Various local mediators, such as adenosine diphosphate (ADP), thromboxane A_2 (TXA$_2$), and thrombin are then produced and amplify platelet activation *(2)*. This sequence provides multiple opportunities to pharmacologically interfere with platelet activation, and antiplatelet therapies are a central component in the treatment of all acute coronary syndromes (ACS).

Whether the reperfusion strategy employed for ST-segment elevation myocardial infarction (STEMI) is pharmacologic or catheter-based, the use of adjunctive antiplatelet therapy is crucial to reduce the rate of death and ischemic complications. The focus of this chapter will be antiplatelet therapies, including aspirin, thienopyridines, and glycoprotein (GP) IIb/IIIa inhibitors, in the management of STEMI.

ASPIRIN

Aspirin irreversibly inhibits platelet cyclooxygenase 1 (COX-1) through acetylation of the amino acid serine at position 529, thereby preventing the formation of prostaglandin H_2 from the precursor arachidonic acid. This blocks the subsequent formation of TXA$_2$, a potent mediator of platelet aggregation *(3)*.

In 1988, the use of aspirin in the ISIS-2 (Second International Study of Infarct Survival) trial conferred a 23% reduction in vascular mortality compared with placebo alone in patients with STEMI *(4)*. In this trial, over 17,000 patients were randomized to SK versus placebo and aspirin versus placebo in a 2×2 factorial design. The mortality benefit for aspirin was similar to the 25% reduction in death with SK alone. Furthermore, the combination of aspirin and SK provided additive benefit, with a 42% reduction in mortality rate (8.0% for the combination vs. 13.2% for placebo; $p < 0.001$; Fig. 1).

It has been hypothesized that fibrinolysis may in itself promote platelet aggregation, possibly by exposure of the clot's platelet-rich core or through the release of thrombin. A meta-analysis demonstrated that aspirin reduced coronary reocclusion and recurrent ischemic events after fibrinolytic therapy with either streptokinase or alteplase *(5)*. Long-term follow-up data have demonstrated that the early survival advantage of SK and aspirin therapy is maintained over 10 years *(6)*.

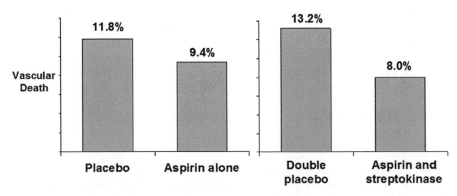

Fig. 1. Incidence of vascular death for patients in the ISIS-2 trial randomized to treatment with placebo, aspirin, or a combination of streptokinase and aspirin after 5 weeks' follow-up.

American Heart Association/American College of Cardiology (AHA/ACC) practice guidelines give a Class I (evidence that treatment is beneficial and effective) recommendation for aspirin to be chewed by patients who have not taken the medication before presentation with STEMI (7). The initial dose should be between 162 and 325 mg and continued indefinitely at a daily dose of 75–162 mg (8). For initial dosing, non-enteric-coated formulations are favored due to more rapid buccal absorption (9). The main contraindication to aspirin use is a hypersensitivity to salicylate. In patients with true aspirin allergy (hives, nasal polyps, bronchospasm, or anaphylaxis), clopidogrel or ticlopidine may be substituted, although likely a thienopyridine may already be indicated itself as adjunctive therapy (see below).

Failure to respond to aspirin may be caused by an inadequate primary pharmacological effect, known as "aspirin resistance." Depending on the population studied, the assay used, and the definition applied, the prevalence of aspirin resistance has ranged from 5% to 65% (10). Aspirin resistance, as defined by an aggregation-based rapid platelet function assay, was associated with an increased risk of adverse clinical outcomes in stable patients with coronary artery disease (11). Furthermore, in high-risk aspirin-treated patients, urinary concentrations of 11-dehydro thromboxane B2 (a marker of in vivo thromboxane generation and therefore aspirin resistance) predicted the future risk of myocardial infarction (MI) or cardiovascular death (12). The clinical ramifications of aspirin resistance in STEMI management have not yet been clearly defined, although it is unlikely to play a major role (13). Monitoring of antiplatelet activity is mainly done for investigational purposes at the present time (14).

THIENOPYRIDINES

As more has become known about the pathogenesis of plaque rupture and clot formation, there has been increasing interest in evaluating more potent antiplatelet agents. The thienopyridine derivative clopidogrel is an oral antiplatelet agent that inhibits platelet activation and aggregation by targeting the $P2Y_{12}$ ADP receptor (15). Ticlopidine, another thienopyridine and quite similar chemically to clopidogrel, can cause the adverse effects of neutropenia and thrombotic thrombocytopenic purpura. Both agents are prodrugs requiring hepatic metabolism to form their active metabolites that irreversibly bind to the $P2Y_{12}$ receptor. Given the fewer side effects, lack of need for laboratory monitoring, and once-daily dosing clopidogrel is the preferred agent (16).

Dual antiplatelet treatment, with aspirin and a thienopyridine, decreases the incidence of death or ischemic complications in the setting of percutaneous coronary intervention (PCI) (17) and when given upstream in patients presenting with non ST-segment elevation (NSTE) ACS (18).

Pharmacologic Reperfusion

The CLARITY-TIMI 28 (Clopidogrel as Adjunctive Reperfusion Therapy – Thrombolysis in Myocardial Infarction 28) trial was a placebo-controlled, double blinded trial that enrolled 3,491 patients worldwide, aged 18–75 years, within 12 h of STEMI symptom onset (19). Patients were randomly assigned to receive either clopidogrel (300 mg loading dose, followed by 75 mg once daily) or placebo at presentation. All patients were to be treated with aspirin (150–325 mg on the first day and 75–162 mg daily thereafter) and a fibrinolytic. Patients who received a fibrin-specific lytic (69% of patients) were to receive heparin (unfractionated or low-molecular weight). As per trial protocol, all patients were to undergo coronary angiography during the index hospitalization (48–192 h after randomization) in order to assess for late patency of the infarct-related artery.

The primary efficacy endpoint was the composite of an occluded infarct-related artery (defined by a TIMI flow grade of 0 or 1) at angiography or death or recurrent MI prior to angiography. The last two served as surrogate markers for failed reperfusion or reocclusion of the infarct-related artery. The rates of the primary efficacy endpoint were 21.7% in the placebo group and 15.0% in the clopidogrel group, representing an absolute risk reduction of 6.7% and an odds reduction of 36% with treatment with clopidogrel ($p < 0.001$; Fig. 2). Among the individual components of the primary endpoint, clopidogrel had the greatest effect on reducing the rate of an occluded infarct-related artery (18.4% to 11.7%; $p < 0.001$) and the rate of recurrent MI prior to angiography (3.6% to 2.5%; $p = 0.08$). The benefit of clopidogrel in reducing the risk of the primary endpoint was observed across all prespecified subgroups including age, sex, type of heparin, type of fibrinolytic, and infarct location. At 30 days' follow-up treatment with clopidogrel prior to angiography had significantly reduced the odds of cardiovascular death, recurrent MI, or recurrent ischemia leading to urgent revascularization by 20% (from 14.1% to 11.6%; $p = 0.03$; Fig. 3).

The addition of clopidogrel to fibrinolytic therapy did not significantly increase the risk of TIMI major bleeding (1.3% with clopidogrel vs. 1.1% with placebo; $p = 0.64$), including a similar risk of intracranial hemorrhage (ICH), (0.5% with clopidogrel vs. 0.7% with placebo; $p = 0.38$). Importantly, of the 136 patients who underwent coronary artery bypass graft (CABG) surgery during their index

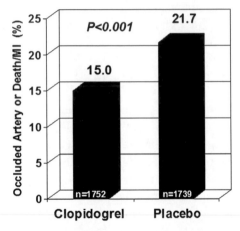

Fig. 2. Incidence of the primary endpoint, a composite of an occluded infarct-related artery (defined as a TIMI flow grade of 0 or 1), or death or recurrent MI prior to coronary angiography, in the CLARITY-TIMI 28 trial.

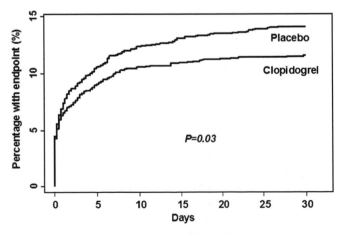

Fig. 3. Cumulative incidence curves in the CLARITY-TIMI 28 trial for the endpoint of death from cardiovascular causes, recurrent MI, or recurrent ischemia leading to the need for urgent revascularization through 30 days' follow-up.

hospitalization, there was no excess in major bleeding through 30 days (7.5% with clopidogrel vs. 7.2% with placebo; $p = 1.00$), and there was a trend toward reduction in 30-day ischemic events *(20)*.

In the CLARITY-TIMI 28 trial, clopidogrel therapy did not significantly improve the mean degree of ST-segment elevation (a non-invasive marker of early reperfusion) at 180 min. However, clopidogrel was found to improve late angiographical outcomes, including a 36% increase in the odds of optimal epicardial flow (a TIMI flow grade of 3; $p < 0.0001$), a 21% increase in the odds of optimal microvascular perfusion (a TIMI myocardial perfusion grade of 3; $p = 0.008$), and a 27% reduction in the odds of intracoronary thrombus ($p < 0.001$), when angiography was performed 2–8 days after randomization. Furthermore, the largest treatment benefit with clopidogrel was observed in patients who achieved initial vessel reperfusion, as suggested by either partial (30–70%) or complete (>70%) ST-segment resolution at 90 min, whereas angiographical or clinical benefit with clopidogrel was not apparent in patients in the absence of initial ST-segment resolution (p for interaction 0.003) *(21)*. These data suggest that clopidogrel appears to improve late coronary patency and clinical outcomes by preventing reocclusion of the infarct-related artery rather than by facilitating reperfusion.

The second major trial examining the role of clopidogrel in the setting of pharmacologic reperfusion for STEMI was COMMIT/CCS-2 (the Clopidogrel and Metoprolol Infarction Trial/the Second Chinese Cardiac Study) *(22)*. This was a randomized trial that used a 2×2 factorial design to evaluate the addition of clopidogrel (75 mg daily, without a loading dose) and metoprolol, both compared with placebo, in patients with a suspected STEMI within 24 h of symptom onset. The trial enrolled 45,852 patients in China and had two prespecified co-primary endpoints: the composite of death, reinfarction, or stroke; and death from any cause. Patients were followed until hospital discharge or day 28, whichever occurred sooner. Ninety-three percent of patients had evidence of ST-segment elevation or left bundle branch block on their electrocardiogram at the time of randomization. In comparison with the CLARITY-TIMI 28 trial, there was no upper age limit to the trial and 26% of enrolled patients were greater than 70 years old. All patients were treated with aspirin 162 mg daily; only 54% received a fibrinolytic, 75% received an anticoagulant, and less than 5% of patients underwent PCI.

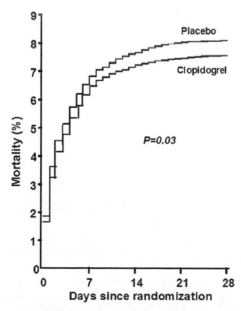

Fig. 4. Cumulative incidence curves for the endpoint of death prior to discharge in COMMIT/CCS-2.

In COMMIT/CCS-2, treatment with clopidogrel resulted in a significant 9% reduction in the incidence of death, reinfarction, or stroke (10.1% vs. 9.2%; p=0.002) and a significant 7% reduction in the risk of death alone (8.1% to 7.5%; p=0.03; Fig. 4). The benefit of clopidogrel on the incidence of the composite primary endpoint was observed independent of age, sex, or the use of fibrinolytic therapy. Despite the absence of a loading dose, the clinical benefit of clopidogrel emerged rapidly, with a significant 11% reduction in the incidence of death, reinfarction, or stroke by the end of the second hospital day (p=0.014), driven predominantly by an 11% reduction in the risk of death (3.2% vs. 3.6%; p=0.019).

The rates of major bleeding (defined as requiring transfusion, fatal, or cerebral) in COMMIT/CCS-2 were low and similar in the two treatment groups (0.58% with clopidogrel vs. 0.55% with placebo; p=0.59), including participants receiving concomitant fibrinolytic therapy and older patients. The rates of ICH were identical across treatment arms (0.2%). Treatment with clopidogrel was associated with a higher incidence of minor bleeding, including bruising and dental bleeding (3.6% vs. 3.1%; p=0.005).

The CLARITY-TIMI 28 trial and COMMIT/CCS-2 demonstrate that the addition of clopidogrel to aspirin in patients with STEMI receiving fibrinolytic therapy helps to maintain infarct-related artery patency and reduce the rate of ischemic complications, including mortality. The trials had several differences, including the use of a loading dose of clopidogrel and the performance of angiography (Table 1), yet both studies support the use of clopidogrel as adjunctive therapy in the setting of pharmacologic reperfusion for STEMI.

The duration of treatment in these trials was brief (up to and including the day of coronary angiography or day 8/hospital discharge in CLARITY-TIMI 28; until hospital discharge or up to 4 weeks

Table 1
Comparison of the CLARITY-TIMI 28 trial and COMMIT/CCS-2

	CLARITY-TIMI 28	COMMIT/CCS-2
Number of patients	3,491	45,852
Primary endpoint	Occluded infarct-related artery or death or recurrent MI before angiography	Death, reinfarction or stroke; mortality
Inclusion	STEMI < 12 h, age ≤ 75	Acute MI < 24 h, no age limit (maximum age was 99 years)
Trial location	International (predominantly North America and Europe)	China
Percentage receiving fibrinolysis	99%	54% (Predominantly urokinase)
Clopidogrel dosing	Loading dose (300 mg), followed by 75 mg daily	75 mg Daily (no loading dose)
Angiography	Routine (94%)	Rare
Percentage undergoing PCI	53.4%	<5%
Results	Clopidogrel improves patency rate of infarct-related artery and reduces ischemic complications	Clopidogrel reduces *mortality* and major vascular events
Safety	No increase in TIMI major bleeding or ICH	No increase in major bleeding or ICH

CLARITY-TIMI 28: Clopidogrel as Adjunctive Reperfusion Therapy – Thrombolysis in Myocardial Infarction 28
COMMIT/CCS-2: the Clopidogrel and Metoprolol in Myocardial Infarction Trial/the Second Chinese Cardiac Study
MI myocardial infarction, *TIMI* thrombolysis in myocardial infarction, *ICH* intracranial hemorrhage, *CABG* coronary artery bypass grafting

in the hospital in COMMIT/CCS-2). Thus, there is a lack of long-term data regarding the duration of clopidogrel therapy in STEMI patients receiving thrombolysis. However, extrapolation of data from patients with NSTE ACS treated with clopidogrel over 12 months (18) and a subset of patients with prior MI, ischemic stroke, or symptomatic peripheral arterial disease (PAD) treated with long-term therapy (23) indicate that extended treatment can reduce ischemic complications or death.

The most recent iteration of the STEMI practice guidelines (7) is several years old and predates the CLARITY-TIMI 28 trial and COMMIT/CCS-2. However, based on those trials, a clopidogrel loading dose of 300 mg would be reasonable for patients aged less than 75 years receiving fibrinolytic therapy, followed by a daily dose of 75 mg. For patients aged greater than 75 years, the addition of clopidogrel 75 mg daily (without a loading dose) to fibrinolytic therapy appears to be well tolerated and improves clinical outcomes without any significant excess in bleeding. These recommendations are supported by the 2007 STEMI focused update (24). Determination of the optimal duration of therapy will require further study, although, as noted above, data from other patient populations suggest that 12 months of therapy may be beneficial.

Mechanical Reperfusion

Although not focused on patients with STEMI, there is data to support the use of thienopyridines with PCI. Several initial trials examined the use of ticlopidine in conjunction with aspirin in patients treated with PCI (17,25) and demonstrated the synergistic benefit of thienopyridine and aspirin therapy. The aspirin–ticlopidine combination, as compared to aspirin–warfarin, demonstrated a decrease in a combined primary endpoint of death, MI, angiographically evident thrombosis, or revascularization of the target lesion within 30 days (0.5% for aspirin–ticlopidine vs. 2.7% for aspirin–warfarin; $p < 0.001$) (26). Studies have shown clopidogrel to have comparable if not better efficacy and a superior safety profile compared with ticlopidine (27,28). Thus, clopidogrel is the preferred thienopyridine and the use of clopidogrel is considered the standard of care in patients undergoing primary PCI for STEMI (7), despite a lack of clinical trial data specific to this population.

However, a key question is when to initiate clopidogrel therapy relative to the timing of PCI: upstream or at the start of PCI. Even when a 300-mg loading dose is used, it requires at least 4–6 h for clopidogrel to approach its maximal antiplatelet effect (29). Although CLARITY-TIMI 28 enrolled patients receiving pharmacologic reperfusion therapy rather than primary PCI, the upstream initiation of clopidogrel and the protocol-mandated coronary angiography 2–8 days thereafter permitted the assessment of the benefit of pretreatment in the 53.4% of all randomized patients who underwent PCI, who thereafter were to receive open-label clopidogrel (30). In PCI-CLARITY, pretreatment with clopidogrel was found to significantly reduce the odds of cardiovascular death, recurrent MI, or stroke by 46% following PCI through 30 days from randomization (3.6% vs. 6.2%; adjusted $p = 0.008$), without a significant increase in bleeding rate. The Kaplan-Meier estimated event rate curves for the two treatment groups separated soon after PCI and continued to diverge over time (Fig. 5). The benefit of clopidogrel pretreatment was observed across all patient subgroups, including patients who received a GP IIb/IIIa receptor inhibitor at the time of PCI (31). Analogously, the benefit of clopidogrel pretreatment has also been demonstrated in patients with NSTE ACS undergoing PCI (32). Some clinicians are reluctant to administer clopidogrel before angiography because of concerns that the patient will be found to have disease requiring coronary artery bypass grafting (CABG). Nonetheless, data from both CLARITY-TIMI 28 and CURE suggest that even for patients requiring CABG there is a benefit to upstream clopidogrel initiation and minimal risk of bleeding, especially if one waits 5 days after discontinuing clopidogrel (20,33).

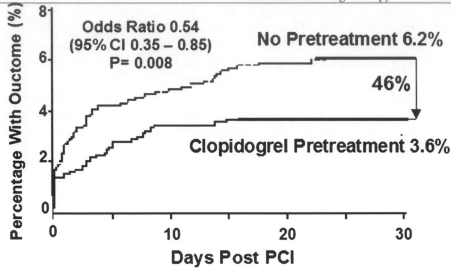

Fig. 5. Cumulative incidence curves of cardiovascular death, recurrent MI, or stroke following PCI through 30 days' follow-up in the PCI-CLARITY-TIMI 28 study.

Determination of the optimal loading dose of clopidogrel with PCI is under active investigation. Higher loading doses of clopidogrel have been shown to achieve more rapid and consistent platelet inhibition as compared with the standard 300-mg loading dose *(29,34–36)*. In the ARMYDA-2 (Antiplatelet Therapy for Reduction of Myocardial Damage during Angioplasty) trial, a 600-mg loading dose of clopidogrel, as compared to 300 mg, significantly reduced the incidence of periprocedural MI by 50% in patients undergoing PCI for indications other than STEMI ($p=0.041$) *(37)*. The 600 mg loading dose had an acceptable safety profile during short-term follow-up. Data also suggest that a 600 mg loading dose may improve cardiovascular outcomes at 1 month of follow-up in NSTE ACS patients undergoing PCI *(38)*. Whether any additional benefit is gained with the use of loading doses higher than 600 mg is yet to be determined as trials have revealed somewhat discordant results *(29,35)*. Evidence also suggests that a higher maintenance dose of clopidogrel with 150 mg daily provides more effective platelet inhibition than the currently recommended dose of 75 mg daily *(39)*. Whether this will reduce complications, including late stent thrombosis, has not yet been determined. The clinical effects of higher loading and early maintenance doses of clopidogrel in patients with unstable angina and NSTE ACS undergoing early invasive therapy is being evaluated in the CURRENT/OASIS 7 (Clopidogrel Optimal Loading Dose Usage to Reduce Recurrent Events/ Optimal Antiplatelet Strategy for Interventions) trial.

For patients with STEMI proceeding directly to primary PCI, the ACC/AHA guidelines recommend a clopidogrel loading dose of 300 mg after diagnostic angiography and prior to PCI *(7)*. The 2005 ACC/AHA/SCAI (Society for Cardiovascular Angiography and Interventions) guidelines recommend a 300 mg loading dose of clopidogrel at least 6 h before PCI and support a loading dose of greater than 300 mg for patients undergoing PCI who need to achieve a greater degree of platelet inhibition more rapidly, as would be the case in primary PCI for STEMI *(40)*. Most recently, the 2007 guidelines from the European Society of Cardiology suggest a 600-mg loading dose of clopidogrel in patients with STEMI undergoing primary PCI *(41)*.

As is the case with pharmacologic reperfusion, the optimal duration of clopidogrel therapy following mechanical reperfusion in STEMI remains unknown. Extrapolation of data from patients undergoing elective PCI suggests that 12 months of therapy is beneficial *(42)*. The type of stent (bare metal stent

[BMS] or drug eluting stent [DES]) deployed at the time of PCI affects arterial healing by several mechanisms (43). Data suggest that premature discontinuation of clopidogrel after DES implantation can be associated with an increase in late cardiac death or nonfatal MI, possibly related to late stent thrombosis (44). Observational data suggest a benefit of dual antiplatelet therapy for more than 1 year following DES placement (45). A current scientific advisory document stresses the importance of 12 months of dual antiplatelet therapy after placement of a DES, and education of the patient and health care provider about hazards of premature discontinuation (46). ACC/AHA/SCAI guidelines recommend daily clopidogrel for at least 1 month following BMS implantation (40).

Similar to aspirin resistance, the concept of "clopidogrel resistance" has been gaining interest. The definition of clopidogrel resistance and assay specifications varies from study to study and nonstandardized methods and use of varying doses of ADP makes comparison of study results difficult (10). However, it is believed that several factors, typically divided into those intrinsically or extrinsically related to the platelet, are responsible for the phenomenon of clopidogrel resistance (47). Intrinsic mechanisms include variability of $P2Y_{12}$ receptor affinity for the active metabolite of clopidogrel, variable receptor number, and variability in the response to binding (internal signaling, secondary messenger release). Several genetic mutations that modulate both $P2Y_{12}$ function and expression have been identified (48,49). Extrinsic mechanisms include any factor that affects platelet aggregation response other than the direct interaction of the active metabolite of clopidogrel with the $P2Y_{12}$ receptor and the subsequent downstream signaling. Examples include noncompliance, drug–drug interactions, and variability in absorption or metabolism. Potential for interaction exists with clopidogrel and the 3-hydroxy-3-methyl-glutaryl-CoA (HMG-CoA) reductase inhibitors (statins), as in vitro, clopidogrel metabolism is inhibited by more than 90% when clopidogrel and atorvastatin are present at equimolar concentrations (50). However, there was no evidence of an interaction clinically in a large placebo-controlled trial with long-term follow-up (51).

Patient variability in platelet response to clopidogrel has been demonstrated, and resistance portends worse clinical outcomes in patients, particularly in those who undergo coronary stenting (52–55). Furthermore, incomplete inhibition of ADP-induced platelet aggregation has been demonstrated after stent thrombosis has occurred (55).

The optimal management strategy for patients deemed to have response variability to clopidogrel is not well defined. The possibility of higher loading or maintenance doses, as discussed previously, may be a reasonable treatment strategy. Alternatively, other $P2Y_{12}$ receptor antagonists are under development and may provide more predictable levels of ADP inhibition. There are also reports of ticlopidine serving as an alternative therapy in cases of clopidogrel resistance (56).

GLYCOPROTEIN (GP) IIB/IIIA RECEPTOR INHIBITORS

The platelet GP IIb/IIIa receptor mediates platelet aggregation induced by all physiologic agonists. Activation of intracellular signaling pathways within the platelet causes the resting GP IIb/IIIa receptor to undergo a conformational change allowing it to bind to fibrinogen. Platelet aggregation then occurs via the cross-linking of two separate platelets by fibrinogen. Blockade of the receptor, either by monoclonal antibodies or by small molecules patterned after the arginine glycine-aspartic acid (RGD) cell recognition domain, prevents arterial thrombosis in animal models better than aspirin (57).

The first of these inhibitors to be developed was abciximab, a chimeric monoclonal antibody that binds nonspecifically to the GP IIb/IIIa receptor (58). With concerns relating to irreversibility, nonspecificity for the GP IIb/IIIa receptor and immunogenicity, small molecule GP IIb/IIIa receptor inhibitors were developed, including eptifibatide and tirofiban.

Pharmacologic Reperfusion

The role of GP IIb/IIIa receptor inhibitors as an adjunct to pharmacologic reperfusion for STEMI has been evaluated. Combination therapy of GP IIb/IIIa receptor inhibitors and reduced-dose fibrinolytic therapy has been the subject most extensively studied. Early studies showed encouraging findings that GP IIb/IIIa receptor inhibition might offer incremental benefit and it was believed that it may help to minimize the risk of bleeding by allowing reduction in the dose of the co-administered lytic (59–62). The GUSTO-V (Global Utilization of Strategies to Open Occluded Coronary Arteries – V) trial was a randomized, open-label trial to compare the effect of reteplase alone with reteplase plus abciximab in patients with STEMI (63). A total of 16,588 patients in the first 6 h of evolving STEMI were randomly assigned standard-dose reteplase or half-dose reteplase and full-dose abciximab. The primary endpoint was 30-day mortality, and secondary endpoints included various complications of MI. The combination of reteplase and abciximab did not offer a significant survival benefit (5.6% mortality in the combined group vs. 5.9% in the reteplase group; $p=0.43$), but it did decrease the risk of nonfatal reinfarction, as well as other complications of MI (including ventricular tachycardia and fibrillation, high-grade atrioventricular block, and septal or free wall rupture). However, this occurred at the cost of twice the rate of major bleeding, including an increased risk of ICH in patients over the age of 75 years (2.1% vs. 1.1%; $p=0.069$). Furthermore, the ASSENT-3 (Assessment of the Safety and Efficacy of a New Thrombolytic Regimen – 3) trial evaluated abciximab and half-dose tenecteplase as compared with standard dose thrombolytics. The findings were consistent with GUSTO-V as this trial showed reduced MI, but doubled bleeding, and had no effect on mortality (64).

Based on the available data, ACC/AHA practice guidelines provide a Class IIb (usefulness/efficacy less well established) recommendation for the consideration of combination pharmacological reperfusion with abciximab and half-dose reteplase or tenecteplase for prevention of reinfarction and other complications of STEMI in selected patients (anterior location of MI, age less than 75 years, and no risk factors for bleeding) (7). Specific mention is given to the lack of a mortality benefit at both 30 days and 1 year with this treatment strategy. A Class III (evidence that treatment is not effective or harmful) recommendation is given to the combination of abciximab and half-dose reteplase or tenecteplase in patients aged greater than 75 years, due to the increased risk of ICH (7).

Mechanical Reperfusion

In the management of STEMI, the role of GP IIb/IIIa receptor inhibitors in primary PCI was evaluated in the ADMIRAL (Abciximab Before Direct Angioplasty and Stenting in Myocardial Infarction Regarding Acute and Long Term Follow-up) trial (65). Of the 300 patients, those randomized to abciximab and PCI as compared with PCI alone had a significant 59% reduction in the rate of death, recurrent MI, or urgent target vessel revascularization at 30 days (6.0% vs. 14.6%; $p=0.01$). At 6 months, the corresponding figures were 7.4% and 15.9% ($p=0.02$; Fig. 6). The better clinical outcomes in the abciximab group were related to the greater frequency of a TIMI flow grade of 3 before the procedure (16.8% vs. 5.4%, $p=0.01$), immediately afterward (95.1% vs. 86.7%, $p=0.04$), and 6 months afterward (94.3% vs. 82.8%, $p=0.04$). One major bleeding event occurred in the abciximab group and none occurred in the placebo group. A significant mortality benefit in the ADMIRAL trial persisted at 3-year follow-up (66).

The beneficial results of the ADMIRAL trial were not replicated in the larger CADILLAC (Controlled Abciximab Device Investigation to Lower Late Angioplasty Complications) trial, as abciximab did not produce a significant additive benefit to primary stenting (67). However, in a meta-analysis, in which 11 trials involving 27,115 patients were analyzed, a significant benefit with the use of adjunctive abciximab therapy during primary PCI for STEMI was demonstrated, and this was not seen when abciximab was used as an adjunct to fibrinolysis (68). When compared with the control

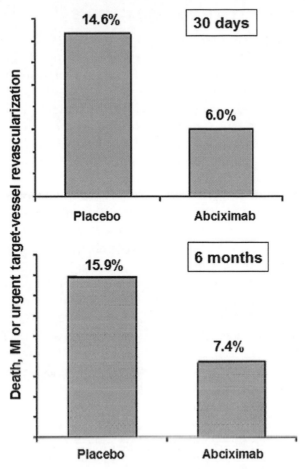

Fig. 6. Incidence of death, reinfarction, and urgent target-vessel revascularization at 30 days and at 6 months after randomization to abciximab or placebo in patients with acute MI undergoing primary PCI in the ADMIRAL trial.

group, abciximab was associated with a significant reduction in short-term (30 days) mortality (2.4% vs. 3.4%, $p=0.047$) and long-term (6–12 months) mortality (4.4% vs. 6.2%; $p=0.01$) in patients undergoing primary angioplasty but not in those treated with fibrinolysis.

ACC/AHA guidelines state that it is reasonable to start treatment with abciximab as early as possible before primary PCI (with or without stenting) in patients with STEMI (Class IIa, weight of evidence is in favor of efficacy) (7). The data on eptifibatide and tirofiban are more limited than for abciximab, but given the common mode of action and general clinical experience these agents are given a Class IIb indication to support primary PCI in STEMI (7).

The timing of adjunctive GP IIb/IIIa receptor inhibitor administration relative to PCI has been an area of recent investigation. In the RELAx-AMI (Randomized Early versus Late Abciximab in Acute Myocardial Infarction treated with primary coronary intervention) trial early abciximab administration improved pre-PCI angiographic findings, post-PCI tissue perfusion, and 1-month left ventricular function recovery (69). Furthermore, in the TITAN (Time to Integrilin Therapy in Acute Myocardial Infarction) – TIMI 34 trial, initiation of eptifibatide in the emergency department was shown to improve myocardial perfusion without a significant increase in major bleeding (70).

However, neither facilitation of PCI with reteplase plus abciximab nor facilitation with abciximab alone significantly improved clinical outcomes in the much larger FINESSE (Facilitated Intervention with Enhanced Reperfusion Speed to Stop Events) trial (71,72).

FUTURE DIRECTIONS

The issues of variability in response, irreversibility of inhibitor effects and length of time required for maximum platelet inhibition has fostered the search for newer antiplatelet agents. The third generation oral thienopyridine, prasugrel, was shown to be ten times more potent than clopidogrel in animal studies (73). The JUMBO-TIMI 26 (Joint Utilization of Medications to Block Platelets Optimally – TIMI 26) trial, was a phase 2, randomized, dose-ranging, double-blinded safety trial of prasugrel versus clopidogrel in 904 patients undergoing elective or urgent percutaneous coronary intervention (74). A loading dose followed by 1 month of maintenance therapy with prasugrel was just as safe as clopidogrel. Although not specifically designed to assess efficacy, prasugrel-treated patients had a non-significant decrease in the incidence of death, MI, stroke, or target vessel thrombosis at 30-day follow-up. The TRITON-TIMI 38 (Trial to Assess Improvement in Therapeutic Outcomes by Optimizing Platelet Inhibition with Prasugrel) trial was a phase III study evaluating prasugrel against clopidogrel in patients presenting with ACS with PCI as the planned management strategy (75). In this trial, prasugrel therapy was associated with significantly reduced rates of ischemic events, including stent thrombosis, but with an increased risk of major bleeding (76).

AZD6140 is an orally active, non-thienopyridine reversible inhibitor of the platelet $P2Y_{12}$ receptor. This agent is a cyclopentyl triazolopyrimidine that provides more rapid and complete antiplatelet effect than clopidogrel (77). The PLATO (Platelet Inhibition and Patient Outcomes) trial will compare the efficacy of AZD6140 and clopidogrel in patients with STEMI and NSTE ACS.

Cangrelor is an intravenous non-thienopyridine reversible inhibitor of the $P2Y_{12}$ receptor. The very short half-life of this agent makes it an attractive alternative and it has been shown to be safe and well tolerated in patients with acute coronary syndromes (78).

Other novel classes of agents being explored include protease-activated receptor antagonists and platelet adhesion antagonists (16).

Adjunctive antiplatelet therapy in pharmacologic or catheter-based reperfusion for STEMI has produced improved cardiovascular outcomes, including mortality benefits. The novel agents under investigation will likely better refine the role of antiplatelet therapy in this clinical setting and lead to further improvement in patient outcomes.

REFERENCES

1. Ruggeri ZM (2002) Platelets in atherothrombosis. Nat Med 8(11):1227–1234
2. Offermanns S (2006) Activation of platelet function through G protein-coupled receptors. Circ Res 99(12):1293–1304
3. Campbell CL, Smyth S, Montalescot G et al (2007) Aspirin dose for the prevention of cardiovascular disease: a systematic review. JAMA 297(18):2018–2024
4. ISIS-2 (second international study of infarct survival) Collaborative Group (1988) Randomised trial of intravenous streptokinase, oral aspirin, both, or neither among 17,187 cases of suspected acute myocardial infarction: ISIS-2. Lancet 2(8607):349–360
5. Roux S, Christeller S, Ludin E (1992) Effects of aspirin on coronary reocclusion and recurrent ischemia after thrombolysis: a meta-analysis. J Am Coll Cardiol 19(3):671–677
6. Baigent C, Collins R, Appleby P et al (1998) ISIS-2: 10 year survival among patients with suspected acute myocardial infarction in randomised comparison of intravenous streptokinase, oral aspirin, both, or neither. The ISIS-2 (Second International Study of Infarct Survival) Collaborative Group. BMJ 316(7141):1337–1343
7. Antman EM, Anbe DT, Armstrong PW et al (2004) ACC/AHA guidelines for the management of patients with ST-elevation myocardial infarction: a report of the American College of Cardiology/American Heart Association Task Force on Practice Guidelines (Committee to Revise the 1999 Guidelines for the Management of Patients with Acute Myocardial Infarction). Circulation 110(9):e82–e292
8. Antithrombotic Trialists' Collaboration (2002) Collaborative meta-analysis of randomised trials of antiplatelet therapy for prevention of death, myocardial infarction, and stroke in high risk patients. BMJ 324(7329):71–86

9. Sagar KA, Smyth MR (1999) A comparative bioavailability study of different aspirin formulations using on-line multidimensional chromatography. J Pharm Biomed Anal 21(2):383–392

10. Maree AO, Fitzgerald DJ (2007) Variable platelet response to aspirin and clopidogrel in atherothrombotic disease. Circulation 115(16):2196–2207

11. Chen WH, Cheng X, Lee PY et al (2007) Aspirin resistance and adverse clinical events in patients with coronary artery disease. Am J Med 120(7):631–635

12. Eikelboom JW, Hirsh J, Weitz JI et al (2002) Aspirin-resistant thromboxane biosynthesis and the risk of myocardial infarction, stroke or cardiovascular death in patients at high risk for cardiovascular events. Circulation 105(14):1650–1655

13. Barnes GD, Li J, Kline-Rogers E et al (2007) Dual antiplatelet agent failure: a new syndrome or clinical nonentity? Am Heart J 154(4):732–735

14. Cattaneo M (2007) Resistance to antiplatelet drugs: molecular mechanisms and laboratory detection. J Thromb Haemost 5(Suppl 1):230–237

15. Quinn MJ, Fitzgerald DJ (1999) Ticlopidine and clopidogrel. Circulation 100(15):1667–1672

16. Meadows TA, Bhatt DL (2007) Clinical aspects of platelet inhibitors and thrombus formation. Circ Res 100(9):1261–1275

17. Leon MB, Baim DS, Popma JJ et al (1998) A clinical trial comparing three antithrombotic-drug regimens after coronary-artery stenting. Stent Anticoagulation Restenosis Study Investigators. N Engl J Med 339(23):1665–1671.

18. Yusuf S, Zhao F, Mehta SR et al (2001) Effects of clopidogrel in addition to aspirin in patients with acute coronary syndromes without ST-segment elevation. N Engl J Med 345(7):494–502

19. Sabatine MS, Cannon CP, Gibson CM et al (2005) Addition of clopidogrel to aspirin and fibrinolytic therapy for myocardial infarction with ST-segment elevation. N Engl J Med 352(12):1179–1189

20. McLean DS, Sabatine MS, Guo W et al (2007) Benefits and risks of clopidogrel pretreatment before coronary artery bypass grafting in patients with ST-elevation myocardial infarction treated with fibrinolytics in CLARITY-TIMI 28. J Thromb Thrombolysis 24(2):85–91

21. Scirica BM, Sabatine MS, Morrow DA et al (2006) The role of clopidogrel in early and sustained arterial patency after fibrinolysis for ST-segment elevation myocardial infarction: the ECG CLARITY-TIMI 28 Study. J Am Coll Cardiol 48(1):37–42

22. Chen ZM, Jiang LX, Chen YP et al (2005) Addition of clopidogrel to aspirin in 45, 852 patients with acute myocardial infarction: randomised placebo-controlled trial. Lancet 366(9497):1607–1621

23. Bhatt DL, Flather MD, Hacke W et al (2007) Patients with prior myocardial infarction, stroke, or symptomatic peripheral arterial disease in the CHARISMA trial. J Am Coll Cardiol 49(19):1982–1988

24. Antman EM, Hand M, Armstrong PW et al (2008) 2007 Focused update of the ACC/AHA 2004 guidelines for the management of patients with ST-elevation myocardial infarction: a report of the American College of Cardiology/American Heart Association Task Force on Practice Guidelines. Circulation 117:296–329

25. Schomig A, Neumann FJ, Kastrati A et al (1996) A randomized comparison of antiplatelet and anticoagulant therapy after the placement of coronary-artery stents. N Engl J Med 334(17):1084–1089

26. Berger PB, Bell MR, Grill DE et al (1998) Frequency of adverse clinical events in the 12 months following successful intracoronary stent placement in patients treated with aspirin and ticlopidine (without warfarin). Am J Cardiol 81(6):713–718

27. Bertrand ME, Rupprecht HJ, Urban P et al (2000) Double-blind study of the safety of clopidogrel with and without a loading dose in combination with aspirin compared with ticlopidine in combination with aspirin after coronary stenting: the clopidogrel aspirin stent international cooperative study (CLASSICS). Circulation 102(6):624–629

28. Bhatt DL, Bertrand ME, Berger PB et al (2002) Meta-analysis of randomized and registry comparisons of ticlopidine with clopidogrel after stenting. J Am Coll Cardiol 39(1):9–14

29. Montalescot G, Sideris G, Meuleman C et al (2006) A randomized comparison of high clopidogrel loading doses in patients with non-ST-segment elevation acute coronary syndromes: the ALBION (Assessment of the Best Loading Dose of Clopidogrel to Blunt Platelet Activation, Inflammation and Ongoing Necrosis) trial. J Am Coll Cardiol 48(5):931–938

30. Sabatine MS, Cannon CP, Gibson CM et al (2005) Effect of clopidogrel pretreatment before percutaneous coronary intervention in patients with ST-elevation myocardial infarction treated with fibrinolytics: the PCI-CLARITY study. JAMA 294(10):1224–1232

31. Sabatine MS (2006) Benefit of clopidogrel pretreatment before PCI regardless of GP IIb/IIIa inhibitor use. Eur Heart J 27(Abstract Suppl):862

32. Mehta SR, Yusuf S, Peters RJ et al (2001) Effects of pretreatment with clopidogrel and aspirin followed by long-term therapy in patients undergoing percutaneous coronary intervention: the PCI-CURE study. Lancet 358(9281):527–533

33. Fox KA, Mehta SR, Peters R et al (2004) Benefits and risks of the combination of clopidogrel and aspirin in patients undergoing surgical revascularization for non-ST-elevation acute coronary syndrome: the clopidogrel in unstable angina to prevent recurrent ischemic events. Circulation 110(10):1202–1208

34. Muller I, Seyfarth M, Rudiger S et al (2001) Effect of a high loading dose of clopidogrel on platelet function in patients undergoing coronary stent placement. Heart 85(1):92–93

35. von Beckerath N, Taubert D, Pogatsa-Murray G et al (2005) Absorption, metabolization, and antiplatelet effects of 300-, 600-, and 900-mg loading doses of clopidogrel: results of the ISAR-CHOICE (Intracoronary Stenting and Antithrombotic Regimen: Choose Between 3 High Oral Doses for Immediate Clopidogrel Effect) Trial. Circulation 112(19):2946–2950

36. Gurbel PA, Bliden KP, Zaman KA (2005) Clopidogrel loading with eptifibatide to arrest the reactivity of platelets: results of the clopidogrel loading with eptifibatide to arrest the reactivity of platelets (CLEAR PLATELETS) study. Circulation 111(9):1153–1159

37. Patti G, Colonna G, Pasceri V et al (2005) Randomized trial of high loading dose of clopidogrel for reduction of periprocedural myocardial infarction in patients undergoing coronary intervention: results from the ARMYDA-2 (antiplatelet therapy for reduction of myocardial damage during angioplasty) study. Circulation 111(16):2099–2106

38. Cuisset T, Frere C, Quilici J et al (2006) Benefit of a 600-mg loading dose of clopidogrel on platelet reactivity and clinical outcomes in patients with non-ST-segment elevation acute coronary syndrome undergoing coronary stenting. J Am Coll Cardiol 48(7):1339–1345

39. von Beckerath N, Kastrati A, Wieczorek A et al (2007) A double-blind, randomized study on platelet aggregation in patients treated with a daily dose of 150 or 75 mg of clopidogrel for 30 days. Eur Heart J 28(15):1814–1819

40. Smith SC Jr, Feldman TE, Hirshfeld JW Jr et al (2006) ACC/AHA/SCAI 2005 guideline update for percutaneous coronary intervention-summary article: a report of the American College of Cardiology/American Heart Association Task Force on Practice Guidelines (ACC/AHA/SCAI Writing Committee to update the 2001 guidelines for percutaneous coronary intervention). J Am Coll Cardiol 47(1):216–235

41. Silber S, Albertsson P, Aviles FF et al (2005) Guidelines for percutaneous coronary interventions. The Task Force for Percutaneous Coronary Interventions of the European Society of Cardiology. Eur Heart J 26(8):804–847

42. Steinhubl SR, Berger PB, Mann JT III (2002) Early and sustained dual oral antiplatelet therapy following percutaneous coronary intervention: a randomized controlled trial. JAMA 288(19):2411–2420

43. Joner M, Finn AV, Farb A et al (2006) Pathology of drug-eluting stents in humans: delayed healing and late thrombotic risk. J Am Coll Cardiol 48(1):193–202

44. Pfisterer M, Brunner-La Rocca HP, Buser PT et al (2006) Late clinical events after clopidogrel discontinuation may limit the benefit of drug-eluting stents: an observational study of drug-eluting versus bare-metal stents. J Am Coll Cardiol 48(12):2584–2591

45. Eisenstein EL, Anstrom KJ, Kong DF et al (2007) Clopidogrel use and long-term clinical outcomes after drug-eluting stent implantation. JAMA 297(2):159–168

46. Grines CL, Bonow RO, Casey DE Jr et al (2007) Prevention of premature discontinuation of dual antiplatelet therapy in patients with coronary artery stents: a science advisory from the American Heart Association, American College of Cardiology, Society for Cardiovascular Angiography and Interventions, American College of Surgeons, and American Dental Association, with representation from the American College of Physicians. J Am Coll Cardiol 49(6):734–739

47. Wiviott SD (2006) Clopidogrel response variability, resistance, or both? Am J Cardiol 98(10A):18N–24N

48. Cattaneo M, Zighetti ML, Lombardi R et al (2003) Molecular bases of defective signal transduction in the platelet P2Y12 receptor of a patient with congenital bleeding. Proc Natl Acad Sci USA 100(4):1978–1983

49. Hollopeter G, Jantzen HM, Vincent D et al (2001) Identification of the platelet ADP receptor targeted by antithrombotic drugs. Nature 409(6817):202–207

50. Clarke TA, Waskell LA (2003) The metabolism of clopidogrel is catalyzed by human cytochrome P450 3A and is inhibited by atorvastatin. Drug Metab Dispos 31(1):53–59

51. Saw J, Brennan DM, Steinhubl SR et al (2007) Lack of evidence of a clopidogrel-statin interaction in the CHARISMA trial. J Am Coll Cardiol 50(4):291–295

52. Gurbel PA, Bliden KP, Hiatt BL et al (2003) Clopidogrel for coronary stenting: response variability, drug resistance, and the effect of pretreatment platelet reactivity. Circulation 107(23):2908–2913

53. Serebruany VL Steinhubl SR, Berger PB et al (2005) Variability in platelet responsiveness to clopidogrel among 544 individuals. J Am Coll Cardiol 45(2):246–251

54. Matetzky S, Shenkman B, Guetta V et al (2004) Clopidogrel resistance is associated with increased risk of recurrent atherothrombotic events in patients with acute myocardial infarction. Circulation 109(25):3171–3175

55. Gurbel PA, Bliden KP, Samara W et al (2005) Clopidogrel effect on platelet reactivity in patients with stent thrombosis: results of the CREST Study. J Am Coll Cardiol 46(10):1827–1832

56. Aleil B, Rochoux G, Monassier JP et al (2007) Ticlopidine could be an alternative therapy in the case of pharmacological resistance to clopidogrel: a report of three cases. J Thromb Haemost 5(4):879–881

57. Coller BS, Anderson KM, Weisman HF (1996) The anti-GPIIb-IIIa agents: fundamental and clinical aspects. Haemostasis 26(Suppl 4):285–293

58. Coller BS (2001) Anti-GPIIb/IIIa drugs: current strategies and future directions. Thromb Haemost 86(1):427–443

59. Antman EM, Giugliano RP, Gibson CM et al (1999) Abciximab facilitates the rate and extent of thrombolysis: results of the thrombolysis in myocardial infarction (TIMI) 14 trial. The TIMI 14 Investigators. Circulation 99(21):2720–2732

60. Giugliano RP, Roe MT, Harrington RA et al (2003) Combination reperfusion therapy with eptifibatide and reduced-dose tenecteplase for ST-elevation myocardial infarction: results of the integrilin and tenecteplase in acute myocardial infarction (INTEGRITI) phase II angiographic trial. J Am Coll Cardiol 41(8):1251–1260

61. Strategies for Patency Enhancement in the Emergency Department (SPEED) Group (2000) Trial of abciximab with and without low-dose reteplase for acute myocardial infarction. Circulation 101(24):2788–2794

62. Brener SJ, Zeymer U, Adgey AA et al (2002) Eptifibatide and low-dose tissue plasminogen activator in acute myocardial infarction: the integrilin and low-dose thrombolysis in acute myocardial infarction (INTRO AMI) trial. J Am Coll Cardiol 39(3):377–386

63. Topol EJ (2001) Reperfusion therapy for acute myocardial infarction with fibrinolytic therapy or combination reduced fibrinolytic therapy and platelet glycoprotein IIb/IIIa inhibition: the GUSTO V randomised trial. Lancet 357(9272):1905–1914

64. Assessment of the Safety and Efficacy of a New Thrombolytic Regimen (ASSENT)-3 Investigators (2001) Efficacy and safety of tenecteplase in combination with enoxaparin, abciximab, or unfractionated heparin: the ASSENT-3 randomised trial in acute myocardial infarction. Lancet 358(9282):605–613

65. Montalescot G, Barragan P, Wittenberg O et al (2001) Platelet glycoprotein IIb/IIIa inhibition with coronary stenting for acute myocardial infarction. N Engl J Med 344(25):1895–1903

66. Admiral Investigators (2005) Three-year duration of benefit from abciximab in patients receiving stents for acute myocardial infarction in the randomized double-blind ADMIRAL study. Eur Heart J 26(23):2520–2523

67. Stone GW, Grines CL, Cox DA et al (2002) Comparison of angioplasty with stenting, with or without abciximab, in acute myocardial infarction. N Engl J Med 346(13):957–966

68. De Luca G, Suryapranata H, Stone GW et al (2005) Abciximab as adjunctive therapy to reperfusion in acute ST segment elevation myocardial infarction: a meta-analysis of randomized trials. JAMA 293(14):1759–1765

69. Maioli M, Bellandi F, Leoncini M et al (2007) Randomized early versus late abciximab in acute myocardial infarction treated with primary coronary intervention (RELAx-AMI Trial). J Am Coll Cardiol 49(14):1517–1524

70. Gibson CM, Kirtane AJ, Murphy SA et al (2006) Early initiation of eptifibatide in the emergency department before primary percutaneous coronary intervention for ST-segment elevation myocardial infarction: results of the Time to Integrilin Therapy in Acute Myocardial Infarction (TITAN)-TIMI 34 trial. Am Heart J 152(4):668–675

71. Ellis SG, Armstrong P, Betriu A et al (2004) Facilitated percutaneous coronary intervention versus primary percutaneous coronary intervention: design and rationale of the Facilitated Intervention with Enhanced Reperfusion Speed to Stop Events (FINESSE) trial. Am Heart J 147(4):E16

72. Ellis SG, Tendera M, de Belder MA et al (2008) Facilitated PCI in patients with ST-elevation myocardial infarction. N Engl J Med 358(21):2205–2217

73. Niitsu Y, Jakubowski JA, Sugidachi A et al (2005) Pharmacology of CS-747 (prasugrel, LY640315), a novel, potent antiplatelet agent with in vivo P2Y12 receptor antagonist activity. Semin Thromb Hemost 31(2):184–194

74. Wiviott SD, Antman EM, Winters KJ et al (2005) Randomized comparison of prasugrel (CS-747, LY640315), a novel thienopyridine P2Y12 antagonist, with clopidogrel in percutaneous coronary intervention: results of the Joint Utilization of Medications to Block Platelets Optimally (JUMBO)-TIMI 26 trial. Circulation 111(25):3366–3373

75. Wiviott SD, Antman EM, Gibson CM et al (2006) Evaluation of prasugrel compared with clopidogrel in patients with acute coronary syndromes: design and rationale for the trial to assess improvement in therapeutic outcomes by optimizing platelet inhibition with prasugrel thrombolysis in myocardial infarction 38 (TRITON-TIMI 38). Am Heart J 152(4):627–635

76. Wiviott SD, Braunwald E, McCabe CH et al (2007) Prasugrel versus clopidogrel in patients with acute coronary syndromes. N Engl J Med 357(20):2001–2015

77. Husted S, Emanuelsson H, Heptinstall S et al (2006) Pharmacodynamics, pharmacokinetics, and safety of the oral reversible P2Y12 antagonist AZD6140 with aspirin in patients with atherosclerosis: a double-blind comparison to clopidogrel with aspirin. Eur Heart J 27(9):1038–1047

78. Storey RF, Oldroyd KG, Wilcox RG (2001) Open multicentre study of the P2T receptor antagonist AR-C69931MX assessing safety, tolerability and activity in patients with acute coronary syndromes. Thromb Haemost 85(3):401–407

12

Antithrombin Therapy for Acute ST-Segment Elevation Myocardial Infarction

John M. Galla and Arman T. Askari

CONTENTS

ABSTRACT Thrombus formation at the site of plaque rupture has long been recognized as the inciting event in the pathophysiology of ST-segment elevation myocardial infarction (STEMI). Fibrinolysis remains the most common mode of revascularization worldwide and has the recognized limitation of creating large amounts of activated thrombin as a byproduct of its mechanism of action. Several antithrombin agents have been developed as adjuncts to either pharmacologic or mechanical revascularization strategies for this patient population. Unfractionated heparin remains a very important agent although low-molecular weight heparins and direct thrombin inhibitors have been developed and studied in these patients. How each class of antithrombin therapies will be optimally utilized for patients with STEMI remains to be defined. At the core of any antithrombin therapy rests the goals of minimizing ischemic complications while simultaneously avoiding any bleeding complications.

Key words: Acute myocardial infarction; Direct thrombin inhibitor; Fibrinolysis; Low molecular weight heparin; Percutaneous coronary intervention; Revascularization; ST-segment elevation myocardial infarction; Unfractionated heparin

INTRODUCTION

Acute ST-segment elevation myocardial infarction (STEMI) is associated with substantial morbidity and mortality. Estimated to account for almost 8 million annual deaths worldwide, considerable research has been conducted to refine both mechanical and pharmacologic reperfusion strategies in order to improve outcomes in patients with STEMI *(1)*. While primary percutaneous coronary intervention (PCI) has been shown superior to fibrinolysis in STEMI *(2)*, fibrinolysis remains the primary

From: *Contemporary Cardiology: Antithrombotic Drug Therapy in Cardiovascular Disease*
Edited by: A.T. Askari and A.M. Lincoff (eds.), DOI 10.1007/978-1-60327-235-3_12
© Humana Press, a part of Springer Science+Business Media, LLC 2010

reperfusion approach worldwide due to lack of timely access to primary PCI. Nevertheless, the benefits of antithrombin therapy in the management of patients with STEMI have been demonstrated when used as an adjunct to both pharmacologic and mechanical reperfusion with the primary purpose of preventing thromboembolic complications (i.e. left ventricular thrombus formation) and maintaining patency of the infarct-related artery (IRA).

HEPARINS

Unfractionated heparin is a heterogenous mixture of polysulfated glycosaminoglycans that exert its antithrombotic effect through catalysis of antithrombin III mediated inhibition of factor Xa and thrombin *(3)*. Unfractionated heparin (UFH) was the first antithrombin therapy tested for the management of patients with STEMI. While there are data suggesting a potential benefit as a stand-alone therapy in the management of these patients, this is not reflective of current practice standards of prompt and complete restoration of IRA patency.

The initial experience with both subcutaneous and intravenous UFH revealed an improvement in infarct-related artery patency and prevention of left ventricular thrombus formation when used as an adjunct to nonspecific fibrinolytic agents *(4,5)*.

The importance of adjunctive antithrombin therapy as well as the route of administration was more clearly demonstrated in a randomized trial comparing nonspecific to fibrin-specific fibrinolytics. The Global Use of Streptokinase and Tissue Plasminogen Activator for Occluded Coronary Arteries (GUSTO)-1 trial enrolled over 41,000 patients and compared streptokinase to accelerated t-PA and included subcutaneous and intravenous UFH arms in the SK treatment group *(6)*. When tested in this head-to-head fashion, IV UFH was not superior to subcutaneous UFH as an adjunct to streptokinase *(7)*.

Early studies that specifically evaluated strategies of antithrombin therapy with heparin in patients undergoing fibrinolysis were individually underpowered to detect differences in their primary outcomes and even in aggregate include less than 2000 patients *(8–12)*. Not surprisingly, UFH failed to significantly reduce the risk of death or recurrent myocardial infarction and was associated with increased bleeding events. Despite these limited data, adjunctive UFH became the standard antithrombin therapy for fibrinolysis, especially when using a fibrin-specific agent such as t-PA *(13–16)*.

Throughout the comparisons of UFH to both placebo and low-molecular-weight heparin, investigators have evaluated differing strategies in the route of administration, timing and dosage in an attempt to reduce recurrent ischemic events and simultaneously minimize bleeding complications. While differing strategies of UFH have not been compared in a head-to-head fashion, current recommendations have arisen through the formation of expert consensus from clinical investigations. Subcutaneous heparin, which was evaluated primarily in three large trials, failed to provide sufficient reduction in ischemic events to continue as a viable strategy *(4,5,17)*. Concerns over the timing of the initiation of antithrombin therapy arose with the recognition of the prothrombotic state following fibrinolysis. While there is ample support for fibrinolysis in the setting of established antithrombotic milieu, a reduction of recurrent ischemic events with the concurrent administration of UFH has not definitively been established *(6)*. Regardless of these results, simultaneous administration of UFH with fibrinolytics has become standard practice. Monitoring the therapeutic effect of UFH dosing through the calculation of activated partial thromboplastin time (aPTT) has been prescribed throughout evaluations of UFH as an adjunct to fibrinolysis. Therapeutic aPTT limits have varied from trial to trial, observations that patients with shorter times were less likely to demonstrate benefit *(12)* while those with higher times were more likely to suffer a morbid bleeding or mortal event *(18)*. Current guideline recommendations incorporate these lessons within the recommendation that patients receive weight-based UFH with an IV bolus followed by continuous infusion to achieve an aPTT that is 1.5 to 2.0 times the control value *(19)*.

Low-Molecular-Weight Heparin

Low-molecular weight heparins (LMWH) are derived through the chemical or enzymatic fragmentation of UFH with resultant varying chain lengths and anticoagulant properties. Compared to UFH, LMWH have a more predictable response, longer half-life, better bioavailability and dose-independent clearance *(20)*. (Table 1). These benefits, in addition to obviating the need for laboratory monitoring, led to investigations of LMWH for patients presenting with STEMI in the setting of both fibrinolysis and percutaneous intervention.

When compared to placebo in patients receiving fibrinolysis, LMWH has been shown to be superior in reducing in-hospital and 30-day death and reinfarction. Two small trials conducted shortly after the commercial introduction of LMWH evaluated the benefit of dalteparin in patients receiving streptokinase for AMI. After treatment for an average of 9 days, delayed subcutaneous LMWH was associated with a 37% decrease in the incidence of left ventricular thrombus formation at the expense of increased rates of hemorrhage *(21)*. Subsequently, short-term benefits of upstream LMWH administration were assessed utilizing a reduced LMWH dose aimed at minimizing bleeding *(22)*. After two doses of dalteparin, rates of TIMI-3 flow within the infarct related artery (IRA) were not significantly different 24 hours after fibrinolysis but trended toward benefit in the LMWH group without a significant difference in bleeding outcomes compared to placebo.

Short-term IRA patency has been evaluated following early administration of intravenous enoxaparin with a short-term course of subcutaneous therapy in patients receiving fibrinolysis for STEMI *(23)*. After a median treatment duration of five days with enoxaparin or placebo, significant improvements were seen in favor of LMWH for TIMI-3 flow at 8-day follow-up catheterization and in the clinical composite of death, myocardial infarction or recurrent angina. The composite was primarily driven by a 3-fold reduction in recurrent myocardial infarction.

The Clinical Trial of Reviparin and Metabolic Modulation in Acute Myocardial Infarction Treatment Evaluation (CREATE) trial was planned as the definitive evaluation of short-term LMWH for patients presenting with STEMI. In this trial of over 15,000 patients LMWH was compared to placebo with the reperfusion strategy left to the discretion of the enrolling physician (approximately 75% fibrinolysis; less than 10% primary PCI). Following 7 days of treatment, patients randomized to LMWH showed a 13% relative reduction in death, recurrent MI or stroke with an absolute risk reduction of 1.4%, a benefit that was durable through the 30-day follow-up period. In addition to showing superiority in the combined endpoint, preplanned secondary analyses were able to demonstrate significant reductions in the individual components of death (NNT=67) and reinfarction (NNT=167).

Table 1
Properties of low-molecular-weight heparins

Name	Dosing	Anti-Xa-IIa ratio	$T_{1/2}$	Mean MW	FDA approved for STEMI?
Enoxaparin	30-mg IV bolus and 1 mg/kg SC dose q 12° dose adjusted if >75 y	3.8	4.5	4,200	Yes
Reviparin	<50 kg – 3436 IU SC q12°; <80 kg – 5153 IU SC q 12°; >80 kg – 6871 IU SC q12°	3.5	2.5–5.3	4,000	No
Dalteparin	30 IU/kg IV bolus then 90I U/kg SC then 120 IU/kg q 12°	2.7	2.3	6,000	No
Nadroparin	86 IU/kg IV then 86 IU/kg SC q 12°	3.6	2.5–5.5	4,500	No

Following the initial positive results of LMWH in patients receiving fibrinolysis for STEMI, multiple comparisons were made in trials of adjunctive unfractionated versus low-molecular-weight heparin. Many of these head-to-head comparisons also incorporated assessments of emerging therapies in the dynamic field of medical therapies for acute coronary syndromes. (Table 2)

The Assessment of the Safety and Efficacy of a New Thrombolytic Regimen (ASSENT)-3 trial compared the use of enoxaparin (until hospital discharge or 7 days) to UFH (48 h) in over 4,000 patients receiving weight-adjusted tenecteplase for STEMI *(24)*. A third arm of the trial received tenecteplase in addition to the glycoprotein IIb/IIIa inhibitor, abciximab. Enoxaparin was associated with a significant 26% reduction in the primary endpoint of 30-day mortality, in-hospital refractory ischemia or reinfarction (11.4% vs. 15.4%, $p=0.0001$). Of significant note, these improvements in adverse cardiac events came without significant increases in major bleeding or intracranial hemorrhage even with the longer duration of enoxaparin therapy.

Two smaller contemporary trials of ASSENT-3 compared alternate fibrinolytic strategies in the setting of either UFH or enoxaparin. The HART II study evaluated early angiographic outcomes in 400 patients receiving t-PA for STEMI *(25)*. Antithrombin therapy was continued for at least 3 days in both arms and patients underwent diagnostic angiography at both 90 minutes and 5-7 days following administration of fibrinolysis. Designed to test noninferiority, enoxaparin met its prespecified criteria with 80.1% of patients with TIMI-2 or 3 flow compared to 75.1% receiving UFH. Safety and 30-day mortality were similar between both groups.

The safety and efficacy of adjunctive LMWH compared with UFH was also demonstrated in a "real-world" environment *(26)*. Three hundred patients received one of three fibrinolytics (streptokinase, anistreplase or recombinant t-PA) at the discretion of the admitting physician and were then randomized to 4 days of either UFH of enoxaparin unadjusted for weight. At 90 days, enoxaparin-treated patients demonstrated significant reductions in death, recurrent myocardial infarction or readmission for unstable angina (26% vs. 36%, $p=0.04$). There was no observed difference in major bleeding between the UFH and LMWH groups.

In a comparison of both antithrombin strategies and adjunctive IIb/IIIa inhibitors, the ENTIRE-TIMI-23 trial compared LMWH to UFH in patients receiving either full-dose tenecteplase or half-dose tenecteplase with abciximab *(27)*. UFH dosing was reduced in the abciximab group and allowances were made for patients who underwent PCI. For the primary endpoint of TIMI-3 flow at 60 min following fibrinolysis, enoxaparin had similar efficacy to UFH. The enoxaparin group did show a robust decrease in 30-day ischemic endpoints primarily driven by reductions in nonfatal MI in patients receiving full-dose tenecteplase. As was seen in the previous trials, there were no important distinctions in safety observed between the UFH or LMWH groups.

In an attempt to improve the short-term outcomes of patients receiving fibrinolysis for STEMI, the ASSENT investigators sought to capitalize on the comparative ease of prolonged LMWH administration in ASSENT-Plus *(28)*. After receiving tenecteplase, 439 patients were randomized to receive either 48 hours of UFH or 4-7 days of dalteparin. The primary endpoint was the rate of TIMI 3 flow in the infarct related artery as assessed by in-hospital angiography. Dalteparin failed to produce any significant difference in TIMI 3 flow rates, but was associated with significantly less TIMI 0-1 flow and intraluminal thrombus.

Recognizing the benefits of reducing the time from symptom onset to fibrinolysis the ASSENT group conducted a larger trial of pre-hospital therapy in ASSENT-3 PLUS *(29)*. Enrolling over 1600 patients, they tested whether UFH or LMWH, in addition to tenecteplase administered by first-responders, would reduce 30-day adverse cardiac endpoints. The modest benefits seen in the patients in the enoxaparin failed to achieve significance (14.2% vs. 17.4%, $p=0.08$) and were associated with higher rates of stroke (2.9% vs. 1.3%, $p=0.026$) and intracranial hemorrhage (ICH) (2.2% vs. 0.97%,

Table 2
Trials of LMWH in STEMI

Trial	n	LMWH	Control	Primary outcome active vs. control	Fibrinolytic agent	Result
FRAMI, 1997	776	Dalteparin 150 IU/kg BID×8–11 days	Placebo	14.2% vs. 21.9% LV thrombus or arterial embolism	SK	37% Decrease in LV thrombus but increased bleeding
BIOMACS II, 1999	101	Dalteparin 100 then 120 IU/kg	Placebo	68% vs. 51% TIMI-3 flow	SK	Trend toward improved TIMI flow, bleeding similar to placebo
ASSENT-3, 2001	4,078	Enoxaparin 1 mg/kg BID, ≤7 days	UFH 60/12 for 48°	11.4% vs. 15.4% Death, MI or refractory ischemia	TNK	26% Reduction in 30-day MACE, no significant increase in bleeding
HART II, 2001	400	Enoxaparin 1 mg/kg BID, ≥3 days	UFH 4-5k/12 ≥3 days	80.1% vs. 75.1% TIMI-2 or 3 flow	t-PA	Enoxaparin noninferior to UFH in early angiographic outcomes
Baird, 2002	300	Enoxaparin 40-mg TID	UFH 5k/30k ≥4 days	36% vs. 26% Death, MI or unstable angina	SK, APSAC, t-PA	Significant reduction in 90-day MACE, no increase in bleeding
AMI-SK, 2002	496	Enoxaparin 30 mg	Placebo	70% vs. 58% TIMI-3 flow	SK	Improved TIMI-3 flow at 8 days and 90-day MACE
ENTIRE-TIMI-23, 2003	242	Enoxaparin 1 mg/kg BID, ≥8 days	UFH 50/12 ≥4 days	51% vs. 50% TIMI-3 flow	TNK±GP IIb/IIIa	Reduced 30-day ischemic endpoints, no significant safety issues
ASSENT Plus, 2003	439	Dalteparin 90 then 120 IU/kg BID, 4–7 days	UFH 4-5k/800–1,000 IU/h, 48°	69.3% vs. 62.5% TIMI-3 Flow	t-PA	No difference in in-hospital TIMI-3 flow
ASSENT-3 Plus, 2003	1,639	Enoxaparin 1 mg/kg BID ≤7 days	UFH 60/12 ≥3 days	14.2% vs. 17.4% Death, MI or refractory ischemia	TNK	Increased rates of stroke and ICH, especially ≥75 years
CREATE, 2005	15,570	Reviparin BID, ≥7 days	Placebo	9.6% vs. 11.0% Death, MI or stroke	SK, UK	13% Reduction in 7 and 30-day MACE
CLARITY-TIMI-28, 2005	3,491	Various	UFH 60/12 for ≤8°	13.5% vs. 22.5% Closed infarct artery, death or MI	Various	Significant reductions in in-hospital and 30-day death/MI
ExTRACT-TIMI-25, 2006	20,506	Enoxaparin weight and age-adjusted ≤8 days	UFH 60i 12 ≥48°	9.9% vs. 12.0% Death or MI	Numerous	17% Reduction in 30-day death/MI, but increased major bleeding

SK streptokinase, LV left Ventricle, UFH unfractionated heparin, TNK tenecteplase, APSAC anisoylated, t-PA tissue plasminogen activator, UK urokinase, MACE major adverse cardiac events, GP IIb/IIIa glycoprotein IIb/IIIa inhibitor, UFH dosing listed as bolus/drip in IU/kg

$p = 0.047$). The increase in ICH seen with enoxaparin was particularly evident in patients older than 75 years, with rates more than 5 times that of younger patients.

Synthesizing the lessons learned from these comparisons of LMWH to UFH, the TIMI trialists conducted the definitive trial on this issue, ExTRACT-TIMI-25 *(30)*. Enrolling over 20,000 patients, they compared a strategy of 48 hours of UFH to enoxaparin for the duration of hospitalization or a maximum of 7 days. Dosing adjustments were made for patients over 75 years or with significant renal impairment. Choice of fibrinolytic was left to the discretion of the treating physician. For the primary endpoint of death or recurrent MI at 30 days, enoxaparin was associated with a very significant, clinically relevant 17% reduction (9.9% vs. 12.0%, $p < 0.001$). Enoxaparin was associated with an increase in major bleeding events (2.1% vs. 1.4%, $p < 0.001$), but as a measure of net clinical benefit, it remained superior to UFH in the endpoint of 30-day death, MI or nonfatal ICH (10.1% vs. 12.2%, $p < 0.001$).

Concurrent to TIMI-25 was a large Chinese trial of patients with STEMI that convincingly demonstrated the benefit of clopidogrel therapy, thus an additional investigation was begun to validate both the safety and efficacy of LMWH as part of a more contemporary anti-thrombotic regimen. The CLARITY-TIMI-28 trial included 2,860 patients undergoing fibrinolysis who at the discretion of their treating physician received LMWH or UFH in addition to clopidogrel or placebo. Heparin therapy was administered for 48 hours after which patients underwent coronary angiography to assess the primary outcome of an occluded IRA or pre-angiography death or recurrent MI. Treatment with LMWH was associated with a 24% reduction in primary endpoint (13.5% vs. 22.5, $p = 0.027$) and 32% reduction in 30-day rates of death or recurrent MI (6.9% vs. 11.5%, $p = 0.030$) without any signal for safety concern. Patients randomized to both LMWH and clopidogrel had excellent clinical outcomes with a primary endpoint composite of 15.3% with a similar rate of major bleeding.

While patients presenting within 12 hours of symptom onset are eligible for reperfusion therapy, a significant number present late and are thus left to medical therapy at the discretion of the treating physician. It is in this setting that enoxaparin was compared to UFH in over 1,200 patients ineligible for reperfusion. The Treatment with Enoxaparin and Tirofiban in Acute Myocardial Infarction (TETAMI) trial was a two-by-two randomization to either enoxaparin or UFH and the IIb/IIIa inhibitor, tirofiban or placebo *(31)*. There was no observed benefit of enoxaparin over UFH. In addition, adjunctive IIb/IIIa inhibition with tirofiban was not effective in improving the primary combined endpoint of 30-day death, reinfarction or recurrent angina. Enoxaparin did exhibit similar safety to UFH suggesting it as a viable strategy in these patients.

These trials of LMWH compared to placebo and UFH have been reported in aggregate *(32)*. Compared to placebo, LMWH has been demonstrated to produce significant reductions in both in-hospital and 30-day reinfarction and death ranging from 10 to 28%. When tested against UFH, LMWH was shown to reduce in-hospital (43%) and 30-day reinfarction (35%). These benefits did come with some important safety concerns. In the placebo-controlled trials, LMWH was associated with significant increases in in-hospital ICH (0.3% vs. 0.1%), major (1.1% vs. 0.4%) and minor bleeding (15.1% vs. 5.2%). When compared to UFH, only in-hospital minor bleeding (22.8% vs. 19.4%) remained significantly increased for patients receiving LMWH

FONDAPARINUX

Fondaparinux is a synthetic pentasaccharide with daily subcutaneous dosing that selectively increases the antithrombin-mediated inactivation of factor Xa and as such shares many beneficial aspects of LMWH over UFH in patients with ACS. In an initial dose-finding trial, 333 patients undergoing fibrinolysis with alteplase for STEMI were randomized to fondaparinux or UFH *(33)*. Fondaparinux was found to be as safe as UFH with a trend toward improvement of clinical outcomes with observed reductions in reocclusions and need for revascularization through the 30-day follow-up period.

As part of a planned development effort to evaluate fondaparinux across the spectrum of ACS, a trial powered to compare clinical outcomes was conducted in the setting of STEMI. Enrolling over 12,000 patients, the Organization for the Assessment of Strategies for Ischemic Syndromes (OASIS)-6 trial compared an initial 2.5mg dose of fondaparinux administered intravenously followed by daily subcutaneous injections to UFH or placebo (34). Active therapy was continued for up to 8 days and compared to placebo or up to 48 hours of UFH depending on the treating physician's perceived need for adjunctive heparin therapy. Three-quarters of enrolled patients received reperfusion therapy with slightly less than 30% undergoing PCI. Powered to assess death and recurrent MI at 30 days, OASIS-6 demonstrated overall benefit in favor of fondaparinux with a 14% reduction in the primary endpoint (9.7% vs. 11.2%, $p=0.008$). Similar findings were observed for a preplanned analysis at 9 and 180 days. With regard to safety, fondaparinux was equivalent to control therapy with a prespecified subgroup analysis suggesting benefit over control in patients receiving fibrinolytics. There was significant heterogeneity for the treatment effect based on choice of initial reperfusion strategy. Fondaparinux was associated with lower rates of death or MI compared with control in medically treated or thrombolysed patients while there was no benefit observed in those who underwent primary PCI. In patients undergoing primary PCI fondaparinux was associated with a trend toward worse outcome including problems with catheter thrombosis. These concerns with fondaparinux bring into question its widespread acceptance in regions where primary PCI is the prevailing mode of reperfusion.

DIRECT THROMBIN INHIBITORS

Encompassing a class of medications that can inactivate thrombin without need for intermediary, the direct thrombin inhibitors (DTI) have received much interest in the treatment of STEMI and have been investigated as primary treatment in addition to adjuncts for both fibrinolysis and percutaneous intervention in this setting (Table 3). These compounds are predominantly polypeptides that achieve their activity by binding to catalytic sites on thrombin. During fibrinolysis, a large amount of thrombin bound to fibrin is created and since the catalytic center of thrombin is separate from its fibrin-binding domain, thrombin bound to fibrin remains enzymatically active (35). Thrombin bound to fibrin has been shown resistant to the effects of heparins and other agents that exert their antithrombotic effects through an antithrombin -mediated process (36). Thus, the ability of DTI to bind clot-bound thrombin generated during fibrinolysis provides a mechanistic benefit over heparins as adjuncts in the pharmacologic treatment of STEMI (37).

The first major trials to evaluate DTI in STEMI compared hirudin to UFH in patients undergoing fibrinolysis with either streptokinase (SK) or t-PA. Initially begun as large-scale trials with hard clinical primary endpoints, the TIMI-9 (38) and GUSTO-II (39) were terminated early due to an excessive rate of hemorrhagic stroke in both control and actively treated patients. The trials were restarted after adjustments were made in both heparin and hirudin dosing and completed enrollment of just over 7,000 patients (40,41). Following the dose decreases, neither trial reported an excess of intracranial or major bleeding. TIMI-9B evaluated the composite of death, reinfarction, cardiac failure or cardiogenic shock at 30 days as its primary endpoint and found rates of 11.9% and 12.9% (OR 1.09, p=0.4) for the hirudin and UFH groups, respectively. GUSTO-IIB was similarly unable to demonstrate a difference between hirudin and UFH for the prevention of death or recurrent myocardial infarction at 30 days (9.9% vs. 11.3%, (OR 0.86, $p=0.13$)) While the overall trial results were negative, the finding that patients receiving SK and hirudin had similar outcomes to patients receiving t-PA provided motivation to test in HERO-2 whether the effects of DTI might be most beneficial with SK rather than a fibrin-specific agent.

Table 3
Major trials of direct thrombin inhibitors in STEMI

Trial	n	DTI	Control	Fibrinolytic agent	Results
TIMI-9B, 1996	3,002	Hirudin 0.1 mg/kg IV bolus then 0.1 mg/kg/h gtt for 96°	UFH 50/10 IV for 96°	t-PA	Equivalence in efficacy and safety outcomes between agents
GUSTO-IIb, 1996 (STEMI only)	4,131	Hirudin 0.1 mg/kg IV bolus then 0.1 mg/kg/h gtt for 72°	UFH 50/10 IV for 72°	SK or t-PA	Similar rates of death or MI and no difference in safety outcomes
HERO, 1997	412	Hirulog, two regimens of bolus + infusion for up to 60°	UFH weight-based for up to 60°	SK	Absolute TIMI 3 flow improvement of 11–13% with hirulog
HIT-4, 1999	1,208	Lepirudin 0.2 mg/kg IV bolus then 0.5 mg/kg SC BID for 5–7 days	UFH IV bolus then SC BID for 5–7 days	SK	Benefit in favor of lepirudin for complete ST resolution at 90 min
ARGAMI, 2000	127	Argatroban (100 μg/kg bolus then 3 μg/kg/min gtt) for 72°	UFH 5k/1k for 72°	Alteplase	No significant difference in IRA TIMI 2/3 flow at 90 min or bleeding outcomes
HERO-2, 2001	17,073	Bivalirudin (0.25 mg/kg IV bolus then 0.5 mg/kg/h for 12° then 0.25 mg/kg/h to 48°	UFH 5k bolus then 1k or 0.8k gtt	SK	No reduction in 30-day mortality, but 30% reduction in recurrent MI at 96°
HORIZONS-AMI, 2008	3,602	Bivalirudin (0.75 mg/kg IV bolus then 1.75 mg/kg/h for the duration of PCI	UFH 60 U/kg bolus then to ACT goal of 250–300	n/a	In patients undergoing primary PCI for STEMI, bivalirudin significantly reduced bleeding and adverse clinical events

IV intravenous, *UFH* unfractionated heparin, *t-PA* tissue type plasminogen activator, *SK* streptokinase, *TIMI* thrombolysis in myocardial infarction, *SC* subcutaneous, *IRA* infarct related artery, *PCI* percutaneous coronary intervention, *ACT* activated clotting time

A contemporary investigation to GUSTOII and TIMI-9 conducted in Europe which studied recombinant hirudin as adjunct to alteplase fibrinolysis faced similar challenges. The Hirudin for the Improvement of Thrombolysis (HIT)-3 trial utilized UFH as control in an appropriately sized clinical event trial, but was halted due to an excessive rate (3.4% vs. 0%) of ICH in the hirudin arm *(42)*. This was followed by several years later with HIT-4 which examined a recombinant form of hirudin, lepirudin in 1,210 STEMI patients treated with SK and evaluated death, MI, stroke, rescue PCI and refractory angina at 30 days as its primary endpoint *(43)*. Lepirudin treated patients were not significantly different from those receiving UFH (22.7% vs. 24.3%, p=NS) with regard to the combined endpoint. Major bleeding and ICH rates were similar between groups.

Following the benefits of upstream administration of DTI seen in small pilot trials *(44–46)*, a large clinical events investigation of the 20 amino acid DTI, bivalirudin, was begun in patients receiving SK for STEMI. The Hirulog and Early Reperfusion of Occlusion (HERO)-2 trial enrolled over 17,000 patients who were randomized to a bolus of bivalirudin or UFH followed immediately by an infusion of SK *(47)*. Infusion of the assigned antithrombin agent was continued through at least 48 hours to evaluate the primary endpoint of 30-day mortality with preplanned secondary analyses of reinfarction and safety endpoints. For its primary endpoint, HERO-2 was neutral with no significant difference in mortality between groups; however, there was a 30% relative reduction in reinfarction at 96 hours seen in favor of the bivalirudin group. There were no reported serious safety concerns with bivalirudin in the overall population; however, in patients older than 75, there was a concerning increase in bleeding and intracranial hemorrhage which has restricted its use in this setting. Prior to the publication of HERO-2, a pooled reporting of the major trials of DTI in STEMI was included in a meta-analysis of DTI in ACS *(48)*. Overall, results similar to HERO-2, with no significant change in mortality and 25% reduction in reinfarction were seen.

With the acceptance of an initial strategy of mechanical reperfusion as superior to pharmacologic reperfusion in STEMI *(2)*, questions arose regarding the best pharmacologic adjuncts in the setting of primary PCI. Building on the lessons learned from investigations of DTI in mechanically reperfused patients with non-ST-segment elevation myocardial infarction, in which bivalirudin was compared to UFH and a GP IIb/IIIa inhibitor *(49,50)*, a similar trial was conducted in primary PCI for STEMI.

The Harmonizing Outcomes with Revascularization and Stents in Acute Myocardial Infarction (HORIZONS-AMI) trial randomized just over 3,600 patients with a planned intervention for STEMI to heparin or bivalirudin *(51)*. Both were infused for the duration of the intervention following a bolus dose. A glycoprotein IIb/IIIa inhibitor was administered to all patients in the heparin arm and was available on a provisional basis for those receiving bivalirudin. At 30 days, bivalirudin was found superior at reducing the co-primary endpoints of major bleeding (4.9% vs. 8.3%, RR=0.60, 95% CI 0.46–0.77, $p<0.001$) and net adverse clinical events which included death, reinfarction, target vessel revascularization, stroke and major bleeding (9.2% vs. 12.1%, RR=0.76, 95% CI 0.63–0.92, $p<0.005$). In addition to the contribution made by the decrease in bleeding, a significant reduction in cardiac mortality contributed to the improved rate of net adverse clinical events seen with bivalirudin. These benefits were slightly offset by an 1% absolute increase in acute (≤24 hr) stent thrombosis seen in the bivalirudin group.

RECOMMENDATIONS

The ACC/AHA practice guidelines currently provide specific instructions regarding the use of antithrombin therapy in patients presenting with STEMI *(19)*. UFH receives the strongest support with the following class I indications including patients undergoing percutaneous or surgical revascularization. For patients who undergo pharmacologic reperfusion with alteplase, reteplase or tenecteplase, IV UFH should be administered as a 60 U/kg bolus (maximum 4000 U) followed by an infusion of 12 U/kg/hr (maximum 1000 U/hr) to achieve an activated partial thromboplastin time (aPTT) of 1.5-2.0 time control (usually 50-70 sec). For patients who receive streptokinase, anistreplase or urokinase, IV UFH should be given to patients at high-risk for embolic complication including those with anterior MI, atrial fibrillation or known LV thrombus. Given its increased prothrombotic potential IV UFH (or bivalirudin in patients with a history of heparin-induced thrombocytopenia, 0.25 mg/kg IV bolus followed by 0.5 mg/kg/h for 12 h then 0.25 mg/kg/h for the subsequent 36 h with reduced dose if the aPTT exceeds 75 sec) may be reasonable for all patients undergoing fibrinolysis with streptokinase, and receives a class IIb recommendation from the ACC/AHA. With regard to newer therapies, the guidelines give a IIb recommendation to consideration of LMWH (enoxaparin, 30mg IV followed by 1mg/kg SC every 12 h until hospital discharge) as an alternative to patients undergoing fibrinolysis provided they are less than 75 years old and have normal renal function. The use of LMWH should be avoided in patients older than 75 years or with significant renal dysfunction (serum creatinine clearance < 30 ml/min) undergoing fibrinolysis.

CONCLUSIONS

Thrombus formation at the site of plaque rupture has been long recognized as the inciting event in the pathophysiology of STEMI. Fibrinolysis remains the most common mode of revascularization worldwide and has the recognized limitation of creating large amounts of activated thrombin as a byproduct of it mechanism of action. Antithrombin therapy at the time of fibrinolysis has been extensively evaluated with early trialists adopting UFH as an unproven, yet recognized standard. Subsequent evaluations of LMWH, particularly enoxaparin, have demonstrated its superiority in reducing major adverse cardiac endpoints following fibrinolysis with some concern over increases in major bleeding events. Fondaparinux, a synthetic antithrombin compound was found superior to enoxaparin in reducing clinical endpoints with fewer bleeding concerns among patients treated pharmacologically, but does not appear to provide sufficient anticoagulation for patients undergoing mechanical percutaneous revascularization. Direct thrombin inhibitors, in the setting of fibrinolysis, have been found to have an unacceptable safety profile with limited benefit in efficacy when compared to UFH. For patients who undergo mechanical reperfusion, bivalirudin has demonstrated yet incipient benefits which will require further development. The treatment of STEMI remains a dynamic environment where new agents will continue to challenge the validity of proven therapies.

REFERENCES

1. Yusuf S, Reddy S, Ounpuu S, Anand S (2001) Global burden of cardiovascular diseases: part I: general considerations, the epidemiologic transition, risk factors, and impact of urbanization. Circulation 104:2746–2753
2. Keeley EC, Boura JA, Grines CL (2003) Primary angioplasty versus intravenous thrombolytic therapy for acute myocardial infarction: a quantitative review of 23 randomised trials. Lancet 361:13–20
3. Rosenberg RD, Bauer KA (1994) The heparin-antithrombin system: a natural anticoagulant mechanism. In: Colman RW, Hirsh J, Marder VJ, Salzman EW (eds) Hemostasis and thrombosis: basic principles and clinical practice, 3rd edn. J.B. Lippincott, Philadelphia
4. GISSI-2: a factorial randomised trial of alteplase versus streptokinase and heparin versus no heparin among 12,490 patients with acute myocardial infarction. Gruppo Italiano per lo Studio della Sopravvivenza nell'Infarto Miocardico (1990) Lancet 336:65–71
5. ISIS-3: a randomised comparison of streptokinase vs tissue plasminogen activator vs anistreplase and of aspirin plus heparin vs aspirin alone among 41,299 cases of suspected acute myocardial infarction. ISIS-3 (Third International Study of Infarct Survival) Collaborative Group (1992) Lancet 339:753–770
6. An international randomized trial comparing four thrombolytic strategies for acute myocardial infarction. The GUSTO investigators. N Engl J Med 1993;329:673-82.
7. The effects of tissue plasminogen activator, streptokinase, or both on coronary-artery patency, ventricular function, and survival after acute myocardial infarction. The GUSTO Angiographic Investigators (1993) N Engl J Med 329:1615–1622
8. Randomized factorial trial of high-dose intravenous streptokinase, of oral aspirin and of intravenous heparin in acute myocardial infarction. ISIS (International Studies of Infarct Survival) pilot study (1987) Eur Heart J 8:634–642
9. de Bono DP, Simoons ML, Tijssen J et al (1992) Effect of early intravenous heparin on coronary patency, infarct size, and bleeding complications after alteplase thrombolysis: results of a randomised double blind European Cooperative Study Group trial. Br Heart J 67:122–128
10. Col J DO, Hanique G, Delligne B, Boland J, Pirenne B, Cheron P, Renkin J (1992) Infusion of heparin conjunct to streptokinase accelerates reperfusion of acute myocardial infarction: results of a double blind randomized study (OSIRIS). Circulation 86:259a
11. O'Connor CM, Meese R, Carney R et al (1994) A randomized trial of intravenous heparin in conjunction with anistreplase (anisoylated plasminogen streptokinase activator complex) in acute myocardial infarction: the Duke University Clinical Cardiology Study (DUCCS) 1. J Am Coll Cardiol 23:11–18

12. Hsia J, Hamilton WP, Kleiman N, Roberts R, Chaitman BR, Ross AM (1990) A comparison between heparin and low-dose aspirin as adjunctive therapy with tissue plasminogen activator for acute myocardial infarction. Heparin–Aspirin Reperfusion Trial (HART) Investigators. N Engl J Med 323:1433–1437

13. Chesebro JH, Knatterud G, Roberts R et al (1987) Thrombolysis in Myocardial Infarction (TIMI) Trial phase I: a comparison between intravenous tissue plasminogen activator and intravenous streptokinase. Clinical findings through hospital discharge. Circulation 76:142–154

14. Neuhaus KL, Tebbe U, Gottwik M et al (1988) Intravenous recombinant tissue plasminogen activator (rt-PA) and urokinase in acute myocardial infarction: results of the German Activator Urokinase Study (GAUS). J Am Coll Cardiol 12:581–587

15. Califf RM, Topol EJ, Stack RS, et al. (1991) Evaluation of combination thrombolytic therapy and timing of cardiac catheterization in acute myocardial infarction. Results of thrombolysis and angioplasty in myocardial infarction – phase 5 randomized trial. TAMI Study Group. Circulation 83:1543–1556

16. Neuhaus KL, von Essen R, Tebbe U et al (1992) Improved thrombolysis in acute myocardial infarction with front-loaded administration of alteplase: results of the rt-PA-APSAC patency study (TAPS). J Am Coll Cardiol 19:885–891

17. In-hospital mortality and clinical course of 20,891 patients with suspected acute myocardial infarction randomised between alteplase and streptokinase with or without heparin. The International Study Group (1990) Lancet 336:71–75

18. Granger CB, Hirsch J, Califf RM et al (1996) Activated partial thromboplastin time and outcome after thrombolytic therapy for acute myocardial infarction: results from the GUSTO-I trial. Circulation 93:870–878

19. Antman EM, Hand M, Armstrong PW et al (2008) 2007 Focused update of the ACC/AHA 2004 guidelines for the management of patients with ST-elevation myocardial infarction: a report of the American College of Cardiology/American Heart Association Task Force on Practice Guidelines. J Am Coll Cardiol 51:210–247

20. Weitz JI (1997) Low-molecular-weight heparins. N Engl J Med 337:688–698

21. Kontny F, Dale J, Abildgaard U, Pedersen TR (1997) Randomized trial of low molecular weight heparin (dalteparin) in prevention of left ventricular thrombus formation and arterial embolism after acute anterior myocardial infarction: the Fragmin in Acute Myocardial Infarction (FRAMI) Study. J Am Coll Cardiol 30:962–969

22. Frostfeldt G, Ahlberg G, Gustafsson G et al (1999) Low molecular weight heparin (dalteparin) as adjuvant treatment of thrombolysis in acute myocardial infarction–a pilot study: biochemical markers in acute coronary syndromes (BIOMACS II). J Am Coll Cardiol 33:627–633

23. Simoons M, Krzeminska-Pakula M, Alonso A et al (2002) Improved reperfusion and clinical outcome with enoxaparin as an adjunct to streptokinase thrombolysis in acute myocardial infarction. The AMI-SK study. Eur Heart J 23:1282–1290

24. Efficacy and safety of tenecteplase in combination with enoxaparin, abciximab, or unfractionated heparin: the ASSENT-3 randomised trial in acute myocardial infarction (2001) Lancet 358:605–613

25. Ross AM, Molhoek P, Lundergan C et al (2001) Randomized comparison of enoxaparin, a low-molecular-weight heparin, with unfractionated heparin adjunctive to recombinant tissue plasminogen activator thrombolysis and aspirin: second trial of Heparin and Aspirin Reperfusion Therapy (HART II). Circulation 104:648–652

26. Baird SH, Menown IB, McBride SJ, Trouton TG, Wilson C (2002) Randomized comparison of enoxaparin with unfractionated heparin following fibrinolytic therapy for acute myocardial infarction. Eur Heart J 23:627–632

27. Antman EM, Louwerenburg HW, Baars HF et al (2002) Enoxaparin as adjunctive antithrombin therapy for ST-elevation myocardial infarction: results of the ENTIRE-Thrombolysis in Myocardial Infarction (TIMI) 23 trial. Circulation 105:1642–1649

28. Wallentin L, Bergstrand L, Dellborg M et al (2003) Low molecular weight heparin (dalteparin) compared to unfractionated heparin as an adjunct to rt-PA (alteplase) for improvement of coronary artery patency in acute myocardial infarction – the ASSENT Plus study. Eur Heart J 24:897–908

29. Wallentin L, Goldstein P, Armstrong PW et al (2003) Efficacy and safety of tenecteplase in combination with the low-molecular-weight heparin enoxaparin or unfractionated heparin in the prehospital setting: the Assessment of the Safety and Efficacy of a New Thrombolytic Regimen (ASSENT)-3 PLUS randomized trial in acute myocardial infarction. Circulation 108:135–142

30. Antman EM, Morrow DA, McCabe CH et al (2006) Enoxaparin versus unfractionated heparin with fibrinolysis for ST-elevation myocardial infarction. N Engl J Med 354:1477–1488

31. Cohen M, Gensini GF, Maritz F et al (2003) The safety and efficacy of subcutaneous enoxaparin versus intravenous unfractionated heparin and tirofiban versus placebo in the treatment of acute ST-segment elevation myocardial infarction patients ineligible for reperfusion (TETAMI): a randomized trial. J Am Coll Cardiol 42:1348–1356

32. Eikelboom JW, Quinlan DJ, Mehta SR, Turpie AG, Menown IB, Yusuf S (2005) Unfractionated and low-molecular-weight heparin as adjuncts to thrombolysis in aspirin-treated patients with st-elevation acute myocardial infarction. Circulation 112:3855–3867

33. Coussement PK, Bassand JP, Convens C et al (2001) A synthetic factor-Xa inhibitor (ORG31540/SR9017A) as an adjunct to fibrinolysis in acute myocardial infarction. The PENTALYSE study. Eur Heart J 22:1716–1724

34. Yusuf S, Mehta SR, Chrolavicius S et al (2006) Effects of fondaparinux on mortality and reinfarction in patients with acute ST-segment elevation myocardial infarction: the OASIS-6 randomized trial. JAMA 295:1519–1530

35. Kaminski M, McDonagh J (1987) Inhibited thrombins. Interactions with fibrinogen and fibrin. Biochem J 242: 881–887

36. Hogg PJ, Jackson CM (1989) Fibrin monomer protects thrombin from inactivation by heparin-antithrombin III: implications for heparin efficacy. Proc Natl Acad Sci USA 86:3619–3623

37. Weitz JI, Hudoba M, Massel D, Maraganore J, Hirsh J (1990) Clot-bound thrombin is protected from inhibition by heparin-antithrombin III but is susceptible to inactivation by antithrombin III-independent inhibitors. J Clin Invest 86:385–391

38. Antman EM (1994) Hirudin in acute myocardial infarction. Safety report from the Thrombolysis and Thrombin Inhibition in Myocardial Infarction (TIMI) 9A Trial. Circulation 90:1624–1630

39. Randomized trial of intravenous heparin versus recombinant hirudin for acute coronary syndromes. The Global Use of Strategies to Open Occluded Coronary Arteries (GUSTO) IIa Investigators (1994) Circulation 90:1631–1637

40. Antman EM (1996) Hirudin in acute myocardial infarction. Thrombolysis and Thrombin Inhibition in Myocardial Infarction (TIMI) 9B trial. Circulation 94:911–921

41. Metz BK, White HD, Granger CB, et al. (1998) Randomized comparison of direct thrombin inhibition versus heparin in conjunction with fibrinolytic therapy for acute myocardial infarction: results from the GUSTO-IIb Trial. Global Use of Strategies to Open Occluded Coronary Arteries in Acute Coronary Syndromes (GUSTO-IIb) Investigators. J Am Coll Cardiol 31:1493–1498

42. Neuhaus KL, von Essen R, Tebbe U, et al. (1994) Safety observations from the pilot phase of the randomized r-Hirudin for Improvement of Thrombolysis (HIT-III) study. A study of the Arbeitsgemeinschaft Leitender Kardiologischer Krankenhausarzte (ALKK). Circulation 90:1638–1642

43. Neuhaus KL, Molhoek GP, Zeymer U et al (1999) Recombinant hirudin (lepirudin) for the improvement of thrombolysis with streptokinase in patients with acute myocardial infarction: results of the HIT-4 trial. J Am Coll Cardiol 34: 966–973

44. Cannon CP, McCabe CH, Henry TD et al (1994) A pilot trial of recombinant desulfatohirudin compared with heparin in conjunction with tissue-type plasminogen activator and aspirin for acute myocardial infarction: results of the Thrombolysis in Myocardial Infarction (TIMI) 5 trial. J Am Coll Cardiol 23:993–1003

45. Lidon RM, Theroux P, Lesperance J et al (1994) A pilot, early angiographic patency study using a direct thrombin inhibitor as adjunctive therapy to streptokinase in acute myocardial infarction. Circulation 89:1567–1572

46. Theroux P, Perez-Villa F, Waters D, Lesperance J, Shabani F, Bonan R (1995) Randomized double-blind comparison of two doses of Hirulog with heparin as adjunctive therapy to streptokinase to promote early patency of the infarct-related artery in acute myocardial infarction. Circulation 91:2132–2139

47. White HD, Aylward PE, Frey MJ et al. (1997) Randomized, double-blind comparison of hirulog versus heparin in patients receiving streptokinase and aspirin for acute myocardial infarction (HERO). Hirulog Early Reperfusion/Occlusion (HERO) Trial Investigators. Circulation 96:2155–2161

48. Direct thrombin inhibitors in acute coronary syndromes: principal results of a meta-analysis based on individual patients' data (2002) Lancet 359:294–302

49. Stone GW, Ware JH, Bertrand ME et al (2007) Antithrombotic strategies in patients with acute coronary syndromes undergoing early invasive management: one-year results from the ACUITY trial. JAMA 298:2497–2506

50. Lincoff AM, Kleiman NS, Kereiakes DJ et al (2004) Long-term efficacy of bivalirudin and provisional glycoprotein IIb/IIIa blockade vs heparin and planned glycoprotein IIb/IIIa blockade during percutaneous coronary revascularization: REPLACE-2 randomized trial. JAMA 292:696–703

51. Stone GW, Guagliumi G, Peruga JZ, Brodie BR, Dudek D, Kornowski R, Hartman F, Gersh BJ, Pocock SJ, Dangas G, Wong SC, Kirtane AJ, Parise J, Mehran R for the HORIZONS-Trial Investigators (2008) Bivalirudin during primary PCI in acute myocardial infarction. N Engl J Med 358:2218–2230

13 Fibrinolysis and Facilitated PCI

Ryan D. Christofferson and Sorin J. Brener

Contents

ABSTRACT Early and effective reperfusion is the primary treatment goal in acute myocardial infarction. The use of fibrinolytic (lytic) therapy to achieve early infarct vessel patency is well established and recommended where primary percutaneous coronary intervention (PCI) is not available. Several lytic agents are available with differing advantages and disadvantages. Contraindications to lytic therapy are important to appreciate as the major complication, intracranial hemorrhage, is potentially devastating. Rescue angioplasty is necessary if reperfusion is not achieved by lytic therapy. After lytic therapy, early transfer to a PCI-capable facility for angiography may be beneficial in high-risk patients regardless of reperfusion status. The routine use of lytics with planned primary PCI is not recommended, however, as adverse outcomes may result. A strategy of facilitated PCI with half-dose lytics and GP IIb/IIIa is also currently not recommended.

Key words Fibrinolytics; Time-to-treatment; Primary PCI; Rescue angioplasty; Facilitated angioplasty

INTRODUCTION

The pathophysiology of the majority of acute myocardial infarctions (MI) is characterized by atherosclerotic plaque erosion or rupture with subsequent platelet adhesion and aggregation, and simultaneous activation of the coagulation cascade, as described in previous chapters. The end result is thrombin generation and fibrin clot formation, partially or completely occluding the infarct artery. The major difference between non-ST elevation myocardial infarction (NSTEMI) and ST-elevation myocardial infarction (STEMI) is the location of the infarct artery and the degree of arterial occlusion, with STEMI usually representing complete occlusion of a major epicardial artery lacking significant collateral flow. Stuttering symptoms may represent temporary occlusion.

From: *Contemporary Cardiology: Antithrombotic Drug Therapy in Cardiovascular Disease*
Edited by: A.T. Askari and A.M. Lincoff (eds.), DOI 10.1007/978-1-60327-235-3_13
© Humana Press, a part of Springer Science+Business Media, LLC 2010

Early reperfusion following symptom onset (within 12–24 h) is the primary goal of any acute MI therapy as timely patency of the infarct-related artery has been shown to correlate with improved clinical outcomes. The primary goal of reperfusion therapy, irrespective of the type (mechanical or pharmacologic) is to restore sufficient blood flow in order to preserve as much myocardium as possible. The secondary goal, perhaps better achieved by primary (when timely), rescue or late PCI, is prevention of recurrent ischemia and infarction. However, when used appropriately in an early reperfusion strategy, lytics have been shown to be safe and effective in select patients where timely primary PCI is not available. Early transfer to a PCI-capable facility is then recommended.

The purpose of this chapter is to review the appropriate use of lytic therapy as a primary reperfusion strategy, and as a part of a facilitated PCI strategy.

APPROPRIATE DIAGNOSIS AND EARLY TREATMENT OF STEMI

Acute STEMI remains a significant cause of morbidity and mortality. The accurate diagnosis of STEMI requires the appropriate clinical scenario in the setting of a diagnostic electrocardiogram (Table 1). Assuming the appropriate diagnosis is made, the risk of morbidity and mortality depends heavily on the size of the jeopardized myocardium and the duration of occlusion. A significant reduction in mortality may be achieved by early and effective restoration of antegrade flow in the infarct-related artery. The optimal method used to achieve reperfusion has been a matter of some debate. However, the patients treated within the first hour appear to have the highest mortality benefit. It has been demonstrated that there is an inverse relationship between time to treatment and survival benefit which extends to 12 h when lytic therapy is used (1). Recent data indicate that this time dependency may extend beyond 12–24 h in patients who receive primary PCI (Brave-2) (2). All patients with ST-segment elevation or new left bundle branch block MI presenting within this time period from onset of symptoms should be considered for reperfusion therapy.

FIBRINOLYSIS VERSUS DIRECT PCI

Following diagnosis, rapid decision-making is necessary to appropriately manage patients with STEMI. The assessment of availability of primary PCI and the contraindications to lytic therapy are essential factors when choosing a reperfusion strategy. In facilities where coronary angiography and PCI are available within 90 min of medical contact, primary PCI has been

Table 1
Differential diagnostic considerations for STEMI

Comorbid ischemia	ST elevation but no ischemia	Chest pain but no ischemia
Aortic dissection	Early repolarization	Aortic dissection
Systemic arterial embolism	Left ventricular hypertrophy	Myopericarditis
Hypertensive crisis	Left bundle branch block	Pleuritis
Aortic stenosis	Hyperkalemia	Pulmonary embolism
Cocaine use	Brugada syndrome	Costochondritis
Arteritis		GI disorders

Adapted from Christofferson RD (2008) Acute ST-elevation myocardial infarction. In: Shishehbor MH, Wang TH, Askari AT, Penn MS, Topol EJ (eds) Management of the patient in the coronary care unit. Lippincott Williams and Wilkins, New York deemed to be the preferred therapy (3). Several large, randomized trials have demonstrated a pooled 22% short-term mortality reduction for patients treated with primary PCI compared to lytic therapy within this early treatment window (4). In addition, significant reductions in death, MI, and recurrent ischemia at long-term follow-up have been demonstrated (Fig. 1). However, practical limitations often prevent timely administration of primary PCI. An analysis of 21 trials showed that the mortality reduction from primary PCI over lytics decreased with each 10 min increase in time delay, with the therapies becoming equivalent after a PCI-related delay of 62 min (5). Therefore, in facilities where PCI is not available and transfer is not likely within the appropriate time window [medical contact-to-balloon time > 90 min, lytic therapy is preferred unless contraindicated (Table 2)].

The use of primary PCI with prolonged transfer times is controversial. Several trials have addressed the question of primary PCI with modest transfer times (DANAMI-2, AIR-PAMI, and PRAGUE) and have found favorable outcomes, although these studies have been criticized regarding broad applicability due to practical limitations on transfer times in the US, in particular (3). As a result, current guidelines emphasize early reperfusion, regardless of the method. If a contraindication to lytic therapy is present or in the setting of cardiogenic shock or prior bypass surgery, arrangement should be made for immediate transfer for primary PCI.

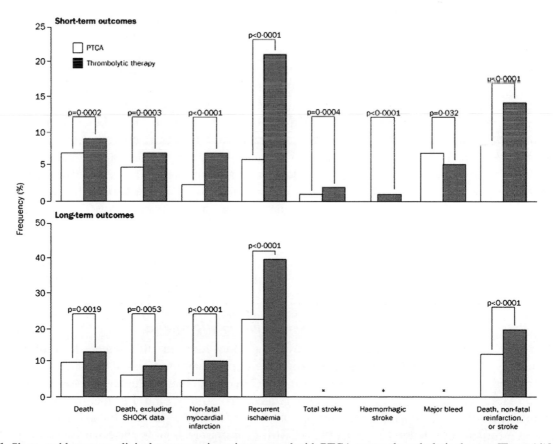

Fig. 1. Short- and long-term clinical outcomes in patients treated with PTCA versus thrombolytic therapy [From (4)].

Table 2
Decision-making algorithm for acute MI

Step 1: Assess *time* and *risk*
  Time since symptom onset
  Risk of STEMI
  Risk of fibrinolysis
  Time required for transport to PCI
Step 2: Determine if *fibrinolysis* or *invasive strategy* is preferred
  Fibrinolysis is preferred if:
    Invasive strategy is not an option (lack of access to skilled PCI laboratory)
    Delay present for invasive strategy (prolonged transport > 60 min, or delayed laboratory activation time)
  Invasive strategy is preferred if:
    Skilled PCI laboratory available immediately (door to balloon < 90 min, or transfer < 60 min)
    High risk from STEMI (cardiogenic shock, Killip class ≥ 3)
    Contraindications to fibrinolysis (bleeding, ICH)
    Late presentation (symptom onset > 3 h)
    Diagnosis of STEMI in doubt

Adapted from Boden WE, Eagle K, Granger CB (2007) Reperfusion strategies in acute ST-segment elevation myocardial infarction: a comprehensive review of contemporary management options. JACC 50:917–929

FIBRINOLYTIC AGENTS

Fibrinolysis is mediated by a non-specific protease called plasmin, which exerts its effect by degrading clot-associated fibrin and fibrinogen. Lytic agents are all plasminogen activators, leading to the direct or indirect conversion of plasminogen to plasmin. There are currently several approved lytic agents (Table 3). These agents differ in their fibrin specificity and dosing regimen, with reduced bleeding complications from enhanced fibrin specificity, and improved ease of delivery from bolus dose agents, allowing prehospital treatment by emergency medical personnel.

Streptokinase is a 415-amino acid bacterial protein. It differs greatly from the newer recombinant lytic agents in that it is produced by bacteria, is antigenic, and has little fibrin specificity. It can cause substantial systemic lytic effects at clinical doses. Because of the antigenicity, it cannot be administered twice in the same patient as antibodies are developed against the protein. The major advantage to streptokinase however is low cost. Much of the data derived for lytic use in MI has been obtained for alteplase, the naturally occurring version of human tissue plasminogen activator. The drug, alteplase, in clinical use contains no genetic modification but is produced by recombinant DNA technology. The most commonly used agent in the United States is tenecteplase (TNK t-PA), a genetically modified version of alteplase (t-PA). It contains a triple substitution that allows a longer plasma half-life, better fibrin binding, and single-bolus administration. The major limitation to TNK t-PA is high cost.

Data for the Use of Fibrinolytic Agents

The GISSI study was the initial landmark trial to demonstrate mortality benefit for thrombolytics in acute MI *(6)*. The GUSTO I (Global Utilization of Streptokinase and Tissue Plasminogen Activator for Occluded Coronary Arteries) trial, comparing the use of accelerate alteplase versus streptokinase, showed that accelerated alteplase significantly reduced the 30-day mortality rate by 15% relative to streptokinase, when used with subcutaneous or intravenous heparin *(7)*. In addition, accelerated alteplase afforded significantly higher rates of TIMI (Thrombolysis in Myocardial Infarction) 3 flow at 90 min compared with SK (54% vs. 31%, $p < 0.001$). The accelerated protocol consisted of an

Table 3
Summary of properties of fibrinolytic agents used in clinical practice

	Streptokinase	t-PA	r-PA	TNK
Source	Group C strep	Recombinant	Recombinant	Recombinant
Fibrin specificity	None	++	+	+++
Fibrin affinity	None	+++	+	++++
Antigenic	Yes	No	No	No
Allergic reaction	Yes	No	No	No
Half-life (minute)	18–23	3–4	14	20–24
Dose	Drip	Weight-based bolus and drip	Bolus X 2	Weight-based bolus
Cost	+	+++	++	++
Rate of ICH (%)	~0.4	~0.4–0.7	~0.8–0.9	~0.9
Advantages	Low cost	Short half-life, effective	Bolus admin	Bolus admin

t-PA alteplase, r-PA reteplase, TNK tenecteplase, ICH intracranial hemorrhage

intravenous bolus dose of 15 mg followed by 0.75 mg/kg (up to 50 mg) over 30 min followed by 0.5 mg/kg (up to 35 mg) over 60 min.

The first of the third-generation fibrinolytic agents approved for use in the United States, reteplase is less fibrin-specific than alteplase. Also, reteplase has a longer half-life than alteplase and can be administered in a double bolus (10 U each, 30 min apart). The GUSTO III trial (8), however, failed to show a mortality benefit of reteplase over alteplase, although its ease of use was thought to potentially reduce time to administration.

Tenecteplase (TNK) is another third-generation fibrinolytic, and is characterized by its improved fibrin specificity, enhanced resistance to plasminogen activator inhibitor (PAI-1), and decreased plasma clearance, properties allowing it be administered as a single bolus. The ASSENT 2 (Assessment of the Safety and Efficacy of a New Thrombolytic) trial found no mortality difference between TNK and t-PA at 30 days (9). However, TNK was associated with significantly less non-cerebral bleeding and improved mortality in patients treated more than 4 h after symptom onset.

As a result of the various properties, advantages and disadvantages of each lytic, there remains a role for each in clinical practice. However, the most commonly used lytic in the United States is TNK, likely due to its fibrin specificity, lower bleeding rates, and improved mortality in late presenters. In some locations worldwide, cost limits the use of newer agents, and streptokinase still may have a role. In addition, the lower ICH rates with streptokinase may make it more attractive in patients at risk for this complication.

Complications

BLEEDING AND HYPERSENSITIVITY

The most feared complication of lytic therapy is intracranial hemorrhage (ICH). This complication appears to occur at a rate of 0.5–0.7% of patients receiving lytic therapy. The diagnosis of ICH should be considered when there is severe headache, acute confusional state, new neurological deficits, or seizures. The risk factors for ICH include female gender, age > 75 years, hypertension, low body weight, and coagulopathy. When the clinical suspicion of ICH is high, all antithrombotic therapies should be held while emergent CT scan is performed. When ICH is present, emergent neurosurgery to evacuate the hematoma may be lifesaving, so early diagnosis is paramount. Even with prompt recognition and treatment, mortality from ICH is as high as 60%. Additional bleeding complications may occur in the gastrointestinal tract, retroperitoneum, or at intravenous or intra-arterial access sites. Hypersensitivity reaction to lytic agents occurs only with streptokinase, as it is a bacterial protein and is antigenic. These events are usually not life threatening if recognized and treated promptly.

Lytic Use in the Elderly

Elderly patients represent a high-risk group for thrombolytic therapy as the rate of ICH is higher among patients > 75 years of age and the mortality rate from ICH in these patients is as high as 90%. There is controversy in the literature, however, regarding just how much higher the risk is among elderly patients, as reports are conflicting. An observational study *(10)* from the Medicare database found patients older than 75 years had an increased risk of death at 30 days with fibrinolytic therapy (RR = 1.38, 95% CI: 1.12–1.71, p = 0.003). However, an updated meta-analysis of nine randomized trials *(11)* found the risk reduction with fibrinolysis in patients older than 75 years was 16% (OR = 0.84, 95% CI: 0.72–0.98, p < 0.05). The only randomized trial to specifically address management of STEMI in the elderly found that elderly patients treated with PCI had significantly lower 30-day and 1-year mortality rates than elderly patients treated with fibrinolysis *(12)*. However, a recent study suggested that fibrinolytic therapy may be safe in the elderly if a reduced dose of enoxaparin is used *(13)*. Nevertheless, it appears reasonable to conclude that wherever available, primary PCI should be the treatment of choice in the elderly.

Contraindications

Recent cerebrovascular accident (including hemorrhagic stroke), intracranial neoplasm, active internal bleeding, and suspected aortic dissection are the only absolute contraindications to lytic therapy. There are a number of relative contraindications, including severe hypertension, remote ischemic stroke, non-compressible vascular puncture sites, among others (see Table 4). The presence of one absolute contraindication or one or more relative contraindications should favor PCI, even if this means delaying reperfusion.

Adjunctive Therapies

ANTIPLATELET AGENTS

The benefits of aspirin in the treatment of acute MI are well established. Aspirin should be administered as quickly as possible when the diagnosis of STEMI is made. Aspirin should be given by mouth, chewable if possible, and non-enteric coated, in a dose of at least 162–325 mg. The evidence for this practice is founded on the landmark ISIS-2 trial (International Studies of Infarct Survival) which showed a significant mortality benefit for aspirin *(14)*. Since that study numerous others in acute MI and NSTEMI have shown benefit.

More recently, trials have been completed evaluating the use of clopidogrel in addition to aspirin. The CLARITY trial compared clopidogrel to placebo in 3,491 patients, finding a 36% reduction in a composite endpoint of death, recurrent MI, or occluded infarct artery at early angiography *(15)*. The larger COMMIT trial had a similar finding, with 9% reduction in death, reinfarction, or stoke with the addition of clopidogrel to aspirin *(16)*. Therefore, early administration of clopidogrel, with an oral loading dose of 300 mg except in those older than 75 years of age, is recommended for patients with STEMI.

Table 4
Contraindications and cautions for use of fibrinolytic agents to manage myocardial infarction

Absolute contraindications
  Previous hemorrhagic stroke at any time; ischemic stroke within 3 months
  Known intracranial neoplasm, structural cerebral vascular lesion or closed-head injury within 3 months
  Active bleeding or bleeding diathesis (excluding menses)
  Suspected aortic dissection
Relative contraindications
  Severe, uncontrolled hypertension at presentation (blood pressure > 180/110 mmHg) or history of chronic severe hypertension
  History of ischemic stroke > 3 months, dementia, or known intracerebral pathologic condition not covered in contraindications
  Current use of anticoagulants, the risk increases with increasing INR
  Traumatic or prolonged (>10 min) CPR or major surgery (<3 wk)
  Noncompressible vascular punctures
  Recent (within 2–4 wk) internal bleeding
  For streptokinase or anistrepeplase: prior exposure (more than 5 days prior) or prior allergic reaction
  Pregnancy
  Active peptic ulcer

CPR cardiopulmonary resuscitation, *INR* international normalized ratio
Adapted from Antman EM, Anbe DT, Armstrong PW, et al. (2004) ACC/AHA guidelines for the management of patients with ST-elevation myocardial infarction: a report of the American College of Cardiology/American Heart Association Task Force on Practice Guidelines (Committee to Revise the 1999 Guidelines for the Management of Patients with Acute Myocardial Infarction). J Am Coll Cardiol 44:E1–E211

ANTITHROMBOTIC AGENTS

When used as an adjunct to t-PA, intravenous *unfractionated heparin* (UFH) has been shown to improve late patency. This is likely due to its antithrombin effects, as thrombin activity is paradoxically increased after fibrinolysis. Intravenous heparin was used successfully in conjunction with accelerated t-PA in the GUSTO I trial to improve infarct artery patency and outcomes. However, in the same trial, there was no benefit to intravenous heparin with streptokinase. The use of unfractionated heparin as adjunctive therapy with reteplase and tenecteplase was validated in the the GUSTO III and ASSENT 2 trials, respectively. The dose of heparin recommended in the AHA/ACC guidelines is a bolus of 60 U/kg bolus (maximum, 4,000 units), followed by 12 U/kg/h (maximum, 1,000 U/h). The goal activated partial thromboplastin time (aPTT) should be adjusted to 50–70 s.

LOW-MOLECULAR-WEIGHT HEPARINS

Low-molecular-weight heparin (LMWH) has recently been shown to improve upon outcomes obtained with adjunctive UFH use. Because UFH is neutralized by activated platelets, it cannot inhibit clot-bound thrombin. However, enoxaparin, a low-molecular-weight heparin, overcomes this disadvantage due to consistent bioavailability and diminished inhibition by platelet factor 4. In addition, there is a reduced incidence of heparin-induced thrombocytopenia with LMWH. Table 5 summarizes the observations from trials of anticoagulants in STEMI.

The ASSENT 3 trial *(17)* found that patients treated with full-dose TNK and enoxaparin had a lower 30-day risk of death or MI compared to full-dose TNK and UFH (6.8% vs. 9.1%; $p=0.02$). The ENTIRE-TIMI 23 (Enoxaparin as Adjunctive Antithrombin Therapy for ST-Elevation Myocardial Infarction) demonstrated that patient enoxaparin was superior to UFH in a similar trial design to

Table 5
Summary of findings from trials of enoxaparin and fondaparinux for STEMI

Pharmacologic agent	30-Day efficacy	Safety	Use during PCI
Enoxaparin	Appears superior to UFH with fibrinolysis	Increased risk of serious bleeds	Can be used to support PCI after fibrinolysis
Fondaparinux	Appears superior to placebo/UFH in fibrinolysis. Trend toward worse outcomes with primary PCI	Trend toward decreased risk of serious bleeds	Increased risk of catheter thrombosis when used alone

PCI percutaneous coronary intervention, UFH unfractionated heparin
Adapted from (3)

ASSENT 3. The rate of major hemorrhage was slightly less with adjunctive enoxaparin compared to UFH. However, the EXTRACT-TIMI 25 trial showed that the primary benefit of enoxaparin was in prevention of reinfarction, rather than in survival. Although the EXTRACT-TIMI 25 trial did not have a primary PCI group, among patients who had subsequent PCI after lytics, enoxaparin appeared to be superior to UFH without increased bleeding events (13).

Fondaparinux

Fondaparinux is a synthetic factor X inhibitor that has been studied in acute MI. The OASIS-6 trial evaluated fondaparinux with fibrinolytics and appeared to demonstrate benefit versus placebo/UFH in terms of death and re-infarction at 30 days (9.7% vs. 11.2%; HR = 0.86) without an increased risk in bleeding (18). However, in the primary PCI subset, there was no benefit and a significant increase in guiding catheter thrombosis was noted which has limited its widespread use.

Glycoprotein IIb/IIIa Inhibitors and Direct Thrombin Inhibitors

Sustained tissue-level reperfusion occurs in only 25% of patients who receive lytics. In addition, there is paradoxically increased activity of platelets after lytic therapy, and this activation may be an important mediator in vessel reocclusion. Glycoprotein IIb/IIIa (GPIIb/IIIa) inhibitors are potent antiplatelet agents which block the final common pathway of platelet aggregation, and so may be useful in conjunction with lytics. The GUSTO V trial found that the addition of abciximab to half-dose r-PA did not reduce mortality, but did reduce the rate of reinfarction and complications after MI (19). The ASSENT 3 trial also found similar reduction in reinfarction with abciximab and half-dose TNK (17). However, this reduction in reinfarction came at a high cost in the elderly, with almost twice the level of ICH among patients receiving combination therapy. Therefore, age > 75 can be considered a contraindication to combination GP IIb/IIIa and lytics.

Direct thrombin inhibitors have failed to show a significant benefit over heparin during fibrinolysis in acute MI, and outside of the realm of heparin-induced thrombocytopenia, do not appear to play a significant role in the treatment of acute MI with lytics.

RESCUE ANGIOPLASTY

The use of PCI in the setting of failed reperfusion with fibrinolytic therapy has been called rescue angioplasty. The clinical determination of successful reperfusion can be difficult to determine as resolution of chest pain can occur for reasons other than reperfusion, such as blunting of pain with narcotic analgesics. Serial 12-lead ECGs can be a more reliable measure of reperfusion, with resolution of

ST-segment elevation by more than 70% correlating with effective tissue level reperfusion and clinical outcomes. In a small number of patients, resolution of chest pain with an accompanied run of accelerated idioventricular rhythm (AIVR) indicated successful reperfusion.

Infarct-related artery patency at 90 min following lytic administration has been shown to correlate with long-term survival. If reperfusion is not evident after 90 min, a prompt decision should be made regarding the use of emergency angiography and PCI. High-risk patients with large infact size, severe congestive heart failure, or unstable cardiac rhythms after lytic administration should not await clinical assessment of reperfusion, but instead should be taken to immediate PCI.

The RESCUE (Randomized Evaluation of Salvage Angioplasty with Combined Utilization of Endpoints) trial (20) showed that patients with a large anterior MI and unsuccessful thrombolysis (TIMI 0 or 1 flow) can benefit from rescue PCI. The REACT trial showed that when lytics fail, treatment with rescue PCI is associated with a 50% reduction in death, reinfarction, stroke, and severe heart failure (21). Although not technically "rescue angioplasty," the strategy of early invasive approach among STEMI patients treated with lytic therapy has been evaluated in several small trials, including GRACIA I, Capital AMI, and SIAM III (22–24). These trials showed a reduction in revascularization events in the early invasive group, and a trend toward fewer deaths and reinfarctions.

The conclusion which may be drawn from these trials is that an early angiography strategy (within 24 h) may be a reasonable approach in all patients who undergo lytic treatment, with emergent PCI in those patients where reperfusion at 90 min is not achieved or hemodynamic or electrical instability are present.

FACILITATED PCI

Evidence from PCI trials has shown that a patent infarct artery at the time of presentation to the catheterization laboratory is associated with improved procedural success and decreased mortality (25). The success of lytics in improving infarct artery patency created interest in combining the use of lytic therapy with immediate PCI. The combination of an initial pharmacologic regimen with planned primary PCI has been termed "facilitated PCI." The theoretical advantages include earlier reperfusion, improved hemodynamic stability, enhanced procedural success, smaller infarct size, and, hopefully, improved survival. The disadvantages may include increased bleeding risk when combining lytics with PCI. A number of different facilitated PCI strategies have been proposed, including high-dose heparin, early glycoprotein IIb/IIIa inhibitor use, full-dose or reduced-dose fibrinolytics, and combination fibrinolytics and glycoprotein IIb/IIIa inhibitors.

Full-Dose Lytics

Although previously studied in a smaller number of patients, the largest study to date to evaluate full-dose fibrinolytic therapy was ASSENT-4 PCI (Assessment of Safety and Efficacy of a New Treatment Strategy with PCI). This trial evaluated tenecteplase plus PCI versus primary PCI alone. Higher in-hospital mortality (6% vs. 3%; $p=0.01$) and higher primary composite endpoints (18.6% vs. 13.4% ; $p=0.0045$) with full-dose fibrinolytics led to premature termination of this trial (26). As a result of this trial the practice of full-dose thrombolytic therapy prior to PCI is not recommended. The reason for the excess mortality and other endpoints was appeared to be an excess in stroke and reinfarction, possibly representing a prothrombotic, post-fibrinolytic milieu.

Half-Dose Lytics + Glycoprotein IIb/IIIa Inhibitor or Glycoprotein IIb/IIIa Inhibitor Alone

The first combination therapy trial, ADVANCE-MI, evaluated eptifibatide, a glycoprotein IIb/IIIa inhibitor, together with bolus-dose TNK. This trial included 146 patients and evaluated 30-day outcomes. The result was better initial TIMI 3 flow with facilitated PCI, but no improvement in final ST-segment resolution and a non-significant increase in mortality *(27)*. Subsequently, a large meta-analysis of multiple, small randomized trials confirmed that primary PCI is a superior strategy to facilitated PCI with respect to the endpoints of death, reinfarction, target vessel revascularization *(28)*. This meta-analysis recommended that use of such regimens be limited to the setting of randomized trials.

The most definitive randomized control trial to date designed to answer the questions about facilitated PCI was recently published. The FINESSE (Facilitated Intervention with Enhanced Speed to Stop Events) *(29)* trial assessed the effects of half-dose reteplase plus abciximab, abciximab alone, or placebo on outcomes in patients undergoing PCI for STEMI. The lytic plus glycoprotein IIb/IIIa arm had greater infarct-related artery patency at the time of cardiac catheterization, although the composite primary endpoint of death or complications of MI at 90 days was no different between the three strategies (9.8% half-dose fibrinolytic + GP IIB/IIIA inhibitor, 10.5% GP IIb/IIIa inhibitor alone, and 10.7% placebo; P=NS). Although the endpoints were similar, bleeding rates were higher with the half-dose lytic + IIB/IIIA inhibitor strategy.

Although not technically "facilitated PCI" per se, there is evidence that early administration of a glycoprotein IIb/IIIa inhibitor may be beneficial. The On-TIME 2 trial evaluated the prehospital initiation of tirofiban in patients with STEMI undergoing primary PCI *(30)*. This trial documented improved residual ST-segment elevation at one hour post-PCI. There was also a trend toward improved survival at 30 days with early tirofiban but the study was not powered for clinical endpoints.

As a result of the lack of data showing benefit for facilitated PCI regimens, current guidelines recommend the use of facilitated PCI only with regimens other than full-dose lytics when patients are at high risk but PCI is not immediately available within 90 min and bleeding risk is low *(3)*. The current emphasis for research and resources allocation should now be placed on improving transfer times and overall door-to-balloon times, as facilitated PCI, although intellectually appealing, has not solved the dilemma of prolonged PCI times.

REFERENCES

1. Boersma E, Maas AC, Deckers JW, Simoons ML (1996) Early thrombolytic treatment in acute myocardial infarction: reappraisal of the golden hour. Lancet 348(9030):771–775
2. Schomig A, Mehilli J, Antoniucci D et al (2005) Mechanical reperfusion in patients with acute myocardial infarction presenting more than 12 hours from symptom onset: a randomized controlled trial. JAMA 293(23):2865–2872
3. Antman EM, Hand M, Armstrong PW et al (2008) 2007 focused update of the ACC/AHA 2004 guidelines for the management of patients with ST-elevation myocardial infarction: a report of the American College of Cardiology/American Heart Association Task Force on Practice Guidelines. J Am Coll Cardiol 51(2):210–247
4. Keeley EC, Boura JA, Grines CL (2003) Primary angioplasty versus intravenous thrombolytic therapy for acute myocardial infarction: a quantitative review of 23 randomised trials. Lancet 361(9351):13–20
5. Nallamothu BK, Bates ER (2003) Percutaneous coronary intervention versus fibrinolytic therapy in acute myocardial infarction: is timing (almost) everything? Am J Cardiol 92(7):824–826
6. Long-term effects of intravenous thrombolysis in acute myocardial infarction: final report of the GISSI study. Gruppo Italiano per lo Studio della Streptochi-nasi nell'Infarto Miocardico (GISSI) (1987) Lancet 2(8564):871–874
7. An international randomized trial comparing four thrombolytic strategies for acute myocardial infarction. The GUSTO investigators (1993) N Engl J Med 329(10):673–682

8. A comparison of reteplase with alteplase for acute myocardial infarction. The Global Use of Strategies to Open Occluded Coronary Arteries (GUSTO III) Investigators (1997) N Engl J Med 337(16):1118–1123

9. Van De Werf F, Adgey J, Ardissino D et al (1999) Single-bolus tenecteplase compared with front-loaded alteplase in acute myocardial infarction: the ASSENT-2 double-blind randomised trial. Lancet 354(9180):716–722

10. Thiemann D (2000) Primary angioplasty vs thrombolysis in elderly patients. JAMA 283(5):601–602

11. Indications for fibrinolytic therapy in suspected acute myocardial infarction: collaborative overview of early mortality and major morbidity results from all randomised trials of more than 1000 patients. Fibrinolytic Therapy Trialists' (FTT) Collaborative Group (1994) Lancet 343(8893):311–322

12. de Boer MJ, Ottervanger JP, van't Hof AW, Hoorntje JC, Suryapranata H, Zijlstra F (2002) Reperfusion therapy in elderly patients with acute myocardial infarction: a randomized comparison of primary angioplasty and thrombolytic therapy. J Am Coll Cardiol 39(11):1723–1728

13. Antman EM, Morrow DA, McCabe CH et al (2006) Enoxaparin versus unfractionated heparin with fibrinolysis for ST-elevation myocardial infarction. N Engl J Med 354(14):1477–1488

14. Randomised trial of intravenous streptokinase, oral aspirin, both, or neither among 17,187 cases of suspected acute myocardial infarction: ISIS-2. ISIS-2 (Second International Study of Infarct Survival) Collaborative Group (1988) Lancet 2(8607):349–360

15. Sabatine MS, Cannon CP, Gibson CM et al (2005) Addition of clopidogrel to aspirin and fibrinolytic therapy for myocardial infarction with ST-segment elevation. N Engl J Med 352(12):1179–1189

16. Chen ZM, Jiang LX, Chen YP et al (2005) Addition of clopidogrel to aspirin in 45, 852 patients with acute myocardial infarction: randomised placebo-controlled trial. Lancet 366(9497):1607–1621

17. Efficacy and safety of tenecteplase in combination with enoxaparin, abciximab, or unfractionated heparin: the ASSENT-3 randomised trial in acute myocardial infarction (2001) Lancet 358(9282):605–613

18. Yusuf S, Mehta SR, Chrolavicius S et al (2006) Effects of fondaparinux on mortality and reinfarction in patients with acute ST-segment elevation myocardial infarction: the OASIS-6 randomized trial. JAMA 295(13):1519–1530

19. Topol EJ (2001) Reperfusion therapy for acute myocardial infarction with fibrinolytic therapy or combination reduced fibrinolytic therapy and platelet glycoprotein IIb/IIIa inhibition: the GUSTO V randomised trial. Lancet 357(9272):1905–1914

20. Ellis SG, da Silva ER, Heyndrickx G et al (1994) Randomized comparison of rescue angioplasty with conservative management of patients with early failure of thrombolysis for acute anterior myocardial infarction. Circulation 90(5):2280–2284

21. Gershlick AH, Stephens-Lloyd A, Hughes S et al (2005) Rescue angioplasty after failed thrombolytic therapy for acute myocardial infarction. N Engl J Med 353(26):2758–2768

22. Fernandez-Aviles F, Alonso JJ, Castro-Beiras A et al (2004) Routine invasive strategy within 24 hours of thrombolysis versus ischaemia-guided conservative approach for acute myocardial infarction with ST-segment elevation (GRACIA-1): a randomised controlled trial. Lancet 364(9439):1045–1053

23. Scheller B, Hennen B, Hammer B et al (2003) Beneficial effects of immediate stenting after thrombolysis in acute myocardial infarction. J Am Coll Cardiol 42(4):634–641

24. Le May MR, Wells GA, Labinaz M et al (2005) Combined angioplasty and pharmacological intervention versus thrombolysis alone in acute myocardial infarction (CAPITAL AMI study). J Am Coll Cardiol 46(3):417–424

25. Stone GW, Cox D, Garcia E et al (2001) Normal flow (TIMI-3) before mechanical reperfusion therapy is an independent determinant of survival in acute myocardial infarction: analysis from the primary angioplasty in myocardial infarction trials. Circulation 104(6):636–641

26. Primary versus tenecteplase-facilitated percutaneous coronary intervention in patients with ST-segment elevation acute myocardial infarction (ASSENT-4 PCI): randomised trial (2006) Lancet 367(9510):569–578

27. ADVANCE MI Investigators (2005) Facilitated percutaneous coronary intervention for acute ST-segment elevation myocardial infarction: results from the prematurely terminated ADdressing the Value of facilitated ANgioplasty after Combination therapy or Eptifibatide monotherapy in acute Myocardial Infarction (ADVANCE MI) trial. Am Heart J 150(1):116–122

28. Keeley EC, Boura JA, Grines CL (2006) Comparison of primary and facilitated percutaneous coronary interventions for ST-elevation myocardial infarction: quantitative review of randomised trials. Lancet 367(9510):579–588

29. Ellis SG, Tendera M, de Belder MA et al (2008) Facilitated PCI in patients with ST-elevation myocardial infarction. N Engl J Med 358(21):2205–2217

30. Van't Hof AW, Ten Berg J, Heestermans T et al (2008) Prehospital initiation of tirofiban in patients with ST-elevation myocardial infarction undergoing primary angioplasty (On-TIME 2): a multicentre, double-blind, randomised controlled trial. Lancet 372(9638):537–546

Antithrombotic Therapy in Interventional Cardiology

14

Antithrombotic Therapy in Percutaneous Coronary Intervention

Adrian W. Messerli

CONTENTS

INTRODUCTION
ANTIPLATELET THERAPY
ANTITHROMBIN THERAPY
FONDAPARINUX
SPECIAL POPULATIONS
FUTURE DIRECTIONS
REFERENCES

ABSTRACT A comprehensive understanding of periprocedural anticoagulation is an important component of interventional cardiovascular medicine. Rapid and ongoing advancement in adjunctive pharmacotherapy has made percutaneous coronary intervention (PCI) considerably safer, thereby facilitating the rapid international growth. Nevertheless, debate regarding the optimal pharmacologic ingredients and potency of anticoagulation for PCI persists. This chapter will review the specific value of antiplatelet and anticoagulant therapy to prevent thrombotic complications during PCI, targeting the most contemporary evidence available for each. The focus will be on agents that are routinely available and commonly used.

Key words: Antiplatelet; Antithrombotic; Antithrombin; Intervention; Platelets; Stents; Thrombosis

INTRODUCTION

For good reason, there are no universally accepted guidelines for periprocedural anticoagulation. Logically a number of variables must be taken into account prior to prescribing an antithrombotic regimen for any individual procedure. Patients undergoing PCI in the midst of an acute coronary syndrome (ACS) frequently require more aggressive antithrombotic and platelet aggregation inhibition than lower-risk patients undergoing elective PCI for stable angina pectoris. Similarly, generalizing antithrombotic regimen to a wide spectrum of catheter-based therapeutic devices is unreasonable. A level of anticoagulation that is safe and effective for routine angioplasty and stent placement may not be sufficient for devices with longer intracoronary dwell times such as brachytherapy or atherectomy

From: *Contemporary Cardiology: Antithrombotic Drug Therapy in Cardiovascular Disease*
Edited by: A.T. Askari and A.M. Lincoff (eds.), DOI 10.1007/978-1-60327-235-3_14
© Humana Press, a part of Springer Science+Business Media, LLC 2010

catheters. Perhaps most importantly, risk is a relatively subjective metric; different interventional cardiologists will have different definitions of high-risk lesions and high-risk patients. Nonetheless, the compilation of recently released randomized clinical trial data does provide for several broader recommendations.

ANTIPLATELET THERAPY

Aspirin

Aspirin, or acetylsalicylic acid (ASA), is the stalwart antiplatelet therapy for any percutaneous catheter-based procedure. Approximately, 35 million patients in the United States take ASA chronically (1). The Antithrombotic Trialists meta-analysis (2), which included over 200,000 ASA-treated patients, confirmed definitively that ASA is protective in patients specifically at risk for atheroembolic events, those with a prior history of stable or unstable angina, myocardial infarction, peripheral arterial disease, ischemic stroke, and/or atrial fibrillation. The ISIS-2 study affirmed the cardioprotective role of ASA in the setting of acute STEMI; a 23% reduction in mortality was observed versus placebo (3). Numerous other randomized controlled trials noted decreased mortality rates when ASA (75–325 mg) was given to hospitalized patients with an ACS (4–7).

Aspirin exerts its antiplatelet effect by acetylating and inactivating a key moiety of cyclooxygenase-I (COX-I), thereby preventing the formation of thromboxane A2 from arachidonic acid (1). In platelets, this effect is irreversible and persists for the circulating lifespan of the mature platelet, or roughly seven days. Although no trials have been published that specifically compare low dose versus higher doses of ASA in the setting of PCI, the ability of ASA to inhibit platelet aggregation and prevent thrombotic cardiovascular events makes its administration essential from both risk-benefit and cost-benefit standpoints. The available studies examining ASA administration in the setting of percutaneous coronary intervention are older, frequently included dipyridamole as a comparator or adjunct therapy (8), and revealed a significant reduction in their respective primary endpoints (ST-elevation myocardial infarction or acute vessel closure) in patients administered ASA. As such, an ASA is and should be routinely given to any nonallergic patient undergoing PCI.

Oral ASA achieves an appreciable antiplatelet effect within 60 min of administration (1). Chewed nonenteric-coated ASA has a more rapid bioavailability than swallowed tablets (1). While a lower-dose regimen is entirely effective and appropriate in the chronic condition, in an acute setting at least 325 mg should be given 2 h before intervention whenever possible (9). For elective PCI, ASA 325 mg should be administered at least 24 h before the proposed procedure (9).

The issue of ASA resistance (10,11) has recently confused physicians, specifically regarding appropriate dosing and loading time. Data suggest that between 5 and 60% of patients demonstrate some ASA antiplatelet resistance. In most of these studies, ASA efficacy was determined by effect on bleeding times, or by ability to inhibit platelet aggregation measured by whole blood aggregometry or a rapid platelet function assay. A recent study suggests, however, that aspirin resistance in platelets may be overestimated by these relatively nonspecific methods (12). Arachidonic-acid-induced light transmittance platelet aggregation (LTA) and thromboelastography (TEG) were performed in 223 patients (n=203 undergoing PCI; n=20 with a history of stent thrombosis) reportedly compliant with long-term daily ASA therapy. ASA resistance, defined as >20% aggregation by LTA or >50% aggregation by TEG, was noted in only one patient, suggesting that the true incidence may be quite low. Until the clinical impact and definition of ASA resistance are better defined, the subject has to be considered largely academic (see Chap. 24).

Thienopyridines

The two thienopyridines FDA-approved for clinical use are ticlopidine (Ticlid) and clopidogrel (Plavix) *(13)*. Thienopyridines inhibit the platelet P_{2Y12} type ADP receptor at the adenyl cyclase-coupled receptor site, leading to attenuation of platelet aggregation in response to ADP excreted by activated platelets *(13)* (Fig. 1). ASA and clopidogrel have been studied in comparison with one another, but thienopyridines and ASA most likely exert complementary and synergistic antiplatelet effects *(13)*.

Clopidogrel is preferentially prescribed both in and outside of the catheterization laboratory for several reasons. First, ticlopidine has a more toxic side effect profile, including agranulocytopenia (1% of patients) or thrombotic thrombocytopenic purpura (0.01%) *(14)*. Due to these potential adverse effects, white blood cell count monitoring is advisable for patients taking ticlopidine. In addition, clopidogrel loading, either with 300 mg or 600 mg oral boluses, is generally better tolerated than ticlopidine loading. Finally, ticlopidine is conventionally prescribed as a twice-daily drug, while clopidogrel needs to be taken once daily.

Dual antiplatelet therapy utilizing both ASA and a thienopyridine is currently the most effective regimen for prevention of acute thrombosis after coronary stent placement. The benefit of dual antiplatelet therapy in reducing stent thrombosis was initially demonstrated in a trial of 517 patients undergoing acute or elective stenting *(15)*. Patients who received ASA and ticlopidine were significantly less likely to experience a primary endpoint (death, MI, CABG or repeat PCI) than those receiving ASA, intravenous unfractionated heparin, and phenprocoumon (1.5% vs. 6.2%, respectively). These data were confirmed in a subsequent randomized clinical trial that compared ASA alone, ASA and ticlopidine, or ASA and coumadin in 1,653 low-risk patients undergoing stent placement *(16)*. The primary endpoint, comprising death, target lesion revascularization, subacute stent thrombosis, or MI, was only 0.5% in the ASA and ticlopidine group, versus 3.6% in the ASA alone group, and 2.7% in the ASA and coumadin group solidifying the role of post-PCI dual antiplatelet therapy

Clopidogrel: Dosing and Timing Prior to PCI

A growing body of evidence indicates that high loading doses of clopidogrel (300–600 mg) given two or more hours prior to an interventional procedure may reduce acute ischemic events at the time

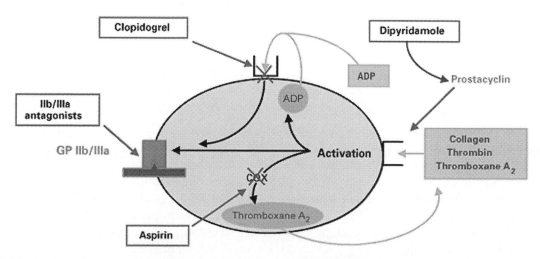

Fig. 1. Mechanism of action of antiplatelet drugs

of PCI. A 600-mg loading bolus appears to exert a more rapid early in vitro benefit than a 300-mg bolus (see later) *(17)*, and is informally being adopted as standard acute therapy in many emergency rooms and catheterization laboratories. Of note, the official AHA/ACC loading dose recommendation remains 300 mg *(9)*.

The foundation for the use of clopidogrel in ACS patients, the CURE trial *(18)*, randomized 12,562 patients with NSTEMI to either clopidogrel 300 mg loading bolus in the emergency room, followed by 75 mg daily for the subsequent year, or matching placebo. The primary endpoint, comprising death, MI, and stroke, was decreased by 20% at 1 year for those patients receiving clopidogrel. The effect of clopidogrel pretreatment and maintenance therapy on outcomes following stent placement was assessed in the PCI-CURE substudy *(19)*. Pretreatment with ASA, and clopidogrel significantly lowered the combined endpoint of death, MI, or target vessel revascularization at 30 days compared to matching placebo (4.5% vs. 6.4%, respectively) A significant benefit was also conferred in patients who received long-term clopidogrel therapy (31% reduction in cardiovascular death or MI was noted at 1 year).

The effect of preprocedural clopidogrel administration and the efficacy of long-term (12 months) treatment were examined among patients undergoing elective PCI in CREDO *(20)* where a 26.9% relative risk reduction (RRR) (8.5% vs. 11.5%; $p<0.02$) in the primary endpoint (composite of death, MI, stroke) was seen among patients randomized to receive clopidogrel for 1 year following PCI compared with those on placebo. The benefit of clopidogrel was at the expense of a significant increase in the number of major bleeding complications. CREDO post hoc subgroup analyses *(21)* also suggested that only those patients pretreated more than 6 h prior to elective PCI derived benefit (RRR 36.8%).

A subsequent series of trials have been published assessing the role of a higher loading dose of clopidogrel in various groups of patients undergoing PCI *(22–25)*. The ISAR-REACT trial *(22)* randomized over 2,000 stable angina patients who received a 600-mg dose of clopidogrel at least 2 h before PCI to periprocedural abciximab or placebo. The addition of abciximab to pretreatment with 600 mg of clopidogrel was not associated with any benefit with respect to the primary endpoint of death, myocardial infarction, and urgent TVR at 30 days; however, it was associated with a statistically significant increased incidence of thrombocytopenia and need of blood transfusions (1.9% vs. 0.7%) compared with placebo.

The first prospective, randomized trial (ARMYDA-2) *(23)* to evaluate the safety and efficacy of pretreatment with a 600-mg versus a 300-mg loading dose of clopidogrel in improving ischemic complications during elective PCI compared these loading doses (given 4–8 h before intervention) in 255 patients scheduled for PCI. The primary endpoint, death, myocardial infarction (MI), or target vessel revascularization at 30 days, occurred in 4% of patients in the high loading dose versus 12% of those in the conventional loading dose group ($p<0.041$), primarily due to decreased periprocedural MI. The absolute benefit was greatest in those patients taking statins. No difference in bleeding was appreciated.

Given the benefit of a 600-mg loading dose over a 300-mg loading dose, the logical next step was to ascertain whether or not even higher loading doses would exert additional or more rapid suppression of platelet function. The ISAR-CHOICE trial *(24)* measured the plasma concentrations of the active thiol metabolite, unchanged clopidogrel, and the inactive carboxyl metabolite of clopidogrel in 60 patients randomized to one of three clopidogrel loading doses (300, 600, or 900 mg) undergoing coronary angiography. Optical aggregometry, performed before and 4 h after administration, revealed that a 600-mg clopipdogrel loading dose was associated with higher plasma concentrations of the active metabolite, clopidogrel, and the carboxyl metabolite compared to a 300-mg dose translating into more potent inhibition of platelet aggregation 4 h after drug ingestion. No further incremental benefit was seen with the 900-mg loading dose. These data were corroborated in a higher-risk population as well *(26)*. However, given the modest size of both these trials, the clinical benefit of a 600-mg loading dose compared with a 300-mg loading dose remains to be more fully established. Accordingly, current guidelines recommend pretreatment with a 300-mg (or 600-mg) loading dose of clopidogrel at least 6 h before the procedure in those undergoing elective intervention, and those presenting with ACS whenever possible. In low- to intermediate-risk patients, clopidogrel pretreatment and a maintenance dose of aspirin and clopidogrel for at least 1 year after PCI are supported by the data, although the optimal duration of clopidogrel treatment beyond 1 year remains contested. It is reasonable to preload appropriately selected patients with clopidogrel prior to transfer for PCI at another facility, or if PCI is planned at a future time. If staged PCI is scheduled for a later date, clopidogrel 75 mg daily should be initiated least 3–5 days prior to the procedure, in order to ascertain maximal inhibition of platelet aggregation. In addition, all patients not at high risk for bleeding complications who undergo ad hoc PCI should receive at least a 300-mg loading dose just prior to stent deployment.

Pretreatment has certain clinical risk. For patients who undergo CABG surgery within five days after being treated with clopidogrel, there is an increased risk of bleeding, a greater need for transfusions, and an increased length of hospital stay (27). Therefore, open heart surgery should be delayed whenever possible while clopidogrel is withheld for the recommended 5–7 days.

Thienopyridine Therapy after Stent Deployment. After bare-metal stent (BMS) placement, a minimum of 4–6 weeks of thienopyridine therapy in addition to aspirin is recommended. Patients undergoing brachytherapy are at particularly high risk of acute and late thrombosis, and should be given a thienopyridine daily indefinitely (28).

Drug-eluting stents (DES) have reduced restenosis rates and the need for revascularization, but stent thrombosis, specifically subacute and late, remains an important limitation (29). While many of the specific clinical and angiographic variables that account for later stent thrombosis have yet to be defined, it appears that early termination of dual antiplatelet therapy poses substantial risk (Fig. 2). Appropriately, considerable attention has been devoted to defining guidelines for the optimal duration of dual antiplatelet therapy for patients receiving DES, specifically within the "vulnerable" period.

While recently published meta-analyses have not shown significant differences in stent thrombosis between DES and BMS (30,31), these studies largely incorporated cohorts that had undergone DES placement per "on-label" recommendations. However, other multicenter studies (32–34) noted appreciably higher cumulative stent thrombosis rates compared with BMS when DES were implanted in unselected patients with more complex coronary stenoses. Virmani et al (35) were among the first to suggest that delayed and incomplete endothelialization of DES could account for sudden cardiac death in select patients, based on their pathological postmortem examination. Subsequent intravascular ultrasound and angioscopic reports have corroborated that late stent thrombosis is likely due to inadequate endothelialization.

With the potential, but as of yet poorly defined, risk of late stent thrombosis, current consensus is to maintain dual antiplatelet therapy for at least 1 year in the absence of clinical or economic contraindications (9). Operators are advised to preferentially consider BMS in patients who are at increased risk of bleeding, have a pending surgical procedure, or have a history of medical nonadherence. If the thienopyridine needs to be discontinued before 1 year, a minimum of 3 months is advised after sirolimus DES implantation, and a minimum of 6 months after paclitaxel DES implantation (9).

Glycoprotein IIb/IIIa Receptor Inhibitors

Given that ASA and thienopyridines are relatively weak platelet antagonists the development of pharmaceuticals targeting the glycoprotein (GP) IIb/IIIa receptor, considered the final and "ultimate" pathway for platelet aggregation, logically ensued (36). There are three FDA-approved GP IIb/IIIa receptor antagonists available: abciximab (Reopro), eptifibatide (Integrilin), and tirofiban (Aggrastat). Abciximab is a chimeric (human/murine) monoclonal antibody (c7E3 Fab) that binds nonselectively to the GP IIb/IIIa receptor (37). The remaining two, eptifibatide and tirofiban, are small molecule

PROPOSED ALGORITHM:
PERIPROCEDURAL ANTICOAGULATION - ELECTIVE PCI

Before procedure:

- Aspirin 80-325 mg once daily; first dose at least 2 hours before procedure.
- Clopidogrel 75 mg once daily at least 3-5 days before the procedure[*]. A 300 mg loading dose is currently recommended prior to the procedure. A 600 mg oral bolus at least 2 hour before the procedure may be administered if PCI is planned on the same day.

During procedure:

- Unfractionated heparin bolus to achieve activated clotting time (ACT) 250-300 seconds. Give 70-100 U/kg or 7000U for women and 8000U for men. If ACT target is not achieved give extra bolus of 2500-5000 U. When GP IIb/IIIa receptor antagonists are added, the target ACT is reduced to 200-250 seconds; the recommended initial bolus is 50-70 U/kg.
- Enoxaparin may be selected in replacement of UFH. A preprocedural 0.75 mg/kg IV bolus is arguably better validated than a 0.5 mg/kg IV bolus.
- Bivalirudin may also be used as a foundation antithrombotic. It is indicated for patients with a history of HIT/HITTS. In addition, it should be considered preferentially in elderly patients (especially women), in patients with a history of renal failure, and in patients not adequately pretreated with clopidogrel.
- For high-risk patients, high-risk stenosis, or multivessel PCI consider adding a GP IIb/IIIa receptor blocker. If indicated, the bolus should be initiated at least 10 minutes before balloon inflation/stent deployment.

After procedure:

- Remove femoral sheath as soon as ACT falls below 150-180 seconds. Heparin infusions postprocedure should not be necessary for uncomplicated PCI.
- Bivalirudin may be discontinued at time of procedure completion.
- GP IIb/IIa inhibitor infusions conclude within 12-24 hours.
- ASA 325 mg should be continued for one month after bare-metal stent implantation, and for three months after sirolimus-eluting stent implantation, and for 6 months after paclitaxel-eluting stent implantation. Thereafter, 81 mg daily should be continued indefinitely.
- Clopidogrel 75 mg daily should be given for at least one month after bare-metal stent implantation, and for at least one year after drug-eluting stent implantation.

[*] Patients who are clopidogrel intolerant may be preloaded with ticlopidine 500mg orally bid X 48 hours;

Fig. 2. Proposed algorithm: periprocedural anticoagulation – elective PCI

inhibitors that bind the receptor selectively. As a result, they are associated with lower incidences of clinically meaningful thrombocytopenia.

Abciximab

The initial GP IIb/IIIa inhibitor trials tested abciximab, the most thoroughly studied agent in its class. The first large clinical trial testing the efficacy of GP IIb/IIIa antagonists was the EPIC trial *(38)*, randomized 2,099 high-risk patients to periprocedural abciximab bolus alone (0.25 mg/kg), abciximab bolus followed by 12-h infusion (0.1 mcg/min), or placebo. All patients received ASA and nonweight-adjusted unfractionated heparin (UFH) (10,000–12,000 IU). The cohort receiving abciximab bolus and infusion enjoyed a significant reduction in the combined endpoint of death, nonfatal MI, procedural failure, or repeat target vessel revascularization (TVR) (12.8% vs. 8.3% placebo; $p<0.008$)

at 30 days. This benefit was at the expense of increased bleeding complications *(39)*. Compared with placebo, the bolus and infusion of abciximab resulted in a doubling in the rates of major bleeding (7% vs. 14%, $p = 0.001$) and red blood cell transfusions (7% vs. 15%, $p < 0.001$). Adjunctive UFH therapy appeared to have played a key role in the pathogenesis of bleeding among these patients. In addition, femoral artery vascular access sheaths were left in place for the 12-h abciximab infusion, requiring ongoing UFH during that period.

EPILOG *(40)* addressed the issues of heparin dosing and time to sheath removal that plagued the EPIC trial. This trial randomized 2,972 lower-risk patients undergoing PCI to weight-adjusted UFH (100 IU/kg with a targeted ACT of 300 s); the same UFH dose with abciximab bolus and infusion, or UFH (70 IU/kg with a targeted ACT of 200 s) with abciximab. Again, compared with placebo, the 30-day composite endpoint (death, MI, urgent revascularization) was significantly lower for those patients receiving abciximab. The need for transfusion was significantly lower in the patients receiving lower-dose UFH, thereby making this weight-adjusted regimen of UFH the standard of care. All subsequent GP IIb/IIIa inhibitor trials have utilized low-dose weight-adjusted heparin regimens (60–70 U/kg bolus, adjusted as necessary to maintain ACT > 200–225 s), and the ACC/AHA guidelines *(9,41)* reflect these target doses. Of note, earlier sheath removal was also shown to impact positively on bleeding complications.

A wealth of data supports the use of a GP IIb/IIIa antagonist in patients presenting with ACS, especially those with high-risk features such as elevated cardiac biomarkers or dynamic electrocardiographic changes. Overall, the use of GP IIb/IIIa inhibitors reduces the incidence of thrombotic complications following PCI, is associated with a mortality benefit, but has no impact on the risk of restenosis. Building on the EPIC results, the CAPTURE investigators *(42)* assessed the role of periprocedural abciximab, given for 24 h prior to and for 1 h after PCI, in patients with refractory unstable angina. The rate of MI was significantly lower for those patients receiving abciximab both before and after PCI, as was the composite 30-day endpoint of death, MI, or urgent revascularization.

The role of abciximab in the setting of PCI for acute STEMI has been evaluated in several trials with conflicting results. The ADMIRAL trial *(43)* randomized 300 patients to either abciximab or placebo with stent deployment for the treatment of STEMI. The most noteworthy finding was that prehospital abciximab initiation led to better infarct-related artery patency, left ventricular function, and a reduction in reinfarction and recurrent ischemia. Utilizing an intention-to-treat analysis, the investigator reported that the cohort receiving abciximab had a 25% relative risk reduction in all-case mortality at 3 years. The CADILLAC trial *(44)* randomized 2,082 patients with STEMI were randomized to undergo balloon angioplasty alone, balloon angioplasty plus abciximab, BMS alone, or BMS plus abciximab. At 6 months, the composite primary endpoint of death, recurrent MI, stroke, or TVR occurred in 20% after balloon angioplasty, 16.5% balloon angioplasty with abciximab, 11.5% BMS alone, and 10.2% BMS with abciximab ($p < 0.001$). Importantly, there were no significant differences in mortality, stroke, or revascularization; the primary endpoint was powered mostly by the difference in ischemia-driven TVR. Conceivably, the routine administration of "upstream" abciximab in ADMIRAL accounted for the more robust clinical benefit.

Even patients with ACS who are preloaded with a thienopyridine seem to derive benefit from periprocedural abciximab. The ISAR-REACT 2 trial *(45)* randomized 2,022 patients with ACS undergoing PCI and preloaded with clopidogrel (600 mg at least 2 h prior to procedure) to abciximab or placebo. Specifically in those patients with elevated troponins, abciximab administration still significantly reduced the risk of adverse events at 30 days.

The GUSTO-IV trial *(46)* randomized 7,800 patients with ACS who were not undergoing rapid revascularization to placebo, abciximab bolus plus 24 h infusion, or abciximab bolus plus 48 h infusion. No significant clinical benefit was noted in those patients receiving either abciximab regimen compared to placebo; in fact the incidence of bleeding complications was increased in patients receiving abciximab compared with those receiving placebo. Based on these results, abciximab is not recommended in patients with ACS unless PCI is planned within 24 h.

Eptifibatide and Tirofiban

The initial trials to test eptifibatide did not note statistically significant differences in clinical outcomes when compared to placebo, likely due to inadequate dosing. The PURSUIT investigators *(47)* tested a relatively higher dose in patients with ACS. Specifically, 10,948 patients were randomized into one of three arms: eptifibatide180 mcg/kg bolus followed by 1.3 mcg/kg/min infusion, eptifibatide 180 mcg/kg bolus followed by 2.0 mcg/kg/min infusion, or placebo. The cohort receiving the highest infusion dose of eptifibatide derived the greatest clinical benefit, namely a significant 30-day reduction in death or MI when compared to placebo (14.2% vs. 15.7%; $p<0.04$). Just as important, those patients receiving higher-dose eptifibatide and who underwent rapid revascularization (PCI$<$72 h) derived an even greater benefit (11.6% vs. 16.7% placebo).

ESPRIT *(48)* was subsequently designed to test an even more aggressive dose of eptifibatide. In this trial, 2,064 patients undergoing PCI were randomized to either eptifibatide, administered in two boluses (180 mcg/kg) given 10 min apart followed by an 18–24 h infusion (2.0 mcg/kg), or placebo. The primary endpoint, comprising death, MI, or urgent TVR ,at 30 days was lower in the eptifibatide arm versus placebo (6.8% vs. 10.5%; $p<0.0035$). As a result, this dose and infusion remains the recommended and standard regimen to date.

The PRISM-PLUS trial *(49)* randomized 1,915 patients with ACS to either UFH and tirofiban (0.4 mcg/kg/min bolus given over 30 min, followed by 0.1 mg/kg/min infusion) or UFH alone. A reduction in the composite endpoint (death, MI, recurrent ischemia) was noted in the tirofiban arm, both at 1 week (12.9% vs. 17.9%; $p<0.005$) and 6 months (27.7% vs. 32.1%; $p=0.02$). Again, the greatest clinical benefit was derived in those patients who underwent early revascularization.

In PURSUIT and PRISM-PLUS the majority of patients did not undergo PCI during their initial hospitalization. However, these patients still derived clinical benefit from receiving GP IIb/IIIa antagonists. A meta-analysis *(50)* of PRISM-PLUS, PURSUIT, CAPTURE revealed a statistically significant absolute risk reduction in death/MI of 1.4% was observed with GP IIb/IIIa inhibition during the period of pharmacologic therapy initiated "upstream" before PCI. As a result of these data, eptifibatide or tirofiban administration is reasonable for the medical management of high-risk patients regardless of whether intervention is planned.

The subset of patients who appear to derive no benefit from GP IIb/IIIa inhibition are those who need aortocoronary saphenous vein graft intervention. A pooled analysis of five trials *(51)* including 627 patients undergoing graft intervention did not observe a benefit in terms of adverse event reduction with routine administration of GP IIb/IIIa antagonist either at 30 days or at 6 months. Vein graft disease mostly comprises friable plaque at specifically high risk for embolization, and platelet inhibition may be of secondary importance compared to routine application of distal protection. Instead, these interventions should be performed under cover of aggressive boluses of antithrombotic agents (UFH for a target ACT$>$300 s).

ANTITHROMBIN THERAPY

Unfractionated Heparin

Unfractionated heparin (UFH) is the most widely used anticoagulant during PCI and has served as the backbone anticoagulant for nearly 50 years *(52)*. UFH is a heterogeneous mixture of polysaccharide chains, ranging in size from 5,000 to 40,0000 daltons that potentiate the ability of antithrombin to inactivate thrombin (Factor IIa) and Factor Xa. Although UFH is nearly universally utilized, it has several important pharmacokinetic and clinical limitations. Only about 33% of UFH chains have the appropriate pentasaccharide antithrombin-binding sequence, and UFH binds unpredictably to different plasma proteins, accounting for variable anticoagulation. Additional important limitations, especially for an interventional cardiologist, include UFH's ability to paradoxically stimulate platelet aggregation and inability to neutralize fibrin-bound thrombus. Also, platelet factor 4 binding may blunt its efficacy, and it confers a significant risk of heparin-induced thrombocytopenia (HIT) and/or thrombosis syndrome (HITTS) (53).

UFH administration should be carefully monitored, although the ideal level of anticoagulation, as determined by activated clotting time (ACT), has yet to be consensually defined (see later). According to the guidelines (9) for antithrombotic therapy in patients undergoing PCI recently published by the American College of Cardiology and American Heart Association, target ACT values are 250–300 s with the HemoTec (Medtronics, Minneapolis, Minn) device and 300–350 s with the Hemachron (International Technidyne, Edison, NJ) device (54). A weight-adjusted initial bolus of 60–100 U/kg UFH is recommended. When GP IIb/IIIa receptor antagonists are added, the target ACT is reduced to 200–250 s with either device; the recommended initial bolus is 50–70 U/kg UFH.

Weight-adjusted UFH dosing became the standard after trials utilizing fixed-dose boluses of UFH had inconsistent results. Most notably, the landmark EPIC trial (38) observed that routine administration of higher-dose boluses (10,000 IU) of UFH was associated with higher rates of hemorrhagic complications. In contradistinction, several observational series using fixed low-dose UFH have demonstrated relatively consistent efficacy and safety (55–59). One group used a conservative bolus, 2,500 IU (achieving a mean ACT of 185 s), in a relatively high-risk cohort (>50% had unstable angina) and reported a high angiographic success rate (96%) coupled with low in-hospital mortality/myocardial infarction (<1%) and abrupt closure (2%) (56). Only 16% of these patients received a GP IIb/IIIa inhibitor. A third series administered only 1,000 IU bolus to those patients undergoing PCI, or for those patients already on heparin, had the infusion stopped upon arrival in the catheterization laboratory (58). All patients received aspirin and a thienopyridine, as well as routine abciximab. Seventy-five percent of the 500 patients enrolled had either unstable angina or a history of recent MI. The reported procedural success was 99.8%, while the incidence of major bleeding complications was only 0.2%. Importantly, none of these series were randomized or controlled, but the results challenge the concept that high doses of UFH are routinely necessary to achieve therapeutic benefit.

A recent meta-analysis (60), comprising the CREDO (20), CAPTURE (42), REPLACE-1 (61) and 2 (62) data, examined the relationship between ACT and ischemic or bleeding complications. Of the 9,974 patients in the four trials, ACT data were available in 8,369 (84%); all patients received aspirin, and pretreatment with clopidogrel was encouraged. Final analysis noted that ACT across all levels did not correlate with ischemic complications and had only a modest association with bleeding complications, mostly driven by minor bleeding. Importantly, lower values, defined as 5,000 U total dose or 60–90 U/kg, did not compromise efficacy, but were safer. Another analysis (63) of 2,064 patients in the ESPRIT trial, all of whom received a stent, noted that an ACT target of 200–250 s was safe and effective, regardless of whether or not an adjunctive IIb/IIIa was administered. Approximately 97% of ESPRIT patients received a thienopyridine, and the vast majority had a stent deployed, making these results particularly applicable to contemporary PCI. As such, in current-day practice, a target ACT of 200–250 s may be sufficient, especially if the patient has been appropriately preloaded with clopidogrel. A more conservative UFH bolus of 50–70 IU/kg is advised whenever the use of a GP IIb/IIIa inhibitor is anticipated.

As would be expected, the risk of UFH-associated bleeding increases with dose and with concomitant GP IIb/IIIa inhibitor therapy. Because of the evidence that the PTT is related to patient outcomes, and that the predominant variable mediating the effect of UFH is weight, it is important to administer the initial dose as a weight-adjusted bolus. One important advantage of UFH is it generally does not require dose adjustment for renal dysfunction. In contrast, LMWH, danaparoid sodium, hirudin, and bivalirudin all undergo renal clearance and need to be adjusted accordingly in patients with renal failure.

Low Molecular Weight Heparins

LMWHs are derived from UFH through either chemical or enzymatic depolymerization, resulting in shorter molecules weighing 4,000–5,000 daltons (64). The LMWHs also bind antithrombin via the same pentasaccharide sequence as UFH, but only about 25–50% of the chains are long enough to do so. Therefore, the majority of anticoagulant effect is due to Factor X inhibition; the LMWHs have anti-Xa to anti-IIa ratios between 2:1 and 4:1. The LMWHs bind less strongly to protein, which allows for enhanced and relatively predictable bioavailability. They also activate platelets to a lesser extent, and are more resistant to platelet factor 4 inhibition. Finally, immune-mediated thrombocytopenia is rarely associated with short-term use of LMWH. The relative disadvantages of LMWH compared to UFH include cost, lack of an easily interpretable and standardized point-of care-test, and inability to rapidly reverse its anticoagulant effect. Protamine sulfate only reverses about 60% of LMWH's anti-Xa activity.

A growing body of evidence supports the use of LMWH during PCI, although concerns remain regarding bleeding complications, especially with enoxaparin (Lovenox). LMWH has gained particularly wide acceptance in patients with ACS. The larger randomized trials to date have been conducted using enoxaparin and, more recently, fondaparinux.

The current ACC/AHA guidelines (9) suggest that enoxaparin may be preferable (Class IIa) to UFH in setting of UA/NSTEMI. However, many proceduralists continue to use LMWH reluctantly, perhaps because, until recently, the majority of trial evidence included patients who were largely managed conservatively. In contrast, formal guidelines had increasingly advocated an early invasive therapy, followed by rapid revascularization whenever possible. Two large, randomized trials recently completed addressed the role of LMWH in ACS patients destined for an early invasive strategy; SYNERGY (65), comparing UFH versus enoxaparin for high-risk ACS patients undergoing early invasive strategy, and the A branch (66) of the A-to- Z, compared UFH versus enoxaparin in the context of NSTEMI patients also treated with tirofiban. SYNERGY noted essentially no differences in outcomes or bleeding, while the A-to-Z trial investigators reported a 1% absolute risk reduction in the risk of death/MI/recurrent ischemia at 7 days with enoxaparin. In SYNERGY, enoxaparin was associated with a statistically significant increase in TIMI major bleeding (9.1% vs. 7.6%). In A-to-Z, TIMI major or minor bleeding occurred in 3% versus 2.2% in the enoxaparin and UFH groups, respectively, a statistically insignificant difference.

An accompanying large meta-analysis (67), incorporating the results of SYNERGY and A-to-Z along with four older trials, noted a 0.9% absolute reduction in the combined risk of death/MI at 30 days. This benefit was completely driven by a reduction in MI; the rate of death after 30 days was 3% for both enoxaparin and UFH. No significant difference in major bleeding was appreciated; minor bleeding was increased in the LMWH group. The authors concluded that LMWH was an effective substitute for UFH, with a trend toward nonfatal MI with a modest increase in bleeding risk.

In the ESSENCE (68) and TIMI-11B (69) trials, LMWH therapy was discontinued before catheterization, and interventional procedures were performed using UFH. Rates of major hemorrhage were similar in patients receiving either LMWH or UFH. Perhaps as a result, many interventionalists became comfortable with a "crossover" strategy when anticoagulating their own patients. This may explain why, in the SYNERGY trial *(65)*, nearly 800 patients received postrandomization "crossover" therapy before PCI. Surprisingly, this group experienced a markedly elevated risk of adverse events; the risk of receiving a blood transfusion more than doubled (15.2% vs. 31.5%) while the 30-day incidence of death/ MI increased from 13.9% to 18.5%. GP IIb/IIIa inhibitors may be coadministered with LMWH as clinically indicated without concern for increased bleeding. The NICE-3 registry *(70)* specifically examined the safety of enoxaparin in conjunction with GP IIb/IIIa administration in patients 661 presenting with ACS. The specific GP IIb/IIIa used was left to the discretion of the operator. If enoxaparin had been given within the prior 8 h, no additional dose was administered. If a dose had been given more than 8 h prior, an additional 0.3 mg/kg IV was intravenously injected. For those patients undergoing PCI, the researchers reported an observed primary endpoint (major bleeding) of 1%, which compared favorably to historical controls. However, event rates for transfusion, minor bleeding, or death/MI in PCI patients were not reported.

The role of LMWH in elective PCI is evolving, although support for its utilization is growing. The REDUCE trial *(71)* was a large, randomized trial that compared LMWH and UFH specifically during elective cardiac catheterization. In this trial, 612 patients undergoing single vessel PCI were randomly assigned to receive either reviparin (7,000 IU IV followed by an 18- to 24-h infusion) or UFH (10,000 IU followed by an IV infusion). Reviparin was subsequently continued as a twice-daily SQ injection for 28 days, with the UFH-treated group receiving matching placebo injections. In reviparin-treated patients, the requirement for bailout intervention was significantly reduced (2.0% vs. 6.9% with UFH treatment, $p=0.003$), as was the occurrence of major ischemic complications during the first few days of the trial. At 30 weeks, the composite endpoint of death, MI, or need for repeat intervention was similar in both groups (33% for reviparin vs. 32% for UFH), as was the incidence of major hemorrhage (2.5% for reviparin vs. 2.6% for UFH). A small study *(72)* examined the efficacy and safety of a prespecified low dose of intravenous enoxaparin (0.5 mg/kg) in 242 patients undergoing elective PCI. They enrolled these patients consecutively, regardless of age, weight, renal function, or use of GP IIb/IIIa inhibitors (26%). Sheaths were pulled immediately after the procedure in those patients receiving only enoxaparin, and 4 h after the procedure in those also treated with eptifibatide. A consistent prespecified anticoagulation level was achieved, regardless of advanced age, renal failure, obesity, and eptifibatide use. In addition, the incidence of bleeding complications was relatively low, as was the incidence of ischemic complications.

These results paved the road for the STEEPLE trial *(73)*, which enrolled 3,528 patients undergoing nonurgent PCI and randomized to one of two doses of IV weight-adjusted enoxaparin (0.5 or 0.75 mg/kg) or ACT-directed UFH. The concomitant use of GP IIb/IIIa inhibitors was left to the discretion of the operators; sheaths were removed immediately after the procedure. The primary endpoint of the trial was the incidence of major and minor bleeding at 48 h after the index PCI (excluding bypass graft [CABG] bleeding). The main secondary endpoint was the achievement of therapeutic anticoagulation at the beginning and end of the procedure. Enoxaparin was associated with reduced bleeding. The incidence of major and minor bleeding (primary endpoint) was 31% lower in the enoxaparin 0.5-mg/kg group (5.9% vs. 8.5%, $p=0.01$), which was statistically significant for superiority, while the enoxaparin 0.75-mg/kg group was noninferior to UFH (6.5% vs. 8.5%, $p=0.051$). Major bleeding was also reduced by 57% in both enoxaparin groups versus UFH. The study also showed that enoxaparin is associated with a fourfold increase in the rate of patients achieving target anticoagulation levels compared with UFH (79% for enoxaparin 0.5 mg/kg and 92% for enoxaparin 0.75 mg/kg versus 20% for UFH [$p<0.001$]). Based on the available data, LMWH appear at least as safe and efficacious as UFH for patients undergoing elective PCI *(74)*, although the STEEPLE trial was not adequately powered to demonstrate noninferiority of low-dose enoxaparin regimens with UFH with regard to ischemic endpoints.

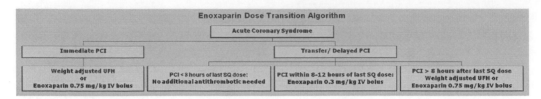

Fig. 3. Enoxaparin dose transition algorithm

In short, LMWHs have a more predictable anticoagulant effect than UFH and may be preferred in NSTEMI/UA patients. Factor Xa levels are effectively inhibited within 30 min and remain so for at least 8 h after injection of a single 1 mg/kg subcutaneous dose of enoxaparin. Therefore, in ACS patients who have received enoxaparin, PCI may be safely performed within this 8-h window without additional dosing. If the procedure takes place within 8–12 h, an additional 0.3 mg/kg intravenous injection is advised. "Crossover" anticoagulation from UFH to LMWH or vice versa should be avoided; the anticoagulant that the patient received prior arriving in the catheterization laboratory should be continued (Fig. 3). Elderly patients, or patients with impaired renal function, should preferentially receive UFH or bivalirudin. Elective PCI with LMWH anticoagulation appears to be safe and effective. However the available data have yet to conclusively demonstrate a clinical advantage for LMWH over UFH.

FONDAPARINUX

Fondaparinux (Arixtra) binds specifically to antithrombin, giving a very specific inhibition of Xa without interfering with other clotting factors, and is already established as an effective therapy in the prevention of asymptomatic and symptomatic venous thromboembolic events *(75)*. The OASIS 5 trial *(76)* was a large, randomized, double-blind, multicenter study designed to evaluate the safety and efficacy of fondaparinux compared with enoxaparin in patients with ACS. The study included 20,078 patients enrolled from 576 sites in 41 countries and randomized them to either fondaparinux 2.5 mg ($n = 10,057$) or enoxaparin 1 mg/kg twice daily ($n = 10,021$). Fondaparinux was associated with a significant reduction in 30-day mortality as well as a decreased incidence of major bleeding compared with enoxaparin. Furthermore, the beneficial effect of fondaparinux appeared to be durable with a 9% reduction in the risk of death or MI and a 13% reduction in the risk of death, MI, refractory ischemia, or major bleeding at 6 months. Despite the apparent benefit of fondaparinux, it currently cannot be endorsed as an adequate antithrombin therapy for the contemporary management of patients with ACS because of the increased incidence of catheter thrombosis seen in patients undergoing PCI.

In the OASIS-6 trial *(77)*, 12,092 patients with STEMI were randomized to receive fondaparinux (2.5 mg daily) or usual care for up to 8 days. Usual care was PTT-directed IV UFH for up to 48 h followed by placebo, or just placebo when UFH was not indicated. Of the entire cohort, 45% received fibrinolysis (mostly streptokinase), 29% underwent primary PCI, and 24% did not receive reperfusion therapy. The incidence of death or reinfarction at 30 days was significantly lower with fondaparinux than with usual care (9.7% vs. 11.2%), with significant benefits also at 9 days and at final follow up (3–6 months). Fondaparinux recipients also had significantly lower mortality rates throughout the study and a trend toward less major bleeding. Notably, the benefits of fondaparinux did not extend specifically to patients who underwent primary PCI secondary to significantly more catheter thromboses in this subgroup (1.2% vs. 0%).

Bivalirudin

Direct-acting thrombin inhibitors, namely hirudin and its analogs, have several important conceptual advantages over heparin. These agents bind specifically and reversibly to both fibrin-bound and unbound thrombin, do not require a cofactor such as antithrombin III, and have no known natural inhibitors, such as platelet factor 4, thereby allowing for a more predictable and uniform anticoagulation *(78)*. Bivalirudin (Angiox, Angiomax) is a synthetic 20-amino acid peptide analog of hirudin. The drug demonstrates linear pharmacokinetics, allowing for a direct correlation between dose and anticoagulation activity, and is cleared through a combination of proteolytic cleavage and renal elimination. Bivalirudin is dialyzable; approximately 25% is cleared by hemodialysis. Accordingly, dosage adjustments are recommended in patients with moderate-to-severe renal impairment and in dialysis-dependent patients.

It has been approved in Europe for use as an anticoagulant in patients undergoing PCI. In the United States, bivalirudin is approved in patients undergoing PCI in conjunction with ASA administration and has recently been approved for use with provisional GP IIb/IIIa inhibition. To date, bivalirudin has been tested in large elective PCI, ACS, and STEMI cohorts.

REPLACE-2 *(62)*, a randomized, double-blinded study, sought to determine whether the use of bivalirudin plus provisional GPIIb/IIIa use ($n = 2,994$) during elective or urgent PCI would reduce the incidence of major adverse ischemic complications compared with UFH and GP IIb/IIIa inhibitors. A total of 6,010 patients (6,002 for follow-up) were recruited in 233 hospitals in 9 countries; the study's primary endpoint consisted of a quadruple composite measure of death, MI, urgent revascularization, and major hemorrhage at 30 days. All patients were treated with aspirin therapy, and more than 85% received pretreatment with a thienopyridine. For bivalirudin, dosing was a 0.75-mg/kg bolus before PCI, then a 1.75-mg/kg-h infusion for the duration of PCI; the pre-PCI bolus of UFH was 65 U/kg. The anticoagulation strategy of bivalirudin and provisional GP IIb/IIIa inhibitor resulted in a numerically reduced incidence of the composite endpoint compared to UFH and routine GP IIb/IIIa inhibition, while the incidence of NSTEMI was higher in the former group. Neither of these differences reached statistical significance. The incidence of major bleeding, need for transfusion, and thrombocytopenia was significantly lower in the bivalirudin cohort however. At 1 year follow-up, the death rate was numerically, but not significantly, lower in the bivalirudin group.

In the ACUITY trial *(79)*, the largest study yet performed in patients with ACS undergoing an invasive strategy, 13,819 patients with ACS (randomized at 448 centers in 17 countries) were prospectively randomized to UFH or enoxaparin plus GPIIb/IIIa inhibition, versus bivalirudin plus GPIIb/IIIa inhibition, versus bivalirudin and provisional GPIIb/IIIa inhibition. All patients underwent cardiac catheterization within 72 h, followed by percutaneous or surgical revascularization when appropriate. In a second random assignment, patients assigned to receive IIb/IIIa inhibitors were subrandomized to upstream drug initiation versus GPIIb/IIIa inhibitor administration during angioplasty only. The primary study endpoint was the composite of death, myocardial infarction, unplanned revascularization for ischemia, and major bleeding at 30 days.

Compared with the UFH/enoxaparin plus GPIIb/IIIa inhibition, treatment with bivalirudin alone was associated with a significant reduction in the 30-day clinical outcome from 11.7% to 10.1% ($p = 0.015$). However, the bivalirudin plus GPIIb/IIIa inhibitor group was only noninferior to UFH/enoxaparin plus GPIIb/IIIa inhibition at 11.8%. The 30-day composite ischemic outcome was similar in all three groups at approximately 7.5%. Major bleeding was significantly lower in the bivalirudin alone group at 3% compared with 5.7% in the UFH or enoxaparin plus GPIIb/IIIa inhibitor group. Patients given bivalirudin plus a GPIIb/IIIa inhibitor had a 5.3% rate of major bleeding, which was noninferior to the rate seen in the UFH or enoxaparin plus a GPIIb/IIIa inhibitor.

ACUITY-PCI *(80)* was made up of the 7,789 patients from the ACUITY trial who underwent PCI during the trial. Drug-eluting-stent use in these patients was roughly 60% in all three groups: those receiving UFH/enoxaparin plus GP IIb/IIIa inhibitors; those receiving bivalirudin plus GP IIb/IIIa inhibitors; and those receiving bivalirudin monotherapy, with randomization roughly equal among the three groups. In an intention-to-treat analysis, the 30-day primary endpoints – composite ischemia (death, MI, or unplanned revascularization for ischemia), major bleeding or net clinical outcomes (major bleeding or composite ischemia) –were not significantly different between the groups receiving bivalirudin plus GP IIb/IIIa inhibitor or a heparin plus GP IIb/IIIa inhibitors. Composite ischemia rates were similar between the two groups; however, major bleeding was significantly lower in the bivalirudin-only group at 30 days, as compared with the group receiving either heparin plus GP IIb/IIIa inhibitors. Unlike the main ACUITY trial, the net clinical benefit (combining ischemic and bleeding events) was no different between the UFH/enoxaparin plus GP-IIb/IIIa-inhibitor and the bivalirudin-only groups. However, in troponin-positive patients, and in patients who received clopidogrel pretreatment, rates of composite ischemic events tended to be higher in the bivalirudin-only group versus the UFH/enoxaparin plus GP-IIb/IIIa-inhibitor group.

HORIZONS AMI *(81)* randomized more than 3,600 patients (123 centers in 11 countries) with STEMI with symptom onset <12 h in a 1:1 fashion to UFH 60 U/kg IV, with subsequent boluses titrated by nomogram to ACT of 200–250 s, plus a GP IIb/IIIa inhibitor (abciximab or eptifibatide), or to bivalirudin monotherapy (0.75 mg/kg bolus; infusion 1.75 mg/kg per h), stopped at the end of the procedure, plus provisional GP IIb/IIIa inhibitors for large thrombus or refractory no-flow. Only 7.2% of patients in the bivalirudin-treated group received provisional GP IIb/IIIa inhibitors in the cath lab. Bivalirudin significantly reduced net adverse clinical events by 24% at 30 days (a composite of major bleeding and MACE) as well as major bleeding alone by 40%, as compared with UFH plus a GP IIb/IIIa inhibitor.

Bivalirudin has not consistently demonstrated superiority to heparins in providing protection against cardiovascular ischemic events, but it has reduced bleeding complications. In fact, a recent meta-analysis *(82)* incorporating five randomized controlled trials comparing bivalirudin to the heparins in 25,457 patients with ACS, including those patients undergoing PCI, demonstrated a significantly lower risk of major bleeding (defined as intracranial, intraocular, or retroperitoneal hemorrhage; clinically overt blood loss leading to a hemoglobin drop exceeding 3 g/dL or transfusion of 2 or more units of whole blood or packed red blood cells) with bivalirudin. Compared to the heparins, the risk of death, MI, revascularization, and composite ischemic endpoints were similar with bivalirudin monotherapy.

Bivalirudin may be particularly appropriate in higher-risk populations, specifically women, the elderly (>65 years), and in patients with renal impairment (serum creatinine >1.2 mg/dL). It may be an alternative to heparin plus planned GP IIb/IIIa inhibition in any patient undergoing urgent or elective PCI, especially in any patient with a high risk of bleeding complications. In addition, bivalirudin is usually the anticoagulant of choice in patients with a history of HIT/HITTS *(83)*. Up to 5% of patients administered UFH develop HIT/HITTS, which is associated with a dramatic increase in morbidity and mortality *(52)*. The ATBAT trial *(84)* evaluated the safety and efficacy of direct thrombin inhibition with bivalirudin during PCI in patients with HIT or HITTS. Over 4 years, this multicenter trial recruited 52 patients; the investigators reported a low incidence of major (1 patient) and minor (7 patients) bleeding complications. None of the patients developed thrombocytopenia. In December 2005 the U.S. Food and Drug Administration (FDA) approved the use of bivalirudin in patients with or at risk of HIT/HITTS undergoing PCI *(83)*.

SPECIAL POPULATIONS

Women

Even though more women than men die each year from heart disease *(85)*, women tend to be referred less frequently for diagnostic cardiac catheterization *(86)*. As a result, only about one-third of the 1.2 million patients undergoing PCIs annually in the United States are women *(87)*. More worrisome yet, women tend to have higher rates of complications and in-hospital mortality after PCI *(88)*, both elective and emergent, albeit much of this difference is attributable to higher-risk clinical characteristics. Fortunately, once beyond the acute hospitalization, adjusted long-term mortality rates after PCI are roughly equivalent *(89–91)*.

Compared to men, women have a twofold to fourfold increased risk of vascular complications such as arteriotomy-associated hematomas, retroperitoneal bleeds, and need for blood transfusions *(92)*. Proceduralists are generally aware of this discrepancy and attempt to attenuate bleeding risk by whatever means possible. Paradoxically, in an effort to prevent major bleeding, especially intracranial hemorrhage, women might receive subtherapeutic antiplatelet and antithrombotic dosing, thereby increasing their risk for ischemic complications.

The ACC/AHA guidelines *(9)* advise that lower doses of UFH should be used in patients undergoing PCI at high risk of bleeding, including women and older adults. Although LMWH and UFH have not been formally compared in an exclusively female population, about 30% of the patients enrolled in the SYNERGY *(65)* and A-to-Z *(66)* ACS trials were female. Again, neither study noted a benefit for either therapy in either men or women, but LMWH was associated with a small increase in risk of bleeding.

Similarly, bivalirudin has not been evaluated in an exclusively female cohort, but about 26% of the patients in the REPLACE-2 trial *(62)* were women. The use of bivalirudin was associated with a significant reduction in major bleeding complications in women. Both major and minor bleeding was significantly reduced ($p<0.0001$) from 34.1% with UFH plus GP IIb/IIIa inhibitor to 19.7% with bivalirudin.

Antiplatelet therapy should not be specifically modified for women undergoing PCI. The CREDO trial *(20)* ($n=2,116$, 29% female) which treated patients undergoing PCI with clopidogrel for up to 1 year noted a nonsignificant 32% relative risk reduction in the combined endpoint of stroke, MI, or death in women. In the ISAR-REACT trial *(22)* ($n=2,159$, 24% women), no additional benefit for the GP IIb/IIIa inhibitor abciximab was found among low-risk PCI patients pretreated with a 600-mg loading dose of clopidogrel. The combined endpoint, comprising of death, MI, and target vessel revascularization at 30 days, did not differ between the two groups in either the entire cohort or specifically in the female subset.

As in the general population, GP IIb/IIIa inhibitor administration is usually beneficial in women undergoing PCI. A meta-analysis *(93)* of ten randomized, placebo-controlled trials of GP IIb/IIIa inhibitors as periprocedural antiplatelet therapy ($n=13\,166$, 26% women) noted a significant reduction in the combined endpoint of death or nonfatal MI 6 months after PCI. Importantly higher-risk patients, including elderly women, appeared to derive the greatest benefit. Contrary to conventional belief, GP IIb/IIIa inhibitors are not associated with an increase in major bleeding or vascular complications in women *(94,95)*. They do confer increased risk for minor bleeding, however.

Renal Failure

Patients with renal failure are at increased risk of both thrombotic and bleeding complications *(96–98)*. Whenever these patients undergo primary PCI in the setting of an acute MI, they incur an increased risk of acute reocclusion and major hemorrhage, thereby increasing their risk of mortality significantly. As such, a creatinine clearance should be calculated as a matter of routine for every patient who presents for a catheterization laboratory procedure. Estimation of renal function is needed when prescribing certain drugs to any patient with renal dysfunction. Specifically, dose adjustment of many anticoagulants is indicated when the creatinine clearance falls below 30 mL/min. While dosing is usually appropriately made in patient with elevated serum creatinine, elderly patients, due to age-related renal dysfunction and smaller body mass index, often have reduced creatinine clearance and may be inadvertently overlooked.

UFH generally does not require dose adjustment. Careful monitoring of ACT level is recommended, however, because these patients are vulnerable to bleeding complications with higher levels of anticoagulation. By contrast, LMWH, danaparoid sodium, hirudins, and bivalirudin all undergo renal clearance. Conservative dosing is advised whenever these agents are used in patients with renal failure. LMWHs are excreted nearly completely via the kidneys. The serum half-life of LMWH averages about 2–4 h after IV injection, and 3–6 h following a SC injection. Dosing of the subcutaneous LMWH enoxaparin in ACS patients undergoing coronary angiogram and coronary angioplasty should be reduced by at least 50% (1 mg/kg per 24 h) in patients with severe renal failure (99).

A modestly sized ($n=170$) single hospital pharmacokinetic study (100) attempted to adjust enoxaparin dosing in response to serum anti-Xa levels. After a bolus of enoxaparin 1 mg/kg SC, patients with a creatinine clearance of 30–60 mL received subsequent boluses of 0.75 mg/kg SC every 12 h, while those with a creatinine clearance < or = 30 mL/min received a 0.50 mg/kg per dose SC every 12 h. The investigators noted that about 80% of percent of patients with moderate renal failure and 60% of the patients with severe renal failure were in the therapeutic anti-Xa range after the third dose. A dose-adjustment ratio New dose=[(Current dose)×(Goal anti-Xa level)]/(Current anti-Xa level) was used to adjust doses in patients whose levels were outside the therapeutic range. This formulation reliably placed patients in the therapeutic range established by consensus guidelines; the incidence of bleeding was noted to be equivalent to normal controls. Obviously, this cleverly designed protocol will need to be validated in larger studies, but the concept of pharmacokinetic-based adjustments based on renal failure seems logical.

Clinical trials specifically addressing the efficacy of aspirin among patients with renal failure undergoing PCI have not been performed. Aspirin is largely hepatically metabolized, but a fraction is also renally excreted (1). Given aspirin's proven track record, however, one should refrain from adjusting the dose in renally impaired patients. Importantly, ASA is dialyzed significantly. Postdialysis dosing is recommended in patient acutely requiring consistent aspirin therapy (i.e., recent stent placement). Clopidogrel and ticlopidine are hepatically metabolized; dose adjustment is not required (13).

There exist few data supporting the efficacy and safety of GP IIb/IIIa inhibitors use in patients with significant renal failure. The small molecule agents (i.e., tirofiban and eptifibatide) are excreted predominantly via the kidneys, and randomized trials have largely excluded patients with renal dysfunction. In contrast, abciximab, a monoclonal antibody fragment, undergoes almost no renal excretion and is eliminated through platelet degradation by the reticuloendothelial system. In the EPIC (38) and EPISTENT (101) trials, abciximab therapy did not confer a significant bleeding risk for patients with mild renal dysfunction; however, safety data among patients with marked reductions in creatinine clearance are not available from these trials. A retrospective analysis of the TARGET trial (102) noted that both ischemic and bleeding complications are highest in the lowest creatinine clearance quartile of patients treated with either tirofiban or abciximab. Of particular interest, no interaction between these GP IIb/IIIa inhibitors and creatinine clearance on ischemic or bleeding events was appreciated.

Bivalirudin undergoes partial elimination through renal excretion; dose adjustment is required in patients with moderate-to-severe renal failure (creatinine clearance < 60 mL/dL) (78). The half-life of bivalirudin is about 25 min in patients with normal renal function, about 34 min in those with moderate renal failure, and 57 min in those with severe renal failure. Clinical support for the use of bivalirudin in patients with renal failure may be derived from a retrospective analysis of the Bivalirudin Angioplasty Trial (BAT) *(103)* in which bivalirudin was compared with UFH therapy among 4,312 patients undergoing angioplasty. Nearly 75% of the enrolled patients had some degree of renal failure. No matter the degree, bivalirudin-treated patients experienced both fewer bleeding complications and fewer ischemic complications than patients treated with UFH. Considering the pathological derangements associated with renal impairment, including evidence of ongoing thrombin generation, a particular emphasis on direct thrombin inhibition seems justified in the renal failure patient.

FUTURE DIRECTIONS

The last decade has seen a remarkable increase in the clinical evaluation and therapeutic application of varied platelet inhibitor pharmaceuticals. Prasugrel is a novel platelet inhibitor that has been tested in patients with ACS planned for PCI. The TRITON-TIMI 38 study *(104)* randomized 13,608 patients with moderate-to-high-risk ACS and planned PCI to receive prasugrel (a 60-mg loading dose and a 10-mg daily maintenance dose) or clopidogrel (a 300-mg loading dose and a 75-mg daily maintenance dose), for 6–15 months. The primary efficacy endpoint was death from cardiovascular causes, nonfatal myocardial infarction, or nonfatal stroke. The key safety endpoint was major bleeding. The investigators found that, as a more potent antiplatelet agent, prasugrel reduced the combined rate of death from cardiovascular causes, acute stent thrombosis, nonfatal myocardial infarction, or nonfatal stroke (12.1% for clopidogrel vs. 9.9% for prasugrel); however, this was at the expense of increased major (1.4%, vs. 0.9% in the clopidogrel group) and fatal bleeding (0.4% vs. 0.1%). Overall, a net clinical benefit in favor of prasugrel remained. Nonetheless, uncertainty remains about the optimal duration and dosing of this agent.

Cangrelor (AR-C69931MX) is a potent, selective, reversible inhibitor of ADP-induced platelet aggregation *(105)*. It is being studied for ACS as an ultrafast acting IV antithrombotic agent. A distinct theoretical advantage is the agent's short plasma half-life, which yields a rapid loss of activity following discontinuation of the infusion and may allow for a significant safety advantage. Phase II trials have shown safety and a greater inhibition of platelet aggregation over clopidogrel. Phase III trials should provide more definitive information on clinical efficacy and safety; preliminary results are due in late 2008.

In the antithrombotic arena, there is intense interest in the development and application of newer antithrombotics that inhibit upstream targets in the coagulation cascade. A number of direct factor Xa inhibitors (DX-9065a and otamixiban), as well as other novel antithrombin inhibitors, are in clinical development; whether or not they will lend themselves to periprocedural anticoagulation remains to be seen *(106–108)*.

REFERENCES

1. Patrono C, Rocca B (2008) Aspirin: promise and resistance in the new millennium. Arterioscler Thromb Vasc Biol 28:s25–s32
2. Antiplatelet Trialists' Collaboration (1994) Collaborative overview of randomised trials of antiplatelet therapy – I: prevention of death, myocardial infarction, and stroke by prolonged antiplatelet therapy in various categories of patients. BMJ 308:81–106
3. (1988) ISIS-2 (Second International Study of Infarct Survival) Collaborative Group. Randomised trial of intravenous streptokinase, oral aspirin, both, or neither among 17,187 cases of suspected acute myocardial infarction: ISIS-2. Lancet 2(8607):349–360
4. Antithrombotic Trialists' Collaboration (2002) Collaborative meta-analysis of randomised trials of antiplatelet therapy for prevention of death, myocardial infarction, and stroke in high risk patients. BMJ 324:71–86

5. Savage MP, Goldberg S, Bove AA, Deutsch E, Vetrovec G, Macdonald RG et al (1995) Effect of thromboxane A$_2$ blockade on clinical outcome and restenosis after successful coronary angioplasty: Multi-hospital eastern Atlantic restenosis trial (M-HEART II). Circulation 92:3194–3200

6. Eisenberg MJ, Topol EJ (1996) Prehospital administration of aspirin in patients with unstable angina and acute myocardial infarction. Arch Intern Med 156:1506–1510

7. Peters RJ, Mehta SR, Fox KA, Zhao F, Lewis BS, Kopecky SL et al (2003) Effects of aspirin dose when used alone or in combination with clopidogrel in patients with acute coronary syndromes: observations from the Clopidogrel in Unstable angina to prevent Recurrent Events (CURE) study. Circulation 108(14):1682–1687

8. Schwartz L, Bourassa MG, Lesperance J, Aldridge HE, Kazim F, Salvatori VA et al (1988) Aspirin and dipyridamole in the prevention of restenosis after percutaneous transluminal coronary angioplasty. N Engl J Med 318(26):1714–1719

9. King SB III, Smith SC Jr, Hirshfeld JW Jr et al (2008) 2007 Focused update of the ACC/AHA/SCAI 2005 guideline update for percutaneous coronary intervention: 2007 Writing Group to review new evidence and update the ACC/AHA/SCAI 2005 guideline update for percutaneous coronary intervention. Circulation 117:261–295

10. Krasopoulos G, Brister SJ, Beattie WS, Buchanan MR (2008) Aspirin "resistance" and risk of cardiovascular morbidity: systematic review and meta-analysis. BMJ 336:195–198

11. Hankey GJ, Eikelboom JW (2006) Aspirin resistance. Lancet 367:606–617

12. Tantry US, Bliden KP, Gurbel PA (2005) Overestimation of platelet aspirin resistance detection by thrombelastograph platelet mapping and validation by conventional aggregometry using arachidonic acid stimulation. J Am Coll Card 46(9):1705–1709

13. Kam PC, Nethery CM (2003) The thienopyridine derivatives (platelet adenosine diphosphate receptor antagonists), pharmacology and clinical developments. Anaesthesia 58(1):28–35

14. Hass WK, Easton JD, Adams HP Jr et al (1989) A randomized trial comparing ticlopidine hydrochloride with aspirin for the prevention of stroke in high-risk patients. N Engl J Med 321:501–507

15. Schühlen H, Hadamitzky M, Walter H et al (1997) Major benefit from antiplatelet therapy for patients at high risk for adverse cardiac events after coronary Palmaz-Schatz stent placement: analysis of a prospective risk stratification protocol in the Intracoronary Stenting and Antithrombotic Regimen (ISAR) trial. Circulation. 95:2015–2021

16. Leon MB, Baim DS, Popma JJ et al (1998) A clinical trial comparing three antithrombotic-drug regimens after coronary-artery stenting. Stent Anticoagulation Restenosis Study Investigators. N Engl J Med 339:1665–1671

17. Kandzari DE, Berger PB, Kastrati A, Steinhubl SR, Mehilli J, Dotzer F et al (2004) Influence of treatment duration with a 600-mg dose of clopidogrel before percutaneous coronary revascularization. J Am Coll Cardiol 44(11):2133–2136

18. Yusuf S, Zhao F, Mehta SR et al (2001) Effects of clopidogrel in addition to aspirin in patients with acute coronary syndromes without ST-segment elevation. N Engl J Med. 345:494–502

19. Mehta SR, Yusuf S, Peters RJ, Bertrand ME, Lewis BS, Natarajan MK et al (2001) Effects of pretreatment with clopidogrel and aspirin followed by long-term therapy in patients undergoing percutaneous coronary intervention: the PCI-CURE study. Lancet 358(9281):527

20. Steinhubl SR, Berger PB, Mann JT III, Fry ET, DeLago A, Wilmer C, Topol EJ, CREDO Investigators (2002) Clopidogrel for the reduction of events during observation. Early and sustained dual oral antiplatelet therapy following percutaneous coronary intervention: a randomized controlled trial. JAMA 288(19):2411–2420

21. Steinhubl SR, Darrah S, Brennan D, McErlean E, Berger PB, Topol EJ (2003) Optimal duration of pretreatment with clopidogrel prior to PCI: data from the CREDO trial. Circulation 108:IV–374 (Abstract)

22. Mehilli J, Kastrati A, Schuhlen H, Dibra A, Dotzer F, Von Beckerath N et al (2004) Randomized clinical trial of abciximab in diabetic patients undergoing elective percutaneous coronary interventions after treatment with a high loading dose of clopidogrel. Circulation 110(24):3627–3635

23. Patti G, Colonna G, Pasceri V, Pepe LL, Montinaro A, Di Sciascio G (2005) Randomized trial of high loading dose of clopidogrel for reduction of periprocedural myocardial infarction in patients undergoing coronary intervention: results from the ARMYDA-2 (Antiplatelet therapy for Reduction of MYocardial Damage during Angioplasty) study. Circulation 111(16):2099–2106

24. von Beckerath N, Taubert D, Pogatsa-Murray G, Schomig E, Kastrati A, Schomig A (2005) Absorption, metabolization, and antiplatelet effects of 300, 600-, and 900-mg loading doses of clopidogrel: results of the ISAR-CHOICE (Intracoronary Stenting and Antithrombotic Regimen: Choose Between 3 High Oral Doses for Immediate Clopidogrel Effect) Trial. Circulation 112(19):2946–2950

25. Mehilli J, Kastrati A, Schühlen H, et al, for the ISAR-SWEET study investigators (2004) Randomized clinical trial of abciximab in diabetic patients undergoing elective percutaneous coronary interventions after treatment with a high loading dose of clopidogrel. Circulation 110:3627–3635

26. Montalescot G, on behalf of the Albion investigators (2005) Assessment of the best loading dose of clopidogrel to blunt platelet activation, inflammation, and ongoing necrosis. Oral presentation EuroPCR Congress. May 24, 2005.

27. Chu MW, Wilson SR, Novick RJ, Stitt LW, Quantz MA (2004) Does clopidogrel increase blood loss following coronary artery bypass surgery? Ann Thor Surg 78(5):1536–1541

28. Costa MA, Sabaté M, van der Giessen WJ et al (1999) Late coronary occlusion after intracoronary brachytherapy. Circulation 100:789–792

29. Lüscher TF, Steffel J, Eberli FR et al (2007) Drug-eluting stent and coronary thrombosis: Biological mechanisms and clinical implications. Circulation 115:1051–1058

30. Moreno R, Fernández C, Hernández R et al (2005) Drug-eluting stent thrombosis: Results from a pooled analysis including 10 randomized studies. J Am Coll Cardiol 45:954–959

31. Stone GW, Ellis SG, Colombo A et al (2007) Offsetting impact of thrombosis and restenosis on the occurrence of death and myocardial infarction after paclitaxel-eluting and bare metal stent implantation. Circulation 115(22):2842–2847

32. Stettler C, Wandel S, Allemann S et al (2007) Outcomes associated with drug-eluting and bare-metal stents: a collaborative network meta-analysis. Lancet 370:937–948

33. Mauri L, Hsieh W, Massaro JM et al (2007) Stent thrombosis in randomized clinical trials of drug-eluting stents. N Engl J Med 356(10):1020–1029

34. Bavry AA, Kumbhani DJ, Helton TJ et al (2006) Late thrombosis of drug-eluting stents: a meta-analysis of randomized clinical trials. Am J Med 119(12):1056–1061

35. Virmani R, Guagliumi G, Farb A et al (2004) Localized hypersensitivity and late coronary thrombosis secondary to a sirolimus-eluting stent: should we be cautious? Circulation 109(6):701–705

36. Topol EJ, Byzova TV, Plow EF (1999) Platelet GPIIb-IIIa blockers. Lancet 353:227–231

37. Kleiman NS (1999) Pharmokinetics and pharmacodynamics of glycoprotein IIb/IIIa inhibitors. Am Heart J 138: S263–S275

38. EPIC Investigators (1994) Use of a monoclonal antibody directed against the platelet glycoprotein IIb/IIIa receptor in high-risk coronary angioplasty. N Engl J Med 330(14):956–961

39. Moliterno DJ, Califf RM, Aguirre FV, Anderson K, Sigmon KN, Weisman HF, Topol EJ (1995) Effect of platelet glycoprotein IIb/IIIa integrin blockade on activated clotting time during percutaneous transluminal coronary angioplasty or directional atherectomy (the EPIC trial). Evaluation of c7E3 Fab in the Prevention of Ischemic Complications trial. Am J Cardiol 75(8):559–562

40. EPILOG Investigators (1997) Platelet glycoprotein IIb/IIIa blockade with abciximab with low-dose heparin during percutaneous coronary revascularization. N Engl J Med 336:1689–1696

41. Chew DP, Bhatt DL, Lincoff AM, Moliterno DJ, Brener SJ, Wolski KE, Topol EJ (2001) Defining the optimal activated clotting time during percutaneous coronary intervention: aggregate results from 6 randomized, controlled trials. Circulation 103(7):961–966

42. Hamm CW, Heeschen C, Goldmann B et al (1999) Benefit of abciximab in patients with refractory unstable angina in relation to serum troponin T levels. c7E3 Fab Antiplatelet Therapy in Unstable Refractory Angina (CAPTURE) Study Investigators. N Engl J Med 340:1623–1629

43. Montalescot G, Barragan P, Wittenberg O et al (2001) Platelet glycoprotein IIb/IIIa inhibition with coronary stenting for acute myocardial infarction. N Engl J Med 344:1895–1903

44. Stone GW, Grines CL, Cox DA et al (2002) Comparison of angioplasty with stenting, with or without abciximab, in acute myocardial infarction. N Engl J Med 346:957–963

45. Kastrati A, Mehilli J, Neumann FJ et al (2006) Abciximab in patients with acute coronary syndromes undergoing percutaneous coronary intervention after clopidogrel pretreatment. The ISAR-REACT 2 Randomized Trial. JAMA 295(13):1531–1538

46. Simoons ML, GUSTO IV-ACS Investigators (2001) Effect of glycoprotein IIbIIIa receptor blocker abciximab on outcome in patients with acute coronary syndromes without early coronary revascularisation: the GUSTO IV-ACS randomised trial. Lancet 357(9272):1915–1924

47. PURSUIT Trial Investigators (1998) Inhibition of platelet glycoprotein IIb/IIIa with eptifibatide in patients with acute coronary syndromes. N Engl J Med 339:436–443

48. ESPRIT Investigators (2002) Long-term efficacy of platelet glycoprotein IIb/IIIa integrin blockade with eptifibatide in coronary stent intervention. JAMA 287(5):618–621

49. PRISM-PLUS Study Investigators (1998) Inhibition of the platelet glycoprotein IIb/IIIa receptor with tirofiban in unstable angina and non-Q-wave myocardial infarction. N Engl J Med 338:1488–1497

50. Boersma E, Akkerhuis KM, Theroux P et al (1999) Platelet glycoprotein IIb/IIIa receptor inhibition in non-ST-elevation acute coronary syndromes: early benefit during medical treatment only, with additional protection during percutaneous coronary intervention. Circulation 100:2045–2048

51. Roffi M, Mukherjee D, Chew DP et al (1991) Lack of benefit from intravenous platelet glycoprotein IIb/IIIa receptor inhibition as adjunctive treatment for percutaneous interventions of aortocoronary bypass grafts: a pooled analysis of five randomized clinical trials. Circulation 2002;106(24):3063-7.Hirsh J. Heparin. N Engl J Med 324:1565–1574

52. Hirsh J (1991) Heparin. N Engl J Med 324(22):1565–1574
53. Bartholomew JR (2008) Heparin-induced thrombocytopenia: 2008 update. Curr Treat Options Cardiovasc Med 10(2): 117–127
54. Avendano A, Ferguson JJ (1994) Comparison of Hemochron and HemoTec activated coagulation time target values during percutaneous transluminal coronary angioplasty. J Am Coll Cardiol 23:907–910
55. Koch KT, Piek JJ, de Winter RJ et al (1997) Safety of low dose heparin in elective coronary angioplasty. Heart 77:517–522
56. Kaluski E, Krakover R, Cotter G et al (2000) Minimal heparinization in coronary angioplasty–how much heparin is really warranted? Am J Cardiol 85:953–956
57. Godon P, Rioufol G, Finet G et al (2001) Efficacy and safety of low-dose heparin (30 IU/kg) during coronary angioplasty. Arch Mal Coeur Vaiss 94:984–988
58. Denardo SJ, Davis KE, Reid PR, Tcheng JE (2003) Efficacy and safety of minimal dose (< or = 1, 000 units) unfractionated heparin with abciximab in percutaneous coronary intervention. Am J Cardiol. 91:1–5
59. Denardo SJ, Davis KE, Tcheng JE (2005) Elective percutaneous coronary intervention using broad-spectrum antiplatelet therapy (eptifibatide, clopidogrel, and aspirin) alone, without scheduled unfractionated heparin or other antithrombin therapy. Am Heart J 149(1):138–144
60. Brener SJ, Moliterno DJ, Lincoff AM et al (2004) Relationship between activated clotting time and ischemic or hemorrhagic complications. Circulation 110:994–998
61. Lincoff AM, Bittl JA, Kleiman NS, for the REPLACE-1 Investigators et al (2004) Comparison of bivalirudin versus heparin during percutaneous coronary intervention (the Randomized Evaluation of PCI Linking Angiomax to Reduced Clinical Events [REPLACE]-1 trial). Am J Cardiol 93:1092–1096
62. Lincoff AM, Bittl JA, Harrington RA et al (2003) Bivalirudin and provisional glycoprotein IIb/IIIa blockade compared with heparin and planned glycoprotein IIb/IIIa blockade during percutaneous coronary intervention. The REPLACE-2 trial. JAMA 289:853–863
63. Tolleson TR, O'Shea JC, Bittl JA et al (2003) Relationship between heparin anticoagulation and clinical outcomes in coronary stent intervention: observations from the ESPRIT trial. J Am Coll Cardiol 41:386–393
64. Hirsh J, Levine M (1992) Low molecular weight heparin. Blood 79:1–17
65. Mahaffey KW, Cohen M, Garg J, Antman E, Kleiman NS, Goodman SG et al (2005) High-risk patients with acute coronary syndromes treated with low-molecular-weight or unfractionated heparin: outcomes at 6 months and 1 year in the SYNERGY trial. JAMA 294(20):2594–2600
66. Blazing MA, de Lemos JA, White HD, Fox KA, Verheugt FW, Ardissino D et al (2004) Safety and efficacy of enoxaparin vs unfractionated heparin in patients with non-ST-segment elevation acute coronary syndromes who receive tirofiban and aspirin: a randomized controlled trial. JAMA 292(1):55–64
67. Petersen JL, Mahaffey KW, Hasselblad V, Antman EM, Cohen M, Goodman SG et al (2004) Efficacy and bleeding complications among patients randomized to enoxaparin or unfractionated heparin for antithrombin therapy in non-ST-Segment elevation acute coronary syndromes: a systematic overview. JAMA 292(1):89–96
68. Goodman SG, Cohen M, Bigonzi F, Gurfinkel EP, Radley DR, Le Iouer V et al (2000) Randomized trial of low molecular weight heparin (enoxaparin) versus unfractionated heparin for unstable coronary artery disease: one-year results of the ESSENCE Study. Efficacy and Safety of Subcutaneous Enoxaparin in Non-Q Wave Coronary Events. J Am Coll Cardiol 36(3):693–698
69. Antman EM, McCabe CH, Gurfinkel EP, Turpie AG, Bernink PJ, Salein D et al (1999) Enoxaparin prevents death and cardiac ischemic events in unstable angina/non-Q-wave myocardial infarction. Results of the thrombolysis in myocardial infarction (TIMI) 11B trial. Circulation 100 (15):1593–1601
70. NICE-3 Investigators (2003) Combining enoxaparin and glycoprotein IIb/IIIa antagonists for the treatment of acute coronary syndromes: final results of the National Investigators Collaborating on Enoxaparin-3 (NICE-3) study. Am Heart J 146(4):628–634
71. Karsch KR, Preisack MB, Baildon R, Eschenfelder V, Foley D, Garcia EJ et al (1996) Low molecular weight heparin (reviparin) in percutaneous transluminal coronary angioplasty. Results of a randomized, double-blind, unfractionated heparin and placebo-controlled, multicenter trial (REDUCE trial). Reduction of Restenosis After PTCA, Early Administration of Reviparin in a Double-Blind Unfractionated Heparin and Placebo-Controlled Evaluation. J Am Coll Cardiol 28(6):1437–1443
72. Choussat R, Montalescot G, Collet JP et al (2002) A unique, low dose of intravenous enoxaparin in elective percutaneous coronary intervention. J Am Coll Cardiol 40(11):1943–1950
73. Montalescot G, White HD, Gallo R, for the STEEPLE Investigators et al (2006) Enoxaparin versus unfractionated heparin in elective percutaneous coronary intervention. N Engl J Med 355(10):1006–1017

74. Borentain M, Montalescot G, Bouzamondo A, Choussat R, Hulot JS, Lechat P (2005) Low-molecular-weight heparin vs. unfractionated heparin in percutaneous coronary intervention: a combined analysis. Catheter Cardiovasc Interv 65(2):212–215

75. Gross PL, Weitz JI (2008) New anticoagulants for treatment of venous thromboembolism. Arterioscler Thromb Vasc Biol 28(3):380–386

76. The Fifth Organization to Assess Strategies in Acute Ischemic Syndromes Investigators (2006) Comparison of fondaparinux and enoxaparin in acute coronary syndromes. N Engl J Med 354(14):1464–1476

77. Yusuf S, Mehta SR, Chrolavicius S et al (2006) Effects of fondaparinux on mortality and reinfarction in patients with acute ST-segment elevation myocardial infarction: the OASIS-6 randomized trial. JAMA 295(13):1519–1530

78. White CM (2005) Thrombin-directed inhibitors: pharmacology and clinical use. Am Heart J 149(1 Suppl):S54–S60

79. Stone GW, McLaurin BT, Cox DA et al (2006) Bivalirudin for patients with acute coronary syndromes. N Engl J Med 355:2203–2216

80. Stone GW, White HD, Ohman EM et al (2007) Bivalirudin in patients with acute coronary syndromes undergoing percutaneous coronary intervention: a subgroup analysis from the Acute Catheterization and Urgent Intervention Triage strategy (ACUITY) trial. Lancet 369:907–919

81. Stone, GW on behalf of the HORIZONS AMI Investigators (2007) HORIZONS AMI: a prospective, randomized comparison of bivalirudin vs. heparin plus glycoprotein IIb/IIIa inhibitors during primary angioplasty in acute myocardial infarction: 30-day results. Oral presentation, 19th annual Transcatheter Cardiovascular Therapeutics Symposium, October 2007

82. Singh S, Molnar J, Arora R (2007) Efficacy and safety of bivalirudin versus heparins in reduction of cardiac outcomes in acute coronary syndrome and percutaneous coronary interventions. J Cardiovasc Pharmacol Ther 12(4):283–291

83. Dang CH, Durkalski VL, Nappi JM (2006) Evaluation of treatment with direct thrombin inhibitors in patients with heparin-induced thrombocytopenia. Pharmacotherapy 26(4):461–468

84. Mahaffey KW, Lewis BE, Wildermann NM, Berkowitz SD, Oliverio RM, Turco MA et al (2003) The anticoagulant therapy with bivalirudin to assist in the performance of percutaneous coronary intervention in patients with heparin-induced thrombocytopenia (ATBAT) study: main results. J Invasive Cardiol 15(11):611–616

85. American Heart Association (2004) Heart Disease and Stroke Statistics—2005 Update. American Heart Association, Dallas, Tex

86. Ayanian JZ, Epstein AM (1991) Differences in the use of procedures between men and women hospitalized for coronary disease. N Engl J Med 325:221–225

87. Mehilli J, Kastrati A, Dirschinger J, Bollwein H, Neumann FJ, Schomig A (2000) Differences in prognostic factors and outcomes between women and men undergoing coronary artery stenting. JAMA 284:1799–1805

88. Watanabe CT, Maynard C, Ritchie JL (2001) Comparison of short-term outcomes following coronary artery stenting in men versus women. Am J Cardiol 88:848–852

89. Mehilli J, Kastrati A, Dirschinger J, Pache J, Seyfarth M, Blasini R et al (2002) Sex-based analysis of outcome in patients with acute myocardial infarction treated predominantly with percutaneous coronary intervention. JAMA 287:210–215

90. Glaser R, Herrmann HC, Murphy SA, Demopoulos LA, DiBattiste PM, Cannon CP, Braunwald E (2002) Benefit of an early invasive management strategy in women with acute coronary syndromes. JAMA 288:3124–3129

91. Mueller C, Neumann FJ, Roskamm H, Buser P, Hodgson JM, Perruchoud AP, Buettner HJ (2002) Women do have an improved long-term outcome after non-ST-elevation acute coronary syndromes treated very early and predominantly with percutaneous coronary intervention: a prospective study in 1, 450 consecutive patients. J Am Coll Cardiol 40:245–250

92. Peterson ED, Lansky AJ, Kramer J, Anstrom K, Lanzilotta MJ, National Cardiovascular Network Clinical Investigators (2001) Effect of gender on the outcomes of contemporary percutaneous coronary intervention. Am J Cardiol 88:359

93. Kong DF, Califf RM, Miller DP, Moliterno DJ, White HD, Harrington RA et al (1998) Clinical outcomes of therapeutic agents that block the platelet glycoprotein IIb/IIIa integrin in ischemic heart disease. Circulation 98:2829–2835

94. Cho L, Topol EJ, Balog C, Foody JM, Booth JE, Cabot C et al (2000) Clinical benefit of glycoprotein IIb/IIIa blockade with Abciximab is independent of gender: pooled analysis from EPIC, EPILOG and EPISTENT trials. Evaluation of 7E3 for the Prevention of Ischemic Complications. Evaluation in Percutaneous Transluminal Coronary Angioplasty to Improve Long-Term Outcome with Abciximab GP IIb/IIIa blockade. Evaluation of Platelet IIb/IIIa Inhibitor for Stent. J Am Coll Cardiol 36:381–386

95. ESPRIT investigators (2002) Is glycoprotein IIb/IIIa antagonism as effective in women as in men following percutaneous coronary intervention? Lessons from the ESPRIT study. J Am Coll Cardiol 40:1085–1091

96. Vasu S, Gruberg L, Brown DL (2007) The impact of advanced chronic kidney disease on in-hospital mortality following percutaneous coronary intervention for acute myocardial infarction. Catheter Cardiovasc Interv 70(5):701–705

97. Papafaklis MI, Naka KK, Papamichael ND et al (2007) The impact of renal function on the long-term clinical course of patients who underwent percutaneous coronary intervention. Catheter Cardiovasc Interv 69(2):189–197

98. Attallah N, Yassine L, Fisher K, Yee J (2005) Risk of bleeding and restenosis among chronic kidney disease patients undergoing percutaneous coronary intervention. Clin Nephrol 64(6):412–418

99. Mosenkis A, Berns JS (2004) Use of low molecular weight heparins and glycoprotein IIb/IIIa inhibitors in patients with chronic kidney disease. Semin Dial 17(5):411–415

100. Kruse MW, Lee JJ (2005) Retrospective evaluation of a pharmacokinetic program for adjusting enoxaparin in renal impairment. Am Heart J 149(3):567

101. Investigators EPISTENT (1998) Randomised placebo-controlled and balloon-angioplasty-controlled trial to assess safety of coronary stenting with use of platelet glycoprotein IIb/IIIa blockade. Lancet 352:87–92

102. Berger PB, Best PJ, Topol EJ et al (2005) The relation of renal function to ischemic and bleeding outcomes with 2 different glycoprotein IIb/IIIa inhibitors: the do Tirofiban and ReoPro Give Similar Efficacy Outcome (TARGET) trial. Am Heart J 149(5):869–875

103. Bittl JA, Chaitman BR, Feit F et al (2001) Bivalirudin versus heparin during coronary angioplasty for unstable or post infarction angina: Final report reanalysis of the Bivalirudin Angioplasty Study. Am Heart J 142:952–959

104. Wiviott SD, Braunwald E, McCabe CH, for the TRITON-TIMI 38 Investigators et al (2007) Prasugrel versus clopidogrel in patients with acute coronary syndromes. N Engl J Med 357(20):2001–2015

105. Michelson AD (2008) P2Y12 antagonism: promises and challenges. Arterioscler Thromb Vasc Biol 28(3):s33–s38

106. Haas S (2008) New oral Xa and IIa inhibitors: updates on clinical trial results. J Thromb Thrombolysis 25(1):52–60

107. Giugliano PR, Wiviott SD, Stone PH, for the ANTHEM-TIMI-32 Investigators et al (2007) Recombinant nematode anticoagulant protein c2 in patients with non-ST-segment elevation acute coronary syndrome: the ANTHEM-TIMI-32 trial. J Am Coll Cardiol 49(25):2398–2407

108. Cohen M, Bhatt DL, Alexander JH, For the SEPIA-PCI Trial Investigators et al (2007) Randomized, double-blind, dose-ranging study of otamixaban, a novel, parenteral, short-acting direct factor Xa inhibitor, in percutaneous coronary intervention: the SEPIA-PCI trial. Circulation 115:2642–2651

15 Antithrombotic Therapy in Carotid and Peripheral Intervention

Thomas J. Helton and Samir R. Kapadia

CONTENTS

ABSTRACT Peripheral arterial disease is a spectrum of disease processes involving the non-coronary arterial system that is primarily the result of atherothrombosis. Although the field of peripheral intervention is older than coronary intervention, the evolution of this field has lagged behind that of its coronary counterpart. Adjunctive therapies demonstrated to be beneficial in the realm of percutaneous coronary interventions (PCI) have not been as systematically assessed within the peripheral arena. Nevertheless, current opinion rests with the belief that adjunctive antiplatelet and antithrombotic agents improve outcomes for patients undergoing peripheral interventional procedures. Future studies will foster a better understanding of the idiosyncrasies related to peripheral interventions and the optimal utilization of currently available and developing antithrombotic agents in order to further advance this field.

Key words: Antiplatelet; Antithrombin; Carotid; Intervention; Peripheral; Renals

INTRODUCTION

Peripheral arterial disease is a spectrum of disease processes involving the non-coronary arterial system that is primarily the result of atherothrombosis. In 1964, Dotter and Judkins pioneered "transluminal angioplasty" for the treatment of peripheral arterial disease (1). Early procedures were fraught with complications (distal emboli and puncture site hematomas). After a decade of growing skepticism and mounting complications Andreas Gruentzig was able to refine the multiple catheter system of Dotter to a single double-lumen catheter with a low compliance balloon. This new system allowed for smaller bore catheters and thus reduced the number of puncture site hematomas prompting the emergence of percutaneous intervention (2). Although reasonably successful at the time (initial patency rate of 86%), there were still many problems with reocclusions and embolic complications (2). The catheters were felt to be thrombogenic and it was speculated that anticoagulation might improve outcomes.

From: *Contemporary Cardiology: Antithrombotic Drug Therapy in Cardiovascular Disease*
Edited by: A.T. Askari and A.M. Lincoff (eds.), DOI 10.1007/978-1-60327-235-3_15
© Humana Press, a part of Springer Science+Business Media, LLC 2010

PERIPHERAL INTERVENTION (NON-CAROTID)

Anticoagulation

INDIRECT THROMBIN INHIBITORS

Heparin

Since its discovery in 1916, heparin's ability to inhibit blood coagulation has led to a variety of clinical uses *(3)*. Heparin is naturally found intracellular in mast cells and is released into the circulation by mast cell degranulation. Under normal circumstances heparin's anti-thrombotic effects are not detectable because it is immediately taken up and degraded by macrophages. Heparin sulfate molecules can be found in vivo on the surface of vascular endothelial cells as well as in the subendothelial extracellular matrix. Through a series of complex interactions heparin functions as a cofactor to accelerate anti-thrombin III inhibition of thrombin (factor IIa) thus playing a pivotal role in maintaining coagulation homeostasis primarily via the intrinsic pathway.

Heparin's ability to inhibit clot formation and its rapid reversibility has made it the mainstay of anticoagulation for coronary and non-coronary intervention since the inception of coronary angioplasty *(4)*. Heparin is used to prevent catheter-related thromboses and clot formation at iatrogenic sites of vascular injury during cardiac catheterization *(5)*. To date, there have been no randomized placebo-controlled trials demonstrating heparin's effectiveness in this setting; however, it would now be considered unethical for such a study to take place. Although heparin has been used as the benchmark to which many new therapies are compared, the data supporting its use in peripheral intervention are sparse and primarily based on outcomes with coronary intervention.

Early retrospective studies demonstrated improved procedural success and decreased post-procedure abrupt vessel closure with pre-procedural intravenous heparin administration in patients with acute coronary syndromes *(6)*. Improved outcomes in acute coronary syndromes led to the widespread use of heparin in percutaneous interventions. There are no standardized dosing guidelines for the use of intravenous heparin during peripheral arterial interventions; however, at our institution dosing protocols are modeled after those of coronary intervention. An initial bolus of 40–60 IUs/kg (maximum 5,000 IU) is given intravenously prior to intervention with periodic monitoring of ACT. Based on the response to the initial bolus dose an additional 1,000–3,000 IUs heparin may be given to achieve an ACT of 300–400 s. The duration of anticoagulation is tailored to the underlying disease process, that is, patients presenting with acute limb ischemia are anticoagulated immediately with therapeutic doses of intravenous unfractionated heparin and transitioned to oral warfarin indefinitely (if the etiology of embolism cannot be corrected).

Warfarin

Routine use of long-term anticoagulation with warfarin has not been shown to reduce the risk of adverse cardiovascular events in patients with chronic peripheral arterial disease. The American Heart Association/American College of Cardiology (AHA/ACC) guidelines on peripheral arterial disease currently give warfarin a class III indication for the prevention of future adverse cardiovascular events in patients with peripheral arterial disease, in the absence of atrial fibrillation. There are limited data for the use of warfarin following peripheral intervention but may be useful in select situations. Post-procedural anticoagulation with warfarin is frequently used for arterial revascularization in patients with HIT *(7)*, recanalization of closed peripheral arterial bypass grafts *(8,9)*, and percutaneous intervention of the superior vena cava (SVC) for SVC syndrome (especially if pacer wires are present) *(10)*.

Low-Molecular Weight Heparins

Low-molecular weight heparins (LMWH) are smaller molecules that primarily act within the coagulation cascade at the factor Xa level to accelerate the anti-thrombin III inhibition of thrombin thus are considered indirect thrombin inhibitors. LMWHs do have varying degrees of selectivity for factor Xa depending on the drug formulation; however, as a group they have several obvious advantages over unfractionated heparin: (1) more predictable dose response and clearance (2) longer half-lives (3) better bioavailability (4) uniform dosing strategy. Many LMWHs exist; however, enoxaparin is the only one studied extensively for percutaneous intervention.

Enoxaparin

Enoxaparin binds preferentially to factor Xa giving it more predictable levels of anticoagulation and in most circumstances, it does not require monitoring.

Favorable pharmacokinetics of enoxaparin evoked interest in using it for percutaneous coronary and non-coronary interventions. The use of LMWHs in percutaneous interventions today are largely driven by data from several studies demonstrating superiority of LMWHs (18–20% reductions in death and nonfatal myocardial infarction) compared to unfractionated heparin in the medical management of acute coronary syndromes (11–16). However, LMWHs have not proven to be superior to unfractionated heparin in the catheterization laboratory. Four large randomized trials enrolled over 12,000 patients to compare outcomes with enoxaparin versus unfractionated heparin in patients with non-ST elevation acute coronary syndromes (NSTE-ACS) (13–16). The largest of these trials is the SYNERGY (Superior Yield of the New strategy of Enoxaparin, Revascularization and GlYcoprotein IIb/IIIa inhibitors) trial, which enrolled 10,027 patients with high-risk NSTE-ACS with an intended early invasive strategy to receive intravenous unfractionated heparin (60 IU/kg bolus followed by 12 IU/kg/h infusion) or enoxaparin (1 mg/kg subcutaneous twice daily) plus a glycoprotein IIb/IIIa inhibitor. Patients who were treated with percutaneous coronary intervention were randomly assigned to receive either intravenous unfractionated heparin or subcutaneous enoxaparin prior to intervention. If patients had previously received enoxparin within 8 h of coronary intervention then no additional enoxaparin was given during the procedure; however, if more than 8 h elapsed since the last dose, a bolus of 0.3 mg/kg intravenous enoxaparin was given prior to balloon inflation. The primary end point (composite of all-cause death or nonfatal myocardial infarction at 30 days after) occurred in 14% of patients treated with enoxaparin compared to 14.5% of patients treated with unfractionated heparin (odds ratio [OR]=0.96, 95% confidence interval [CI] 0.86–1.06). In this setting enoxaparin was neither inferior nor superior to unfractionated heparin. The enoxaparin group experienced a significant increase in TIMI (Thrombolysis in Myocardial Infarction) major bleeding 9.1% compared to the unfractionated heparin group 7.6%, $p=0.008$ (16).

It is difficult to translate these outcomes to peripheral interventions and the role of LMWH in peripheral intervention remains ill defined. In one small group of 56 patients who underwent 93 procedures, intravenous enoxaparin (0.75 mg/kg) plus eptifibatide (180 mcg/kg bolus followed by 2 mcg/kg) appears to have similar efficacy and safety as unfractionated heparin when used for elective non-carotid coronary and peripheral vascular interventions. Procedural success was achieved in 99% of patients with no vascular complications and a 2% incidence of major bleeding (17). Enoxaparin dosing for non-coronary intervention has not been standardized, although this strategy seems to have demonstrated reasonable results. At our institution the use of LMWH for peripheral intervention is uncommon; however, data from coronary literature suggest that a dosing strategy of 1 mg/kg subcutaneous twice daily would be a rational choice if one were inclined to use LMWH.

Table 1
Pharmacokinetics and indications for direct thrombin inhibitors (103)

Drug	Half-life (minutes)	Metabolism	Approved indications
Lepirudin	60	Renal	HIT
Argatroban	53	Hepatic	HIT or PCI with HIT
Bivalirudin	25	Renal/enzymatic	PCI with/without UA or HIT
Ximelegatran	240–300	Renal	None

HIT heparin-induced thrombocytopenia; PCI percutaneous coronary intervention; UA unstable angina

Other studies have suggested lower rates of major bleeding with similar ischemic outcomes for patients treated with LMWHs (18,19), but noted an increased incidence of catheter-related thrombosis when fondaparinaux was compared to enoxaparin (20). Moreover, patients treated with fondaparinaux prior to percutaneous intervention should also be given intravenous unfractionated heparin prior to balloon inflation to reduce the likelihood of this untoward outcome.

Direct Thrombin Inhibitors

Heparin has been the dominant anticoagulant used since the inception of peripheral vascular intervention. However, even when performed with therapeutic doses of heparin complications of peripheral intervention remain relatively frequent: early occlusion 3.1%, limb loss 1.9%, death 1.6%, and major bleeding 2.1% (21). Direct thrombin inhibitors have the potential to reduce such complications. There are currently four direct thrombin inhibitors available for clinical use: bivalirudin, lepirudin, argatroban, and ximelagatran. Only bivalirudin and argatroban (in the setting of HIT) have been approved for angioplasty. Approved indications for the currently available direct thrombin inhibitors are outlined in Table 1.

Bivalirudin

Bivalirudin is a 21 amino acid synthetic peptide that directly binds thrombin to exert its very predictable anticoagulant effects. The half-life of bivalirudin is approximately 25 min and it is renally eliminated. Although it has a very short half-life there is no specific antidote for bivalirudin or any of the direct thrombin inhibitors. Initially this raised concern for a higher incidence of bleeding complications but this has not been demonstrated in clinical trials. The largest study using bivalirudin as the sole anticoagulant was the Angiomax Peripheral Procedure Registry of Vascular Events (APPROVE) registry (22). The APPROVE registry was an open label study that enrolled 505 patients from 26 centers undergoing peripheral intervention to be treated with 0.75 mg/kg bolus of bivalirudin followed by a 1.75 mg/kg/h infusion. Procedural success (defined as a residual stenosis less than 20%) was achieved in 95% of patients. Thirty-day event rates were low: zero deaths, amputation rate 0.4%, unplanned, revascularization 0.8%, and major bleeding 2.2%. Concomitant use of glycoprotein inhibitors (4.4% of patients) was found to be a predictor of bleeding complications. Neither activated clotting time nor the degree of renal impairment was associated with increased bleeding complications.

From the coronary literature, the Randomized Evaluation of PCI Linking Angiomax to Reduced Clinical Events (REPLACE) (23), REPLACE-2 (24), and Harmonizing Outcomes with Revascularization and Stents In Acute Myocardial Infarction (HORIZONS-AMI) (25) trials have demonstrated the efficacy of bivalirudin in both the ST elevation and non-ST elevation acute coronary syndromes. Of note, there was an increased incidence of acute stent thrombosis in the bivalirudin group (1.3% vs. 0.3%, $p = 0.0009$) of the HORIZONS-AMI trial. Several small single center studies have shown similarly low rates of complications and major bleeding with the use of bivalirudin (26–29). Although bivalirudin appears to be a promising anticoagulant for use in peripheral intervention; randomized controlled trials comparing it to unfractionated heparin are needed.

The other direct thrombin inhibitors, argatroban, lepirudin, have been used in patients with heparin-induced thrombocytopenia (HIT) but they have not been adequately studied for use in the treatment of occlusive peripheral arterial disease in the absence of HIT.

Thrombolytics

Acute thrombotic limb ischemia is the abrupt loss of arterial perfusion to a limb typically as a result of an embolic event, either spontaneous or iatrogenic. Early outcomes with surgical thrombectomy were dismal. In 1978, Blaisdell and colleagues reported amputation and mortality rates of more than 25% each in patients undergoing surgical thrombectomy for acute limb ischemia (30). These less than desirable outcomes sparked interest in new treatment strategies. Two strategies emerged (pharmacologic with thrombolytics/anti-thrombotics and percutaneous intervention) to the forefront and eventually merged to improve outcomes in this typically very ill population.

STREPTOKINASE

Streptokinase was the first thrombolytic agent to be discovered and approved for clinical use. In 1933, Tillet and Garner discovered fibrinolytic activity of ß-hemolytic streptococci, although it was not until 1956 that Cliffton and Grunett reported the intravenous use of streptokinase in humans (31). Streptokinase remains the only FDA-approved fibrinolytic drug for the treatment of peripheral arterial occlusions (Table 2) (32).

Table 2
Approved indications and suggested doses for fibrinolytics in PAOD

Drug	Dose[a] 104	Approved indications (46)
Streptokinase	N/A	AMI, PE, DVT, Arterial thrombosis or embolism, Arterial-venous fistulae thrombosis
Urokinase	240,000 IU/h UK for 4 h, then 120,000 IU/h up to 48 h`	PE
Prourokinase	N/A	None
Reteplase	0.25–1.0 IU/h Total dose and infusion time should not exceed 20 U and 24 h, respectively	AMI
Alteplase	0.001–0.02 mg/kg/h or a non–weight-adjusted dose of 0.12–2.0 mg/h Total dose should not exceed 40 mg for catheter-directed administration	AMI, PE, ischemic stroke
Tenecteplase	N/A	AMI
Staphylokinase	N/A	None

PAOD peripheral arterial occlusive disease; AMI acute myocardial infarction; PE pulmonary embolism; DVT deep venous thrombosis; N/A no recommendation available from the current guidelines
[a] Dosage recommendations for acute limb ischemia only

Table 3
Contraindications to thrombolysis *(31,40)*

Absolute	Relative
Active bleeding	SBP>180 mmHg or DBP>110 mmHg
Recent GI bleed (<10 days)	Major nonvascular surgery (<10 days)
Intracranial or spinal surgery (<3 months)	Recent major trauma (<10 days)
Intracranial trauma (3 months)	CPR (<10 days)
Intracranial aneurysm or AVM	Intracranial tumor
Recent stroke or TIA (2 months)	Non-compressible arterial puncture (<2 days)
	Recent eye surgery
	Pregnancy
	Liver failure
	Hemorrhagic diabetic retinopathy

GI gastrointestinal; *SBP* systolic blood pressure; *DBP* diastolic blood pressure; *TIA* transient ischemic attack

Although intravenous administration of fibrinolytics was used initially, today this strategy has been replaced by catheter facilitated intra-arterial injection of the fibrinolytic directly into the thrombus. Early studies with streptokinase demonstrated initial success rates ranging from 70% to 90% and 2 year cumulative patency rates of 81% after treatment with low-dose intra-arterial catheter-directed thrombolytic therapy *(33–35)*. Moreover, these studies and others from the coronary literature alluded to potential serious complications related to the antigenicity of streptokinase with allergic reactions (urticaria, bronchospasm, periorbital edema) in approximately 2% of the treated population *(31,36–38)*. True anaphylaxis with streptokinase is extremely rare, less than 0.1% *(36–38)* and the greatest concern with the administration of streptokinase is similar to that of any thrombolytic agent, that is, major bleeding (approximately 3.7%, with intravenous heparin as the only adjunctive anticoagulant) *(35)*. Accordingly, patients should be screened diligently for contraindications to thrombolysis (Table 3) and appropriate dosing guidelines should be followed.

Dosing regimens for thrombolytics vary widely depending on the route of administration and the drug used. The initial studies with streptokinase for peripheral arterial thrombolysis used 1,000–3,000 IUs with a stepwise infusion (drug was directly injected into the thrombus every 5 min with catheter advancement every 15 min between injections) until successful thrombolysis. Heparin (2,500 IU) was given intermittently to prevent catheter thrombosis during lengthy procedures *(34,35)*. The stepwise method of thrombolytic therapy was quickly replaced by continuous infusion, which remains the most commonly used method. Continuous infusions required that 5,000–10,000 IUs/h of streptokinase for varying lengths of time (11 h to 8 days), tailored to the clinical response (Table 4). Infusions were stopped if most of the thrombi had been lysed by angiogram, a significant complication occurred, or no significant change was noted at 24 h *(39,40)*. Given the limitations (resistance, antigenicity, non-standardized dosing) of streptokinase, its use has largely been abandoned.

UROKINASE

Concurrently with the development of streptokinase, was the discovery of urokinase. Sobel and colleagues first isolated urokinase (UK) from human urine in 1952 and its clinical use followed soon after *(41)*. In the United States, urokinase was originally used for the treatment of pulmonary embolism and it was not the until the 1970s with publication of the Urokinase Pulmonary Embolism Trial (UPET) and Urokinase-Streptokinase Pulmonary Embolism Trial (USPET) that its relative safety compared to streptokinase became obvious *(42,43)*. These trials led to the FDA approval of urokinase for the treatment of pulmonary embolism and the widespread use of urokinase for thrombolytic

Table 4

Fibrinolytic trials in peripheral arterial disease

Study	Drug	N	Recanalization (%)/primary endpoint	Major bleeding (%)
Katzen (33)	SK	12	92	17
Lammer (34)	SK	47	75	4
Lammer (35)	SK, UK, SK-PLG	136	78	3.7
Pilger (105)	SK versus SK-PLG versus UK	98	SK 86; SK-PLG 85; UK 80	NA
Totty (39)	SK/UK	22	36	9
PURPOSE (44)	UK versus Pro-UK	241	UK 45; Pro-UK(8 mg) 56	UK 16.7; Pro-UK 23.1
TOPAS[a] (45)	UK versus surgery	544	Native 60; grafts 75	Fibrinolytics 12.5; surgery 5.5
Meyerovitz (50)	UK versus rt-PA	32	UK 38; rt-PA 50	UK 31 rt-PA 13
STILE[b] (52)	r-PA versus UK versus surgery	393	Native 69; Grafts 81 rt-PA versus UK – no difference	Fibrinolytics 5.6; Surgery 0.7 rt-PA versus UK – no difference
Arepally (106)	rt-PA	35	86	11
Ouriel (56)	rt-PA	26	89	19
Davidian (55)	rt-PA	15	87	6
APART (107)	rt-PA+abciximab versus UK+abciximab	120	rt-PA+abciximab 68 UK+abciximab 61	rt-PA+abciximab 10 UK+abciximab 6
RELAX (75)	rt-PA versus abciximab+rt-PA	74	rt-PA (1 U/h) 50 abciximab –rt-PA (1 U/h) 80	rt-PA 15 Abciximab+ rt-PA 20
Burkart (61)	TNK-t-PA	13	85	6.5
Burkart (108)	TNK-t-PA+eptifibatide	11	82	6.3
Heymans (62)	r-SAK	191	83; Clinical outcomes:1-year amputation-free survival 84;1 year mortality 6.9	12

SK streptokinase; VS versus; UK urokinase; SK-PLG streptokinase-plasminogen; rt-PA alteplase; TNK-t-PA tenecteplase; r-SAK staphylokinase

[a] 6-month operative procedures: 43% reduction 1-year amputation free survival: thrombolytics 65% Surgery 70%, $p=0.23$

[b] 6-month death, ongoing/recurrent ischemia, major morbidity: thrombolytics 36.1%, Surgery 61.7%, $p<0.001$

therapy in the United States. Ironically, in 1999 the FDA issued a warning regarding the safety of urokinase. Urokinase was being produced by human kidney cells harvested from post-mortem neonates, and the FDA was concerned that a less than rigorous screening process may have allowed contamination of the cells with viral and other infectious diseases that could be transmitted during drug administration *(32)*. Although this was only a theoretical concern, the manufacturer temporarily suspended urokinase production until these issues could be corrected and returned the agent safely to the market in October 2002. Recombinant urokinase (r-UK), which has a shorter half-life than urokinase, was also being investigated at this time and was subsequently found to have little clinical difference when compared to urokinase. Another member of the urokinase family of thrombolytics is prourokinase. Prourokinase is a relatively fibrin-specific precursor of urokinase that is derived using recombinant *Escherichia* coli technology. The fibrin specificity of prourokinase allows it to preferentially activate fibrin bound plasminogen in thrombus giving it a higher specificity for formed thrombus. Despite hopes of higher success rates and lower bleeding complications the only proven advantage of prourokinase over urokinase is its non-human origin *(44)*.

At present, the only FDA-approved indication for the use of urokinase is the treatment of massive pulmonary embolism; however, there is considerable descriptive literature supporting its use in peripheral arterial thrombolysis. One trial sought to prove the efficacy of r-UK in peripheral thrombolysis compared to surgical revascularization in an effort to obtain FDA approval. The Thrombolysis or Peripheral Arterial Surgery (TOPAS) trial was a multicenter randomized study that enrolled 548 patients to be treated initially with r-UK or surgery (Table 3) *(45)*. Unlike prior studies TOPAS did not demonstrate a significant advantage for thrombolytic therapy with regards to limb salvage or survival in patients with acute ischemic limbs (symptoms <14 days) at average follow-up of 1 year. Amputation-free survival was 61% and 71% ($p=0.1$) for the thrombolytic and surgery groups respectively in patients with native peripheral arterial disease versus 68% and 69% ($p=0.91$) for patients with bypass graft occlusions at one year. One-year mortality rates were not significantly different among the groups: 24.6% for r-UK versus 19.6% for surgery with native peripheral arterial disease and 16.2% for r-UK versus 15% for surgery in patients bypass graft occlusions. One important lesson learned from TOPAS was that full-dose anticoagulation with heparin plus r-UK is associated with significantly higher major bleeding rates (19%) versus sub-therapeutic heparin (9%), $p=0.02$. The overall rate of major bleeding for the trial was 12.5% for the thrombolytic group versus 5.5% for the surgical group, $p=0.005$. Although TOPAS demonstrated a significant reduction in the combined endpoint of open surgical procedures, death, and amputation during the index hospitalization (54% vs. 91%), $p=0.005$ for patients treated with thrombolytics, r-UK was never approved for use in peripheral arterial thrombolysis *(45)*. This outcome was obviously driven by the reduction in the number of open surgical procedures, which remained impressive at 1 year, 39% versus 65% in favor of the thrombolytics group.

ALTEPLASE

While the manufacturer was working on the purification of urokinase, a fibrin-specific thrombolytic began to dominate the US market *(46)*. Endogenous tissue plasminogen activator (t-PA) is synthesized by endothelial cells and has little effect on free plasminogen. Because t-PA preferentially binds fibrin, it works at the site of thrombus formation to facilitate conversion of fibrin bound plasmin to plasminogen thus activating the endogenous fibrinolytic system. Recombinant tissue plasminogen activator (rt-PA), also known as alteplase, is derived from hamster ovarian cells and was first produced in the 1980s. Like reteplase, alteplase utilization for peripheral vascular indications increased during the urokinase shortage and was ultimately approved for systemic thrombolysis in acute myocardial infarctions, stroke, and pulmonary embolism *(32,47)*. Although it does not carry FDA approval for the treatment of peripheral arterial thrombosis, many studies have demonstrated its efficacy and safety.

Semba et al. reviewed the literature pertaining to the use of alteplase for peripheral arterial occlusive disease. After reviewing 46 studies, the authors found a paucity of prospective randomized trials to define treatment protocols, although they concluded that alteplase may be beneficial in the treatment of acute limb ischemia (<14 days) to reduce the need for surgical or percutaneous intervention. For patients with chronic limb ischemia (>14 days), advanced diabetic arteriopathy or irreversible acute limb ischemia, the data seemed less convincing, suggesting that thrombolytic therapy with alteplase may not be a viable treatment strategy in this cohort *(48)*. Major bleeding rates were similar (5.1%) to those of urokinase, although the lack of standardized dosing protocols and event definitions induce uncertainty in the reporting of complications *(48)*. Dosing strategies for alteplase were quite variable ranging from 0.05 to 0.1 mg/kg/h or 0.25–10 mg/h for continuous infusion *(40)*. Overall, the higher dose regimens have not been found to be more beneficial and today the most commonly used regimen for catheter directed thrombolysis with alteplase is 0.05mg/kg/h or 1mg/h with or without a bolus *(40)*.

The literature comparing the efficacy among thrombolytics is sparse. Early small open-label randomized studies suggested a trend toward higher rates of initial angiographic success with rt-PA compared to SK or UK. One study with 60 patients compared intra-arterial and intravenous rt-PA to intra-arterial SK for the treatment of acute or subacute limb ischemia and demonstrated an initial success rate of 100% for intra-arterial rt-PA versus 80% with intra-arterial SK ($p<0.04$). Intravenous rt-PA was inferior to both intra-arterial rt-PA and intra-arterial SK with initial success rates of only 45% ($p<0.01$) *(49)*. Thirty-day limb salvage rates were also better for intra-arterial rt-PA and SK than with intravenous rt-PA at 80%, 60%, and 45%, respectively *(49)*. Another small-randomized open-label study of 32 patients also suggested higher rates of early angiographic success (<8 h) for rt-PA compared to UK; however, at 24 h there was no significant difference among the groups. Similarly, the 30-day outcomes of death, limb salvage, surgery, or bleeding complications were not significantly different *(50)*.

The largest randomized trial to date comparing the strategies of catheter-directed thrombolysis and surgical revascularization is the Surgery versus Thrombolysis for Ischemia of the Lower Extremity (STILE) trial (Table 15.3) *(51)*. The STILE trial was a multicenter open-label trial of 393 patients randomized to one of three arms: rt-PA, UK, or surgical revascularization. The initial 30-day results suggested that surgical revascularization was superior to thrombolytic therapy ($p<0.001$). Once stratified by duration of ischemic symptoms, patients with greater than 14 days of symptoms did better with surgical revascularization in regards to ongoing/recurrent ischemia ($p<0.001$) and major amputation ($p<0.01$) with a trend to lower morbidity ($p<0.1$). Patients with less than 14 days of symptoms had lower rates of amputation and shorter hospital stays with thrombolysis. Major bleed was significantly higher in the thrombolytic group (5.6%) but similar (0.7%) among the agents *(52)*. One-year follow-up for patients with native peripheral arterial disease revealed higher rates of recurrent ischemia (64% vs. 35%; $p<0.0001$) and major amputation (10% vs. 0%; $p=0.0024$) for patients randomized to thrombolytic therapy. Superficial femoral-popliteal disease, diabetes, and critical ischemia were factors associated with a poor response to fibrinolytics. Mortality was not different among the groups at 1 year. Both thrombolytic agents had similar efficacy and safety, reducing the extent of the surgical procedure in more than 50% of patients. Alteplase had shorter times to thrombolysis than UK at 8 and 24 h, respectively *(51)*.

STILE also prospectively looked at 124 patients with occluded lower extremity bypass grafts randomized to fibrinolytics or surgical revascularization. The primary outcome was a composite of death, amputation, ongoing/recurrent ischemia, and major morbidity. Catheter placement failed in approximately 40% of patients randomized to fibrinolytics and subsequently required surgical revascularization. Intention-to-treat analysis demonstrated a significant advantage for surgical revascularization with respect to the primary composite outcome at 1 year with an incidence of 61% for the surgical group compared to 78% for the fibrinolytic group ($p=0.04$). Again, ischemic time was a factor in response to therapy. Patients with ischemic symptoms of less than 14 days duration had lower rates of major amputation 48% versus 20% ($p=0.026$) at 1 year ($p=0.074$) and 1 year ($p=0.026$) when treated with fibrinolytics. For those with ischemic symptoms greater than 14 days, thrombolytic therapy was associated with higher rates of ongoing/recurrent ischemia (41% vs. 81%, $p=0.001$) *(53)*.

RETEPLASE

The shortage of urokinase, which had dominated the market in 1990s, spawned the use of many alternative fibrinolytics. Reteplase is a single chain recombinant fibrin-specific plasminogen activator that is derived from *Escherichia coli* and is non-glycosolated mutant of rt-PA. Reteplase (r-PA) has the advantage of a longer half-life (13–16 min) with both hepatic and renal clearance *(54)*. The original intent in the development of r-PA was to prove that the relatively long half-life may obviate the need for a continuous infusion but this would never be proven *(31)*. As such reteplase is currently only approved for use in acute myocardial infarction.

Davidian and colleagues drew inspiration from successful coronary fibrinolytics and demonstrated the feasibility of using catheter-directed r-PA for peripheral arterial thrombolysis. This small study of 15 patients demonstrated successful thrombolysis in 73% of the patients with comparable rates of major bleeding (6%) *(55)*. Similarly, a pilot study by Ouriel et al. involving five centers in the United States evaluated 26 patients with peripheral arterial occlusions treated t-PA at doses ranging from 0.5 to 2.0 U/h for a total average dose of 20.5 U and a mean duration of infusion of 19 h. Complete dissolution of the thrombus occurred in 88.5% and major bleeding complications in 19.2% *(56)*. One of the largest r-PA studies to date, in peripheral arterial disease, prospectively enrolled 87 patients with a 101 lower extremity arterial occlusions for thrombolysis using one of three dosing strategies of r-PA (0.5 U/h, 0.25 U/h, 0.125 U/h) in addition to low-dose intravenous heparin (400–500 IU/h). Successful thrombolysis was achieved in 86.7%, 83.8%, and 85.3% of patients in the 0.5U/h, 0.25 U/h, and 0.125 U/h groups with major bleeding and transfusion rates of 13.3%, 5.4%, and 2.9% in the respective groups. The authors concluded that all three dosing regimens were equally efficacious; however, more major bleeding was seen in the 0.5 U/h cohort and longer infusion times (42 vs. 30 h) necessary for the 0.125 U/h group. Unfortunately, large studies demonstrating the safety and efficacy of r-PA for peripheral arterial thrombolysis are non-existent, although it has been studied extensively for acute myocardial infarction and appears to be safe and efficacious when compared to streptokinase and alteplase in this setting *(57–60)*.

TENECTEPLASE

Tenecteplase (TNK-t-PA), like reteplase, is a mutant of t-PA and was developed with the goal of eliminating continuous infusion therapy for acute myocardial infarction *(31)*.

TNK-t-PA has increased fibrin specificity and less systemic degradation compared to t-PA thus is similarly efficacious with lower rates of bleeding complications when used for acute myocardial infarction. Since the vast majority of the data for TNK-t-PA are in the setting of acute myocardial infarction, this remains the only approved indication. There are minimal data for its use in peripheral arterial thrombolysis. Burkart et al. published their experience in 13 patients treated with TNK-t-PA infusions of 0.25 mg/h for peripheral arterial occlusions and 5 patients for venous thrombosis (Table 15.3) *(61)*. Clinical success was achieved in 85% and 80% of patients treated for arterial and venous thrombosis, respectively. The mean duration of treatment was 21.5 h. Major bleeding occurred in one patient *(61)*. Further details regarding TNK-t-PA will be discussed elsewhere.

STAPHYLOKINASE

Recombinant staphylokinase (r-Sak) is also a fibrin-specific thrombolytic that consists of a 136 amino acid protein secreted by S. aureus and linked to polyethylene glycol to reduce its immunogenicity *(46)*. Staphylokinase is an indirect plasminogen activator that is deactivated by α2-antiplasmin in the

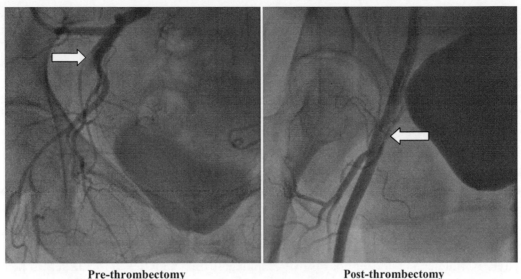

Pre-thrombectomy   Post-thrombectomy

Fig. 1. Iliac thrombus

absence of fibrin. In the presence of thrombus, the staphylokinase-plasminogen complex binds to the clot to induce local thrombolysis. The deactivation of staphylokinase by α2-antiplasmin prevents systemic fibrinolysis (Fig. 1) *(46)*.

There are very little data with regards to the use of r-Sak in either acute myocardial infarction or peripheral arterial thrombolysis. Heymans et al. published their experience in 191 patients with an occlusion (thrombotic or embolic) of either a native peripheral artery or bypass graft of less than 120 days duration using a 2 mg intra-arterial bolus of r-Sak followed by a 1 mg/h infusion overnight (Table 15.3) *(62)*. Alternatively, patients receiving concomitant heparin were treated with an infusion dose of 0.5 mg/h after a 2 mg intra-arterial bolus of r-Sak. The majority of patients (99) had acute/subacute ischemia or severe claudication (57). The remainder of patients had either gangrene or chronic rest pain. Failure of revascularization occurred in 4% of the treated patients and 83% had successful revascularization. Mortality rates at 1 and 12 months were 3.1% and 6.9%, respectively. Major bleeding occurred in 12% with a 2.1% incidence of intracranial hemorrhage. Therapy was discontinued in 2.1% of patients for a suspected allergic reaction *(62)*. R-Sak is not approved for use in the United States.

Antiplatelet Therapy

ASPIRIN

There are no definitive data from large randomized trials to know if aspirin will prevent the progression of atherosclerotic vascular disease. One small angiographic study did demonstrate a delay in progression of atherosclerotic vascular disease (by serial angiography) in patients treated with aspirin alone versus aspirin plus dipyridamole *(63)*. The most likely mechanism by which aspirin delays the progression of atherothrombosis is by prevention of platelet thrombogenesis on the surface of atherosclerotic plaques *(64)*. The clinical relevance of aspirin's beneficial effects are significant when one examines the data from the Antiplatelet Trialists Collaboration meta-analysis of over 100,000 patients from 145 randomized trials, which showed significant reductions (~23%) in the risk of nonfatal stroke, nonfatal myocardial infarction, and vascular death in high-risk patients treated with long-term aspirin therapy *(65)*. In subgroup analyses of 9,214 patients with peripheral arterial occlusive disease, the beneficial effects of aspirin were demonstrated to a similar degree in those with claudication (23%) as well as those with prior peripheral arterial bypass grafts (22%) or angioplasty (29%). In patients with acute limb ischemia, there are no trials to quantify the effects of aspirin therapy and the AHA/ACC guidelines give a class I indication for aspirin (75–325 mg) in the prevention of death, myocardial infarction, and ischemic stroke in patients with peripheral arterial disease *(66)*. For these reasons aspirin is started prior to percutaneous coronary intervention and continued life-long thereafter. Although early randomized trials suggested benefit for percutaneous coronary angioplasty compared to standard medical therapy *(67–69)*, no such data exist for peripheral arterial intervention.

THIENOPYRIDINES

Clopidogrel and its predecessor ticlopidine are thienopyridine derivatives that irreversibly inhibit platelet activation and aggregation by blocking the adenosine diphosphate-induced activation of the glycoprotein IIb-IIIa receptors. Although both drugs are prodrugs and are hepatically cleared, clopidogrel has replaced ticlopidine because of a more favorable side effect profile and once daily administration. Studies supporting the use of clopidogrel or ticlopidine in acute leg ischemia are sparse and most recommendations regarding their use in this arena stem from the long-term beneficial cardiovascular effects in chronic peripheral arterial disease patients.

The efficacy of clopidogrel for reducing future cardiovascular events has been evaluated in several large randomized trials. The first was Clopidogrel versus Aspirin in Patients at Risk of Ischemic Events (CAPRIE), a 19,185 patient study that randomized patients with a recent vascular event to receive aspirin 325 mg daily or clopidogrel 75 mg daily with 1–3 years of follow-up *(70)*. Subgroup analysis suggests that patients with peripheral arterial disease derive the greatest benefit from clopidogrel therapy; this group had 24% relative risk reduction ($p=0.0028$) for myocardial infarction, ischemic stroke, or vascular death. The most frequent side effects with clopidogrel therapy were rash and diarrhea. The incidence of neutropenia with clopidogrel was 0.1% (severe neutropenia 0.05%), similar to that of aspirin.

The ACC/AHA guidelines give a class I recommendation for clopidogrel as an "effective" alternative to aspirin in patients with peripheral arterial disease to reduce the risk of ischemic vascular events *(66)*. Clopidogrel and Acetyl Salicylic Acid in bypass Surgery for Peripheral ARterial disease (CASPAR) is large randomized controlled trial of over 1,400 patients investigating dual antiplatelet therapy (aspirin plus clopidogrel) in patients with peripheral arterial disease undergoing peripheral arterial bypass surgery that was recently completed. A second trial, Clopidogrel and Aspirin in the Management of Peripheral Endovascular Revascularization (CAMPER), is a large randomized trial of 2,000 patients with peripheral arterial disease undergoing percutaneous peripheral intervention which is currently ongoing *(71,72)*. These two trials once published should provide further insight on the utility of dual antiplatelet therapy in this population. Although data regarding dual antiplatelet therapy are still forthcoming, most patients are treated with aspirin indefinitely and clopidogrel for at least 1 month after percutaneous peripheral vascular intervention. For patients who receive a drug eluting stent during a peripheral vascular intervention, clopidogrel is continued for at least 6 months. Prior to the peripheral intervention, patients are typically loaded with 300–600 mg of clopidogrel.

GLYCOPROTEIN IIb-IIIa INHIBITORS

It has been postulated that the addition of antiplatelet therapy, specifically glycoprotein IIb-IIIa inhibitors, may inhibit new thrombus and accelerate thrombus dissolution when used in conjunction with fibrinolytics in patients with atherothrombotic peripheral arterial disease *(73)*. Pathophysiologically, using a combination of fibrinolytics and anti-platelet agents makes sense. Treating a thrombus with fibrinolytics causes the release of thrombin, which enhances platelet aggregation thus leading to more thrombotic occlusions. In vitro, the addition of glycoprotein IIb-IIIa inhibitors interrupts the process of platelet aggregation and prevents thrombus formation. A number of small studies have suggested that glycoprotein IIb-IIIa inhibitors increase the efficacy of peripheral arterial thrombolysis without substantially increasing the risk of major bleeding or death. The largest study randomized 70 patients to either abciximab plus urokinase or urokinase alone. At 90 days of follow-up the abciximab plus urokinase group had an amputation free survival rate of 96% compared to 80% in the urokinase mono-therapy group. This benefit came at an 8% increased risk of nonfatal bleeding *(74)*. Similarly, the reteplase alone versus abciximab plus reteplase (RELAX) study enrolled 74 patients in a non-randomized dose-escalating study to evaluate the safety and efficacy of a glycoprotein IIb-IIIa inhibitor in the treatment of occlusive peripheral arterial disease *(75)*. Major bleeding was not significantly different between the groups, 15% in the reteplase only group versus 20% in the reteplase plus abciximab group and there were no intracranial hemorrhages in the study. There was a trend toward improvement in complete thrombus resolution and patency rates as well as a significant reduction (5% vs. 31%) in distal embolic events, $p=0.014$. These and other smaller studies suggest that glycoprotein IIb-IIIa inhibitors may have potential benefit in the treatment of occlusive peripheral arterial disease; however, larger randomized trials are needed to demonstrate safety and efficacy *(76,77)*.

Mechanical Thrombectomy

Just prior to the publication of Judkins and Dotter's use of percutaneous transluminal angioplasty in 1964 *(1)*, Fogarty et al. described a new method of extraction of arterial and venous thrombus *(78)*. Since the 1960s many thrombectomy devices have been developed for the purpose of eliminating the need for thrombolysis. Instead of antiquating thrombolysis, these thrombectomy devices have helped demonstrate the complementary nature of both treatment modalities. The two most common indications for thrombectomy are in the management of thrombosed arteriovenous dialysis fistulae and acute limb ischemia, although other indications exist (Table 5). Data directly comparing pharmacologic to mechanical thrombectomy are few and primarily limited to case series and non-randomized studies. Limitations of thrombectomy include a propensity for distal embolization and vascular injury. These shortcomings have not been very problematic for the treatment of dialysis fistulae but are limiting in the treatment of peripheral arterial disease. Unlike with dialysis fistulae, the microemboli are not absorbed by the venous system and often result in damage to the microvasculature and prolonged ischemia *(79)*.

The appropriate treatment strategy should be individualized based on the characteristics of the thrombotic occlusion (i.e., location, age of thrombus, thrombus burden), as well as the operative and

Table 5
Indications for mechanical thrombectomy *(109)*

Non-carotid
Iatrogenic or traumatic native vessel thrombotic occlusion
Iatrogenic or traumatic arterial graft thrombotic occlusion
Acute thrombotic occlusion of the SVC, IVC, or ileofemoral system
Massive pulmonary embolus
Thrombotic occlusion of a dialysis arteriovenous fistulae
Carotid
Acute ischemic stroke with contraindications to thrombolysis

SVC superior vena cava; *IVC* inferior vena cava

bleeding risks. Mechanical thrombectomy may be attempted if the lesion can be crossed with a guidewire; this is also an important step for local delivery of fibrinolytics. Alternatively, open surgical thrombectomy may be the treatment of choice. Incomplete mechanical thrombectomy or distal embolization are two situations where local fibrinolytics may be a beneficial adjunctive therapy. Mechanical thrombectomy does not eliminate the need for thrombolytic therapy and is not tremendously effective for chronic adherent thrombus. In patients with acute limb ischemia, mechanical thrombectomy alone does not treat the culprit lesion, often requiring adjunctive endovascular or surgical treatment. The majority of patients with acute limb ischemia require a combination of mechanical and pharmacologic therapies. Mechanical thrombectomy is often used to debulk the thrombus with or without balloon angioplasty to allow the lesion to be crossed with a wire to facilitate intra-thrombus administration of a fibrinolytic. The Angiojet (Possis Medical, Minneapolis, MN) is currently the only device FDA approved for thrombus aspiration in peripheral arterial thrombolysis. This device and others allow for a pulse-spray administration of the thrombolytic agent, this type of therapy is postulated to decrease the lengthy thrombolytic administration times and subsequent hemorrhagic complications.

Carotid Intervention

Stroke is the third leading cause of death in the United States and more than 85% of all strokes are ischemic in etiology *(80,81)*. Stroke risk is coincident with severity and instability of the stenotic lesion. An asymptomatic mild internal carotid stenosis has less than a 1% per year stroke risk whereas a symptomatic severe internal carotid stenosis (70–90%) carries a one year stroke risk as high as 11% *(82)*. Many strokes arise in arterial territories that are approachable with percutaneous intervention. The approach to reducing stroke risk is multi-factorial including risk factor modification and revascularization. At present the mainstay of carotid revascularization remains carotid endarterectomy, and carotid stenting is reserved for patients enrolled in clinical trials or with a high-surgical risk. Irrespective of the modality of revascularization, patients should receive aggressive atherosclerotic risk factor reduction, in addition to antiplatelet therapy.

Anticoagulation

INDIRECT THROMBIN INHIBITORS
Heparin

There are sparse data supporting the use of heparin for acute ischemic strokes and there are no randomized trials to support or refute the use of heparin in percutaneous carotid intervention. Current guidelines recommended the use of heparin for carotid stenting with a targeted activated clotting time of 250–300 s, initiated after sheath insertion for elective carotid stenting. Heparin is usually discontinued immediately after the completion of the procedure *(80)*. There are no data with regards to the use of direct thrombin inhibitors or low-molecular weight heparins in carotid intervention.

In the setting of an acute stroke the utilization of intravenous heparin remains controversial because of the risk of hemorrhagic transformation. The International Stroke Trial enrolled 19,436 patients with an acute ischemic stroke with symptoms less than 48 h duration to be randomized to high (12,500 IU) or low dose (5,000 IU) subcutaneous heparin bid versus placebo. Both groups were also randomized to aspirin 300 mg daily or placebo in a factorial design *(83)*. At 14 days there was a non-significant reduction in deaths (9.0%) in the heparin-treated group compared to the "avoid heparin" group (9.3%). Patients allocated to heparin did experience a significant reduction in stroke at 14 days, 2.9% versus 3.8% for the placebo group. However, this reduction in ischemic stroke was offset by an increase in hemorrhagic stroke of similar magnitude (1.2% for heparin vs. 0.4% for the placebo). The transformation risk was the highest in the 12, 500 IU group and neither group demonstrated a significant clinical advantage at 6 months. Patients receiving aspirin also had a significant reduction in ischemic strokes at 14 days (2.8% vs. 3.9%) without the incremental risk of hemorrhagic stroke. In the aspirin-treated group, the risk of death or nonfatal stroke was also significantly reduced (11.3% vs. 12.4%) at 14 days. At 6 months the aspirin-treated group demonstrated a small non-significant reduction in the primary endpoint of death or dependency (62.2% vs. 63.5%, $p = 0.07$). After adjusting for baseline prognosis this benefit was statistically significant ($p = 0.03$).

Warfarin

As with many instances in carotid intervention there are no data with regards to outcomes in patients treated with warfarin after carotid stenting. There are trials from which we can draw some inferences, albeit not in this population. The Warfarin-Aspirin Symptomatic Intracranial Disease (WASID) was a retrospective multicenter study that enrolled 151 symptomatic patients with a 50–99% carotid stenosis to evaluate the efficacy of aspirin versus warfarin for the prevention of myocardial infarction, ischemic stroke, or sudden death (84). There was a suggestion of benefit in the warfarin-treated group; however, no sound conclusions could be drawn because of its retrospective nature. The Warfarin Aspirin Recurrent Stroke Study (WARSS) was a prospective randomized trial of 2,206 patients with a recent ischemic non-cardioembolic stroke that compared aspirin to warfarin for the prevention of death or recurrent stroke (85). WARSS failed to show any significant difference in stroke, death or, major bleeding between the groups at 2 years; however, the study may have been underpowered to detect excess harm in the warfarin-treated group (86). Another large open-label controlled trial of 2,161 patients, warfarin antiplatelet vascular events (WAVE), randomized patients to antiplatelet therapy (aspirin, ticlopidine, or clopidogrel) alone or antiplatelet therapy plus oral anticoagulation (warfarin) with a targeted INR of 2–3. At a mean of 35 months of follow-up there was no significant difference in the composite outcome of death, myocardial infarction, or stroke between the groups; however, there was an increased risk of life-threatening bleeding (4% vs. 1.2%, $p < 0.001$) in the warfarin group (87).

DIRECT THROMBIN INHIBITORS

Bivalrudin

No randomized trial data exist for the use of bivalirudin in carotid stenting and there is very little evidence of its safety or efficacy in this population. One group of investigators reported their experience using bivalirudin as the sole anticoagulant (1.75 mg/kg bolus followed by 1.75 mg/kg/h drip) in more than 150 patients receiving carotid stents. These patients did receive adjunctive clopidogrel and aspirin as part of the treatment protocol. The investigators reported no major neurologic sequelae or hemorrhagic complications requiring transfusion or surgical procedures (88). Bivalirudin has also been used successfully in a patient with heparin-induced thrombocytopenia undergoing carotid endarterectomy (89).

Although bivalirudin has been used successfully in percutaneous carotid intervention and endarterectomy, concerns for intracranial hemorrhage with an irreversible drug still exist.

FIBRINOLYTICS

Fibrinolytic therapy has no role in elective carotid interventions but may have utility in carotid interventions for acute ischemic or iatrogenic embolic stroke (Fig. 2). Fibrinolytic therapy with intravenous t-PA for reperfusion in acute ischemic stroke has been shown to improve neurologic outcomes at 3 months (patients were 30% more likely to have minimal or no disability) in the National Institute of Neurological Disorders and Stroke (NINDS) trial *(90)*. The benefit of intravenous t-PA for acute ischemic strokes comes at the cost of a 6.4% risk of a symptomatic intracranial hemorrhage within 36 h of administration, compared to a 0.6% risk in the placebo. This risk is even greater when fibrinolytic therapy is used inappropriately (i.e., >3 h from the onset of symptoms).

Intra-arterial fibrinolytic therapy for the treatment of acute ischemic stroke was evaluated in the Prolyse in Acute Cerebral Thromboembolism Trial (PROACT)-II *(91)*. PROACT-II randomized 180 patients with acute angiographically proven acute middle cerebral artery occlusions to intra-arterial

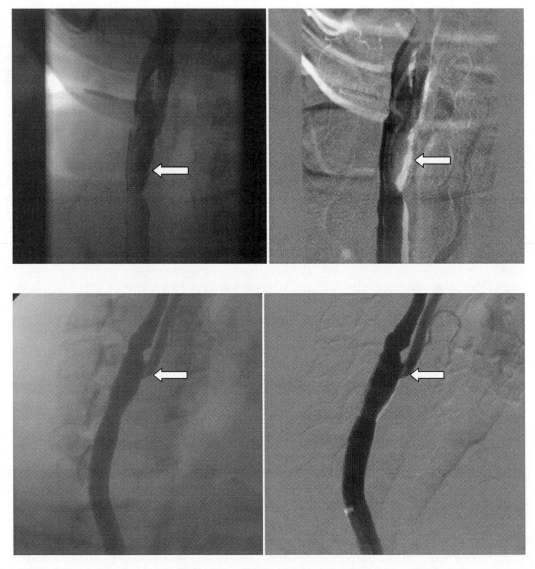

Fig. 2. (a) Carotid stent thrombosis-pre-fibrinolytic. **(b)** Carotid stent thrombosis-post-fibrinolytic.

prourokinase plus heparin or heparin only within 6 h of the onset of symptoms. Neurological outcomes were improved at 90 days (15% increase in patients with a modified Rankin score less than 2, $p=0.04$); however, there was an 8% increase in the risk of intracranial hemorrhage ($p=0.06$). The overall mortality was high and not significantly different among the groups, 25% and 27%, respectively for the prourokinase and control groups *(91)*.

Combination therapy with intravenous and intra-arterial fibrinolytics has been looked at in two small trials. The Emergency Management of Stroke (EMS) was a 35 patient trial where patients were randomized to reduced dose intra-arterial t-PA (0.6 mg/kg) plus intravenous t-PA or intra-arterial t-PA alone within 3 h of symptom onset *(92)*. There was no difference in clinical neurologic outcomes at 90 days between the groups, although there was a higher rate of recanalization in the intra-arterial plus intravenous group (54%) compared to the intra-arterial only group (10%). The 90-day mortality rate was higher in the intra-arterial plus intravenous group (29%) compared to the intra-arterial only group (6%), $p=0.06$. Similarly, the Interventional Management of Stroke (IMS) study enrolled 80 patients in a non-randomized fashion to be treated with intravenous t-PA followed by intra-arterial t-PA if residual thrombus was visualized on angiogram *(93)*. Unlike EMS, IMS demonstrated significantly better clinical neurologic outcomes at 90 days compared to those obtained in the NINDS trial with similar rates of intracranial hemorrhage (6.3% vs. 6.6%, $p=0.91$) and death (16% vs. 21%, $p=0.33$) *(90,93)*. IMS-III is an ongoing clinical trial to evaluate the efficacy of combined intra-arterial t-PA delivered via an ultrasonic EKOS catheter plus intravenous thrombolysis in acute ischemic stroke *(94)*.

Antiplatelet Therapy

ASPIRIN

Aspirin has been the mainstay of antiplatelet therapy for both primary and secondary prevention of adverse cardiovascular events for many years. For secondary prevention aspirin decreases the risk of recurrent nonfatal stroke by 22% irrespective of gender *(65)*. Based on the available data from randomized trials aspirin alone is superior to carotid revascularization for symptomatic carotid stenoses of less than 50% and for asymptomatic carotid stenosis greater than 60% for secondary prevention *(80)*. The AHA/ACC consensus recommends aspirin 81–325 mg daily for patients with carotid artery occlusive disease, especially those undergoing carotid stenting. Aspirin is typically started 3–4 days prior to the procedure and continued indefinitely at doses of 75–325 mg daily. Higher doses of aspirin 650 mg or 1,300 mg daily have been associated with higher rates of death, myocardial infarction, or stroke with 1–3 months of carotid endarterectomy *(80)*.

THIENOPYRIDINES

Clopidogrel and ticlopidine have been proven to reduce future cardiovascular events for secondary prevention but have not been evaluated for use in primary prevention. The Ticlopidine Aspirin Stroke Study (TASS) was a 3,069 patient study that randomized patients with a recent ischemic stroke or transient ischemic attack to aspirin 1,300 mg daily versus ticlopidine 500 mg daily with up to 5 years of follow-up *(95)*.

Ticlopidine was superior to aspirin in reducing death, nonfatal strokes, and reversible ischemic events with a relative risk reduction of 23% and 12% at 1 and 5 years, respectively. The most frequent side effect of ticlopidine was diarrhea, which occurred in approximately 20% of the treated population; however, the more clinically worrisome side effect of neutropenia was seen in 2% (0.9% severe neutropenia) of the ticlopidine group.

Since data from CAPRIE suggest that clopidogrel is superior to aspirin for secondary prevention of cardiovascular events *(70)*, the Management of Atherothrombosis with Clopidogrel in High Risk Patients with Recent Transient Ischemic Attack or Ischemic Stroke (MATCH) trail was designed to evaluate combination therapy (aspirin plus clopidogrel) compared to clopidogrel alone *(96)*. MATCH enrolled 7,599 patients with recent transient ischemic attacks or ischemic stroke to aspirin 75 mg daily versus aspirin 75 mg daily plus clopidogrel 75 mg daily. Data analysis demonstrated a non-significant relative risk reduction of 5.9% ($p=0.360$) for myocardial infarction, ischemic stroke, or vascular death; however, there was an increased risk of life-threatening bleeding with dual antiplatelet therapy (1% vs. 3%), $p=0.0001$.

There are no carotid stent trials comparing aspirin plus clopidogrel versus aspirin or clopidogrel alone. Based on the aforementioned data pertaining to cardiovascular event reduction seen with clopidogrel, specifically in patients with symptomatic carotid occlusive disease, we recommend aspirin 81–325 mg daily starting 3–4 days prior to carotid stenting (if not started at the time of the ischemic event) and plus a loading dose of clopidogrel (300–600 mg) on the day of the procedure. Aspirin should be continued indefinitely and clopidogrel for 4 weeks. Because the carotid vessels are large caliber and most strokes after carotid stenting seem to occur in the peri-procedural period, it seems unlikely that a longer duration of dual antiplatelet therapy would be beneficial.

GLYCOPROTEIN IIB-IIIA INHIBITORS

Currently glycoprotein IIb-IIIa inhibitors are not used in elective carotid interventions because of concerns of increased intracranial hemorrhage, which have been born out in trials with acute ischemic stroke. The Abciximab in Emergency Treatment of Stroke Trial (AbESTT-II) was a large phase III trial that randomized patients who present within 5–6 h of symptom onset (i.e., outside the 3 h window for fibrinolytics) or with signs of stroke upon awakening (presentation must be less than 3 h from awakening) to abciximab versus placebo *(97)*. Patients were treated with abciximab 0.25 mg/kg bolus followed by a drip at 0.125 mcg/kg/min for 12 h. After 808 of the planned 1,900 patients were enrolled, the trial was stopped secondary to an excess intracranial hemorrhage (symptomatic fatal intracranial hemorrhage 6.5% versus 0.5% at 90 days, $p<0.001$) in the abcixmab-treated group and no detectable benefit in any of the cohorts studied. One small non-randomized prospective study of 300 patients compared the use of embolic protection devices to adjunctive glycoprotein IIb-IIIa inhibitors for the prevention of neurologic death, nonfatal stroke, and major bleeding (including intracranial hemorrhage) in patients undergoing elective carotid stenting. Embolic protection demonstrated a favorable decrease in the incidence of the composite outcome (0% vs. 5.1%, $p=0.02$) *(98)*. A second small prospective study compared 128 high-surgical risk patients with severe carotid stenosis undergoing carotid stenting with abciximab to historic controls. Abciximab decreased the risk of peri-procedural stroke (1.6%) compared to the controls (8%, $p=0.05$), without increasing the risk of intracranial hemorrhage *(99)*. Today, carotid stenting is performed exclusively with embolic protection and the combination of glycoprotein IIb-IIIa inhibitors with embolic protection has not been studied.

Other studies using perfusion brain imaging to guide patient selection for combination of intravenous and intra-arterial t-PA, Reperfusion Of Stroke Imaging Evaluation (ROSIE), and Combination Approach to Thrombolysis Utilizing Eptifibatide and rt-PA (CLEAR) are ongoing *(100,101)*.

Mechanical Thrombectomy

Mechanical thrombectomy for carotid intervention was developed with the intent of improving outcomes in acute ischemic stroke and its use remains limited to this population. The Mechanical Embolus Removal in Cerebral Ischemia (MERCI) trial was a non-randomized study that enrolled 151 patients who presented within 8 h of an acute ischemic that were not candidates for thrombolysis to be treated with the Merci Retriever device (Concentric Medical, Mountain View, CA) to open an occluded intracranial carotid, vertebrobasilar or middle cerebral artery *(102)*. Adjunctive fibrinolytic therapy was allowed for incomplete thrombectomy but was considered separate in the final analysis. Mechanical thrombectomy was successful in 46% of patients and was associated with improved neurologic outcomes (modified Rankin < 2) in 46% of patients who had recanalization (compared to 10% with unsuccessful recanalization). Mortality rates at 90 days were also improved with successful recanalization (32% vs. 54%). This device was subsequently FDA approved for the use in patients who present with an acute ischemic stroke and are ineligible for fibrinolytic therapy.

References

1. Dotter CT, Judkins MP (1964) Transluminal treatment of arteriosclerotic obstruction. Description of a new technic and a preliminary report of its application. Circulation 30:654–670
2. Myler R (2005) Coronary and peripheral angioplasty: a historical perspective. In: Topol EJ (ed) Textbook of interventional cardiology, 4th edn. Saunders, Philadelphia, PA, pp 141–157
3. Mc LJ (1959) The discovery of heparin. Circulation 19(1):75–78
4. Gruntzig A (1978) Transluminal dilatation of coronary-artery stenosis. Lancet 1:263
5. Grayburn PA, Willard JE, Brickner ME et al (1991) In vivo thrombus formation on a guidewire during intravascular ultrasound imaging: evidence for inadequate heparinization. Cathet Cardiovasc Diagn 23(2):141–143
6. Laskey MA, Deutsch E, Barnathan E et al (1990) Influence of heparin therapy on percutaneous transluminal coronary angioplasty outcome in unstable angina pectoris. Am J Cardiol 65(22):1425–1429
7. Ahmed I, Majeed A, Powell R (2007) Heparin induced thrombocytopenia: diagnosis and management update. Postgrad Med J 83(983):575–582
8. Brumberg RS, Back MR, Armstrong PA et al (2007) The relative importance of graft surveillance and warfarin therapy in infrainguinal prosthetic bypass failure. J Vasc Surg 46(6):1160–1166
9. LeCroy CJ, Patterson MA, Taylor SM et al (2005) Effect of warfarin anticoagulation on below-knee polytetrafluoroethylene graft patency. Ann Vasc Surg 19(2):192–198
10. Kalra M, Gloviczki P, Andrews JC et al (2003) Open surgical and endovascular treatment of superior vena cava syndrome caused by nonmalignant disease. J Vasc Surg 38(2):215–223
11. Goodman SG, Fitchett D, Armstrong PW et al (2003) Randomized evaluation of the safety and efficacy of enoxaparin versus unfractionated heparin in high-risk patients with non-ST-segment elevation acute coronary syndromes receiving the glycoprotein IIb/IIIa inhibitor eptifibatide. Circulation 107(2):238–244
12. (1999) Invasive compared with non-invasive treatment in unstable coronary-artery disease: FRISC II prospective randomised multicentre study. FRagmin and Fast Revascularisation during InStability in Coronary artery disease Investigators. Lancet 354(9180):708–715
13. Blazing MA, de Lemos JA, White HD et al (2004) Safety and efficacy of enoxaparin vs unfractionated heparin in patients with non-ST-segment elevation acute coronary syndromes who receive tirofiban and aspirin: a randomized controlled trial. JAMA 292(1):55–64
14. Antman EM, McCabe CH, Gurfinkel EP et al (1999) Enoxaparin prevents death and cardiac ischemic events in unstable angina/non-Q-wave myocardial infarction. Results of the thrombolysis in myocardial infarction (TIMI) 11B trial. Circulation 100(15):1593–1601
15. Cohen M, Demers C, Gurfinkel EP et al (1997) A comparison of low-molecular-weight heparin with unfractionated heparin for unstable coronary artery disease. Efficacy and Safety of Subcutaneous Enoxaparin in Non-Q-Wave Coronary Events Study Group. N Engl J Med 337(7):447–452
16. Ferguson JJ, Califf RM, Antman EM et al (2004) Enoxaparin vs unfractionated heparin in high-risk patients with non-ST-segment elevation acute coronary syndromes managed with an intended early invasive strategy: primary results of the SYNERGY randomized trial. JAMA 292(1):45–54
17. Khosla S, Kunjummen B, Guerrero M et al (2002) Safety and efficacy of combined use of low molecular weight heparin (enoxaparin, lovenox) and glycoprotein IIb/IIIa receptor antagonist (eptifibatide, integrelin) during nonemergent coronary and peripheral vascular intervention. Am J Ther 9(6):488–491
18. Klein W, Buchwald A, Hillis SE et al (1997) Comparison of low-molecular-weight heparin with unfractionated heparin acutely and with placebo for 6 weeks in the management of unstable coronary artery disease. Fragmin in unstable coronary artery disease study (FRIC). Circulation 96(1):61–68
19. (1999) Long-term low-molecular-mass heparin in unstable coronary-artery disease: FRISC II prospective randomised multicentre study. FRagmin and Fast Revascularisation during InStability in Coronary artery disease. Investigators. Lancet 354(9180):701–707

20. Mehta SR, Granger CB, Eikelboom JW et al (2007) Efficacy and safety of fondaparinux versus enoxaparin in patients with acute coronary syndromes undergoing percutaneous coronary intervention: results from the OASIS-5 trial. J Am Coll Cardiol 50(18):1742–1751
21. Shammas NW (2005) Complications in peripheral vascular interventions: emerging role of direct thrombin inhibitors. J Vasc Interv Radiol 16(2 Pt 1):165–171
22. Allie DE, Hall P, Shammas NW et al (2004) The Angiomax Peripheral Procedure Registry of Vascular Events Trial (APPROVE): in-hospital and 30-day results. J Invasive Cardiol 16(11):651–656
23. Lincoff AM, Bittl JA, Kleiman NS et al (2004) Comparison of bivalirudin versus heparin during percutaneous coronary intervention (the Randomized Evaluation of PCI Linking Angiomax to Reduced Clinical Events [REPLACE]-1 trial). Am J Cardiol 93(9):1092–1096
24. Lincoff AM, Kleiman NS, Kereiakes DJ et al (2004) Long-term efficacy of bivalirudin and provisional glycoprotein IIb/IIIa blockade vs heparin and planned glycoprotein IIb/IIIa blockade during percutaneous coronary revascularization: REPLACE-2 randomized trial. JAMA 292(6):696–703
25. HORIZONS AMI (2008) http://www.cardiosource.com/img/horizonsami01.ppt. Accessed 23 Feb 2008
26. Shammas NW, Lemke JH, Dippel EJ et al (2003) Bivalirudin in peripheral vascular interventions: a single center experience. J Invasive Cardiol 15(7):401–404
27. Shammas NW, Lemke JH, Dippel EJ et al (2003) In-hospital complications of peripheral vascular interventions using unfractionated heparin as the primary anticoagulant. J Invasive Cardiol 15(5):242–246
28. Grubbs G (2003) Single center experience with bivalirudin anticoagulation in peripheral vascular interventions: possible benefits over unfractionated heparin. Poster presented at: Cardiovascular Revascularization Therapy Conference, Washington, DC, 26–29 Jan, 2003
29. Knopf W, St. Joseph's Hospital experience (2003) Direct thrombin inhibitors in ACS and PCI: the case for bivalirudin replacing unfractionated heparin in PCI. Paper presented at Transcatheter Cardiovascular Therapeutics 14th Annual Scientific Symposium, Washington, DC, 24–28 Sept, 2003
30. Blaisdell FW, Steele M, Allen RE (1978) Management of acute lower extremity arterial ischemia due to embolism and thrombosis. Surgery 84(6):822–834
31. Ouriel K (2005) Peripheral arterial thrombolysis. In: Yadav J (ed) Manual of peripheral vascular intervention. Lippincott Williams & Wilkins, Philadelphia, PA, pp 56–68
32. Zoon K (2007) Important drug warning: safety information regarding the use of abbokinase (urokinase). http://www.fda.gov/cder/biologics/ltr/abb012599.htm. Accessed 10 Dec 2007
33. Katzen BT, van Breda A (1981) Low dose streptokinase in the treatment of arterial occlusions. AJR Am J Roentgenol 136(6):1171–1178
34. Lammer J, Pilger E, Justich E et al (1985) Fibrinolysis in chronic arteriosclerotic occlusions: intrathrombotic injections of streptokinase. Work in progress. Radiology 157(1):45–50
35. Lammer J, Pilger E, Neumayer K et al (1986) Intraarterial fibrinolysis: long-term results. Radiology 161(1):159–163
36. (1998) Randomised trial of intravenous streptokinase, oral aspirin, both, or neither among 17,187 cases of suspected acute myocardial infarction: ISIS-2. ISIS-2 (Second International Study of Infarct Survival) Collaborative Group. Lancet 2(8607):349–360
37. (1986) Effectiveness of intravenous thrombolytic treatment in acute myocardial infarction. Gruppo Italiano per lo Studio della Streptochinasi nell'Infarto Miocardico (GISSI). Lancet 1(8478):397–402
38. (1986) A prospective trial of intravenous streptokinase in acute myocardial infarction (I.S.A.M.). Mortality, morbidity, and infarct size at 21 days. The I.S.A.M. Study Group. N Engl J Med 314(23):1465–1471
39. Totty WG, Gilula LA, McClennan BL et al (1982) Low-dose intravascular fibrinolytic therapy. Radiology 143(1):59–69
40. (2003) Thrombolysis in the management of lower limb peripheral arterial occlusion – a consensus document. J Vasc Interv Radiol 14(9 Pt 2):S337–S349.
41. MS SGW, Jones NW et al (1952) Urokinase: an activator of plasma fribinolysin extracted from urine. Am J Physiol 171:768–769
42. (1973) The urokinase pulmonary embolism trial. A national cooperative study. Circulation 47(2 Suppl):II1–108.
43. (1974) Urokinase–streptokinase embolism trial. Phase 2 results. A cooperative study. JAMA 229(12):1606–1613
44. Ouriel K, Kandarpa K, Schuerr DM et al (1999) Prourokinase versus urokinase for recanalization of peripheral occlusions, safety and efficacy: the PURPOSE trial. J Vasc Interv Radiol 10(8):1083–1091
45. Ouriel K, Veith FJ, Sasahara AA (1998) A comparison of recombinant urokinase with vascular surgery as initial treatment for acute arterial occlusion of the legs. Thrombolysis or Peripheral Arterial Surgery (TOPAS) Investigators. N Engl J Med 338(16):1105–1111
46. Comerota AJ, Carman TL (2005) Thrombolytic agents and their actions. In: Rutherford R (ed) Vascular surgery, vol 1, Sixth edth edn. Elsevier Saunders, Philadelphia, PA, pp 530–545

47. Semba CP, Bakal CW, Calis KA et al (2000) Alteplase as an alternative to urokinase. Advisory Panel on Catheter-Directed Thrombolytic Therapy. J Vasc Interv Radiol 11(3):279–287
48. Semba CP, Murphy TP, Bakal CW et al (2000) Thrombolytic therapy with use of alteplase (rt-PA) in peripheral arterial occlusive disease: review of the clinical literature. The Advisory Panel. J Vasc Interv Radiol 11(2 Pt 1):149–161
49. Berridge DC, Gregson RH, Hopkinson BR et al (1991) Randomized trial of intra-arterial recombinant tissue plasminogen activator, intravenous recombinant tissue plasminogen activator and intra-arterial streptokinase in peripheral arterial thrombolysis. Br J Surg 78(8):988–995
50. Meyerovitz MF, Goldhaber SZ, Reagan K et al (1990) Recombinant tissue-type plasminogen activator versus urokinase in peripheral arterial and graft occlusions: a randomized trial. Radiology 175(1):75–78
51. Weaver FA, Comerota AJ, Youngblood M et al (1996) Surgical revascularization versus thrombolysis for nonembolic lower extremity native artery occlusions: results of a prospective randomized trial. The STILE Investigators. Surgery versus Thrombolysis for Ischemia of the Lower Extremity. J Vasc Surg 24(4):513–521 (discussion 521–513)
52. (1994) Results of a prospective randomized trial evaluating surgery versus thrombolysis for ischemia of the lower extremity. The STILE trial. Ann Surg 220(3):251–266; discussion 266–258
53. Comerota AJ, Weaver FA, Hosking JD et al (1996) Results of a prospective, randomized trial of surgery versus thrombolysis for occluded lower extremity bypass grafts. Am J Surg 172(2):105–112
54. (2007) Retavase: clinical pharmacology. http://www.rxlist.com/cgi/generic/reteplase_cp.htm. Accessed 31 Dec 2007
55. Davidian MM, Powell A, Benenati JF et al (2000) Initial results of reteplase in the treatment of acute lower extremity arterial occlusions. J Vasc Interv Radiol 11(3):289–294
56. Ouriel K, Katzen B, Mewissen M, 7 et al (2000) Reteplase in the treatment of peripheral arterial and venous occlusions: a pilot study. J Vasc Interv Radiol 11:849–854
57. (1995) Randomised, double-blind comparison of reteplase double-bolus administration with streptokinase in acute myocardial infarction (INJECT): trial to investigate equivalence. International Joint Efficacy Comparison of Thrombolytics. Lancet 346(8971):329–336
58. Smalling RW, Bode C, Kalbfleisch J et al (1995) More rapid, complete, and stable coronary thrombolysis with bolus administration of reteplase compared with alteplase infusion in acute myocardial infarction. RAPID Investigators. Circulation 91(11):2725–2732
59. Bode C, Smalling RW, Berg G et al (1996) Randomized comparison of coronary thrombolysis achieved with double-bolus reteplase (recombinant plasminogen activator) and front-loaded, accelerated alteplase (recombinant tissue plasminogen activator) in patients with acute myocardial infarction. The RAPID II Investigators. Circulation 94(5):891–898
60. (1997) A comparison of reteplase with alteplase for acute myocardial infarction. The Global Use of Strategies to Open Occluded Coronary Arteries (GUSTO III) Investigators. N Engl J Med 337(16):1118–1123
61. Burkart DJ, Borsa JJ, Anthony JP et al (2002) Thrombolysis of occluded peripheral arteries and veins with tenecteplase: a pilot study. J Vasc Interv Radiol 13(11):1099–1102
62. Heymans S, Vanderschueren S, Verhaeghe R et al (2000) Outcome and one year follow-up of intra-arterial staphylokinase in 191 patients with peripheral arterial occlusion. Thromb Haemost 83(5):666–671
63. Hess H, Mietaschk A, Deichsel G (1985) Drug-induced inhibition of platelet function delays progression of peripheral occlusive arterial disease. A prospective double-blind arteriographically controlled trial. Lancet 1(8426):415–419
64. Clagett GP, Sobel M, Jackson MR et al (2004) Antithrombotic therapy in peripheral arterial occlusive disease: the Seventh ACCP Conference on Antithrombotic and Thrombolytic Therapy. Chest 126(3 Suppl):609S–626S
65. (2002) Collaborative meta-analysis of randomised trials of antiplatelet therapy for prevention of death, myocardial infarction, and stroke in high risk patients. BMJ 324(7329):71–86
66. Hirsch AT, Haskal ZJ, Hertzer NR et al (2006) ACC/AHA 2005 Practice Guidelines for the management of patients with peripheral arterial disease (lower extremity, renal, mesenteric, and abdominal aortic): a collaborative report from the American Association for Vascular Surgery/Society for Vascular Surgery, Society for Cardiovascular Angiography and Interventions, Society for Vascular Medicine and Biology, Society of Interventional Radiology, and the ACC/AHA Task Force on Practice Guidelines (Writing Committee to Develop Guidelines for the Management of Patients With Peripheral Arterial Disease): endorsed by the American Association of Cardiovascular and Pulmonary Rehabilitation; National Heart, Lung, and Blood Institute; Society for Vascular Nursing; TransAtlantic Inter-Society Consensus; and Vascular Disease Foundation. Circulation 113(11):e463–e654
67. Davies RF, Goldberg AD, Forman S et al (1997) Asymptomatic Cardiac Ischemia Pilot (ACIP) study two-year follow-up: outcomes of patients randomized to initial strategies of medical therapy versus revascularization. Circulation 95(8):2037–2043
68. Hueb WA, Bellotti G, de Oliveira SA et al (1995) The Medicine, Angioplasty or Surgery Study (MASS): a prospective, randomized trial of medical therapy, balloon angioplasty or bypass surgery for single proximal left anterior descending artery stenoses. J Am Coll Cardiol 26(7):1600–1605

69. (1997) Coronary angioplasty versus medical therapy for angina: the second Randomised Intervention Treatment of Angina (RITA-2) trial. RITA-2 trial participants. Lancet 350(9076):461–468

70. (1996) A randomised, blinded, trial of clopidogrel versus aspirin in patients at risk of ischaemic events (CAPRIE). CAPRIE Steering Committee. Lancet 348(9038):1329–1339

71. (2008) CASPAR: Clopidogrel and Acetyl Salicylic Acid in Bypass Surgery for Peripheral ARterial Disease. http://www.clinicaltrials.gov/ct2/show/NCT00174759?term=clopidogrel+and+aspirin&rank=41. Accessed 8 Feb 2008.

72. (2008) Clopidogrel studied in one of the largest clinical trial programs in the fight against atherothrombosis. http://investor.bms.com/phoenix.zhtml?c=106664&p=irol-newsArticle_print&ID=396544&highlight=. Accessed 8 Feb 2008

73. Ouriel K (2004) Use of concomitant glycoprotein IIb/IIIa inhibitors with catheter-directed peripheral arterial thrombolysis. J Vasc Interv Radiol 15(6):543–546

74. Duda SH, Tepe G, Luz O et al (2001) Peripheral artery occlusion: treatment with abciximab plus urokinase versus with urokinase alone – a randomized pilot trial (the PROMPT Study). Platelet Receptor Antibodies in Order to Manage Peripheral Artery Thrombosis. Radiology 221(3):689–696

75. Ouriel K, Castaneda F, McNamara T et al (2004) Reteplase monotherapy and reteplase/abciximab combination therapy in peripheral arterial occlusive disease: results from the RELAX trial. J Vasc Interv Radiol 15(3):229–238

76. Tepe G, Schott U, Erley CM et al (1999) Platelet glycoprotein IIb/IIIa receptor antagonist used in conjunction with thrombolysis for peripheral arterial thrombosis. AJR Am J Roentgenol 172(5):1343–1346

77. Drescher P, Crain MR, Rilling WS (2002) Initial experience with the combination of reteplase and abciximab for thrombolytic therapy in peripheral arterial occlusive disease: a pilot study. J Vasc Interv Radiol 13(1):37–43

78. Fogarty TJ, Cranley JJ, Krause RJ et al (1963) A method for extraction of arterial emboli and thrombi. Surg Gynecol Obstet. 116:241–244

79. Kasirajan K, Haskal ZJ, Ouriel K (2001) The use of mechanical thrombectomy devices in the management of acute peripheral arterial occlusive disease. J Vasc Interv Radiol 12(4):405–411

80. Bates ER, Babb JD, Casey DE et al (2007) ACCF/SCAI/SVMB/SIR/ASITN 2007 clinical expert consensus document on carotid stenting: a report of the American College of Cardiology Foundation Task Force on Clinical Expert Consensus Documents (ACCF/SCAI/SVMB/SIR/ASITN Clinical Expert Consensus Document Committee on Carotid Stenting). J Am Coll Cardiol 49(1):126–170

81. (2008) Heart Disease and Stroke Statistics; 2008 update. http://www.americanheart.org/downloadable/heart/1200078608862HS_Stats%202008.final.pdf. Accessed 23 Feb 2008.

82. (1991) North American Symptomatic Carotid Endarterectomy Trial Collaborators. Beneficial effect of carotid endarterectomy in symptomatic patients with high-grade carotid stenosis. N Engl J Med 325(7):445–453

83. (1997) The International Stroke Trial (IST): a randomised trial of aspirin, subcutaneous heparin, both, or neither among 19435 patients with acute ischaemic stroke. International Stroke Trial Collaborative Group. Lancet 349(9065):1569

84. Chimowitz MI, Kokkinos J, Strong J et al (1995) The Warfarin-Aspirin Symptomatic Intracranial Disease Study. Neurology 45(8):1488–1493

85. Mohr JP, Thompson JL, Lazar RM et al (2001) A comparison of warfarin and aspirin for the prevention of recurrent ischemic stroke. N Engl J Med 345(20):1444–1451

86. Lewis SC, Sandercock PA (2002) Warfarin or aspirin for recurrent ischemic stroke. N Engl J Med 346(15):1169–1171

87. Anand S, Yusuf S, Xie C et al (2007) Oral anticoagulant and antiplatelet therapy and peripheral arterial disease. N Engl J Med 357(3):217–227

88. Bush RL, Lin PH, Mureebe L et al (2005) Routine bivalirudin use in percutaneous carotid interventions. J Endovasc Ther 12(4):521–522

89. Finks SW (2006) Bivalirudin use in carotid endarterectomy in a patient with heparin-induced thrombocytopenia. Ann Pharmacother 40(2):340–343

90. (1995) Tissue plasminogen activator for acute ischemic stroke. The National Institute of Neurological Disorders and Stroke rt-PA Stroke Study Group. N Engl J Med 333(24):1581–1587

91. Furlan A, Higashida R, Wechsler L et al (1999) Intra-arterial prourokinase for acute ischemic stroke. The PROACT II study: a randomized controlled trial. Prolyse in Acute Cerebral Thromboembolism. JAMA 282(21):2003–2011

92. Lewandowski CA, Frankel M, Tomsick TA et al (1999) Combined intravenous and intra-arterial r-TPA versus intra-arterial therapy of acute ischemic stroke: Emergency Management of Stroke (EMS) Bridging Trial. Stroke 30(12):2598–2605

93. (2004) Combined intravenous and intra-arterial recanalization for acute ischemic stroke: the Interventional Management of Stroke Study. Stroke 35(4):904–911

94. (2008) Interventional management of stroke – III. http://www.strokecenter.org/trials/TrialDetail.aspx?tid=747. Accessed 8 Feb 2008.

95. Bellavance A (1993) Efficacy of ticlopidine and aspirin for prevention of reversible cerebrovascular ischemic events. The Ticlopidine Aspirin Stroke Study. Stroke 24(10):1452–1457
96. Diener HC, Bogousslavsky J, Brass LM et al (2004) Aspirin and clopidogrel compared with clopidogrel alone after recent ischaemic stroke or transient ischaemic attack in high-risk patients (MATCH): randomised, double-blind, placebo-controlled trial. Lancet. 364(9431):331–337
97. Adams HP Jr, Effron MB, Torner J et al (2008) Emergency administration of abciximab for treatment of patients with acute ischemic stroke: results of an international phase III trial: Abciximab in Emergency Treatment of Stroke Trial (AbESTT-II). Stroke 39(1):87–99
98. Chan AW, Yadav JS, Bhatt DL et al (2005) Comparison of the safety and efficacy of emboli prevention devices versus platelet glycoprotein IIb/IIIa inhibition during carotid stenting. Am J Cardiol 95(6):791–795
99. Kapadia SR, Bajzer CT, Ziada KM et al (2001) Initial experience of platelet glycoprotein IIb/IIIa inhibition with abciximab during carotid stenting: a safe and effective adjunctive therapy. Stroke 32(10):2328–2332
100. (2008) ReoPro Retavase Reperfusion of Stroke Safety Study – Imaging Evaluation. http://www.strokecenter.org/trials/TrialDetail.aspx?tid=462. Accessed 8 Feb 2008
101. (2008) Combined Approach to Lysis Utilizing Eptifibatide and rt-PA in Acute Ischemic Stroke. http://www.strokecenter.org/trials/TrialDetail.aspx?tid=478. Accessed 8 Feb 2008
102. Smith WS, Sung G, Starkman S et al (2005) Safety and efficacy of mechanical embolectomy in acute ischemic stroke: results of the MERCI trial. Stroke 36(7):1432–1438
103. Stringer KA, Lindenfeld J (1992) Hirudins: antithrombin anticoagulants. Ann Pharmacother 26(12):1535–1540
104. Rajan DK, Patel NH, Valji K et al (2005) Quality improvement guidelines for percutaneous management of acute limb ischemia. J Vasc Interv Radiol 16(5):585–595
105. Pilger E, Lammer J, Bertuch II et al (1986) Intraarterial fibrinolysis: in vitro and prospective clinical evaluation of three thrombolytic agents. Radiology 161(3):597–599
106. Arepally A, Hofmann LV, Kim HS et al (2002) Weight-based rt-PA thrombolysis protocol for acute native arterial and bypass graft occlusions. J Vasc Interv Radiol 13(1):45–50
107. Tepe G, Hopfenzitz C, Dietz K et al (2006) Peripheral arteries: treatment with antibodies of platelet receptors and reteplase for thrombolysis – APART trial. Radiology 239(3):892–900
108. Burkart DJ, Borsa JJ, Anthony JP et al (2003) Thrombolysis of acute peripheral arterial and venous occlusions with tenecteplase and eptifibatide: a pilot study. J Vasc Interv Radiol 14(6):729–733
109. Kapadia SR, Ramee S (2005) Percutaneous mechanical thrombectomy for arterial thrombus. In: Yadav J (ed) Manual of peripheral vascular intervention. Lippincott Williams & Wilkins, Philadelphia, PA, pp 69–82

16 Monitoring of Antithrombotic Therapies in Interventional Cardiology

Kristofer Dosh and Steven Steinhubl

CONTENTS

INTRODUCTION
PLATELET MONITORING
ANTICOAGULANT MONITORING
CONCLUSIONS
BIBLIOGRAPHY

ABSTRACT Percutaneous coronary intervention causes rupture of atherosclerotic plaque, which leads to platelet aggregation and thrombus formation. Antiplatelet and antithrombotic therapies are routine in the catheterization laboratory, but the optimal use of these agents during PCI continues to evolve. Central to the performance of procedures in the catheterization laboratory is the goal of decreasing ischemic complications while simultaneously minimizing bleeding complications. Dosing of medications for most disease processes involves some assessment of physiologic response to the medication. Despite the availability of multiple simple, point-of-care methods to monitor antiplatelet and anticoagulant therapies the utilization of these methods is almost never routinely performed and most anticoagulants are no longer monitored except for unfractionated heparin (UFH). As the use of more unique combinations of antithrombotic agents becomes commonplace, the need for effective monitoring will become even more important, making a thorough understanding of the limitations and benefits of present-day monitoring in the cath lab crucial.

Key words: ACT(ACTIVATED clotting time); APTT (activated partial thromboplastin time); Platelet; Aggregation; Monitoring

INTRODUCTION

It is clear that there is a delicate balance between the antithrombotic efficacy of an agent and its propensity to cause bleeding. While the complications associated with thrombotic events in the cath lab have been well appreciated for decades, it is only recently that the long-term detrimental impact of bleeding events has become better understood. Through the monitoring of antithrombotic therapies it is possible to improve clinical efficacy while minimizing bleeding events. Multiple simple, point-of-care methods are now available to monitor antiplatelet and anticoagulant therapies, but there is no single proven best test for any one

From: *Contemporary Cardiology: Antithrombotic Drug Therapy in Cardiovascular Disease*
Edited by: A.T. Askari and A.M. Lincoff (eds.), DOI 10.1007/978-1-60327-235-3_16
© Humana Press, a part of Springer Science+Business Media, LLC 2010

agent and much less for the cocktail of antithrombotics most frequently used today. This chapter will summarize currently available tests and their current and potential future role in interventional cardiology.

PLATELET MONITORING

Platelet Function Tests

Since the initial description of bleeding time in 1901 (1), multiple tests have been devised to assess platelet function. The following is a description of several testing modalities that have been studied in the cardiac catheterization laboratory. A review of their utility in interventional cardiology will follow.

BLEEDING TIME

Bleeding time provides a crude assessment of primary hemostasis and the ability of platelets to form a thrombus. In the traditional Ivy method (2), a sphygmomanometer is inflated to 40 mmHg on the upper arm, and a standardized superficial incision is made on the volar surface of the forearm. Blood is then blotted gently with filter paper every 30 s until bleeding ceases. Although bleeding time is a point-of-care test, its utility is limited by the need for a dedicated technologist and results demonstrate significant inter- and intraobserver variability (3). The test also lacks data supporting its ability to accurately predict response to antiplatelet therapy (4).

TURBIDIMETRIC AGGREGOMETRY

Conventional turbidimetric aggregometry is a commonly used platelet function assay and has long been considered the gold standard of platelet function testing. As will be described later, turbidimetric aggregometry was used in early trials that led to the current dosing of GPIIb/IIIa inhibitors (5–7). The test is performed by centrifuging whole blood to obtain platelet-rich plasma (PRP). A platelet agonist such as adenosine diphosphate (ADP), collagen, epinephrine, or thrombin receptor-activating peptide (TRAP) is added to the PRP causing platelet aggregation. The device is calibrated by defining the transfer of light through platelet poor plasma (PPP) as 100% aggregation and through preagonist treated PRP as 0% aggregation. As platelets aggregate, the optical density of the solution decreases and transmitted light increases (Fig. 1). Inhibitors of platelet activation or aggregation reduce or eliminate the decrease in optical density, and results are expressed as a percent reduction in light transmission compared to baseline aggregation.

Although turbidimetric aggregometry has remained a gold standard for comparison of newer testing modalities, there are several challenges limiting its clinical use. First, the test has been criticized as being nonphysiologic because platelets aggregate under low shear conditions and in the absence of erythrocytes and leukocytes which poorly replicates in vivo stimulation of platelet aggregation (8). In addition, since some platelets sediment with red blood cells during centrifugation, a percentage of platelets that would otherwise contribute to aggregation are lost. The test is also labor intensive, requiring performance in a central laboratory by a specially trained individual. Finally, various challenges in performing the test make it difficult to compare results between different laboratories (3).

IMPEDANCE WHOLE BLOOD AGGREGOMETRY (WBA)

Electrical impedance aggregometry was developed with the goal of allowing aggregometry to be performed on whole blood (9), hence overcoming several of the problems with turbidimetric aggregometry. The test is performed by placing two electrodes in a solution of PRP or whole blood. Electrical impedance is measured before and after agonist-stimulated platelet aggregation. During aggregation, impedance increases with platelet accretion to the electrodes (Fig. 1). Impedance aggregometry can also be performed on PRP, but whole blood has several advantages including use of smaller sample volumes, reduced time to perform the test, and avoiding potential problems associated

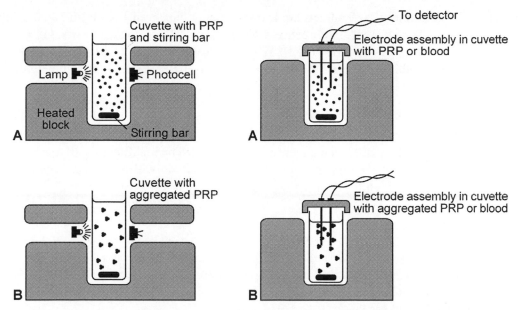

Fig. 1. Diagram comparing conventional turbidimetric aggregometry and electrical impedance aggregometry. The *left panel* demonstrates conventional aggregometry: (**a**) A light source shines through a glass cuvette and transmitted light is monitored by a photocell. (**b**) As platelets aggregate in response to an agonist, the amount of transmitted light increases. The *right panel* demonstrates electrical impedance aggregometry: (**a**) Electrodes are placed into the sample of PRP or whole blood. (**b**) Impedance between the electrodes increases as addition of an agonist causes platelet aggregation and accretion to the electrodes. Reprinted with permission from (9).

with centrifugation as described earlier for turbidimetric aggregometry. Fully computerized instruments are available, reducing the need for specialized training to perform the test. Potential problems with impedance WBA include a dilution step in preparing the whole blood sample, which may affect test results while monitoring low-molecular-weight agents such as tirofiban and eptifibatide that have high dissociation constants (10). Other potential challenges include difficulty in cleaning the electrodes and less reliability of the test at lower hemoglobin concentrations. Impedance WBA has been compared to turbidimetric aggregometry in patients undergoing PTCA with abciximab treatment (11). Comparable results were found between the two tests for degree of platelet inhibition as well as close correlation with GPIIb/IIIa receptor blockade by radioimmune assay.

FLOW CYTOMETRY

Whole blood flow cytometry uses fluorescently labeled monoclonal antibodies to detect activation-dependent changes in the platelet surface proteins. The test is performed by passing fluorescently labeled platelets through a flow chamber at a rate of 1,000 to 10,000 cells per minute (12). As cells pass through the flow chamber they are exposed to a laser beam that activates the fluorophore, and the emitted fluorescence and light scattering properties of each cell are detected. Performing the test on whole blood avoids some potential downfalls of washed platelets or PRP that are susceptible to artifactual platelet activation resulting from the separation process. Use of flow cytometry has been primarily used as a research tool because the high level of technical expertise required to run the test limits its use to specialized laboratories.

The flow cytometry-based vasodilator-stimulated phosphoprotein (VASP) assay (BioCytex, Marseille, France) is designed to evaluate the effect of clopidogrel on platelet function (13,14). In this test, inhibition of the P2Y12 receptor by clopidogrel in the presence of prostaglandin E1 induces phosphorylation of vasodilator-stimulated phosphoprotein (VASP). Increased levels of VASP phosphorylation

310 Antithrombotic Drug Therapy in Cardiovascular Disease

therefore reflect P2Y12 inhibition. Platelets are activated using the agonist ADP, and then using flow cytometry, the difference in VASP fluorescence intensity between resting and activated platelets is expressed as the platelet reactivity index (PRI). While the test is thought to be the most specific for platelet P2Y12 receptor inhibition, it is limited currently by its expense, need for sample preparation, and the requirement for an experienced technician (15).

PLATELET FUNCTION ANALYZER (PFA-100)

The PFA-100 (Dade Behring, Deerfield, IL) is an automated instrument that evaluates primary hemostasis in whole blood flowing in a high shear environment. The instrument uses a disposable test cartridge that includes a sample reservoir, capillary, and membrane with a 150-μm central aperture. The membrane is precoated with either collagen and epinephrine (CEPI) or collagen and ADP (CADP) (Fig. 16.2). A sample of citrated whole blood is drawn through the capillary under constant vacuum and is hence exposed to the membrane and aperture. As platelets adhere and aggregate at the membrane, the aperture eventually closes causing cessation of flow. The test takes about 10 min to complete and the result is reported as closure time (CT). A normal CT has been defined as 60–130 s (16). Maximal CT is defined as 300 s, which indicates nonclosure of the membrane aperture at 300 s. Benefits of the PFA-100 include the ability to use whole blood, simplicity of performing the test, and short time required to obtain results.

The PFA-100 has been compared to turbidimetric aggregometry and receptor occupancy for monitoring GPIIb/IIIa therapy in patients treated with PCI and adjunctive abciximab therapy (16). Results in 27 enrolled patients demonstrated a maximal achieved CT of 300 s for the majority of patients at 10 min, 4 h, and 12 h (96, 100, and 86% respectively). At 24 h, 72% of patients had CT return to normal (≤130 s). Since the majority of patients achieved CT >300 s initially, the results suggest that the PFA-100 may be too sensitive to detect quantitative differences in high levels of platelet inhibition.

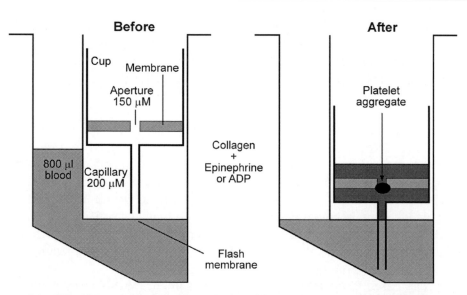

Fig. 2. Diagram of the PFA-100 test principle. Citrated whole blood is drawn through the capillary under a constant vacuum. Platelets aggregate as they are exposed to the membrane and aperture. Cessation of flow occurs when the aperture closes and the instrument records this time as the closure time. Reprinted with permission from (16).

VERIFYNOW RAPID PLATELET FUNCTION ASSAY (RPFA)

The VerifyNow RPFA (formerly known as Ultegra, Accumetrics, San Diego, CA) was initially designed as a point-of-care assay to monitor patients treated with GPIIb/IIIa antagonists (17). The assay is based on the ability of platelets to bind fibrinogen. The test is performed using self-contained cartridges with the contents of the cartridge dependent upon the antiplatelet agent being monitored. For GPIIb/IIIa monitoring, the cartridge contains the platelet activator iso-TRAP (a modified form of thrombin receptor activating peptide) and fibrinogen-coated polystyrene beads (18). A sample of whole blood is collected into a tube containing either citrate or PPACK (Phe-Pro-Arg chloromethyl ketone). The instrument draws the blood into two sample chambers that contain iso-TRAP and the polystyrene beads. The sample is mixed for 70 s by movement of a steel ball in the chamber. As the polystyrene beads agglutinate, they fall out of solution causing an increase in light transmission (Fig. 3). Light absorbance is recorded 16 times per second, allowing the rate of agglutination to be quantified as the slope of change in absorbance over time and is reported as millivolts per 10 s (mV/10s). Following treatment with GPIIb/IIIa antagonist, the test is repeated on a new sample and results are compared to the baseline measurement. The result is reported as raw Platelet Aggregation Units (PAU) and also as a percentage of the baseline PAU. The use of citrate containing tubes has been shown to cause overestimation of the degree of platelet inhibition with the small molecule GPIIb/IIIa inhibitors tirofiban and eptifibatide (19). This can be avoided by use of collection tubes containing PPACK instead of citrate. Benefits of the RPFA include rapid results, simplicity of performing the test, and ability to use whole blood. One disadvantage is the need to obtain a baseline comparison sample.

The VerifyNow was validated as a test for monitoring GPIIb/IIIa antagonists in an early study comparing it to turbidimetric aggregometry (18). Whole-blood RPFA was performed on samples of in vitro treatment with abciximab and correlated well with percentage inhibition by PRP turbidimetric aggregometry ($r^2 = 0.98$) and with receptor occupancy by radiolabeled receptor-binding assay ($r^2 = 0.96$). There was no difference in sensitivity of RPFA to the effect of abciximab when either aspirin or heparin was used.

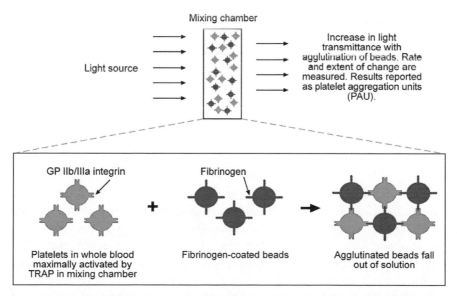

Fig. 3. Diagram of the rapid platelet function assay test principle. The instrument draws a sample of whole blood into two sample chambers that contain iso-TRAP and polystyrene beads. As the sample is mixed, the polystyrene beads agglutinate and fall out of solution causing an increase in light transmission. Reprinted with permission from (10).

Another study compared the VerifyNow to conventional turbidimetric aggregometry and receptor-binding assay in 192 enrolled patients undergoing PCI with adjunctive abciximab therapy (20). Abciximab was administered as a 0.25 mg/kg bolus followed by 0.125 µg/kg/min drip for 12 h. Blood samples were taken at baseline before abciximab administration, within 1 h of abciximab bolus, and 24 h after the abciximab bolus. In the 120 patients able to be evaluated, the Ultegra RPFA correlated well with aggregometry ($r = 0.89$) and with the receptor-binding assay ($r = 0.89$). The degree of correlation was similar to that between conventional aggregometry and receptor-binding assay ($r = 0.87$). The study also demonstrated good correlation between values obtained by point-of-care users and laboratory scientists ($r = 0.80$).

The VerifyNow has more recently been adapted with specialized cartridges containing different platelet agonists to measure the antiplatelet effects of aspirin (VerifyNow Aspirin) and clopidogrel (VerifyNow P2Y12). The VerifyNow Aspirin assay uses arachidonic acid to stimulate platelets. The test is specific for aspirin because arachidonic-acid-induced platelet aggregation requires cyclooxygenase-1 activity, which is directly blocked by aspirin (15). Light transmittance changes as platelets aggregate in response to arachidonic acid, and the change is reported as Aspirin Reaction Units (ARU). A cutoff ARU of ≥550 has a reported sensitivity and specificity of 91.4 and 100%, respectively, for the presence of aspirin (VerifyNow Aspirin package insert). The VerifyNow P2Y12 assay uses ADP as the agonist, which stimulates both P2Y1 and P2Y12 receptors. As with the VASP assay, in order to isolate the effect of clopidogrel on the P2Y12 receptor, prostaglandin E1 is added to block the contribution of ADP binding to the P2Y1 receptor (15). The change in light transmittance from ADP-stimulated platelet aggregation in this assay is reported as P2Y12 Reaction Units (PRU). Since a baseline sample cannot always be taken, a separate channel is tested using the agonist iso-TRAP, which is unaffected by theinopyridine treatment. Final results are reported as raw PRU and as percentage of baseline PRU based on the iso-TRAP sample (21).

THROMBOELASTOGRAPHY

Thromboelastography (TEG, Haemoscope, Niles, IL) measures mechanical properties of a developing clot including time to initial fibrin formation, kinetics of initial fibrin clot to reach maximum strength, and the peak strength and stability of the fibrin clot (22). The test is performed on 0.35 ml of whole blood that is placed in a heated cup. The cup oscillates 4° 45′ in each direction every 4.5 s (Fig. 4). A pin is suspended in the cup from a torsion wire that is connected to a chart recorder or computer. As the clot forms, the torque of the rotating cup is transmitted to the pin, and a tracing is recorded (23). Several characteristics of clot formation can be determined from the tracing. Five that are commonly reported include reaction time (R time), K time, alpha angle, maximum amplitude (MA), and clot lysis index (A60) (23,24) (Fig. 5). The R time is the time of latency between placing blood in the cup and initial clot formation and indicates plasma clotting factor and inhibitor activity. The K time is the time for the blood to achieve an assigned fixed level of viscoelasticity and assesses the rapidity of fibrin clot linking. Alpha angle is the angle formed by the gradient of the initial trace and demonstrates the speed of clot formation. MA is the largest vertical amplitude of the tracing and represents the maximal clot-shear elasticity. The whole blood clot lysis index (A60) is the amplitude 60 min after the MA and is a measure of rapidity of fibrinolysis. One limitation of conventional TEG was that thrombin generation made it impossible to assess the effects of milder platelet inhibitors such as aspirin and clopidogrel. A modified TEG assay has been developed that uses reptilase (batroxobin) and factor XIIIa to form clot without thrombin generation, thus overcoming this limitation. This modified TEG has been shown to correlate closely with optical aggregation for evaluating the antiplatelet effects of clopidogrel and aspirin (25). The test is available as a point-of-care assay and has the benefits of using whole blood and providing information on clot formation and clot lysis.

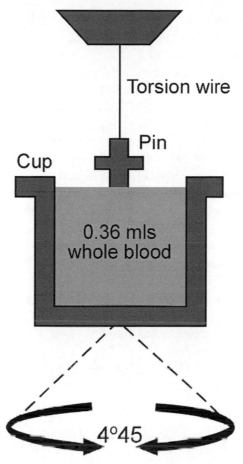

Fig. 4. Diagram of the TEG assay. A pin is suspended in a cup containing heated whole blood. As clot forms, torque in the oscillating cup is transmitted to the pin and a tracing is recorded. Reprinted with permission from (24).

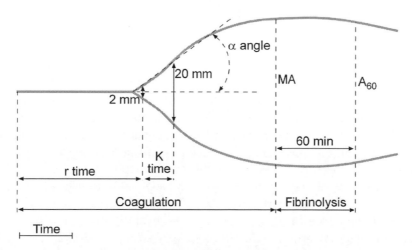

Fig. 5. Schematic showing a thromboelastograph (TEG) tracing. Characteristics of the TEG curve including r time, K time, alpha angle, MA, and A60 are described in the text. Reprinted with permission from (23).

CONE AND PLATE(LET) ANALYZER

The cone and plate(let) analyzer (CPA) exposes whole blood to simulated physiologic shear forces using a rotating Teflon cone in a polystyrene well (26). One early method used 200 µL of citrated whole blood placed in a polystyrene well (27). Constant fluid shear stress was induced by a Teflon cone rotating at 1,875 s^{-1} for 2 min. The well was then washed, stained, and analyzed with an inverted-light microscope connected to a computer analysis system. Results are expressed as the percentage of the well surface covered by platelets (SC) and the average size of the aggregates (AS in µm^2). The instrument has since been automated for use as a point-of-care device (Impact®, DiaMed, Cressier sur Morat, Switzerland) and uses a slightly smaller quantity of blood (120 µL). Benefits include simple operation, fast results (~6 min) (8), lack of need for a baseline platelet function value (27), and the ability to use whole blood. The test may also provide a more relevant physiologic analysis of platelet function in the arterial system because of the high shear forces used as compared to modalities such as platelet aggregometry.

One small trial compared CPA, turbidimetric aggregometry, and the VerifyNow RPFA against receptor occupancy by flow cytometry for monitoring platelet response to abciximab in PCI (27). Results demonstrated that CPA was a better predictor of free GPIIb/IIIa receptors than RPFA when RPFA was expressed in absolute values ($p = 0.0015$), but there was no advantage to CPA when RPFA was expressed as a ratio of baseline PAU. CPA also demonstrated a greater sensitivity to low levels of platelet inhibition as it did not return to baseline between 7 and 30 days post-PCI while patients remained on aspirin and clopidogrel, whereas turbidimetric aggregometry was no different from baseline during this time frame. Other studies have reviewed the CPA for monitoring aspirin and clopidogrel therapy, but additional data are needed to determine its appropriate use in this setting (28). Further studies are also needed to assess the utility of CPA for use in coronary interventions.

PLATELET COUNT RATIOS (PLATELETWORKS®)

The ICHOR Plateletworks® (Helena Laboratories, Beaumont, TX) test is a point-of-care, whole blood assay that is based on platelet aggregation. The test is performed by measuring a standard platelet count from a baseline whole blood sample in which aggregation has been prevented by ethylenediamine tetra-acetic acid (EDTA). A citrated sample is then run after stimulating platelet aggregation with ADP. The clumped platelets exceed threshold limitations for platelet size and will not be counted as platelets when a platelet count is performed on the sample (29). The results are reported as a ratio of the test sample platelet count to the baseline platelet count. The primary advantages of platelet count ratios include the use of whole blood and ability to perform the test at the bedside if the automated ICHOR Plateletworks instrument is used. However, if the instrument is not available, the test requires reagent additions and sample manipulations in a central laboratory.

The Plateletworks assay has been shown to correlate well with conventional turbidimetric aggregometry for evaluating platelet inhibition by clopidogrel (30). A recent trial has also demonstrated a close correlation between the automated ICHOR Plateletworks assay and turbidimetric aggregometry for monitoring platelet inhibition by GPIIb/IIIa inhibitors (31). In this study, blood samples collected in PPACK were treated with increasing concentrations of eptifibatide, tirofiban, or abciximab. Platelet inhibition was measured using conventional turbidimetric aggregometry, VerifyNow, and Plateletworks. This trial notably demonstrated a close correlation between Plateletworks and turbidimetric aggregometry when platelet inhibition levels were <90%. In contrast, the VerifyNow was found to overestimate platelet inhibition at levels <90% as measured by turbidimetric aggregometry (see Figs. 6, 7 and 8). The overall correlation between turbidimetric aggregometry and the Plateletworks was found to be very strong ($r^2 = 0.922$) while VerifyNow less closely correlated ($r^2 = 0.828$). Other recent trials have evaluated the platelet count ratio-based Sysmex K4500 (Sysmex Corp, Kobe, Japan) to evaluate platelet inhibition during PCI with adjunctive GPIIb/IIIa therapy (32,33). These studies will be described later.

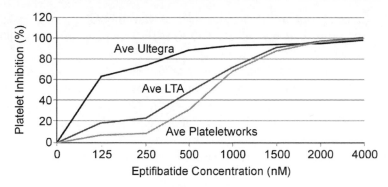

Fig. 6. In vitro comparison of platelet inhibition with increasing concentrations of eptifibatide using light transmission aggregometry, Ultegra RPFA (VerifyNow), and Plateletworks. Reprinted with permission from (31).

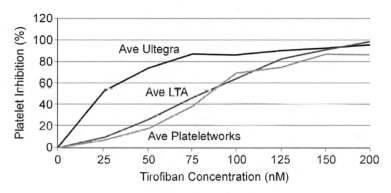

Fig. 7. In vitro comparison of platelet inhibition with increasing concentrations of tirofiban using light transmission aggregometry, Ultegra RPFA (VerifyNow), and Plateletworks. Reprinted with permission from (31).

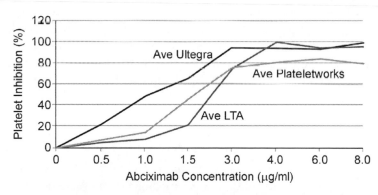

Fig. 8. In vitro comparison of platelet inhibition with increasing concentrations of abciximab using light transmission aggregometry, Ultegra RPFA (VerifyNow), and Plateletworks. Reprinted with permission from (31).

Trials of GPIIb/IIIa Antagonist Monitoring

Initial animal studies helped to establish the necessary level of platelet inhibition required to prevent acute coronary thrombosis. One canine model addressing degree of platelet inhibition used the monoclonal antiplatelet GPIIb/IIIa antibody 7E3 to prevent coronary artery reocclusion following thrombolysis in dogs (34). In this study, coronary reocclusion was prevented only at the highest dose of 7E3 administered (0.8 mg/kg). Using light transmission aggregometry, the authors determined that

>80% of the GPIIb/IIIa receptors on the platelet surface were blocked at this dose. Other studies on animal models also supported that this level of GPIIb/IIIa blockade prevents acute thrombosis in severe coronary stenosis (35,36).

Based on the findings in animal studies, Tcheng et al. performed clinical dosing studies of chimeric monoclonal 7E3 Fab (c7E3 Fab), now called abciximab (Reopro, Centocor, Inc.), in high-risk coronary angioplasty (5). At a dose of 0.25 mg/kg bolus followed by 10 μg/min they were able to block >80% of GPIIb/IIIa receptors and reduce ADP-induced platelet aggregation to ≤20% of baseline, inhibit ex vivo platelet aggregation, and prolong bleeding times throughout infusions up to 24 h. Additional early clinical trials with different GPIIb/IIIa inhibitors continued to use the goal of reducing platelet aggregation to ≤20% of baseline (6,7).

Clinical support for this level of receptor inhibition was provided through a series of clinical trials. The EPIC (Evaluation of 7E3 for the Prevention of Ischemic Complications) (37), EPILOG (Evaluation of PTCA to Improve Long-term Outcome with Abciximab GPIIb/IIIa Blockade) (38), and the EPISTENT (Evaluation of Platelet IIb/IIIa Inhibitor for Stenting) (39) trials all demonstrated significant reductions in periprocedural MIs in patients randomized to doses of abciximab expected to achieve >80% IIb/IIIa receptor blockade compared with placebo.

While the same dose of abciximab was used in all the mentioned trials, indirect evidence regarding the importance of achieving an adequate level of inhibition comes from the comparison of outcomes in the IMPACT-II (40) and ESPRIT (41) trials. Each of these randomized, controlled trials evaluated the use of eptifibatide during percutaneous coronary intervention but evaluated different dosing regimens. The IMPACT-II (Integrilin to Minimize Platelet Aggregation and Coronary Thrombosis) trial compared eptifibatide 135 μg/kg bolus followed by 0.5 μg/kg/min infusion or 135 μg/kg bolus followed by 0.75 μg/kg/min infusion to placebo. Although a treatment-received analysis showed a 22% relative reduction in the 30-day composite event endpoint, the primary intention-to-treat analysis demonstrated no statistically significant difference in the treatment groups when compared to placebo (11.4% vs. 9.2% for 135/0.5 group, $p=0.063$; 11.4% vs. 9.9% for 135/0.75 group, $p=0.22$). This dosing of eptifibatide was later shown to inhibit aggregation by <30% and approach only approximately 50% receptor occupancy (42). By contrast, the ESPRIT (Enhanced Suppression of Platelet Receptor IIb/IIIa Using Integrilin Therapy) trial used two 180 μg/kg boluses with a 2 μg/kg/min infusion and compared to placebo. The trial was terminated early after finding a significant 35% reduction in the 30-day composite event endpoint (10.5% vs. 6.8%, $p=0.0034$). This higher dosing used in ESPRIT was found to reduce platelet aggregation by 20 μM ADP to <10% and to achieve >80% GPIIb/IIIa receptor blockade (43).

The compilation of these studies seemed to validate the initial study results recommending a goal of >80% receptor blockade or reduction in ADP-induced platelet aggregation to ≤20% of baseline. Subsequent studies began to assess the optimal level of GPIIb/IIIa blockade during coronary intervention to optimize clinical endpoints. The GOLD (from the chemical symbol for gold, AU – Assessing Ultegra) trial was the first prospective study comparing clinical outcomes in PCI to levels of platelet inhibition by GPIIb/IIIa inhibitors (44). In this trial, 485 patients undergoing PCI with GPIIb/IIIa inhibitor use had platelet inhibition measured by VerifyNow at 10 min, 1 h, 8 h, and 24 h after initiation of therapy. The majority of patients received abciximab (84%), while 9% received tirofiban and 7% eptifibatide. MACE (including death, MI, or urgent target vessel revascularization) were followed through hospitalization or within 1 week of the PCI and were correlated with the level of platelet inhibition at each time point. Overall, the mean level of platelet inhibition at 10 min was 96±9%, at 1 h was 95±8%, 8 h was 91±11%, and 24 h was 73±20%. The 125 patients who achieved <95% inhibition at 10 min had a significantly higher incidence of an in-hospital MACE compared to those inhibited ≥95% (14.4% vs. 6.4%, $p=0.006$). Data obtained 8 h after the bolus also showed a significant relationship between level of platelet inhibition and occurrence of MACE, with patients having <70% platelet function inhibition experiencing three times the MACE rate compared to those with ≥70% inhibition (25% vs. 8.1%, $p=0.009$) (Fig. 9). The relationship between MACE and level of platelet inhibition was similar for patients treated with tirofiban and eptifibatide as compared to abciximab. There was no correlation between levels of platelet inhibition and bleeding complications. The GOLD trial was the first to demonstrate that the level of platelet inhibition in patients undergoing PCI with adjunctive GPIIb/IIIa inhibitors is significantly associated with the risk of MACE. However, the study was not designed to assess the effect of titrating therapy based on measured levels of platelet inhibition.

Given the finding of the GOLD trial showing lower MACE in patients with ≥95% early platelet inhibition, a recent trial sought to determine the extent of platelet inhibition during and after PCI with the use of current dosing schemes for abciximab, eptifibatide, and tirofiban (45). The authors dosed abciximab as a 0.25 mg/kg bolus followed by 0.125 µg/kg/min infusion for 12 h; eptifibatide was given as 2 boluses of 180 µg/kg followed by a 2 µg/kg/min infusion for 24 h; and tirofiban was dosed as a 25 µg/kg bolus followed by 0.15 µg/kg/min infusion for 18 h. The VerifyNow was used to measure platelet inhibition in 114 patients at baseline, 10 min after bolus administration, and 8 h after start of the infusion. As has been noted in various other trials, considerable variability was noted in the degree of platelet inhibition between different patients at a standard weight-based dosing of GPIIb/IIIa inhibitor. At the 10-min collection, mean inhibition of platelet inhibition was 86±9% for abciximab, 92±6% for eptifibatide, and 95±5% for tirofiban ($p<0.001$). Furthermore, ≥95% platelet inhibition was achieved in only 29% of patients treated with abciximab, 44% of those treated with eptifibatide, and 68% of patients treated with tirofiban ($p=0.02$). No difference was found in 30-day MACE for the three groups according to GPIIb/IIIa agent received. Furthermore, no difference was noted in the extent of 10 min or 8 h platelet inhibition in the MACE or non-MACE groups. Although the study is limited by its small sample size and nonrandomized design, it demonstrates the significant variability in interindividual response to GPIIb/IIIa inhibitors.

As compared to the 80% cutoff for platelet inhibition determined in early trials, the ≥95% level of platelet inhibition required to reduce MACE in the GOLD trial has been suggested to result from overestimation of platelet inhibition by the VerifyNow assay (31). Based on data presented earlier from White et al., ≤90% platelet inhibition by the VerifyNow correlated poorly with turbidimetric aggregometry, while levels >90% roughly correlated to ≥75% inhibition as measured by turbidimetric aggregometry and ICHOR plateletworks. A related platelet count ratio-based test, the Sysmex K4500, was recently used to assess platelet inhibition during PCI for ST-segment elevation myocardial

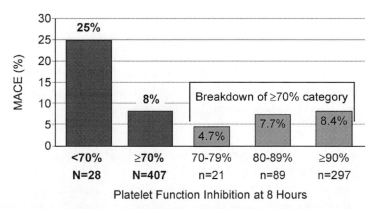

Fig. 9. Incidence of MACE in relation to VerifyNow measured platelet inhibition 8 h following GPIIb/IIIa bolus. Reprinted with permission from (44).

infarction (STEMI) patients treated with GPIIb/IIIa inhibitors (32). Platelet aggregation inhibition was measured immediately before and after PCI, and 1 and 6 h afterward. Patients were randomized to treatment with abciximab 0.25 mg/kg bolus followed by 0.125 µg/kg/min drip, tirofiban 10 µg/kg bolus followed by 0.15 µg/kg/min drip, tirofiban 25 µg/kg bolus followed by 0.15 µg/kg/min drip, or no GPIIb/IIIa inhibitor. Results on 112 patients demonstrated significant variability in interindividual response and suboptimal platelet inhibition for all agents. Only patients in the high-dose tirofiban group achieved >80% periprocedural platelet inhibition. No relationship was found between the level of platelet aggregation and measures of PCI success, including Thrombolysis in Myocardial Infarction (TIMI) flow grade, myocardial blush grade, or TIMI frame count. Another trial using the Sysmex K4500 attempted to compare platelet inhibition with angiographic and clinical endpoints for STEMI patients undergoing PCI with adjunctive tirofiban (33). Results on 412 patients demonstrated no correlation between level of platelet inhibition and angiographic or clinical outcomes. However, even the highest quartile of mean inhibition in the study was less than 80%, suggesting that platelet inhibition may not have been sufficient to demonstrate the benefit of higher levels of inhibition.

Limited other data exist regarding clinical endpoints with other testing modalities. One recent trial evaluating TEG showed an association between high MA and short R time following PCI and 6 month risk of ischemic events (46). The PFA-100 has been evaluated in PCI using GPIIb/IIIa inhibitors and demonstrated that failure to achieve nonclosure following PCI may be associated with an increased incidence of MACE at 6 months (47). Studies have not yet been published evaluating the effect of titrating GPIIb/IIIa inhibitors during PCI based on levels of platelet inhibition.

Aspirin and Clopidogrel Variability in Response

The use of aspirin and clopidogrel in the periprocedural period and subsequent to PCI has been well established to reduce ischemic complications (48–50). Over the last several years, variability in interindividual responses to aspirin and clopidogrel has been observed and is sometimes referred to as a phenomenon of "resistance." Although the exact definition and significance of aspirin and clopidogrel resistance has not been determined, it has been suggested that the term "resistance" should be reserved for the specific scenario when a drug is unable to reach its pharmacological target (50). An individual who experiences an adverse ischemic event following PCI that was not prevented by aspirin or clopidogrel may or may not be "resistant" to either medication, and the definition of resistance should probably not be based on clinical outcomes. Several of the platelet assays described have been evaluated for monitoring the ability of aspirin and clopidogrel to inhibit platelet aggregation (51). Most of the assays are not specific for the action of either aspirin or clopidogrel and may, therefore, not be suitable tests to define threshold levels of "resistance" to these medications. Nevertheless, an assessment of platelet inhibition by aspirin and clopidogrel will provide some measurement of individual response to the medications and allows the opportunity to correlate aspirin and clopidogrel response to clinical outcomes surrounding PCI. A full discussion of aspirin and clopidogrel resistance is out of the scope of this chapter. The following is a brief review of some studies looking at monitoring the antiplatelet effects of aspirin and clopidogrel in the setting of PCI.

ASPIRIN

A recent trial using the VerifyNow Aspirin assay evaluated 151 patients undergoing nonurgent PCI (52). All patients were pretreated with clopidogrel 300 mg between 12 and 24 h before PCI and treated with 80 to 325 mg of aspirin for ≥1 week preprocedure. Using a cutoff ARU ≥ 550 to define aspirin resistance, a significantly higher rate of myonecrosis following PCI was noted in patients who were aspirin resistant. An additional study from the same investigators using the VerifyNow Aspirin assay demonstrated reduced coronary flow reserve after elective PCI in aspirin-resistant patients compared to aspirin-sensitive patients (53). In contrast to these results, a separate recent trial reviewed 330 low-risk patients undergoing elective PCI and found no correlation between post-procedural myonecrosis and aspirin or clopidogrel resistance as measured by the VerifyNow Aspirin and P2Y12 assays (54). Suggested reasons for the different findings between these studies include interindividual variability in platelet response to aspirin and clopidogrel with the same dose, differences in compliance, or underdosing.

The PFA-100 has also been used in trials of aspirin resistance and PCI. One trial prospectively studied 146 patients with acute myocardial infarction who underwent primary PCI (55). PFA-100 closure time was measured 12 to 15 h after revascularization. A cutoff of <203 s was used to define aspirin resistance. After 1 year of follow up, the incidence of MACE was found to be significantly higher in the aspirin-resistant vs. aspirin-sensitive group (39.1 vs. 23.2%, $p < 0.05$). Another recent trial followed 135 patients who had undergone elective PCI and were on aspirin and clopidogrel for ≥1 month (56). Aspirin resistance was assessed by PFA-100 closure time and patients were assessed for platelet aggregation and activation by turbidimetric aggregometry and flow cytometry. Results demonstrated that aspirin resistance was associated with increased platelet reactivity in spite of long-term dual antiplatelet treatment. The PFA-100 has been criticized as an imperfect test for monitoring aspirin-induced platelet inhibition because the closure time is affected by multiple other variables that are not affected by aspirin (50), including von Willebrand Factor (VWF), platelet count and hematocrit, among others (57).

Limited data exist regarding other point-of-care tests for measuring aspirin resistance in the setting of PCI. Both the cone and plate(let) analyzer using arachidonic acid as an agonist (28) and the modified TEG (25) have been shown to correlate well with turbidimetric aggregometry for testing platelet inhibition by aspirin, but further studies are needed to determine their potential role in monitoring aspirin therapy.

Clopidogrel

Testing modalities specific to the effects of clopidogrel are limited and many point-of-care instruments are still in the early stages of determining appropriate use surrounding PCI. As outlined previously, the VerifyNow P2Y12 assay was designed to isolate the effect of the agonist ADP to the activity of P2Y12, which is blocked by clopidogrel. The Verify Thrombosis Risk Assessment (VERITAS) (58) study demonstrated the assay to be sensitive for measuring platelet inhibition with clopidogrel, but VERITAS was not a PCI study. The ongoing Research Evaluation to Study Individuals Who Show Thromboxane or P2Y12 Receptor Resistance (RESISTOR) trial is a double-blind, multicenter trial that will use the VerifyNow P2Y12 and Aspirin assays to determine whether modifying antiplatelet regimens in aspirin and clopidogrel resistance will prevent myonecrosis after PCI.

Although not a point-of-care test, the VASP phosphorylation assay is also specific for the effects of clopidogrel on platelet aggregation, as described earlier. The assay has been shown to identify a greater extent of thienopyridine-induced platelet inhibition than turbidimetric aggregometry (14). This is most likely a result of residual stimulation of ADP-induced aggregation through the P2Y1 receptor in turbidimetry. Two trials using the VASP assay found an increased rate of subacute stent thrombosis in patients with high platelet reactivity despite clopidogrel therapy (59,60). As noted previously, some limitations of the VASP assay include its expense and the need for an experienced technician.

As with aspirin, limited data exist regarding other testing modalities for clopidogrel resistance. The PFA-100 is not recommended as a test for monitoring clopidogrel therapy (61,62). Both the CPA and TEG assays have been shown to correlate well with turbidimetric aggregometry for monitoring clopidogrel therapy (25,28). One trial comparing MACE after stenting for STEMI found an increased risk of MACE in patients with the lowest quartile of aggregate size by CPA (63). Using TEG, high platelet reactivity despite chronic clopidogrel therapy has been shown to correlate with an increased risk of postprocedural ischemic events for patients undergoing nonemergent PCI (64). Further studies are needed to better assess the role of CPA and TEG in monitoring clopidogrel therapy.

ANTICOAGULANT MONITORING

Unfractionated Heparin

Unfractionated heparin has continued to be the most commonly used anticoagulant during PCI as a result of its low price, easy reversibility, and ability to monitor at the bedside. Initial dosing of heparin during PCI used fixed-dose boluses of 10,000 U followed by repeat boluses depending on the length of the procedure (65). Subsequent use of heparin during PCI has shifted toward improving outcomes by using weight-based boluses and monitoring heparin-induced anticoagulation during the procedure. Although the traditional means of monitoring heparin was the activated partial thrombo-plastin time (APTT), at high doses of heparin the APTT is nonlinear, prolonged, and poorly sensitive to heparin level changes (66). The activated clotting time (ACT) performs better at high doses of heparin and has been the primary test used to monitor heparin during PCI.

The ACT was first described by Hattersley in 1966 (67). The test was performed by drawing samples of whole blood into glass tubes containing diatomaceous earth and tilting them back and forth by hand until clot appeared. The applications of ACT for monitoring anticoagulation grew with the develop-ment of extracorporeal bypass support for cardiovascular surgery (68). This created a need for rapid, point-of-care, automated devices to measure the ACT. In 1977, Verska described an automated ACT device that was used successfully to direct heparin therapy in open-heart surgery (69). A number of automated devices to measure ACT have since been developed, most of which are also able to monitor other tests of anticoagulation including APTT and prothrombin time (PT), depending on the cartridge used with the instrument. Several current point-of-care ACT devices are outlined in Table 1.

The ACT test is generally performed using the following steps (70): A discard tube of blood is drawn prior to obtaining the test sample. The sample is then drawn and added to a contact activator,

Table 1
List of several point-of-care devices available for monitoring coagulation. Reprinted with permission from (104)

Instrument	Vendor	Test menu	Clot detection
i-Stat® 1	Abbott	PT/INR, ACT	Amperometry
Actalyte XL	Helena	ACT, Max ACT	Magnet position
Actalyte Mini II	Helena	ACT, Max ACT	Magnet position
GEM PCL Plus	Instrumentation laboratory	PT, PTT, ACT	Fluid movement
Hemochron Signature	ITC	PT, PTT, PTT, ACT	Fluid movement
Hemochron Response	ITC	PT, PTT, PTT, ACT, TT, Protamine dose assay	Magnet displacement
HMS Plus	Medtronic	ACT, Heparin dose response, HeparinProtamine titration	Plunger motion
ACT Plus	Medtronic	ACT	Plunger motion

PT prothrombin time, PTT partial thromboplastin time, ACT activated clotting time, INR international normalized ratio most often celite, silica, kaolin, or glass particles. The ACT is then recorded upon the initiation of clot formation which is detected in different ways depending on the instrument used. Although several instruments are available, the two most commonly cited in PCI literature and specifically mentioned in the 2005 ACC/AHA/SCAI guidelines for PCI include the Hemochron (International Technidyne Corporation, Edison, NJ) and HemoTec (current instrument named ACT Plus) (Medtronic, Minneapolis, MN) instruments. The Hemochron device detects initiation of coagulation by either monitoring for displacement of a magnet in a rotating tube (Hemochron Response) or monitoring for a change in light transmission through blood moving back and forth through a capillary test channel (Hemochron Jr Signature+, Hemochron Signature Elite). The HemoTec instrument uses a mechanical plunger that dips in and out of the activated blood sample and detects a rate change in the movement of the plunger by optical photocells when the fibrin clot begins to form.

The optimal ACT goal during PCI varies depending on the measuring instrument used and concomitant drug therapy. The different methods of measuring ACT are not standardized and so results from different methods cannot be compared (68). The Hemochron device, for example, has been demonstrated to provide ACT values approximately 30% higher than those measured by the HemoTec device (71). Even different devices from the same manufacturer may yield somewhat different results (72). Randomized controlled trials comparing heparin dosing in PCI have not been performed, and current dosing schemes have evolved from the findings of early observational trials. One study reviewed ACTs during PTCA using the HemoTec device and found that ischemic complications occurred in 61% of patients with an ACT <250 s as compared to only 0.3% with an ACT >300 s (73). Another trial comparing ACTs using the Hemochron device found a significant inverse relationship between ACT and abrupt vessel closure following PTCA (74). The rate of abrupt closure fell from 7.9 to 4.5% when comparing the 25th percentile of ACT (324 s) to the 75th percentile (413 s). A pooled analysis of six randomized controlled trials of antithrombotic use in PCI evaluated the control heparin-only groups and found that the lowest rate of ischemic endpoints occurred at an ACT of 350–375 s when using a Hemochron device (75). In the same study, individual analysis of ACTs measured by the HemoTec device identified the most benefit at a range of 300–325 s. The ideal ACT level for PCI remains a matter of debate, but current ACC/AHA/SCAI guidelines recommend a goal of 250–300 s with the HemoTec device and 300–350 s with the Hemochron device.

Lower ACTs are recommended when using the GP IIb/IIIa inhibitors, although the extent of the effect on ACT and the optimal ACT goal with these agents is still a matter of debate. Earlier trials demonstrated a 30–60 s increase in the ACT when abciximab was added to heparin therapy during PCI (76–78). More recent studies found a similar increase in the ACT when either abciximab or tirofiban was used in addition to heparin during PCI (79,80). Alternatively, eptifibatide use with heparin during PCI has been shown to have no significant effect on the ACT (81). Clinical efficacy of lower ACT goals during PCI was first demonstrated in the previously described EPILOG trial, where a goal ACT of 200 s with adjunctive abciximab was associated with no increase in ischemic events while reducing bleeding complications (38). This finding resulted in the recommendation for an ACT goal of 200 s in patients receiving GPIIb/IIIa inhibitor therapy in addition to heparin during PCI. However, a more recent substudy of the TACTICS TIMI-18 (Treat Angina with Aggrestat and Determine Cost of Therapy with an Invasive or Conservative Strategy-Thrombolysis in Myocardial Infarction) trial compared heparin with adjunctive tirofiban for UA and NSTEMI and found that patients with an ACT ≤250 s had an increased risk of thrombotic complications after PCI (82). Based on this finding, the authors recommended a higher goal of 250–300 s when using adjunctive tirofiban for PCI. Current AHA/ACC/SCAI guidelines advise a reduced heparin bolus when GPIIb/IIIa inhibitors are given to achieve a target goal of 200 s with either the HemoTec or Hemochron device. They also specify that the recommended ACT for tirofiban or eptifibatide should be less than 300 s during coronary angioplasty.

Low-Molecular-Weight Heparins

The low-molecular-weight heparins (LMWH) have been increasingly used as an acceptable alternative to UFH in PCI. The most studied LMWH in PCI has been enoxaparin. Several trials evaluating its use in PCI have shown comparable ischemic and bleeding outcomes to UFH (83). Current AHA/ACC/SCAI guidelines allow the use of enoxaparin as an alternative to UFH for patients with NSTEMI who undergo intervention.

The anticoagulant effect of LMWH results primarily from its anti-factor Xa activity, although it has a small inhibitory effect on factor IIa. Studies examining the level of anti-Xa inhibition by enoxaparin in PCI have suggested a target anti-Xa level of 0.6–1.8 IU/ml (84–87). Central laboratory anti-Xa activity tests are available but have poor turnaround time which precludes their use in elective or urgent PCI.

Part of the reluctance of providers to use enoxaparin in the catheterization laboratory has resulted from the lack of a rapid means to assess its anticoagulant activity (88). The ACT has been evaluated as a possible point-of-care test for monitoring LMWH with variable results. In a substudy of the Thrombolysis in Myocardial Infarction (TIMI) 11A trial, peak and trough anti-Xa levels and ACTs were evaluated in patients with UA/NSTEMI who were treated with subcutaneous enoxaparin (89). Results demonstrated that in spite of mean doses of 89 ± 19 mg every 12 h and significant increases in the anti-Xa levels, no change was observed in the ACT measured by the HemoTec device and only small changes were observed in the Hemochron-measured ACT. In contrast, more recent studies evaluating intravenous dosing of enoxaparin and dalteparin during PCI have demonstrated a more significant impact on the ACT. One trial reviewed 67 patients undergoing PCI and compared 1 mg/kg intravenous enoxaparin alone or 0.75 mg/kg intravenous enoxaparin administered with eptifibatide bolus and infusion (90). The ACT was measured just before and 5 min after enoxaparin administration. The mean increase in ACT was 77 ± 26 s for the 1 mg/kg enoxaparin group and 69 ± 23 s in the enoxaparin plus eptifibatide group ($p < 0.0001$ for both groups). A good correlation was noted in this study between the ACT and the ENOX test ($r = 0.86$; $p < 0.0001$), which was a recently designed point-of-care method for monitoring enoxaparin anticoagulant activity that correlated well with anti-Xa activity (91) but never became commercially available. None of the patients in this trial developed complications of transient abrupt closure, thrombus formation, major bleeding, or required urgent revascularization. Additional trials of intravenous enoxaparin have also demonstrated mean increases of ACT in the range of 60–70 s when measured 5 min after 1 mg/kg intravenous enoxaparin (92,93), suggesting that the ACT may have some role in monitoring enoxaparin at the higher intravenous doses used during PCI. Limited data are also available on the effect of dalteparin on ACT. An observational trial using dalteparin found a mean increase in the ACT from 125 to 184 s when measured with a Hemochron device 5 min after patients received an 80 IU/kg bolus (94). A more recent randomized, controlled pilot study compared intravenous dalteparin with UFH using each anticoagulant with and without GPIIb/IIIa inhibitors (95). Dosing for each drug with GPIIb/IIIa inhibitor was 70 U/kg intravenous UFH or 70 IU/kg intravenous dalteparin. In the absence of GPIIb/IIIa inhibitor, 100 U/kg UFH or 100 IU/kg dalteparin was used. Hemochron ACTs were measured 30 min after the bolus and found to be lower and less widely distributed with dalteparin compared to heparin (234 s vs. 344 s, $p < 0.0001$). Mean change from baseline cannot be compared in this study as no baseline samples were measured. Studies have not been reported comparing ACT levels with clinical outcomes for patients treated with LMWH during PCI. Current ACC/AHA/SCAI guidelines for PCI do not recommend using ACT for monitoring LMWH, but further studies are needed.

Direct Thrombin Inhibitors

The direct thrombin inhibitors (DTI) exert their anticoagulant effect by directly blocking the action of thrombin on fibrinogen and also inhibit thrombin-induced platelet activation. While several DTIs are available, the most studied in PCI has been bivalirudin, which has been shown to be equivalent to heparin plus a GPIIb/IIIa receptor antagonist in preventing acute ischemic events while causing fewer bleeding complications (96,97).

A full review of clinical trials on the utility of the DTIs is out of the scope of this chapter, but two recent larger trials that have expanded the use of these agents in PCI include REPLACE-2 and ACUITY. The REPLACE-2 (Randomized Evaluation in PCI Linking Angiomax to Reduced Clinical Events) trial demonstrated noninferiority of bivalirudin to UFH when used with provisional GPIIb/IIIa inhibitor for urgent or elective PCI (96). The ACUITY (Acute Catheterization and Urgent Intervention Triage Strategy) trial evaluated the use of bivalirudin in moderate-to-high-risk ACS patients who were undergoing an early invasive approach (97). Results suggested noninferiority of bivalirudin to UFH or enoxaparin with a lower rate of bleeding complications for the bivalirudin alone group as compared to the group treated with heparin and GPIIb/IIIa inhibitor.

Studies reviewing bivalirudin and other DTI monitoring have not established clear guidelines on how to manage these medications based on monitoring results. The APTT is not considered a useful test for DTI monitoring as the DTI hirudin has been shown to have a linear correlation with APTT only for concentrations in the low to normal therapeutic range (up to 1 mg/L) (98). The ACT has also been evaluated for monitoring DTIs, but poor correlation between hirudin plasma levels and ACT has been observed, with levels >2 mg/L increasing the ACT above the detection limit (99). More recent data have supported such limited utility of the ACT for monitoring DTIs. One recent retrospective analysis assessed 495 patients who underwent PCI using bivalirudin at doses used in the REPLACE-2 trial and compared procedural ACTs (by Hemochron instrument) to clinical endpoints (100). Unlike the relationship between ACT and clinical events with UFH as outlined earlier, no correlation was found between ischemic events or bleeding complications and the periprocedural ACT.

The ecarin clotting time (ECT) was designed to be a more accurate measure of DTI activity. Clotting in the ECT is initiated by a purified metalloprotease from the venom of the saw-scaled viper *Echis carinatus* that specifically activates prothrombin (101). The direct cleavage of prothrombin generates an intermediate serine proteinase called meizothrombin which has procoagulant properties of thrombin but to a lesser degree. Hirudin and other synthetic DTIs are able to inhibit the formation of meizothrombin, while the heparin-antithrombin III complex cannot as a result of steric hindrance. As opposed to the APTT or ACT, ECT-based tests have demonstrated linear relationships throughout a broad range of DTI plasma concentrations (101–103). Two point-of-care monitoring devices for bivalirudin using ECT have been reported, both of which demonstrated good correlation with plasma bivalirudin levels (102,103). One instrument, the thrombin inhibitor management ecarin clotting time (TIM-ECT; PharmaNetics, Morrisville, NC) (103), did not continue commercial development. The other uses thromboelastography, which was described earlier, focusing on the reaction time (R time) to initial clot formation using ECT (102). Further studies are needed to establish the appropriate use of point-of-care ECT tests to monitor or adjust DTI therapy in the catheterization laboratory.

CONCLUSIONS

The inherent variations in how an individual patient responds to treatment with one or, more typically, multiple antithrombotic agents have the potential to mean the difference between life-threatening bleeding or recurrent thrombosis in the PCI patient. The polygenetic and polyenvironment influences on thrombosis make predicting an individual's response to pharmacologic interventions nearly impossible. Therefore the ability to rapidly and effectively monitor a patient's response to treatment with a variety of anticoagulant and antiplatelet agents is critical to optimizing outcomes. Unfortunately, despite the large number of studies and observations highlighted in this chapter there remains no ideal monitoring system. At this time, despite well-proven variability in response to antiplatelet agents no study has yet to show that acting upon those results improves outcomes. Even for something as routine as the ACT, which has been used to monitor UFH in the cath lab for 3 decades, recent studies have found it to have little bearing on thrombotic outcomes.

There are a number of monitoring devices currently available for use in the cath lab and that number continues to grow; a testament to the lack of an accepted standard. At the same time the number of novel antithrombotic agent choices also continues to expand with literally dozens more in advanced clinical testing. As the use of more unique combinations of antithrombotic agents becomes commonplace, the need for effective monitoring will become even more important, making a thorough understanding of the limitations and benefits of present-day monitoring in the cath lab crucial.

BIBLIOGRAPHY

1. Milian M (1901) Influence de la peau sur la coagulabilite du sang. CR Soc Biol (Paris) 53:576–578
2. Ivy A, Nelson D, Bucher G (1941) The standardization of certain factors in the cutaneous "venostasis" bleeding time technique. J Lab Clin Med 26:1812–1822
3. Thompson C, Steinhubl SR (2002) Monitoring of platelet function in the setting of glycoprotein IIb/IIIa inhibitor therapy. J Interv Cardiol 15:61–70
4. Rodgers R, Levin J (1990) A critical reappraisal of the bleeding time. Semin Thromb Hemost 16:1–20
5. Tcheng J, Ellis SG, George BS et al (1994) Pharmacodynamics of chimeric glycoprotein IIb/IIIa integrin antiplatelet antibody Fab 7E3 in high-risk coronary angioplasty. Circulation 90:1757–1764
6. Harrington R, Kleiman NS, Kottke-Marchant K et al (1995) Immediate and reversible platelet inhibition after intravenous administration of a peptide glycoprotein IIb/IIIa inhibitor during percutaneous coronary intervention. Am J Cardiology 76:1222–1227
7. Kereiakes D, Kleiman NS, Ambrose J et al (1996) Randomized, double-blind, placebo-controlled dose-ranging study of tirofiban (MK-383) platelet IIb/IIIa blockade in high risk patients undergoing coronary angioplasty. J Am Coll Cardiol 27:536–542
8. Harrison P et al (2007) Measuring antiplatelet drug effects in the laboratory. Thromb Res 120:323–336
9. Cardinal D, Flower RJ (1980) The electronic aggregometer: a novel device for assessing platelet behavior in blood. J Pharmacol Methods 3(2):135–158
10. Lincoff A (2003) Platelet glycoprotein IIb/IIIa inhibitors in cardiovascular disease. Humana Press, Totowa, NJ
11. Mascelli M, Worley S, Veriabo N et al (1997) Rapid assessment of platelet function with a modified whole-blood aggregometer in percutaneous transluminal coronary angioplasty patients receiving anti-GP IIb/IIIa therapy. Circulation 96:3860–3866
12. Michelson A (1996) Flow cytometry: a clinical test of platelet function. Blood 87:4925–4936
13. Schwarz UR, Geiger J, Walter U, Eigenthaler M (1999) Flow cytometry analysis of intracellular VASP phosphorylation for the assessment of activating and inhibitory signal transduction pathways in human platelets–definition and detection of ticlopidine/clopidogrel effects. Thromb Haemost 82:1145–1152
14. Aleil B, Ravanat C, Cazenave JP, Rochoux G, Heitz A, Gachet C (2005) Flow cytometric analysis of intraplatelet VASP phosphorylation for the detection of clopidogrel resistance in patients with ischemic cardiovascular diseases. J Thromb Haemost 3:85–92
15. Michelson A, Frelinger AL, Furman M (2006) Current options in platelet function testing. Am J Cardio 98(Suppl):4N–10N
16. Madan M, Berkowitz SD, Christie DJ et al (2001) Rapid assessment of glycoprotein IIb/IIIa blockade with the platelet function analyzer (PFA-100) during percutaneous coronary intervention. Am Heart J 141:226–233
17. Coller B, Lang D, Scudder LE (1997) Rapid and simple platelet function assay to assess glycoprotein IIb/IIIa receptor blockade. Circulation 95:860–867
18. Smith J, Steinhubl SR, Lincoff AM et al (1999) Rapid platelet-function assay: an automated and quantitative cartridge-based method. Circulation 99:620–625
19. Simon DI, Liu CB, Ganz P et al (2001) A comparative study of light transmission aggregometry and automated bedside platelet function assays in patients undergoing percutaneous coronary intervention and receiving abciximab, eptifibatide, or tirofiban. Catheter Cardiovasc Interv 52:425–432
20. Wheeler GL, Braden GA, Steinhubl SR et al (2002) The Ultegra rapid platelet-function assay: comparison to standard platelet function assays in patients undergoing percutaneous coronary intervention with abciximab therapy. Am Heart J 143:602–611

21. von Beckerath N, Pogatsa-Murray G, Wieczorek A, Sibbing D, Schomig A, Kastrati A (2006) Correlation of a new point-of-care test with conventional optical aggregometry for the assessment of clopidogrel responsiveness. Thromb Haemost 95:910–911

22. Haemoscope Inc. Homepage, http://www.haemoscope.com. Accessed 7/2009.

23. Salooja N, Perry DJ (2001) Thrombelastography. Blood Coagul Fibrinolysis 12:327–337

24. Hobson AR, Agarwala RA, Swallow RA, Dawkins KD, Curzen NP (2006) Thrombelastography: current clinical applications and its potential role in interventional cardiology. Platelets 17:509–518

25. Craft R, Chavez JJ, Bresee SJ et al (2004) A novel modification of the thrombelastograph assay, isolating platelet function, correlates with optical platelet aggregation. J Lab Clin Med 143:301–309

26. Shenkman B, Savion N, Dardik R et al (2000) Testing of platelet deposition on polystyrene surface under flow conditions by the cone and plate(let) analyzer: role of platelet activation, fibrinogen and von Willebrand factor. Thromb Res 99:353–361

27. Osende J, Fuster V, Lev EI et al (2001) Testing platelet activation with a shear-dependent platelet function test versus aggregation-based tests: Relevance for monitoring long-term glycoprotein IIb/IIIa inhibition. Circulation 103:1488–1491

28. Spectre G, Brill A, Gural A et al (2005) A new point-of-care method for monitoring anti-platelet therapy: application of the cone and plate(let) analyzer. Platelets 16:293–299

29. Lakkis NM, George S, Thomas E et al (2001) Use of ICHOR-platelet works to assess platelet function in patients treated with GP IIb/IIIa inhibitors. Catheter Cardiovasc Interv 53:346–351

30. Craft RM, Chavez JJ, Snider CC, Muenchen RA, Carroll RC (2005) Comparison of modified Thrombelastograph and Plateletworks whole blood assays to optical platelet aggregation for monitoring reversal of clopidogrel inhibition in elective surgery patients. J Lab Clin Med 145:309–315

31. White MM, Krishnan R, Kueter TJ, Jacoski MV, Jennings LK (2004) The use of the point of care Helena ICHOR/Plateletworks and the Accumetrics Ultegra RPFA for assessment of platelet function with GPIIB IIIa antagonists. J Thromb Thrombolysis 18:163–169

32. Ernst NM, Suryapranata H, Miedema K et al (2004) Achieved platelet aggregation inhibition after different antiplatelet regimens during percutaneous coronary intervention for ST-segment elevation myocardial infarction. J Am Coll Cardiol 44:1187–1193

33. Smit JJ, Ernst NM, Slingerland RJ et al (2006) Platelet microaggregation inhibition in patients with acute myocardial infarction pretreated with tirofiban and relationship with angiographic and clinical outcome. Am Heart J 151:1102–1107

34. Gold H, Coller BS, Yasuda T et al (1988) Rapid and sustained coronary artery recanalization with combined bolus injection of recombinant tissue-type plasminogen activator and monoclonal antiplatelet GPIIb/IIIa antibody in a canine preparation. Circulation 77:670–677

35. Yasuda T, Gold HK, Fallon JT et al (1988) Monoclonal antibody against the platelet glycoprotein (GP) IIb/IIIa receptor prevents coronary artery reocclusion after reperfusion with recombinant tissue-type plasminogen activator in dogs. J Clin Invest 81:1284–1291

36. Bates E, McGillem MJ, Mickelson JK et al (1991) A monoclonal antibody against the platelet glycoprotein IIb/IIIa receptor complex prevents platelet aggregation and thrombosis in a canine model of coronary angioplasty. Circulation 84:2463–2469

37. Use of a monoclonal antibody directed against the platelet glycoprotein IIb/IIIa receptor in high-risk coronary angioplasty. The EPIC Investigation. N Engl J Med (1994); 330:956–961.

38. Platelet glycoprotein IIb/IIIa receptor blockade and low-dose heparin during percutaneous coronary revascularization. The EPILOG Investigators (1997). N Engl J Med 336:1689–1696

39. Randomised placebo-controlled and balloon-angioplasty-controlled trial to assess safety of coronary stenting with use of platelet glycoprotein-IIb/IIIa blockade (1998). Lancet 352:87–92

40. Randomised placebo-controlled trial of effect of eptifibatide on complications of percutaneous coronary intervention: IMPACT-II. Integrilin to Minimise Platelet Aggregation and Coronary Thrombosis-II (1997). Lancet 349:1422–1428

41. Novel dosing regimen of eptifibatide in planned coronary stent implantation (ESPRIT): a randomised, placebo-controlled trial (2000). Lancet 356:2037–2044

42. Phillips D, Teng W, Arfsten A (1997) Effect of Ca2+ on GPIIb/IIIa interactions with integrilin. Enhanced GPIIb/IIIa binding and inhibition of platelet aggregation by reductions in the concentration of ionized calcium in plasma anticoagulated with citrate. Circulation 96:1488–1494

43. Gilchrist I, O'Shea JC, Kosoglou T et al (2001) Pharmacodynamics and pharmacokinetics of higher-dose double-bolus eptifibatide in percutaneous coronary intervention. Circulation 104:406–411

44. Steinhubl SR, Talley JD, Braden GA et al (2001) Point-of-care measured platelet inhibition correlates with a reduced risk of an adverse cardiac event after percutaneous coronary intervention: results of the GOLD (AU-Assessing Ultegra) multicenter study. Circulation 103:2572–2578

45. Danzi GB, Capuano C, Sesana M, Mauri L, Sozzi FB (2006) Variability in extent of platelet function inhibition after administration of optimal dose of glycoprotein IIb/IIIa receptor blockers in patients undergoing a high-risk percutaneous coronary intervention. Am J Cardiol 97:489–493

46. Gurbel PA, Bliden KP, Guyer K et al (2005) Platelet reactivity in patients and recurrent events post-stenting: results of the PREPARE POST-STENTING Study. J Am Coll Cardiol 46:1820–1826

47. Madan M, Berkowitz SD, Christie DJ, Smit AC, Sigmon KN, Tcheng JE (2002) Determination of platelet aggregation inhibition during percutaneous coronary intervention with the platelet function analyzer PFA-100. Am Heart J 144:151–158

48. Popma JJ, Ohman EM, Weitz J, Lincoff AM, Harrington RA, Berger P (2001) Antithrombotic therapy in patients undergoing percutaneous coronary intervention. Chest 119:321S–336S

49. Popma JJ, Berger P, Ohman EM, Harrington RA, Grines C, Weitz JI (2004) Antithrombotic therapy during percutaneous coronary intervention: the seventh ACCP conference on antithrombotic and thrombolytic therapy. Chest 126:576S–599S

50. Cattaneo M (2004) Aspirin and clopidogrel: efficacy, safety, and the issue of drug resistance. Arterioscler Thromb Vasc Biol 24:1980–1987

51. Michelson AD (2004) Platelet function testing in cardiovascular diseases. Circulation 110:e489–e493

52. Chen WH, Lee PY, Ng W, Tse HF, Lau CP (2004) Aspirin resistance is associated with a high incidence of myonecrosis after non-urgent percutaneous coronary intervention despite clopidogrel pretreatment. J Am Coll Cardiol 43:1122–1126

53. Chen WH, Lee PY, Ng W et al (2005) Relation of aspirin resistance to coronary flow reserve in patients undergoing elective percutaneous coronary intervention. Am J Cardiol 96:760–763

54. Buch AN, Singh S, Roy P et al (2007) Measuring aspirin resistance, clopidogrel responsiveness, and postprocedural markers of myonecrosis in patients undergoing percutaneous coronary intervention. Am J Cardiol 99:1518–1522

55. Marcucci R, Paniccia R, Antonucci E et al (2006) Usefulness of aspirin resistance after percutaneous coronary intervention for acute myocardial infarction in predicting one-year major adverse coronary events. Am J Cardiol 98:1156–1159

56. Angiolillo DJ, Fernandez-Ortiz A, Bernardo E et al (2006) Influence of aspirin resistance on platelet function profiles in patients on long-term aspirin and clopidogrel after percutaneous coronary intervention. Am J Cardiol 97:38–43

57. Jilma B (2001) Platelet function analyzer (PFA-100): a tool to quantify congenital or acquired platelet dysfunction. J Lab Clin Med 138:152–163

58. Malinin A, Pokov A, Spergling M et al (2007) Monitoring platelet inhibition after clopidogrel with the VerifyNow-P2Y12(R) rapid analyzer: the VERIfy Thrombosis risk ASsessment (VERITAS) study. Thromb Res 119:277–284

59. Barragan P, Bouvier JL, Roquebert PO et al (2003) Resistance to thienopyridines: clinical detection of coronary stent thrombosis by monitoring of vasodilator-stimulated phosphoprotein phosphorylation. Catheter Cardiovasc Interv 59:295–302

60. Gurbel PA, Bliden KP, Samara W et al (2005) Clopidogrel effect on platelet reactivity in patients with stent thrombosis: results of the CREST Study. J Am Coll Cardiol 46:1827–1832

61. Golanski J, Pluta J, Baraniak J, Watala C (2004) Limited usefulness of the PFA-100 for the monitoring of ADP receptor antagonists – in vitro experience. Clin Chem Lab Med 42:25–29

62. Hayward CP, Harrison P, Cattaneo M, Ortel TL, Rao AK (2006) Platelet function analyzer (PFA)-100 closure time in the evaluation of platelet disorders and platelet function. J Thromb Haemost 4:312–319

63. Matetzky S, Shenkman B, Guetta V et al (2004) Clopidogrel resistance is associated with increased risk of recurrent atherothrombotic events in patients with acute myocardial infarction. Circulation 109:3171–3175

64. Bliden KP, DiChiara J, Tantry US, Bassi AK, Chaganti SK, Gurbel PA (2007) Increased risk in patients with high platelet aggregation receiving chronic clopidogrel therapy undergoing percutaneous coronary intervention: is the current antiplatelet therapy adequate? J Am Coll Cardiol 49:657–666

65. Benito B, Masotti M, Betriu A (2005) Advances in adjunctive pharmacological therapy for percutaneous coronary interventions. Rev Esp Cardiol 58:729–743

66. Ravel R (1995) Clinical laboratory medicine. Mosby-Year Book, Inc., St. Louis, pp 85–112.

67. Hattersley PG (1966) Activated coagulation time of whole blood. Jama 196:436–440

68. Bowers J, Ferguson JJ (1993) Use of the activated clotting time in anticoagulation monitoring of intravascular procedures. Tex Heart Inst J 20:258–263

69. Verska JJ (1977) Control of heparinization by activated clotting time during bypass with improved postoperative hemostasis. Ann Thorac Surg 24:170–173

70. Spinler SA, Wittkowsky AK, Nutescu EA, Smythe MA (2005) Anticoagulation monitoring part 2: Unfractionated heparin and low-molecular-weight heparin. Ann Pharmacother 39:1275–1285

71. Avendano A, Ferguson JJ (1994) Comparison of Hemochron and HemoTec activated coagulation time target values during percutaneous transluminal coronary angioplasty. J Am Coll Cardiol 23:907–910

72. Aylsworth CL, Stefan F, Woitas K, Rieger RH, LeBoutillier M 3rd, DiSesa VJ (2004) New technology, old standards: disparate activated clotting time measurements by the Hemochron Jr compared with the standard Hemochron. Ann Thorac Surg 77:973–976

73. Ferguson JJ, Dougherty KG, Gaos CM, Bush HS, Marsh KC, Leachman DR (1994) Relation between procedural activated coagulation time and outcome after percutaneous transluminal coronary angioplasty. J Am Coll Cardiol 23:1061–1065

74. Narins CR, Hillegass WB Jr, Nelson CL et al (1996) Relation between activated clotting time during angioplasty and abrupt closure. Circulation 93:667–671

75. Chew DP, Bhatt DL, Lincoff AM et al (2001) Defining the optimal activated clotting time during percutaneous coronary intervention: aggregate results from 6 randomized, controlled trials. Circulation 103:961–966

76. Moliterno DJ, Califf RM, Aguirre FV et al (1995) Effect of platelet glycoprotein IIb/IIIa integrin blockade on activated clotting time during percutaneous transluminal coronary angioplasty or directional atherectomy (the EPIC trial). Evaluation of c7E3 Fab in the Prevention of Ischemic Complications trial. Am J Cardiol 75:559–562

77. Ammar T, Scudder LE, Coller BS (1997) In vitro effects of the platelet glycoprotein IIb/IIIa receptor antagonist c7E3 Fab on the activated clotting time. Circulation 95:614–617

78. Ambrose JA, Hawkey M, Badimon JJ et al (2000) In vivo demonstration of an antithrombin effect of abciximab. Am J Cardiol 86:150–152

79. Ambrose JA, Doss R, Geagea JM, et al (2001) Effects on thrombin generation of the platelet glycoprotein IIb/IIIa inhibitors abciximab versus tirofiban during coronary intervention. Am J Cardiol 87:1231–1233, A8

80. Casserly IP, Topol EJ, Jia G et al (2003) Effect of abciximab versus tirofiban on activated clotting time during percutaneous intervention and its relation to clinical outcomes – observations from the TARGET trial. Am J Cardiol 92:125–129

81. Dauerman HL, Ball SA, Goldberg RJ, Desourdy MA, Furman MI (2002) Activated clotting times in the setting of eptifibatide use during percutaneous coronary intervention. J Thromb Thrombolysis 13:127–132

82. Pinto DS, Lorenz DP, Murphy SA, et al. Association of an activated clotting time < or = 250 seconds with adverse event rates after percutaneous coronary intervention using tirofiban and heparin (a TACTICS-TIMI 18 substudy). Am J Cardiol 2003; 91:976-8, A4.

83. Levine GN, Berger PB, Cohen DJ et al (2006) Newer pharmacotherapy in patients undergoing percutaneous coronary interventions: a guide for pharmacists and other health care professionals. Pharmacotherapy 26:1537–1556

84. Collet JP, Montalescot G, Lison L et al (2001) Percutaneous coronary intervention after subcutaneous enoxaparin pre-treatment in patients with unstable angina pectoris. Circulation 103:658–663

85. Collet JP, Montalescot G, Fine E et al (2003) Enoxaparin in unstable angina patients who would have been excluded from randomized pivotal trials. J Am Coll Cardiol 41:8–14

86. Martin JL, Fry ET, Sanderink GJ et al (2004) Reliable anticoagulation with enoxaparin in patients undergoing percutaneous coronary intervention: the pharmacokinetics of enoxaparin in PCI (PEPCI) study. Catheter Cardiovasc Interv 61:163–170

87. Montalescot G, Collet JP, Tanguy ML et al (2004) Anti-Xa activity relates to survival and efficacy in unselected acute coronary syndrome patients treated with enoxaparin. Circulation 110:392–398

88. Kereiakes DJ, Montalescot G, Antman EM et al (2002) Low-molecular-weight heparin therapy for non-ST-elevation acute coronary syndromes and during percutaneous coronary intervention: an expert consensus. Am Heart J 144:615–624

89. Henry TD, Satran D, Knox LL, Iacarella CL, Laxson DD, Antman EM (2001) Are activated clotting times helpful in the management of anticoagulation with subcutaneous low-molecular-weight heparin? Am Heart J 142:590–593

90. Lawrence M, Mixon TA, Cross D, Gantt DS, Dehmer GJ (2004) Assessment of anticoagulation using activated clotting times in patients receiving intravenous enoxaparin during percutaneous coronary intervention. Catheter Cardiovasc Interv 61:52–55

91. Saw J, Kereiakes DJ, Mahaffey KW et al (2003) Evaluation of a novel point-of-care enoxaparin monitor with central laboratory anti-Xa levels. Thromb Res 112:301–306

92. Rabah MM, Premmereur J, Graham M et al (1999) Usefulness of intravenous enoxaparin for percutaneous coronary intervention in stable angina pectoris. Am J Cardiol 84:1391–1395

93. Chen WH, Lau CP, Lau YK et al (2002) Stable and optimal anticoagulation is achieved with a single dose of intravenous enoxaparin in patients undergoing percutaneous coronary intervention. J Invasive Cardiol 14:439–442

94. Marmur JD, Anand SX, Bagga RS et al (2003) The activated clotting time can be used to monitor the low molecular weight heparin dalteparin after intravenous administration. J Am Coll Cardiol 41:394–402

95. Natarajan MK, Velianou JL, Turpie AG et al (2006) A randomized pilot study of dalteparin versus unfractionated heparin during percutaneous coronary interventions. Am Heart J 151:175

96. Lincoff AM, Bittl JA, Harrington RA et al (2003) Bivalirudin and provisional glycoprotein IIb/IIIa blockade compared with heparin and planned glycoprotein IIb/IIIa blockade during percutaneous coronary intervention: REPLACE-2 randomized trial. Jama 289:853–863

97. Stone GW, McLaurin BT, Cox DA et al (2006) Bivalirudin for patients with acute coronary syndromes. N Engl J Med 355:2203–2216

98. Hafner G, Roser M, Nauck M (2002) Methods for the monitoring of direct thrombin inhibitors. Semin Thromb Hemost 28:425–430

99. Despotis GJ, Hogue CW, Saleem R et al (2001) The relationship between hirudin and activated clotting time: implications for patients with heparin-induced thrombocytopenia undergoing cardiac surgery. Anesth Analg 93:28–32

100. Cheneau E, Canos D, Kuchulakanti PK et al (2004) Value of monitoring activated clotting time when bivalirudin is used as the sole anticoagulation agent for percutaneous coronary intervention. Am J Cardiol 94:789–792

101. Nowak G (2003) The ecarin clotting time, a universal method to quantify direct thrombin inhibitors. Pathophysiol Haemost Thromb 33:173–183

102. Carroll RC, Chavez JJ, Simmons JW et al (2006) Measurement of patients' bivalirudin plasma levels by a thrombelastograph ecarin clotting time assay: a comparison to a standard activated clotting time. Anesth Analg 102:1316–1319

103. Casserly IP, Kereiakes DJ, Gray WA et al (2004) Point-of-care ecarin clotting time versus activated clotting time in correlation with bivalirudin concentration. Thromb Res 113:115–121

104. Lehman C, Thompson C. (2007) Instrumentation for the coagulation laboratory. Laboratory hemostasis: a practical guide for pathologists. Springer, New York, pp 41–55.

Part VI
Antithrombotic Therapy in Venous Thromboembolism

17

Venous Thromboembolism

Esther S.H. Kim and John R. Bartholomew

CONTENTS

ABSTRACT Venous thromboembolism, a clinical entity which includes deep vein thrombosis (DVT) and pulmonary embolism (PE), is a common, lethal disease that affects both hospitalized and non-hospitalized patients, recurs frequently, is often overlooked, and results in long-term complications. The currently available antithrombin agents, including unfractionated heparin, low molecular weight heparin, direct thrombin inhibitors, vitamin K antagonists, and factor Xa antagonists are employed to prevent and treat this clinical entity. Improved understanding of the optimal dosing, timing of administration, and duration of therapy of the currently available antithrombotic therapies to treat venous thromboembolism will hopefully translate into improved outcomes for these patients.

Key words: Deep vein thrombosis; Pulmonary embolism; Venous; Thromboembolism; Treatment; Prophylaxis

EPIDEMIOLOGY AND PATHOGENESIS

Venous thromboembolism (VTE), a clinical entity which includes deep vein thrombosis (DVT) and pulmonary embolism (PE), is a common, lethal disease that affects both hospitalized and non-hospitalized patients, recurs frequently, is often overlooked, and results in long-term complications including chronic thromboembolic pulmonary hypertension (CTPH) and the post-thrombotic syndrome (PTS). While VTE affects 7.1 persons per 10,000 person-years among community residents *(1)*, two-thirds of all VTE events are related to hospitalization, and most hospitalized patients have at least one or more risk factors for VTE (Table 1).

From: *Contemporary Cardiology: Antithrombotic Drug Therapy in Cardiovascular Disease*
Edited by: A.T. Askari and A.M. Lincoff (eds.), DOI 10.1007/978-1-60327-235-3_17
© Humana Press, a part of Springer Science+Business Media, LLC 2010

Table 1
Risk factors for VTE

Surgery
Trauma (major or lower extremity)
Immobility, paresis
Malignancy
Cancer therapy (hormonal, chemotherapy, or radiotherapy)
Previous VTE
Increasing age
Pregnancy and the postpartum period
Estrogen-containing oral contraception or hormone replacement therapy
Selective estrogen receptor modulators
Acute medical illness
Heart or respiratory failure
Inflammatory bowel disease
Nephrotic syndrome
Myeloproliferative disorders
Paroxysmal nocturnal hemoglobinuria
Heparin-induced thrombocytopenia
Antiphospholipid antibody syndrome
Obesity
Smoking
Varicose veins
Central venous catheterization
Inherited or acquired thrombophilia

Geerts et al. *(5)* Copyright©2004 by Am College of Chest Physicians. Reproduced with permission of Am College of Chest Physicians in the format Textbook via Copyright Clearance Center

Rudolph Virchow's triad, formulated in 1856, still forms the best framework for understanding the pathogenesis of VTE. The triad includes stasis, hypercoagulability, and injury to the vessel wall. There are both inherited and acquired risk factors for hypercoagulability. The most common inherited risk factors include: factor V Leiden (activated protein C resistance), the prothrombin gene mutation 20210A, deficiency of the natural anticoagulants proteins C, S, and antithrombin, hyperhomocystinemia, and elevated factor VIII levels. Acquired risk factors are listed in Table 1 and include immobilization, surgery, trauma, pregnancy, use of oral contraceptives or hormone replacement therapy, malignancy, antiphospholipid antibody syndrome (lupus anticoagulant and/or anticardiolipin antibodies) heparin-induced thrombocytopenia (HIT), myeloproliferative disorders, obesity (BMI>30), inflammatory bowel disease, central venous catheters or pacemakers, and the nephrotic syndrome. Other emerging risk factors include increasing age, gender, persistence of an elevated D-dimer level, and the continued presence of venous thrombosis on compression ultrasonography once anticoagulation treatment is completed. Older patients are at higher risk for VTE *(2)* as are men treated for an idiopathic VTE (compared to women) after cessation of anticoagulation therapy *(3)*. There is also recent evidence linking atherosclerotic arterial disease and VTE *(4)*.

Without appropriate prophylaxis, the incidence of hospital-acquired DVT is 10–20% among medical patients and even higher among surgical patients (15–40%) *(5)*. Surprisingly, while PE is the third most common cause of hospital-related death in the United States [10% of hospital deaths are attributed to PE *(6,7)* and the in-hospital fatality rate for VTE is 12% *(8)*], only 58.5% of surgical

Table 2

Pharmacotherapy for the prevention of DVT in medical patients

Patient characteristics	Medication Options	Contraindications to Anticoagulatior
Acutely ill medical patients with any of the following: – Congestive heart failure – Severe respiratory disease – Bedridden with risk factors for development of VTE	– Unfractionated heparin 5,000 units SC q8–12 h – Enoxaparin (Lovenox®) 40 mg SC daily – Enoxaparin (Lovenox®) 30 mg SC daily for patients with severe renal disease and creatinine clearance <30 mL/min – Dalteparin (Fragmin®) 5,000 units SC daily	– Severe active or major bleeding – Severe thrombocytopenia – Heparin induced thrombocytopenia (HIT) – Hypersensitivity to Heparin or Low Molecular Weight Preparations

patients and 39.5% of hospitalized medical patients at risk for VTE receive ACCP guideline-recommended prophylaxis (9).

PREVENTION OF VENOUS THROMBOEMBOLISM

Primary thromboprophylaxis has been shown in numerous studies to be effective in the prevention of VTE (10–14) and is recommended for all patients at risk for VTE (15). Monitoring for signs or symptoms of DVT is unreliable as a method for prevention as PE can be the first manifestation of VTE. The primary methods of thromboprophylaxis include mechanical compression devices (graduated compression stockings, intermittent pneumatic compression devices, and venous foot pumps) and/or antithrombotic medications including low-dose unfractionated heparin, low molecular weight heparins, fondaparinux, and vitamin K antagonists.

Full recommendations for the prevention of VTE in a wide variety of medical and surgical patients can be found in the report of the Eigth American College of Chest Physicians Conference on Antithrombotic and Thrombolytic Therapy (5). Seventy to eighty percent of fatal PEs occur in non-surgical patients (16), and risk factors for VTE in hospitalized medical patients include (in addition to those outlined in Table 1) advanced heart failure (NYHA Class III or IV), COPD exacerbations, sepsis, and bed rest. The ACCP recommends the use of low-dose unfractionated heparin or low molecular weight heparin in these individuals or those who have one or more additional risk factors (5). The recommended dose of UFH for prophylaxis in medical and most surgical patients is 5,000 units administered subcutaneously every 8–12 h and the recommended dose of the LMWH, enoxaparin, is 40 mg subcutaneously given once daily unless the patient has a creatinine clearance under 30 mL/min (Table 2). Mechanical prophylaxis with graduated compression stockings or intermittent pneumatic compression is recommended in those medical (5) or surgical patients for whome there is a contraindication to anticoagulation.

NON-FATAL COMPLICATIONS OF VTE

While prevention of fatal PE is a major goal of VTE prophylaxis and treatment, prevention of the long-term sequelae of VTE is also imperative. These major complications include recurrent VTE, chronic thromboembolic pulmonary hypertension (CTPH), and the post-thrombotic syndrome (PTS).

Recurrent VTE

Recurrence rates of VTE were investigated in a retrospective cohort study of 1,719 patients with DVT or PE who were followed for a first recurrence. Overall, 404 patients developed a recurrent event during 10,198 person-years of follow-up. The overall cumulative incidence rates of probable or definite recurrence were 1.4% at 1 month, 4.1% at 6 months, 5.6% at 1 year, and 17.6% at 10 years. The greatest risk for recurrence was in the first 6 months to 1 year, and the hazard rate for recurrence never fell to zero during the median follow-up times of 7.4 years for DVT and 6.1 years for PE *(17)*. Potential risk factors for recurrence of VTE include male gender, increasing age, increased BMI, neurologic disease with associated extremity paresis, active malignancy, lupus anticoagulant, antithrombin deficiency, protein C or S deficiency, elevated D-dimer and factor VIII levels, persistent residual DVT on ultrasound, institutionalization, inflammatory bowel disease, previous central venous catheter or permanent pacemaker placement, and the presence of an IVC filter.

Chronic Thromboembolic Pulmonary Hypertension

Chronic thromboembolic pulmonary hypertension results from an unresolved vascular obstruction due to pulmonary embolism and is associated with significant morbidity and mortality. The severity of pulmonary hypertension is determined, in part, by the extent of vascular obstruction and in most patients with CTPH, more than 40% of the vasculature is involved *(18)*. Patients can remain asymptomatic for years after their initial PE event, but the incidence of CTPH after PE without a known prior DVT has been shown to be as high as 1.0% at 6 months, 3.1% at 1 year, and 3.8 % at 2 years *(19)*. Progression to CTPH may be due to recurrent VTE but similar to other forms of pulmonary hypertension, pulmonary vascular remodeling and subsequent hypertensive arteriopathy also play a role *(20,21)*. The rate of survival appears to be related to the degree of pulmonary hypertension at the time of diagnosis and survival is poor when the mean pulmonary artery pressure is >30 mmHg, or when there is evidence of right heart failure. One observational study of 76 patients with pulmonary thromboembolic disease found that the survival rate over a mean of 5 years of follow-up was 30% if the initial mean pulmonary artery pressure was >40 mmHg and only 10% if it was >50 mmHg *(22)*.

Post-thrombotic Syndrome

Post-thrombotic syndrome is caused by venous valvular incompetence due to previous DVT. It is a cause of substantial morbidity *(23)* and usually occurs within the first 2 years after DVT with a reported incidence of 17% at 1 year and up to 28% by 5 years *(24)*. PTS is characterized by a cluster of signs and symptoms including extremity pain, dependent edema, and cramping which is often worse at the end of the day. Severe manifestations of PTS (Fig. 1) are stasis hyperpigmentation, venous ulceration, and venous claudication. One treatment modality which drastically reduces the incidence of PTS is the use of graduated compression stockings and current ACCP guidelines recommend their use at a pressure of 30–40 mmHg (at the ankle) for 2 years after an acute DVT *(25)*.

DEEP VENOUS THROMBOSIS

Physical Examination

DVT most commonly occurs in the lower extremities but other affected sites include the upper extremities, cerebral, mesenteric, portal, renal, and pelvic veins. Untreated proximal lower-extremity DVTs (popliteal vein and above) have an estimated 50% risk for PE, while about 25% of calf vein

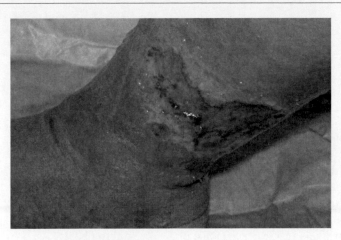

Fig. 1. Venous ulceration is a severe manifestation of the post-thrombotic syndrome. There is associated stasis hyper-pigmentation, edema, and lipodermatosclerosis. Venous ulcers usually occur around the medial malleolus where venous pressure is greatest due to the presence of large perforating veins.

thrombi propagate (in the absence of treatment) to involve a more proximal vein. Patients with DVT may complain of pain and swelling and physical examination may reveal warmth, tenderness, edema, or the presence of dilated veins (collaterals). In extreme situations, cyanosis or gangrene of the limb may be present. Phlegmasia cerulea dolens (a limb-threatening manifestation of DVT in which the thrombus completely occludes venous outflow resulting in severe limb swelling, capillary bed hypertension, and eventually ischemia and necrosis) occurs most frequently in patients with underlying malignancy, heparin-induced thrombocytopenia (HIT), or other hypercoagulable conditions. It is a vascular emergency and treatment includes leg elevation, anticoagulation, and in refractory cases, thrombolysis or mechanical thrombectomy. If present, an associated compartment syndrome requires fasciotomy.

Homans' sign (dorsiflexion of the ankle with knee at 30° flexion causing calf pain), Louvel's sign (worsening of pain with coughing or sneezing), and Lowenberg's sign (pain on the affected leg after inflation of a sphygmomanometer around each calf) may be present in patients with DVT. In general, these signs and clinical examination are unreliable in the diagnosis of DVT (26) because they are often insensitive and nonspecific. Pretest probability scores have been developed to aid in the diagnosis of DVT. For example, patients with a low pretest probability using the Wells score (27,28) (Table 3) have a 96% negative predictive value for DVT (99% if the D-dimer is negative as well). For patients with high pretest probability, however, the Wells score confers a positive predictive value of less than 75%, supporting the need for further diagnostic testing to identify patients with thrombosis (29,30).

Diagnosis

While venography has been the gold standard for the diagnosis of DVT, it is an invasive test which requires the use of intravenous contrast agents. For these reasons, it has largely been replaced as a first-line diagnostic tool by other noninvasive tests such as duplex ultrasonography. When utilized, the presence of DVT on venography is confirmed by the presence of an intraluminal filling defect, although several other clues to the presence of thrombus include an abrupt cutoff, nonfilling of the deep venous system, and/or the demonstration of collateral flow.

Duplex compression ultrasonography is a highly sensitive and specific test for the detection of DVT in symptomatic patients (sensitivity 95% and specificity 98%); however, it is operator dependent and is less sensitive in asymptomatic individuals and for detection of DVT in the calf veins (31,32).

Table 3
Pretest probability of deep venous thrombosis (Wells score)

Clinical feature[a]	Score
Active cancer (treatment ongoing or within previous 6 months of palliative treatment)	1
Paralysis, paresis, or recent plaster immobilization of the lower extremities	1
Recently bedridden for more than 3 days or major surgery, within 4 weeks	1
Localized tenderness along the distribution of the deep venous system	1
Entire leg swollen	1
Calf swelling by more than 3 cm when compared with the asymptomatic leg (measured 10 cm below tibial tuberosity)	1
Pitting edema (greater in the symptomatic leg)	1
Collateral superficial veins (non-varicose)	1
Alternative diagnosis as likely or greater than that of deep-vein thrombosis	−2
Score	
High	3 or more
Moderate	1 or 2
Low	0 or less

[a]In patients with symptoms in both legs, the more symptomatic leg is used
Reproduced from (27) (Copyright©1997 with permission from Elsevier) and (28) (Copyright©2003 Massachusetts Medical Society. All rights reserved)

There are two major assessments performed during duplex ultrasonography for the diagnosis: venous compression using the ultrasound transducer during gray-scale imaging and Doppler assessment of respirophasic flow in the proximal deep veins. Venous incompressibility is diagnostic for DVT (Fig. 2) while venous distension or absent or monophasic venous flow detected by Doppler are suggestive for DVT. The diagnosis of a recurrent DVT is more challenging as veins can remain persistently noncompressible after an initial event. Compression ultrasonography is also limited in its ability to detect isolated thrombi in the iliac veins or superficial femoral veins within the abductor canal. False positives may occur when pelvic abscesses or neoplasms result in isolated noncompressibility of the common femoral veins (33).

Plasma D-dimer is a very sensitive marker for thrombosis but is non-specific. It can be elevated in a variety of conditions including infection, malignancy, trauma, pregnancy, myocardial infarction, and hemorrhage. While a positive D-dimer is of limited clinical utility in the diagnosis of DVT, the combination of a low pretest probability and a negative D-dimer has an extremely high negative predictive value (approximately 99%) (30).

Treatment

Prevention of PE, CTPH, PTS, and recurrent VTE is the goal of therapy in the management of DVT. It is important to emphasize that once a DVT is suspected, anticoagulation should be started immediately and continued once the diagnosis has been confirmed. Unless there is a contraindication to anticoagulation, initial therapy includes unfractionated heparin, low molecular weight heparin (LMWH), or fondaparinux (Table 4). Oral anticoagulation with a vitamin K antagonist is initiated for long-term therapy.

Weight-based regimens of heparin (80 units/kg bolus followed by 18 units/kg/h IV infusion) achieve a therapeutic activated partial thromboplastin time (aPTT) more rapidly than fixed-dose regimens. A therapeutic aPTT corresponds to a heparin level of 0.3–0.7 IU/mL determined by factor

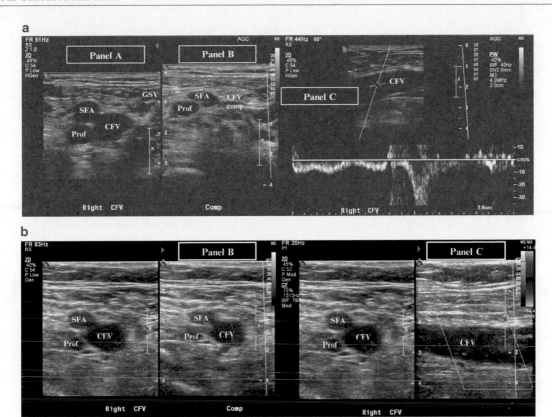

Fig. 2. (**a**) Normal venous ultrasound of the right leg at the level of the common femoral vein (CFV) (*Panel A*). Compression image (*Panel B*) shows normal compressibility of the CFV and greater saphenous vein (GSV). Doppler imaging (*Panel C*) of the same CFV shows normal resplrophasic flow and augmentation. *SFA* superficial femoral artery; *Prof* profunda femoris artery. (**b**) Venous ultrasound of the right leg at the level of the common femoral vein (CFV) showing acute DVT. There is lack of compressibility (*Panel B*), and color Doppler (*Panel C*) of the CFV in long shows lack of blood flow through the vessel. *SFA* superficial femoral artery; *Prof* profunda femoris artery.

Xa inhibition (anti-factor Xa assay) and should be determined by each hospitals' laboratory. The use of the aPTT ratio (1.5–2.5 times the control) is no longer recommended for monitoring treatment. The aPTT is unreliable in patients with an abnormal baseline aPTT (e.g., in patients with a lupus anticoagulant) and in patients who require unusually high doses of heparin, otherwise known as heparin resistance. This can occur in patients with antithrombin deficiency, medications including nitroglycerin and aprotinin, in patients with HIT, an underlying malignancy, or during pregnancy. The anti-factor Xa assay should be used in lieu of the aPTT in these situations.

Subcutaneously administered unfractionated heparin is an alternative to intravenous administration. A 5,000 unit intravenous bolus followed by a subcutaneous dose of 17,500 units twice daily on the first day is the usual recommended starting dose. Subsequent subcutaneous doses are based on the aPTT and adjusted accordingly to achieve an anti-Xa level as reported above. The first aPTT should be drawn 6 h after the initiation dose. A simpler regimen developed recently eliminates the need for aPTT monitoring and uses a nomogram with a subcutaneous loading dose of 333 units/kg followed by fixed doses of 250 units/kg subcutaneously every 12 h (*34*).

LMWHs are easier to administer, have once or twice daily dosing, no monitoring is required (in most patients), are associated with fewer cases of HIT, and cause less osteoclast activation and bone density loss than UFH. There is also evidence that long-term LMWH is more effective in

Table 4
Pharmacotherapy for the treatment of DVT/PE

Medication	Monitoring	Contraindications
Unfractionated heparin 80 units/ kg bolus then 18 units/kg/h IV infusion Unfractionated heparin 5,000 unit IV bolus then 17,500 units SC BID on day 1 Adjust based on aPTT Unfractionated heparin 333 units/kg SC loading dose then 250 units/kg SC q12 hours	Activated Partial Thromboplastin Time (aPTT) Heparin level of 0.3–0.7 IU/ mL determined by factor Xa inhibition (anti-factor Xa assay) No monitoring necessary	Active major bleeding Hypersensitivity to heparin or Heparin induced thrombocytopenia Severe thrombocytopenia Situations where monitoring parameters cannot be obtained
Enoxaparin 1.5 mg/kg SC daily Enoxaparin 1 mg/kg SC q12 h Enoxaparin 1 mg/kg SC daily For patients with severe renal impairment (creatinine clearance <30 mL/min)	(Not required except in obese, pediatric, renal insufficiency, or pregnant patients) Anti-Xa level 0.5–1.0 IU/mL for q12 h dosing Anti-Xa level ≥ 1.0 IU/mL for daily dosing	Active major bleeding Thrombocytopenia or Heparin induced thrombocytopenia Hypersensitivity to enoxaparin, heparin, or pork products
Fondaparinux (Arixtra®) 5 mg SC daily (weight<50 kg) Fondaparinux (Arixtra®) 7.5 mg SC daily (weight 50–100 kg) Fondaparinux (Arixtra®) 10 mg SC daily(weight>100 kg)	Not required for most patients	Active major bleeding Severe renal impairment (creatinine clearance <30 mL/min) Bacterial endocarditis Weight <50 kg undergoing hip fracture, hip or knee replacement, or abdominal surgery Thrombocytopenia associated with a positive in vitro test for anti-platelet antibody in the presence of fondaparinux sodium Hypersensitivity to fondaparinux sodium

preventing recurrent VTE than long-term warfarin therapy in patients with cancer (35). Enoxaparin is the most commonly used LMWH in the United States and is administered as a daily injection (1.5 mg/kg/day) or twice per day (1 mg/kg/q12 h). No monitoring is required except in the obese, pediatric, renal insufficiency, or pregnant patients. The anti-Xa level using LMWH as a reference should be measured 4 h after an injection and the therapeutic range is 0.5–1.0 IU/mL for the 12 h regimen and ≥1.0 IU/mL for the daily dose. LMWH is renally cleared and contraindicated in patients requiring dialysis but can be used in patients with renal insufficiency after dose adjustment.

There have been several randomized-controlled trials which have demonstrated the safety and efficacy of LMWH without monitoring in comparison to intravenous unfractionated heparin with monitoring in patients with acute DVT *(36,37)*. Additionally, outpatient LMWH for the treatment of symptomatic proximal vein DVT has been shown to be safe and efficacious when compared to unfractionated heparin administered in the hospital setting *(38,39)*. As a result of these and other studies, it is recommended that patients with an acute DVT be treated with subcutaneous LMWH as an outpatient if possible, or as an inpatient if necessary without routine monitoring of anti-factor Xa levels. Unfractionated heparin is recommended over LMWH in patients with severe renal failure *(25)*. For patients with DVT and cancer, LMWH is recommended for at least the first 3–6 months of long-term treatment *(25)*.

Vitamin K antagonists are initiated simultaneously with either IV UFH or LMWH. An overlap in therapies should be maintained for a minimum of 5 days and until the international normalized ratio (INR) is ≥2.0–3.0 to permit adequate depletion of vitamin K-dependent coagulation factors *(25)*. The duration of treatment is dependent on the risk of recurrence. Patients with an idiopathic DVT and individuals with persistent risk factors such as select thrombophilias and malignancy require longer therapy. The risk of recurrence decreases with longer durations of anticoagulation; however, clinicians must weigh the risk of bleeding against the risk of new thrombosis.

Current guidelines *(25)* recommend 3 months of anticoagulation with a vitamin K antagonist targeting an INR between 2 and 3 for patients with a first episode of DVT or PE secondary to a transient cause. Anticoagulation with a VKA for at least 3 months is recommended for patients with a first episode of an idiopathic DVT or PE, although consideration should also be given for indefinite anticoagulation in this situation. Long-term (indefinite) anticoagulation is recommended in patients with

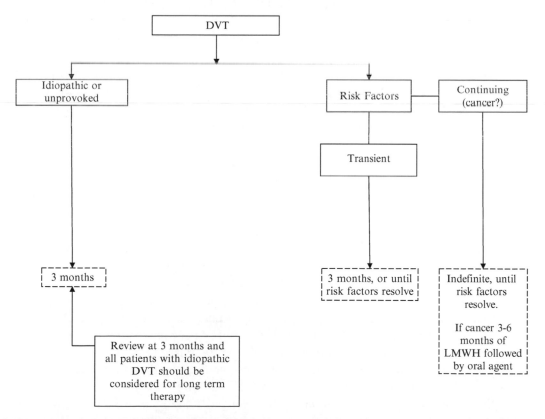

Fig. 3. Long-term treatment algorithm for deep venous thrombosis based on the 8th ACCP Guidelines for Antithrombotic Therapy for Venous Thromboembolic Disease *(25)*.

malignancy as long as the cancer remains active and in select patients with recurrent DVT or PE *(25)* (Fig. 3). Patients with a family history of clotting disorders who have their first VTE event before the age of 50, have thrombosis at unusual locations, have resistance to anticoagulation, or experience recurrent thromboses should be considered for evaluation of an underlying hypercoagulable condition.

Approximately 25% of calf vein DVTs will propagate to involve the proximal (popliteal vein and above) deep veins. Three months of treatment with a VKA is also recommended for patients with a first episode of symptomatic DVT confined to the calf veins secondary to a transient cause *(25)*. Monitoring calf vein thrombosis for propagation into the proximal veins with serial ultrasonography without anticoagulation represents an alternative approach for those individuals with a contraindication to anticoagulation.

Fondaparinux is a synthetic factor Xa inhibitor which has been shown to be efficacious and safe when compared to LMWH for the treatment of acute DVT *(40)* and compared to IV UFH for the treatment of PE *(41)*. It is approved in the United States as treatment for acute DVT and PE when used in combination with oral anticoagulation (administered for at least 5 days and until the INR is >2.0). Fondaparinux is also FDA approved for use as DVT prophylaxis in patients undergoing orthopedic procedures (total hip and knee arthroplasty) and abdominal surgery. It is administered as a once daily subcutaneous injection of 2.5 mg for DVT prophylaxis and 5 mg, 7.5 mg, or 10 mg based on body weight (<50 kg, 50–100 kg, >100 kg, respectively) for the treatment of DVT or PE. Fondaparinux is contraindicated in patients with severe renal impairment (creatinine clearance<30 mL/min) and bacterial endocarditis. Fondaparinux is also contraindicated in patients with a body weight<50 kg who are undergoing hip fracture, hip or knee replacement surgery, and abdominal surgery *(42)*.

The role of thrombolytics in the acute treatment of DVT in the absence of a threatened limb is still unclear. Thrombolytics may promote early recanalization and minimize the incidence of the PTS; however, current ACCP guidelines recommend against their routine use except for patients with a massive ilefemoral DVT at risk of limb gangrene secondary to venous occlusion despite adequate heparin therapy in select patients with acute proximal out *(25)*. For those individuals who qualify, thrombolytic therapy is best administered or under catheter directed therapy. This route carries an increased risk of systemic hemorrhage compared to standard anticoagulation alone.

Inferior Vena Cava Filters

Inferior vena cava (IVC) filters are a mechanical treatment option for the prevention of pulmonary embolism in patients with DVT who have a contraindication or suffer a complication of anticoagulation therapy. Current guidelines recommend against the routine insertion of an IVC filter for the treatment of DVT. IVC filters are also indicated in patients who have experienced recurrent thromboembolization despite adequate anticoagulant therapy *(25)*. Relative indications for IVC filters include: massive PE, iliocaval or free floating proximal DVT, cardiac or pulmonary insufficiency, high risk of complications from anticoagulation (frequent falls, ataxia), or poor compliance.

Complications of IVC filters include migration, organ penetration, recurrent VTE, formation of thrombus above the filter, and caval obstruction. The use of nonpermanent, temporary, or retrievable IVC filters may help to prevent complications. Retrievable filters are removed percutaneously under fluoroscopic guidance within a device-specific window of time and those devices which are not removed can function as permanent filters. Convertible filters are permanent devices which can be structurally altered under fluoroscopic guidance to no longer function as a filter. There are currently no evidence-based recommendations on the use of retrievable filters; however, published consensus guidelines *(43)* advise that their indications are the same as the permanent filters. They should also be considered where anticoagulation is temporarily contraindicated, or there is a short duration of PE risk *(43)*. An IVC filter alone is not effective therapy for DVT alone (as many as 20% of patients with an IVC filter develop a new DVT over a 2-year period) and resumption of anticoagulation as soon as possible after placement of an IVC filter is recommended.

Upper Extremity DVT

– Upper extremity DVT is most often related to central venous catheter placement and/or pacemaker devices. Other less common causes include the thoracic outlet syndrome, Paget–von Schröetter (effort thrombosis), and hypercoagulable conditions. Patients may be asymptomatic but more frequently complain of arm swelling and pain. Anticoagulation is indicated if there are no contraindications. Thrombolysis can be considered in younger patients with low risk of bleeding and symptoms of acute onset *(25)*. The duration of oral anticoagulation should be determined using the same processes described for acute lower extremity DVTs.

Superficial Venous Thrombosis

Superficial venous thrombosis frequently occurs as a complication of an intravenous line, but may occur spontaneously *(25)*. Anticoagulation is generally not required due to the lower risk of pulmonary embolization unless the thrombosis propagates into the deep venous system or if the event is spontaneous. Guidelines recommend intermediate dosages of heparin or LMWH for at least 4 weeks for spontaneous superficial thrombophlebitis *(25)*.

PULMONARY EMBOLISM

Pulmonary embolism is the most common preventable cause of hospital death. Furthermore, an alarming 25% of patients with PE present with sudden death *(44)*. In those patients who do not present with sudden death, the majority of deaths occur due to failure of diagnosis rather than inadequate therapy. Important prognostic variables for mortality after PE as described by the International Cooperative Pulmonary Embolism Registry (ICOPER) (2,454 patients diagnosed with acute PE, overall 3-month mortality 15.3%) are age over 70 years (hazard ratio 1.6 [95% CI 1.1–2.3]), cancer (2.3 [1.5–3.5]), congestive heart failure (2.4 [1.5–3.7]), chronic obstructive pulmonary disease (1.8 [1.2–2.7]), systolic arterial hypotension (2.9 [1.7–5.0]), tachypnea (2.0 [1.2–3.2]), and right ventricular hypokinesis on echocardiography (2.0 [1.3–2.9]) *(45)*.

Physical Examination

In the International Cooperative Pulmonary Embolism Registry (ICOPER), which consists of 2,454 patients diagnosed with acute PE, the most common signs and symptoms were dyspnea (82%), chest pain (49%), cough (20%), syncope (14%), and hemoptysis (7%) *(45)*. Acute cor pulmonale presents with the sudden development of dyspnea, cyanosis, shock, or syncope and signals the presence of a massive PE causing cardiovascular collapse. Physiologically, acute cor pulmonale results from the combination of thrombotic obstruction of the pulmonary vasculature and vasoconstriction due to hypoxia and inflammatory mediators leading to right heart failure, decreased preload, and finally, reduced cardiac output causing hemodynamic collapse. In order to overcome an obstruction of 75% and maintain pulmonary perfusion, the right ventricle must generate a systolic pressure in excess of 50 mmHg and a mean pulmonary artery pressure greater than 40 mmHg *(46)*. A normal right ventricle is unable to generate these pressures and right heart failure and cardiac collapse ensues. Additionally, elevated right ventricular wall tension can lead to decreased right coronary artery flow and ischemia. Cardiopulmonary collapse from pulmonary embolism is more common in patients with coexisting coronary artery disease or underlying cardiopulmonary disease *(47)*.

Diagnosis

Clinical decision rules also known as the wells score have also been developed to determine the pretest probability of PE based on signs and symptoms of a DVT, the presence of tachycardia, hemoptysis, malignancy, or immobilization, a history of previous DVT or PE, and clinical suspicion of PE *(48)*. In a validation study of this clinical decision rule, only 0.5% of patients who were unlikely to have PE and had a negative D-dimer went on to have subsequent nonfatal VTE *(49)*.

The gold standard diagnostic test for PE is pulmonary angiography, but it is not universally available and has in large part been replaced by the use of multi-slice spiral computed tomography. Pulmonary angiography involves the injection of contrast into the pulmonary arteries to assess for intraluminal filling defects. Its major disadvantages include the invasiveness of the procedure, radiation exposure, and the use of potentially nephrotoxic contrast. In experienced centers, associated morbidity and mortality is low.

Computed tomography imaging is widely available and has become the standard imaging technique for the diagnosis of acute PE. It has been especially useful in evaluating patients with a central PE, and with the advent of multislice CT scanners, subsegmental PE can also be detected. Other advantages include the ability to directly image other structures, including the inferior vena cava and lower extremities as well as detect other pathologies which may be mimicking an acute PE. Based on the results of the PIOPED II study *(50)*, CT arteriography (CTA) has a sensitivity of 83% and specificity of 96%. When combined with clinical probability for PE by using the Wells score described above *(48)*, the positive predictive value of CTA is 96% for patients who have high clinical probability but only 58% for those patients with a low clinical probability (i.e., the false positive rate for CTA to diagnose PE in a patient with low clinical probability is 42%). Conversely, the negative predictive value of CTA to exclude PE is 96% in patients with a low clinical probability for PE, but for patients with a high clinical probability and a negative CTA, the false negative rate is 40%. The test is considered nondiagnostic if the results are discordant to the clinical probability *(50)*. Of note, approximately 6% of studies in PIOPED II were inconclusive due to poor image quality.

The safety of withholding anticoagulation in patients with a suspected PE but a negative pulmonary CTA was investigated in a meta-analysis of 23 studies involving 4,657 patients. Only 1.4% of patients with a suspected PE and a normal CTA went on to develop VTE and only 0.51% developed a fatal PE by 3 months *(51)*. These rates are similar to those in patients who had suspected PE but were found to have normal pulmonary angiograms *(52)*. The major disadvantages of CT are its cost, radiation exposure, and the possibility of contrast-induced nephrotoxicity. A diagnostic algorithm based on the results of the PIOPED II study *(53)* is presented in Fig. 4.

Magnetic resonance angiography (MRA) may be an alternative to CT for the diagnosis of PE in patients who have a contrast allergy or for whom avoidance of radiation exposure is desired. Reports of sensitivity and specificity are varied but compared to CT, MRA has been reported to be both less sensitive and specific and limited by inter-observer variability *(54)*.

Ventilation-perfusion (V/Q) scanning remains useful for the diagnosis of PE, but with the increasing availability of spiral CT, it is now a second line imaging modality. A V/Q scan is particularly useful, however, in patients who have normal chest radiography and a contraindication to CT, such as

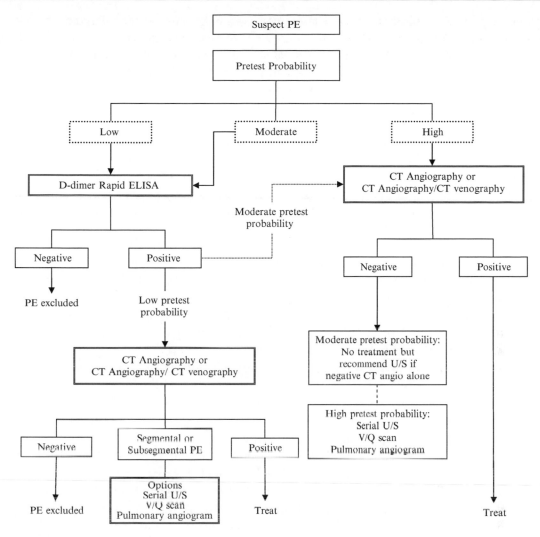

Fig. 4. Diagnostic algorithm for the diagnosis of acute pulmonary embolism: Recommendations of PIOPED II Investigators. Adapted from *(53)* (Copyright©2006 with permission from Elsevier).

those with renal insufficiency, contrast allergy, or pregnancy. The diagnostic ability of V/Q scanning for the detection of PE was evaluated in the original PIOPED study *(55)*. This landmark report showed that while V/Q scanning is helpful if the test is normal or high-probability (87% of patients with high-probability scans had PE but only 4% of patients with normal scans had PE), an intermediate- or low-probability scan was the most common finding and not helpful in making the diagnosis. It is also important to note that the patients in PIOPED who had low-probability scans but for whom there was a high or intermediate clinical suspicion for PE still had a 40 and 16% rate, respectively, of PE diagnosed by pulmonary angiography*(55)*. Thus, for patients with a low-probability V/Q scan but for whom there is a high or intermediate clinical suspicion for PE, additional testing should be performed to confirm or refute the diagnosis.

The major utility of chest radiography is to exclude other diagnoses which could mimic PE and to aid in the interpretation of ventilation-perfusion scans. Findings are generally nonspecific and include cardiomegaly, pleural effusion, an elevated hemidiaphragm, pulmonary artery enlargement, atelectasis, and consolidation. Normal chest radiographs were the second most common finding after cardiomegaly in patients with acute PE in ICOPER *(56)*. Classic signs such as the Westermark sign (regional oligemia), Hampton's hump (pleural based, wedge-shaped shadow), and Palla's sign (enlarged right descending pulmonary artery) are uncommon and have low sensitivity for the diagnosis *(57)*.

Like chest radiography, the major utility of electrocardiography is to exclude other major diagnoses such as acute myocardial infarction. The classic finding on electrocardiogram is the $S_1Q_3T_3$ pattern, but the most common findings are nonspecific ST-segment and T-wave changes *(58)*. Sinus tachycardia, atrial fibrillation, and right bundle-branch block may also be present. In a study of electrocardiograms in patients with acute PE, increased right ventricular end-diastolic dimension, and tricuspid regurgitation, three or more of the following abnormalities were seen in more than three fourths of the patients: (a) incomplete or complete right bundle-branch block; (b) S waves > 1.5 mm in lead I and aVL; (c) shift in transition zone to V_5; (d) Q waves in leads III and aVF but not II; (e) right axis deviation greater than 90 or indeterminate axis; (f) low-voltage QRS in limb leads; and (g) T-wave inversion in leads III and aVF or leads V_1 through V_4 *(59)*. In a study of 90 patients with angiographically proven massive or submassive PE, 6% and 23% of ECGs were normal in these patients, respectively *(58)*.

Transthoracic echocardiography (TTE) can provide rapid bedside assessment for hemodynamically significant PE in the critically ill patient *(53)*. The sensitivity for a massive PE is 97% and the negative predictive value is 98% if any two of the following three findings are present: high clinical probability for PE, echocardiographic evidence of acute right ventricular overload, or positive finding on ultrasonography. Signs of acute cor pulmonale indicative of a massive PE include right ventricular dilatation, right ventricular hypokinesis, tricuspid regurgitation, septal flattening, paradoxical septal motion, diastolic left ventricular impairment secondary to septal displacement, pulmonary artery hypertension, lack of inspiratory collapse of the inferior vena cava, and occasionally direct visualization of the thrombus. McConnel's sign, apical sparing in the setting of moderate or severe right ventricular free-wall hypokinesis, has a specificity of 94% and a positive predictive value of 71% *(60)*. Due to its specificity, McConnel's sign is a useful discriminator for right ventricular dysfunction due to PE versus other causes of right heart dysfunction.

While TTE may be a useful diagnostic tool in the evaluation of the hemodynamically unstable patient with suspected PE, its usefulness as a diagnostic tool has not been as well established in the hemodynamically stable patient as over 60% will not have evidence of right ventricular dysfunction *(61)*. TTE has important prognostic uses, however, in both the hemodynamically stable and unstable patient with PE. Multiple studies using TTE have shown that patients with signs of right ventricular strain have both higher in-hospital and long-term mortalities *(61–64)*. For the 745 patients with acute PE who had TTE performed in ICOPER, right ventricular hypokinesis was associated with a twofold increase in mortality over 3 months *(45)*.

Biomarkers, such as D-dimer, cardiac troponins, and brain natriuretic peptide drawn at the time of diagnosis, can be useful prognostic tools. Elevated cardiac troponins in this setting are associated with echocardiographically confirmed right ventricular dysfunction and are also associated with complicated in-hospital course and overall mortality *(65,66)*. In patients with both right ventricular dysfunction and elevated cardiac troponins, the incidence of death 30 days after diagnosis is as high as 38%. This rate is higher than seen in patients with elevated cardiac troponins or right ventricular dysfunction alone *(67)*. Cardiac troponins can also predict an uncomplicated course as well; cardiac troponins (cTnI and cTnT) have a 92–93% negative predictive value for a complicated in-hospital course following acute PE *(65)*. Similar to cardiac troponins, an elevated BNP can indicate right ventricular dysfunction in patients with PE and similar to elevated troponin levels is a predictor of adverse outcomes *(68)*.

Treatment

The ACCP guidelines *(25)* advocate the initiation of anticoagulation for patients for whom there is a strong suspicion of PE while awaiting the results of diagnostic testing. The mainstays of management for a nonmassive acute PE are initial anticoagulation with heparin, LMWH, or fondaparinux followed by the addition of vitamin K antagonists (Table 4). Unlike the use of LMWH which is approved for the treatment of acute proximal vein DVT on an outpatient basis, the initial treatment of acute PE using these agents should be done in the hospital. The LMWHs are recommended over UFH for the treatment of acute nonmassive PE in patients without renal failure *(25)*. These agents have been shown in several studies to be at least as safe and effective as UFH for the initial treatment of acute nonmassive PE *(37,69,70)*. The initiation of vitamin K antagonists on the first treatment day together with LMWH or UFH is recommended, and overlap treatment should continue for at least 5 days and until the INR is ≥2.0 *(25)*.

Fondaparinux, an indirect factor Xa inhibitor, has been shown to be at least as safe and effective as IV UFH for the treatment of acute nonmassive PE. The Matisse PE Study *(41)* randomized 2,213 hemodynamically stable patients to either IV UFH or once daily subcutaneously administered fondaparinux and followed them for the 3-month composite endpoint of symptomatic, recurrent PE and new or recurrent DVT. The composite endpoint developed in 3.8% of the fondaparinux group compared to 5.0% of the UFH group, and major bleeding rates were similar in the two groups (1.3% in the fondaparinux and 1.1% in the UFH groups, respectively). Fondaparinux is FDA approved for the treatment of acute PE when initial treatment is started in the hospital and when used in conjunction with warfarin sodium *(71)*.

While thrombolytics have been shown to be better than heparin alone for the lysis of pulmonary emboli and improvement in hemodynamic parameters, the risk of major bleeding and the lack of conclusive data showing a mortality benefit have limited its use in patients without massive PE. The first large trial comparing thrombolytics to heparin alone for the treatment of PE was the UPET (Urokinase in Pulmonary Embolism Trial) which included 160 patients with angiographically proven pulmonary embolism *(72)*. Patients were randomly assigned to a 12-h infusion of urokinase followed by heparin treatment versus heparin treatment alone. The results showed that while the urokinase group had improved thrombus resolution on angiography and significant improvement in hemodynamics compared to the heparin group at 24 h, there was no lasting improvement in V/Q scan results or mortality. There was also more bleeding in the urokinase group.

A follow-up study to UPET, USPET (The Urokinase–Streptokinase Pulmonary Embolism Trial) *(73)* randomized 167 patients with acute PE to a 24-h streptokinase infusion or a 12- or 24-h urokinase infusion. All three regimens led to improvement in angiographic and V/Q scan abnormalities as well as improvement in hemodynamic parameters when compared to the heparin only group in UPET with no significant difference among the three regimens in efficacy, mortality, or bleeding. The greatest hemodynamic benefit of thrombolytic therapy was seen in patients with massive pulmonary embolism.

Recombinant tissue-type plasminogen activator (rt-PA) is the third thrombolytic agent studied for the acute treatment of PE. A comparison study of rt-PA and urokinase therapy *(74)*, each followed by heparin therapy, showed greater improvement in angiographic abnormalities and hemodynamic parameters in the rt-PA group after 2 h of therapy, but there was no difference in V/Q scan results between the two groups at 24 h. Similarly, when 50 patients with massive PE were randomized to treatment with rt-PA or streptokinase, each followed by heparin treatment, there was more rapid thrombolysis with rt-PA but no difference between the two regimens in hemodynamic parameters including total pulmonary resistance and right ventricular ejection fraction *(75)*.

Thrombolytic therapy has not been shown to have a clear short-term mortality benefit in patients with PE perhaps largely due to the large number of patients required for a study with mortality as a primary outcome. The all-cause mortality at 3 months of patients who suffer from a PE and who are treated with anticoagulation alone is <10% while the mortality directly due to PE after proper treatment with anticoagulation is 2% (25). A review of thrombolytic therapy for the treatment of acute PE estimates that with a 6.7% death rate from treatment with heparin therapy alone, a study sample of 1,000 patients is needed to have an 80% power to detect a 50% reduction in mortality (76). There have been no large randomized controlled trials on this subject to date, but a recent Cochrane meta-analysis (77) including 679 patients in eight trials comparing thrombolytic agents (streptokinase, urokinase, or rt-PA) followed by heparin to heparin alone or heparin plus placebo for the treatment of PE showed no statistically significant difference in overall mortality (OR 0.89; 95% CI 0.45–1.78), recurrence of PE (OR 0.63, 95% CI 0.33–1.20), major hemorrhagic events (OR 1.61; 95% CI 0.91–2.86), or minor hemorrhagic events (OR 1.98; 95% CI 0.68–5.75). Patients who received thrombolytics did have improved hemodynamic, echocardiographic, V/Q scan, and angiographic outcomes compared to patients who received heparin alone, but this did not translate to improved mortality. Similarly, of 108 patients in ICOPER with massive PE, 33 patients who received thrombolysis received no mortality benefit at 90 days (HR 0.79 [95% CI 0.44–1.43]). The overall 90-day mortality rates were 46.3% (95% CI 31.0–64.8%) with thrombolysis, 55.1% (95% CI 44.3–66.7%) without thrombolysis (78).

Very few studies have been performed regarding the use of thrombolytics in patients with submassive PE who have evidence of right ventricular dysfunction but who are hemodynamically stable. There has been one such randomized controlled trial of 101 hemodynamically stable patients who were given rt-PA followed by heparin or heparin alone and followed with echocardiography at 3 and 24 h after administration. There was a statistically significant improvement in right ventricular wall motion at both 3 and 24 h in the rt-PA group compared to the heparin only group (OR 2.90, 95% CI 0.98–8.6 at 3 h; OR 3.20, 95% CI 1.20–8.57 at 24 h). Worsening of right ventricular motion was seen in 2% of patients in the rt-PA group and 17% of patients in the heparin only group at 24 h ($p = 0.005$). There was also a significant decrease in right ventricular end-diastolic area in the rt-PA group but not in the heparin only group (79).

Only one study has investigated the effect of systemic versus intrapulmonary thrombolytic therapy for the treatment of PE (80). This multicenter study included 34 patients with angiographically proven PE who were randomly assigned to intravenous or intrapulmonary rt-PA in addition to heparin therapy. There were similar decreases in the severity of embolism determined by angiography and in mean pulmonary artery pressures among the two groups leading the authors to conclude that inpulmonary infusion of rt-PA has no benefit over intravenous injection of rt-PA for the treatment of acute PE.

Based on the data available, the 8th ACCP guidelines (25) recommend against the use of systemic thrombolytic therapy in most patients with PE (Grade 1B), but suggest the use of systemic thrombolytic therapy in patients who are hemodynamically unstable (Grade 1B). The guidelines further suggest that catheter-directed local thrombolytic therapy not be administered (Grade 1C). The recommended dose for streptokinase for the treatment of PE is 250,000 IU as a loading dose followed by a 100,000 IU/h infusion for 24 h. The dose of rt-PA is a 100 mg infusion given over 2 h (Table 5). Urokinase is not available in the United States. Heparin therapy should be started following the infusion of thrombolytic therapy.

Pulmonary thromboembolectomy is a complex surgical procedure with an associated mortality of 5–24% (81–84). It is generally offered to symptomatic patients with hemodynamic or ventilatory defects at rest or exercise who have thrombotic material in the main, lobar, or proximal segmental arteries. The only absolute contraindication to the procedure is severe underlying lung disease, and the major complications after surgery are bleeding, reperfusion pulmonary edema, and persistent pulmonary hypertension. Most patients have improvement in NYHA functional class (III or IV before surgery to I or II after surgery) (85) and in their hemodynamic parameters including mean pulmonary artery pressure and pulmonary vascular resistance (86). A recent retrospective study involving 47

Table 5
Thrombolytic Regimens for the Treatment of Acute PE

Medication	Dose	Contraindications to thrombolytic Agents
Streptokinase (Not recommended for use if streptokinase has been used previously)	250,000 IU as a loading dose over 30 min followed by a 100,000 IU/h infusion for 24 h	Active internal bleeding Recent (within 2 months) cerebrovascular accident, intracranial or intraspinal surgery Intracranial neoplasm, arteriovenous malformation, or aneurysm Severe uncontrolled hypertension
Recombinant tissue-type plasminogen activator (rt-PA)	100-mg infusion given over 2 h	

patients described outcomes of surgical pulmonary embolectomy performed for massive PE (hypotension present) and submassive PE (right ventricular dysfunction but normal blood pressure) ($n = 15$). The operative mortality was 6%, and overall survival was 86% at 1 year and 83% at 3 years *(81)*. A similar study involving 13 patients, 9 with submassive PE, described an 8% in-hospital mortality *(87)*. Thus, with progressively decreasing operative morality rates, surgical pulmonary embolectomy may become a viable option for submassive PE to prevent future right ventricular failure, but randomized controlled studies are needed to determine the benefit of surgery over contemporary medical therapy. Currently, pulmonary embolectomy is not recommended for most patients with PE. It is generally reserved for patients with massive PE who are hemodynamically unstable despite maximal medical therapy, including anticoagulation and thrombolytic therapy, or for patients who have a contraindication to thrombolytic therapy or whose critical status does not allow for sufficient time for infusion of thrombolytics *(25)*. The ACCP guidelines recommend lifelong treatment with a vitamin K antagonist (VKA) following surgery, and IVC filter placement before or at the time of pulmonary thromboembolectomy is also suggested *(25)*.

REFERENCES

1. Snow V, Qaseem A, Barry P et al (2007) Management of venous thromboembolism: a clinical practice guideline from the American College of Physicians and the American Academy of Family Physicians. Ann Intern Med 146:204–210
2. Silverstein MD, Heit JA, Mohr DN, Petterson TM, O'Fallon WM, Melton LJ 3rd (1998) Trends in the incidence of deep vein thrombosis and pulmonary embolism: a 25-year population-based study. Arch Intern Med 158:585–593
3. Kyrle PA, Minar E, Bialonczyk C, Hirschl M, Weltermann A, Eichinger S (2004) The risk of recurrent venous thromboembolism in men and women. N Engl J Med 350:2558–2563
4. Prandoni P, Bilora F, Marchiori A et al (2003) An association between atherosclerosis and venous thrombosis. N Engl J Med 348:1435–1441
5. Geerts WH, Berggrist D, Heit JA et al (2008) Prevention of venous thromboembolism: the Seventh ACCP Conference on Antithrombotic and Thrombolytic Therapy. Chest 133:3815–4535
6. Lindblad B, Eriksson A, Bergqvist D (1991) Autopsy-verified pulmonary embolism in a surgical department: analysis of the period from 1951 to 1988. Br J Surg 78:849–852
7. Sandler DA, Martin JF (1989) Autopsy proven pulmonary embolism in hospital patients: are we detecting enough deep vein thrombosis? J R Soc Med 82:203–205
8. Anderson FA Jr, Wheeler HB, Goldberg RJ et al (1991) A population-based perspective of the hospital incidence and case-fatality rates of deep vein thrombosis and pulmonary embolism. The Worcester DVT Study. Arch Intern Med 151:933–938

9. Cohen AT, Tapson VF, Bergmann JF et al (2008) Venous thromboembolism risk and prophylaxis in the acute hospital care setting (ENDORSE study): a multinational cross-sectional study. Lancet 371:387–394

10. Geerts WH, Heit JA, Clagett GP et al (2001) Prevention of venous thromboembolism. Chest 119:132S–175S

11. (1975) Prevention of fatal postoperative pulmonary embolism by low doses of heparin. An international multicentre trial. Lancet 2:45–51.

12. Sagar S, Massey J, Sanderson JM (1975) Low-dose heparin prophylaxis against fatal pulmonary embolism. Br Med J 4:257–259

13. Halkin H, Goldberg J, Modan M, Modan B (1982) Reduction of mortality in general medical in-patients by low-dose heparin prophylaxis. Ann Intern Med 96:561–565

14. Collins R, Scrimgeour A, Yusuf S, Peto R (1988) Reduction in fatal pulmonary embolism and venous thrombosis by perioperative administration of subcutaneous heparin. Overview of results of randomized trials in general, orthopedic, and urologic surgery. N Engl J Med 318:1162–1173

15. Shojania KG, Duncan BW, McDonald KM, Wachter RM, Markowitz AJ (2001) Making health care safer: a critical analysis of patient safety practices. Evid Rep Technol Assess (Summ) 43:i–x, 1–668

16. Lindblad B, Sternby NH, Bergqvist D (1991) Incidence of venous thromboembolism verified by necropsy over 30 years. BMJ 302:709–711

17. Heit JA, Mohr DN, Silverstein MD, Petterson TM, O'Fallon WM, Melton LJ 3rd (2000) Predictors of recurrence after deep vein thrombosis and pulmonary embolism: a population-based cohort study. Arch Intern Med 160:761–768

18. Fedullo PF, Auger WR, Kerr KM, Rubin LJ (2001) Chronic thromboembolic pulmonary hypertension. N Engl J Med 345:1465–1472

19. Pengo V, Lensing AW, Prins MH et al (2004) Incidence of chronic thromboembolic pulmonary hypertension after pulmonary embolism. N Engl J Med 350:2257–2264

20. Moser KM, Bloor CM (1993) Pulmonary vascular lesions occurring in patients with chronic major vessel thromboembolic pulmonary hypertension. Chest 103:685–692

21. Kim H, Yung GL, Marsh JJ et al (2000) Pulmonary vascular remodeling distal to pulmonary artery ligation is accompanied by upregulation of endothelin receptors and nitric oxide synthase. Exp Lung Res 26:287–301

22. Riedel M, Stanek V, Widimsky J, Prerovsky I (1982) Longterm follow-up of patients with pulmonary thromboembolism. Late prognosis and evolution of hemodynamic and respiratory data. Chest 81:151–158

23. Kahn SR, Ginsberg JS (2002) The post-thrombotic syndrome: current knowledge, controversies, and directions for future research. Blood Rev 16:155–165

24. Puggioni A, Kalra M, Gloviczki P (2005) Practical aspects of the postthrombotic syndrome. Dis Mon 51:166–175

25. Kesron C, Kahn SR, Agnell G et al (2008) Antithrombotic therapy for venous thromboembolic disease: the Seventh ACCP Conference on Antithrombotic and Thrombolytic Therapy. Chest 133:4545–5455

26. Sandler DA, Martin JF, Duncan JS et al (1984) Diagnosis of deep-vein thrombosis: comparison of clinical evaluation, ultrasound, plethysmography, and venoscan with X-ray venogram. Lancet 2:716–719

27. Wells PS, Anderson DR, Bormanis J et al (1997) Value of assessment of pretest probability of deep-vein thrombosis in clinical management. Lancet 350:1795–1798

28. Wells PS, Anderson DR, Rodger M et al (2003) Evaluation of D-dimer in the diagnosis of suspected deep-vein thrombosis. N Engl J Med 349:1227–1235

29. Tamariz LJ, Eng J, Segal JB et al (2004) Usefulness of clinical prediction rules for the diagnosis of venous thromboembolism: a systematic review. Am J Med 117:676–684

30. Wells PS, Owen C, Doucette S, Fergusson D, Tran H (2006) Does this patient have deep vein thrombosis? JAMA 295:199–207

31. Lensing AW, Prandoni P, Brandjes D et al (1989) Detection of deep-vein thrombosis by real-time B-mode ultrasonography. N Engl J Med 320:342–345

32. Mattos MA, Londrey GL, Leutz DW et al (1992) Color-flow duplex scanning for the surveillance and diagnosis of acute deep venous thrombosis. J Vasc Surg 15:366–375 discussion 375-6

33. Birdwell BG, Raskob GE, Whitsett TL et al (2000) Predictive value of compression ultrasonography for deep vein thrombosis in symptomatic outpatients: clinical implications of the site of vein noncompressibility. Arch Intern Med 160:309–313

34. Kearon C, Ginsberg JS, Julian JA et al (2006) Comparison of fixed-dose weight-adjusted unfractionated heparin and low-molecular-weight heparin for acute treatment of venous thromboembolism. JAMA 296:935–942

35. Lee AY, Levine MN, Baker RI et al (2003) Low-molecular-weight heparin versus a coumarin for the prevention of recurrent venous thromboembolism in patients with cancer. N Engl J Med 349:146–153

36. Lensing AW, Prins MH, Davidson BL, Hirsh J (1995) Treatment of deep venous thrombosis with low-molecular-weight heparins. A meta-analysis. Arch Intern Med 155:601–607

37. Dolovich LR, Ginsberg JS, Douketis JD, Holbrook AM, Cheah G (2000) A meta-analysis comparing low-molecular-weight heparins with unfractionated heparin in the treatment of venous thromboembolism: examining some unanswered questions regarding location of treatment, product type, and dosing frequency. Arch Intern Med 160:181–188

38. Levine M, Gent M, Hirsh J et al (1996) A comparison of low-molecular-weight heparin administered primarily at home with unfractionated heparin administered in the hospital for proximal deep-vein thrombosis. N Engl J Med 334:677–681

39. Koopman MM, Prandoni P, Piovella F et al (1996) Treatment of venous thrombosis with intravenous unfractionated heparin administered in the hospital as compared with subcutaneous low-molecular-weight heparin administered at home. The Tasman Study Group. N Engl J Med 334:682–687

40. Buller HR, Davidson BL, Decousus H et al (2004) Fondaparinux or enoxaparin for the initial treatment of symptomatic deep venous thrombosis: a randomized trial. Ann Intern Med 140:867–873

41. Buller HR, Davidson BL, Decousus H et al (2003) Subcutaneous fondaparinux versus intravenous unfractionated heparin in the initial treatment of pulmonary embolism. N Engl J Med 349:1695–1702

42. U.S. Food and Drug Administration. Prescribing Information, Arixtra (fondaparinux sodium) Injection 2005; GlaxoSmithKline, Research Triangle Park, NC 27709

43. Kaufman JA, Kinney TB, Streiff MB et al (2006) Guidelines for the use of retrievable and convertible vena cava filters: report from the Society of Interventional Radiology multidisciplinary consensus conference. J Vasc Interv Radiol 17:449–459

44. Heit JA (2005) Venous thromboembolism: disease burden, outcomes and risk factors. J Thromb Haemost 3:1611–1617

45. Goldhaber SZ, Visani L, De Rosa M (1999) Acute pulmonary embolism: clinical outcomes in the International Cooperative Pulmonary Embolism Registry (ICOPER). Lancet 353:1386–1389

46. Benotti JR, Dalen JE (1984) The natural history of pulmonary embolism. Clin Chest Med 5:403–410

47. Moser KM, LeMoine JR (1981) Is embolic risk conditioned by location of deep venous thrombosis? Ann Intern Med 94:439–444

48. Wells PS, Anderson DR, Rodger M et al (2000) Derivation of a simple clinical model to categorize patients probability of pulmonary embolism: increasing the models utility with the SimpliRED D-dimer. Thromb Haemost 83:416–420

49. van Belle A, Buller HR, Huisman MV et al (2006) Effectiveness of managing suspected pulmonary embolism using an algorithm combining clinical probability, D-dimer testing, and computed tomography. JAMA 295:172–179

50. Stein PD, Fowler SE, Goodman LR et al (2006) Multidetector computed tomography for acute pulmonary embolism. N Engl J Med 354:2317–2327

51. Moores LK, Jackson WL Jr, Shorr AF, Jackson JL (2004) Meta-analysis: outcomes in patients with suspected pulmonary embolism managed with computed tomographic pulmonary angiography. Ann Intern Med 141:866–874

52. van Beek EJ, Brouwerst EM, Song B, Stein PD, Oudkerk M (2001) Clinical validity of a normal pulmonary angiogram in patients with suspected pulmonary embolism – a critical review. Clin Radiol 56:838–842

53. Stein PD, Woodard PK, Weg JG et al (2006) Diagnostic pathways in acute pulmonary embolism: recommendations of the PIOPED II investigators. Am J Med 119:1048–1055

54. Blum A, Bellou A, Guillemin F, Douek P, Laprevote-Heully MC, Wahl D (2005) Performance of magnetic resonance angiography in suspected acute pulmonary embolism. Thromb Haemost 93:503–511

55. (1990) Value of the ventilation/perfusion scan in acute pulmonary embolism. Results of the prospective investigation of pulmonary embolism diagnosis (PIOPED). The PIOPED Investigators. JAMA 263:2753–2759

56. Elliott CG, Goldhaber SZ, Visani L, DeRosa M (2000) Chest radiographs in acute pulmonary embolism. Results from the International Cooperative Pulmonary Embolism Registry. Chest 118:33–38

57. Worsley DF, Alavi A, Aronchick JM, Chen JT, Greenspan RH, Ravin CE (1993) Chest radiographic findings in patients with acute pulmonary embolism: observations from the PIOPED Study. Radiology 189:133–136

58. Stein PD, Dalen JE, McIntyre KM, Sasahara AA, Wenger NK, Willis PW 3rd (1975) The electrocardiogram in acute pulmonary embolism. Prog Cardiovasc Dis 17:247–257

59. Sreeram N, Cheriex EC, Smeets JL, Gorgels AP, Wellens HJ (1994) Value of the 12-lead electrocardiogram at hospital admission in the diagnosis of pulmonary embolism. Am J Cardiol 73:298–303

60. Goldhaber SZ (2002) Echocardiography in the management of pulmonary embolism. Ann Intern Med 136:691–700

61. Kucher N, Rossi E, De Rosa M, Goldhaber SZ (2005) Prognostic role of echocardiography among patients with acute pulmonary embolism and a systolic arterial pressure of 90 mm Hg or higher. Arch Intern Med 165:1777–1781

62. Kasper W, Konstantinides S, Geibel A, Tiede N, Krause T, Just H (1997) Prognostic significance of right ventricular after-load stress detected by echocardiography in patients with clinically suspected pulmonary embolism. Heart 77:346–349

63. Ribeiro A, Lindmarker P, Juhlin-Dannfelt A, Johnsson H, Jorfeldt L (1997) Echocardiography Doppler in pulmonary embolism: right ventricular dysfunction as a predictor of mortality rate. Am Heart J 134:479–487

64. Grifoni S, Olivotto I, Cecchini P et al (2000) Short-term clinical outcome of patients with acute pulmonary embolism, normal blood pressure, and echocardiographic right ventricular dysfunction. Circulation 101:2817–2822

65. Konstantinides S, Geibel A, Olschewski M et al (2002) Importance of cardiac troponins I and T in risk stratification of patients with acute pulmonary embolism. Circulation 106:1263–1268
66. Becattini C, Vedovati MC, Agnelli G (2007) Prognostic value of troponins in acute pulmonary embolism: a meta-analysis. Circulation 116:427–433
67. Scridon T, Scridon C, Skali H, Alvarez A, Goldhaber SZ, Solomon SD (2005) Prognostic significance of troponin elevation and right ventricular enlargement in acute pulmonary embolism. Am J Cardiol 96:303–305
68. ten Wolde M, Tulevski II, Mulder JW et al (2003) Brain natriuretic peptide as a predictor of adverse outcome in patients with pulmonary embolism. Circulation 107:2082–2084
69. Hull RD, Raskob GE, Brant RF et al (2000) Low-molecular-weight heparin vs heparin in the treatment of patients with pulmonary embolism. American-Canadian Thrombosis Study Group. Arch Intern Med 160:229–236
70. Simonneau G, Sors H, Charbonnier B et al (1997) A comparison of low-molecular-weight heparin with unfractionated heparin for acute pulmonary embolism. The THESEE Study Group. Tinzaparine ou Heparine Standard: Evaluations dans l'Embolie Pulmonaire. N Engl J Med 337:663–669
71. Food and Drug Administration. Arixtra (fondaparinux sodium) Label Information NDA 21-345/S-010. http://www.fda. gov/cder/foi/label/2005/021345s010lbl.pdf 2005
72. Urokinase pulmonary embolism trial (1970) Phase 1 results: a cooperative study. Jama 214:2163–2172
73. Urokinase-streptokinase embolism trial. Phase 2 results. A cooperative study. Jama 1974;299:1606–13.
74. Goldhaber SZ, Kessler CM, Heit J et al (1988) Randomised controlled trial of recombinant tissue plasminogen activator versus urokinase in the treatment of acute pulmonary embolism. Lancet 2:293–298
75. Meneveau N, Schiele F, Vuillemenot A et al (1997) Streptokinase vs alteplase in massive pulmonary embolism. A randomized trial assessing right heart haemodynamics and pulmonary vascular obstruction. Eur Heart J 18:1141–1148
76. Anderson DR, Levine MN (1992) Thrombolytic therapy for the treatment of acute pulmonary embolism. CMAJ 146:1317–1324
77. Dong B, Jirong Y, Liu G, Wang Q, Wu T. Thrombolytic therapy for pulmonary embolism. Cochrane Database Syst Rev 2006:CD004437
78. Kucher N, Rossi E, De Rosa M, Goldhaber SZ (2006) Massive pulmonary embolism. Circulation 113:577–582
79. Goldhaber SZ, Haire WD, Feldstein ML et al (1993) Alteplase versus heparin in acute pulmonary embolism: randomised trial assessing right-ventricular function and pulmonary perfusion. Lancet 341:507–511
80. Verstraete M, Miller GA, Bounameaux H et al (1988) Intravenous and intrapulmonary recombinant tissue-type plasminogen activator in the treatment of acute massive pulmonary embolism. Circulation 77:353–360
81. Leacche M, Unic D, Goldhaber SZ et al (2005) Modern surgical treatment of massive pulmonary embolism: results in 47 consecutive patients after rapid diagnosis and aggressive surgical approach. J Thorac Cardiovasc Surg 129:1018–1023
82. Jamieson SW, Kapelanski DP (2000) Pulmonary endarterectomy. Curr Probl Surg 37:165–252
83. Miller WT Jr, Osiason AW, Langlotz CP, Palevsky HI (1998) Reperfusion edema after thromboendarterectomy: radiographic patterns of disease. J Thorac Imaging 13:178–183
84. Rubens F, Wells P, Bencze S, Bourke M (2000) Surgical treatment of chronic thromboembolic pulmonary hypertension. Can Respir J 7:49–57
85. Moser KM, Daily PO, Peterson K et al (1987) Thromboendarterectomy for chronic, major-vessel thromboembolic pulmonary hypertension. Immediate and long-term results in 42 patients. Ann Intern Med 107:560–565
86. D'Armini AM, Cattadori B, Monterosso C et al (2000) Pulmonary thromboendarterectomy in patients with chronic thromboembolic pulmonary hypertension: hemodynamic characteristics and changes. Eur J Cardiothorac Surg 18:696–701 discussion 701-2
87. Yalamanchili K, Fleisher AG, Lehrman SG et al (2004) Open pulmonary embolectomy for treatment of major pulmonary embolism. Ann Thorac Surg 77:819–823 discussion 823

18 Fibrinolysis for Pulmonary Embolism

Stavros V. Konstantinides

CONTENTS

ABSTRACT Morbidity and mortality associated with pulmonary embolism (PE) remain high despite important advances in cardiovascular diagnosis and treatment. It is generally estimated that 10% of all patients with PE die during the acute phase of the disease. Overall, 1% of patients admitted to the hospital die of acute PE, and 10% of all hospital deaths are PE-related. Fibrinolytic therapy remains the treatment of choice for those patients at the highest risk of mortality without obvious contraindications. While a consensus opinion exists regarding the management of patients with PE and associated hypotension, controversy surrounds the use of fibrinolysis for the management of normotensive patients with non-massive PE. There is increasing awareness of the need for risk stratification of normotensive patients and the search for an intermediate-risk group. The use of imaging methods to assess for right ventricular dysfunction and the use of cardiac biomarkers may identify the patient with non-massive PE who will benefit from fibrinolysis. Ongoing investigation will hopefully facilitate further risk stratification of patients with PE in order to provide them with optimal therapies which will improve their overall outcome.

Key words: Alteplase; Fibrinolysis; Heparin; PE; Streptokinase

From: *Contemporary Cardiology: Antithrombotic Drug Therapy in Cardiovascular Disease*
Edited by: A.T. Askari and A.M. Lincoff (eds.), DOI 10.1007/978-1-60327-235-3_18
© Humana Press, a part of Springer Science+Business Media, LLC 2010

Morbidity and mortality associated with pulmonary embolism (PE) remain high despite important advances in cardiovascular diagnosis and treatment. The annual incidence rate of venous thromboembolism has been estimated at 100–150 cases per 100,000 population per year, with approximately one third of these patients presenting with acute PE and two thirds with deep vein thrombosis (1). It is generally estimated that 10% of all patients with PE die during the acute phase of the disease. Overall, 1% of patients admitted to the hospital die of acute PE, and 10% of all hospital deaths are PE-related (2–4).

Acute PE covers a wide spectrum of clinical severity, and the mortality rates during the acute, in-hospital phase vary from less than 1% to well over 50% in different studies (5–9). It is now widely acknowledged that the principal clinical factor which determines disease severity, and thus the diagnostic and therapeutic approach to a patient with suspected acute PE, is the presence or absence of acute right ventricular (RV) dysfunction (10). Increased pulmonary artery pressure occurs in 60–70% of patients who have PE and roughly correlates with the anatomic severity of thromboembolic obstruction (11,12). In addition, vasoconstrictive factors released from the thrombus and reaction to hypoxia contribute to the increase in pulmonary vascular resistance. Moreover, pre-existing cardiac or pulmonary disease may exacerbate the hemodynamic impact of an acute thromboembolic event. RV dysfunction, i.e., dilation and hypokinesis, results from the interplay of these factors and may initiate a vicious circle of increased myocardial oxygen demand, myocardial ischemia or infarction, and left ventricular preload reduction (13).

According to the current definition, *high-risk, clinically massive* PE indicates *overt* RV failure which results in refractory arterial hypotension and shock (commonly defined as systolic blood pressure <90 mmHg, or a pressure drop ≥40 mmHg from baseline for at least 15 min). This condition accounts for almost 5% of all cases of acute PE and is associated with a high risk of in-hospital death, particularly during the first few hours after admission. On the other hand, in the absence of overt hemodynamic instability (*non-high-risk or non-massive PE*), patients are generally thought to have a favorable clinical outcome provided that the disease is diagnosed correctly and anticoagulation can be instituted without delay. While consensus exists that fibrinolysis is the treatment of choice in hypotensive patients with high-risk PE, controversy persists regarding the potential clinical benefits of this therapy in selected normotensive patients. Registry data suggests that *subclinical* RV dysfunction in a normotensive patient with acute PE might indicate an elevated risk of death in the acute phase (5,6,14) and therefore, possibly the need for early fibrinolytic treatment (15). These observations were supported by the results of a large multicenter trial (16).

This chapter summarizes our current state of knowledge on the benefits and risks of fibrinolysis in acute PE. It particularly focuses on the recent attempts at risk stratification of normotensive patients with acute PE and the emerging strategies of severity-adjusted treatment beyond arterial hypotension and cardiogenic shock.

ANGIOGRAPHIC AND HEMODYNAMIC BENEFITS OF FIBRINOLYSIS

In 1971, Miller et al. observed that streptokinase infusion over 72 h resulted in a significant reduction of systolic pulmonary artery pressure, total pulmonary resistance, and the angiographic index of PE severity. In comparison, conventional heparin anticoagulation had no appreciable effect on these parameters during the first 3 days. Subsequently, a number of randomized trials performed since the early 1970s (17–24) confirmed that fibrinolytic therapy rapidly resolves thromboembolic obstruction and exerts beneficial effects on hemodynamic indicators of cardiac function. For example, in the Urokinase Pulmonary Embolism Trial (UPET), which enrolled 160 patients and still remains one of the largest randomized fibrinolysis trials in acute PE, urokinase (bolus injection followed by infusion over 24 h) was superior to heparin alone in resolving pulmonary artery thrombi, and in some patients this effect appeared to result in clinical stabilization and reversal of cardiogenic shock (17). Another early study reported an 80% increase in cardiac index and a 40% decrease in pulmonary artery pressure

(PAP) after 72 h of streptokinase (SK) treatment *(18)*. In a more recent trial, follow-up angiograms revealed that 100 mg of recombinant tissue plasminogen activator (alteplase; rtPA) induced a 12% decrease in vascular obstruction at the end of the 2-h infusion period, whereas no change was observed in patients receiving heparin *(23)*. The effect of rtPA was associated with a 30% reduction in mean PAP and a 15% increase in cardiac index. Goldhaber et al. demonstrated a rapid improvement in RV function (on 24-h echocardiographic follow-up) and an absence of PE recurrence in patients with echocardiographic indicators of RV pressure overload and dysfunction who received alteplase (100 mg infusion over 2 h) compared to those who received heparin alone *(24)*. Pathognomonic echocardiographic findings were present in 54% of the patients and patients with a normally functioning right ventricle were not excluded. Registry data suggest that as many as 92% of treated patients can be classified as *responders* to fibrinolysis on the basis of clinical and echocardiographic improvement within the first 36 h *(25)*. The greatest benefit is observed when treatment is initiated within 48 h of symptom onset *(19)*, but fibrinolysis can still be useful in patients who have had symptoms for 6–14 days *(26)*.

The hemodynamic benefits of fibrinolysis are prompt and significant compared to those of heparin, but they do not extend beyond the first few days after the initiation of treatment. In an early observation study, Dalen et al. reported that heparin anticoagulation alone (without fibrinolysis) was capable of reversing pulmonary artery hypertension in most patients, even though improvement required 3 weeks or even longer *(27)*. Trials which directly compared fibrinolytic and heparin treatment and included follow-up studies indeed showed that, 1 week after treatment, the improvement in the severity of vascular obstruction *(17,23)* and the reversal of RV dysfunction *(28)* no longer differed between fibrinolysis-treated and heparin-treated patients. It thus follows that fibrinolysis needs to be considered only in those cases in which a high risk of *early* (i.e., within the first few hours or days after presentation) PE-related death is anticipated.

FIBRINOLYTIC AGENTS AND REGIMENS FOR PE

Validated regimens of the approved fibrinolytic agents SK, UK, and rtPA are shown in Table 1. Heparin should not be infused concurrently with streptokinase or urokinase, while its use during alteplase administration is optional.

It is frequently debated whether all fibrinolytic agents and regimens are equally effective. In this regard, the USPET study documented comparable efficacy of urokinase (UK) and SK infused over a period of 12–24 h *(29)*. In more recent randomized comparison trials *(30,31)*, 100 mg of rtPA infused over 2 h led to faster angiographic and hemodynamic improvement compared to UK infused over 12 or 24 h at the rate of 4,400 U/kg/h. However, the results no longer differed at the end of the UK infusion. Similarly, the 2-h infusion of rtPA appeared to be superior over a 12-h SK infusion (at 100,000 U/h),

Table 1
Validated and approved fibrinolytic regimens for pulmonary embolism

Streptokinase	250,000 IU as a loading dose over 30 min, followed by 100,000 IU/h over 12–24 h[a]
	Alternative dosing: 1.5 million IU over 2 h
Urokinase	4,400 IU/kg as a loading dose over 10 min, followed by 4,400 IU/Kg/h over 12–24 h[a, b]
	Alternative dosing: three million IU over 2 h
rtPA	100 mg over 2 h[a]
	Accelerated dosing: 0.6 mg/kg over 15 min

[a]FDA-approved regimen
[b]Urokinase available in European countries, not in the United States

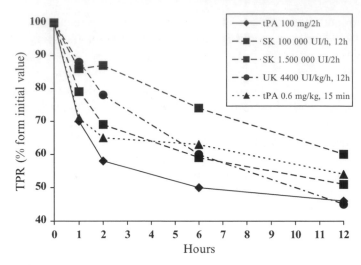

Fig. 1. Reduction of total pulmonary vascular resistance in response to different fibrinolytic regimens evaluated in prospective randomized studies. (Adapted from *(68)*.) *TPR* total pulmonary resistance; *tPA* tissue type plasminogen activator; *SK* streptokinase; *UK* urokinase.

but no difference was observed when the same SK dosage was given over 2 h *(32,33)*. Furthermore, two trials that compared the 2-h, 100-mg rtPA regimen with a short infusion (over 15 min) of 0.6 mg/ kg rtPA reported a slightly faster improvement with the 2-h regimen at the cost of slightly (non-significantly) higher bleeding rates *(34,35)*.

In summary, it can be stated that the fibrinolytic regimens tested to date are more or less comparable with regard to efficacy (Fig. 1), but long infusion periods of SK or UK should generally be avoided.

Recently, satisfactory hemodynamic results were obtained with double-bolus reteplase given as two injections (10 U) 30 min apart *(36)*, although this agent has not yet officially been approved for PE. Preliminary uncontrolled data also appear to support the efficacy and safety of tenecteplase, an agent given by one single rapid bolus injection, in acute PE *(37)*. Tenecteplase is currently being tested in a large randomized multinational trial. On the other hand, direct infusion of a fibrinolytic agent (e.g., rtPA) via a catheter in the pulmonary artery does not offer any advantages over systemic intravenous fibrinolysis *(38)*. This latter approach may be considered in combination with interventional recanalization procedures such as catheter aspiration of thrombi in the pulmonary vessels, but is otherwise not recommended, as it also carries an increased risk of bleeding at the puncture site.

HEMORRHAGIC COMPLICATIONS AND CONTRAINDICATIONS TO FIBRINOLYSIS

Fibrinolytic therapy carries a significant bleeding risk. Data from controlled trials *(16,17,21,23,29–31,35,38–40)* indicate a 13% cumulative rate of major bleeding and a 1.8% rate of intracranial/fatal hemorrhage *(41)*. Despite this, major hemorrhage has been uncommon in the most recent (and largest) trials *(16,24)*, a fact which is in agreement with the observation that fibrinolysis-related bleeding rates are lower when non-invasive imaging methods are used to diagnose PE *(42)*. Non-invasive diagnostic strategies have increasingly been adopted over the past 10 years thanks to the technical advances in computed tomographic (CT) pulmonary angiography. On the other hand, data from retrospective cohort studies and registries suggest a 36% incidence of major bleeding events and a 4% rate of intracranial/fatal hemorrhage *(5,6,43,44)*. These rates may be exaggerated, as registries include patients who received fibrinolysis despite the presence of formal *contraindications* (Table 2). At the same time however,

Table 2
Formal contraindications to fibrinolytic therapy as defined by the
European Society of Cardiology, Task Force on the Management of
Acute Myocardial Infarction (67)

Absolute contraindications
- Hemorrhagic stroke or stroke of unknown origin at any time
- Ischemic stroke in preceding 6 months
- Central nervous system damage or neoplasms
- Recent major trauma/surgery/head injury (within preceding 3 weeks)
- Gastro-intestinal bleeding within the last month
- Known bleeding

Relative contraindications
- Transient ischemic attack in preceding 6 months
- Oral anticoagulant therapy
- Pregnancy or within 1 week post partum
- Non-compressible punctures
- Traumatic resuscitation
- Refractory hypertension (systolic blood pressure >180 mmHg)
- Advanced liver disease
- Infective endocarditis
- Active peptic ulcer

it can be argued that registry data are more realistic (and thus more alarming) with regard to the true risks of fibrinolytic treatment, as they reflect everyday clinical practice. In any case, these results highlight the critical importance of carefully defining the indications for fibrinolysis in acute PE, particularly in patients who appear hemodynamically stable at presentation.

CLINICAL BENEFITS OF FIBRINOLYSIS IN PE: NEED FOR SEVERITY-ADJUSTED MANAGEMENT STRATEGIES

Despite its unequivocal angiographic and hemodynamic benefits, at least during the first days after initiation of treatment, the (presumed) favorable effects of fibrinolysis on the clinical outcome of patients with PE could not be convincingly demonstrated. This partly relies on the fact that the vast majority of fibrinolysis trials in PE neither were designed nor had the statistical power to address clinical end points. Even the most recent and largest of these trials failed to show a survival benefit *(16,24)*, possibly because they included "low-risk" patients whose mortality rate in the acute phase could not (and did not need to) be further reduced by immediate recanalization.

In weighing the risks against the benefits of fibrinolysis and thus the indications for this type of treatment in PE, it is necessary to distinguish between hypotensive, hemodynamically unstable patients with clinically massive PE, and normotensive patients with non-massive PE. Furthermore, within the latter group, the crucial issue is to determine which, if any, patients necessitate prompt relief of pulmonary vascular obstruction and reversal of RV dysfunction.

FIBRINOLYSIS INDICATED IN HIGH-RISK, CLINICALLY MASSIVE PE

Patients with clinically massive PE are those presenting with cardiogenic shock and/or persistent arterial hypotension, generally defined as systolic blood pressure <90 mmHg or a pressure drop of at least 40 mmHg for at least 15 min. This patient group with overt RV failure, representing almost 5%

of all patients with acute PE, is clearly at high risk of in-hospital death *(6,45)*, particularly during the first few hours after admission *(46)*. To date, only one small randomized trial specifically focused on the benefits of fibrinolysis (SK vs. heparin) in massive PE *(47)*. This trial was terminated after only eight patients because of excessively high mortality in the heparin-only group. Overall, meta-analyzed data from five trials which included patients with massive PE appear to suggest a significant reduction of death or PE recurrence after fibrinolysis *(48)*. Despite this weak body of evidence, there is consensus among experts, and in guidelines *(49,50)*, that fibrinolysis should be administered to patients with massive PE in the absence of absolute contraindications (Table 18.2). Uncontrolled data also suggest that fibrinolysis may be a safe and effective alternative to surgery in patients with PE and free-floating thrombi in the right heart *(51,52)*.

FIBRINOLYSIS GENERALLY NOT INDICATED IN NON-HIGH-RISK, NON-MASSIVE PE

A meta-analysis of randomized trials which *excluded* hypotensive patients with high-risk PE suggested that heparin anticoagulation is sufficient as the initial treatment of PE, and that fibrinolysis may have no clinical benefits in this setting *(48)*. Nevertheless, several years ago, registry data generated the hypothesis that the detection of *subclinical* RV dysfunction in a normotensive patient with acute PE may help define an elevated, intermediate death risk in the acute phase *(5,6)*. It was further postulated that these patients may benefit from early fibrinolytic treatment *(15)*.

IDENTIFYING AN INTERMEDIATE-RISK GROUP AMONG NORMOTENSIVE PATIENTS WITH PE

A number of *echocardiographic* findings, including right ventricular enlargement and/or hypokinesis of the free wall, leftward septal shift, and evidence of pulmonary hypertension, have been proposed for non-invasive diagnosis of RV dysfunction at the bedside. Several registries and cohort studies could demonstrate an association between abnormal echocardiographic findings and a poor in-hospital outcome in terms of PE-related death and complications *(7,14,53–55)*. Still, the prognostic value of cardiac ultrasound in *normotensive* patients with PE is not universally accepted *(56)*. Indeed, the echocardiographic studies published to date were characterized by high methodological diversity and a number of important limitations *(57)*. These included, for example, the lack of standardization of the echocardiographic criteria used for assessing the function of the right ventricle, the lack of definitive confirmation of PE in some of the patients, the inclusion of both normotensive and hypotensive patients, and the possible confounding effects of early fibrinolytic treatment. Further limitations related to cardiac ultrasound itself include the need for an experienced echocardiographer on a round-the-clock basis and the poor quality of transthoracic imaging in some individuals, particularly those who are obese, on mechanical ventilation, or have severe pulmonary emphysema. Moreover, differential diagnosis between an episode of acute PE and recurrent thromboembolism (chronic thromboembolic pulmonary hypertension) may be difficult, although some echocardiographic criteria have been proposed to distinguish between acute and chronic cor pulmonale *(58)*.

As an alternative to echocardiography, four-chamber views of the heart on *computed tomography* may detect RV enlargement as a surrogate marker of RV dysfunction due to PE and predict early death. In a large retrospective series of 431 patients, it was found that 30-day mortality was 16% in patients with RV enlargement, defined as right/left ventricular dimension ratio >0.9 on multidetector-row chest CT, compared to 7.7% in those without this finding *(59)*. Multivariate analysis revealed that

RV enlargement independently predicted 30-day mortality (hazard ratio, 5.17). Another retrospective study on 120 patients evaluated the prognostic value of a predefined right/left ventricular short-axis diameter ratio of 1.0 during 3-month follow-up *(60)*. The negative predictive value of a small right ventricle approached 100%, whereas the positive predictive value of an RV/LV ratio >1.0 was rather low with regard to PE-related mortality (10%) and appeared to be inferior to that of a pulmonary artery obstruction index of 40% or higher. In fact, a review of the data available to date reveals that as many as 60% of all patients with PE may have some evidence of RV enlargement on CT scan. It thus appears that detection of an enlarged right ventricle on CT (and possibly on echocardiography) may not, by itself, suffice to indicate an elevated death risk and justify fibrinolysis.

Cardiac biomarkers may assist imaging modalities in identifying intermediate-risk patients. Elevated cardiac troponin I or T levels, a sensitive indicator of myocardial cell damage and microscopic myocardial necrosis, are found in 11–50% of patients with acute PE. A large number of studies, which were included in recent a meta-analysis *(61)*, could show that cardiac troponin elevation correlates with the presence of RV dysfunction on echocardiography and possesses a high (97–100%) negative predictive value with regard to death or complication risk in the acute phase. Thus, normal troponin levels may rule out an adverse outcome in patients with PE. However, the positive predictive value of these biomarkers is probably low. Consequently, troponin elevation alone does not suffice to predict early death or complications in patients with acute PE, and it is unlikely that it could, by itself, identify intermediate-risk patients as potential candidates for fibrinolytic treatment. The natriuretic peptides BNP and NT-proBNP are characterized by extreme prognostic sensitivity and a negative prognostic value, which is probably higher than that of the cardiac troponins. On the other hand, they exhibit a very low specificity and positive prognostic value in the range of 12–25% *(62)*. Furthermore, appropriate threshold levels for distinguishing between a "positive" and a "negative" BNP or NT-proBNP test have not yet been prospectively validated. Heart-type fatty acid-binding protein (H-FABP) is a small cytoplasmatic protein which is abundant in the heart. Following myocardial cell damage, it diffuses rapidly through the interstitial space and appears in the circulation as early as 90 min after symptom onset, reaching its peak within 6 h. It might provide prognostic information superior to that of cardiac troponins in acute pulmonary embolism *(63)*. Finally, very recent data suggest that the novel biomarker Growth-Differentiation Factor (GDF)-15 is a sensitive global indicator of poor outcome in acute PE, and that it can assist imaging studies or myocardium-specific biomarkers in identifying normotensive intermediate-risk patients, as well as those in whom closer long-term follow-up may help prevent late deaths *(64)*.

At present, the existing evidence appears to support the rationale for further risk stratification of normotensive patients with confirmed acute PE. Strategies which combine the information provided by an imaging procedure (echocardiogram or CT) and a biomarker test, preferably troponin I or T, were reported to identify patients with an up to tenfold elevated death or complication risk compared to those with absence of RV dysfunction or myocardial injury *(62,65,66)*. The critical, as yet unanswered question is, of course, whether this information may have therapeutic implications, particularly with regard to a possible indication for early fibrinolysis in this patient group.

IS FIBRINOLYSIS INDICATED IN PATIENTS WITH INTERMEDIATE-RISK PE?

A recent randomized trial randomized 256 normotensive patients with sub-massive PE to heparin vs. rtPA treatment *(16)*. RV dysfunction and/or pulmonary hypertension was diagnosed on the basis of echocardiography, ECG, and right-heart catheterization. The primary combined end point, in-hospital death or clinical deterioration requiring escalation of treatment, was significantly reduced (from 25 to 11%) in the fibrinolysis compared with the heparin group. However, the differences were entirely due to a more frequent need for secondary (emergency) fibrinolysis in the heparin group during the hospital stay, while the overall mortality rate was not affected by the type of treatment. A large multinational trial, initiated in 2007, is currently attempting to resolve the controversy still surrounding the appropriate treatment of the intermediate-risk patient group (ClinicalTrials.gov Identifier: NCT00639743). This study, which plans to randomize more than 1,000 patients by the end of, is using the recently validated risk stratification tools described above (RV imaging and cardiac biomarkers) to diagnose RV dysfunction and myocardial injury in the absence of hypotension and shock.

CONCLUSIONS AND OUTLOOK

Although the diagnostic approach to patients with suspected acute pulmonary embolism has made significant progress in the past years, the indications for fibrinolytic treatment remain partly controversial. Fibrinolysis is clearly indicated in high-risk, clinically massive PE, i.e., in patients with persistent arterial hypotension and shock. Alteplase, given as 100-mg infusion over 2 h, is the most systematically evaluated fibrinolytic regimen and therefore considered as the treatment of choice for patients with PE, although regimens using urokinase or streptokinase also were shown to be efficacious (ClinicalTrials. gov: Identifier: NCT00639743). However, beyond the setting of high-risk PE, there is increasing awareness of the need for risk stratification of normotensive patients and the search for an intermediate-risk group. Recent studies suggested that imaging methods or cardiac biomarkers *alone* may be insufficient for guiding therapeutic decisions, particularly with regard to early fibrinolysis versus heparin alone, in normotensive patients with acute non-massive PE. Instead, the existing evidence appears to support the use of risk assessment algorithms (such as the one proposed in Fig. 2), which combine the information provided by an imaging procedure (RV dysfunction on echocardiography or CT) and a biomarker test (RV myocardial injury indicated by elevated troponin I or T). A large multinational trial is currently investigating whether the indications for fibrinolysis should be extended to intermediate-risk PE.

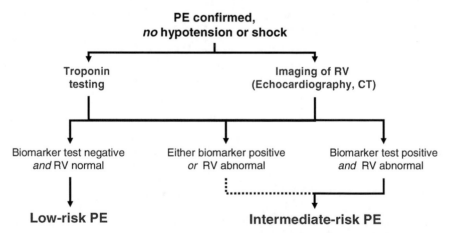

Fig. 2. Contemporary risk stratification of normotensive patients with acute pulmonary embolism, i.e., excluding high-risk, clinically massive PE. (Adapted and slightly modified from *(69)*.) *RV* right ventricle; *CT* computed tomogaphy.

REFERENCES

1. White RH (2003) The epidemiology of venous thromboembolism. Circulation 107:I4–I8
2. Cohen AT, Agnelli G, Anderson FA et al (2007) Venous thromboembolism (VTE) in Europe. The number of VTE events and associated morbidity and mortality. Thromb Haemost 98:756–764
3. Cohen AT, Edmondson RA, Phillips MJ, Ward VP, Kakkar VV (1996) The changing pattern of venous thromboembolic disease. Haemostasis 26:65–71
4. Lindblad B, Sternby NH, Bergqvist D (1991) Incidence of venous thromboembolism verified by necropsy over 30 years. BMJ 302:709–711
5. Goldhaber SZ, Visani L, De Rosa M (1999) Acute pulmonary embolism: clinical outcomes in the International Cooperative Pulmonary Embolism Registry (ICOPER). Lancet 353:1386–1389
6. Kasper W, Konstantinides S, Geibel A et al (1997) Management strategies and determinants of outcome in acute major pulmonary embolism: results of a multicenter registry. J Am Coll Cardiol 30:1165–1171
7. Kasper W, Konstantinides S, Geibel A, Tiede N, Krause T, Just H (1997) Prognostic significance of right ventricular afterload stress detected by echocardiography in patients with clinically suspected pulmonary embolism. Heart 77:346–349
8. British Thoracic Society (1992) Optimum duration of anticoagulation for deep-vein thrombosis and pulmonary embolism. Research Committee of the British Thoracic Society. Lancet 340:873–876
9. Carson JL, Kelley MA, Duff A et al (1992) The clinical course of pulmonary embolism. N Engl J Med 326:1240–1245
10. Konstantinides S (2005) Pulmonary embolism: impact of right ventricular dysfunction. Curr Opin Cardiol 20:496–501
11. McIntyre KM, Sasahara AA (1974) Determinants of right ventricular function and hemodynamics after pulmonary embolism. Chest 65:534–543
12. McIntyre KM, Sasahara AA (1971) The hemodynamic response to pulmonary embolism in patients without prior cardiopulmonary disease. Am J Cardiol 28:288–294
13. Lualdi JC, Goldhaber SZ (1995) Right ventricular dysfunction after acute pulmonary embolism: pathophysiologic factors, detection, and therapeutic implications. Am Heart J 130:1276–1282
14. Kucher N, Rossi E, De Rosa M, Goldhaber SZ (2005) Prognostic role of echocardiography among patients with acute pulmonary embolism and a systolic arterial pressure of 90 mm Hg or higher. Arch Intern Med 165:1777–1781
15. Konstantinides S, Geibel A, Olschewski M et al (1997) Association between thrombolytic treatment and the prognosis of hemodynamically stable patients with major pulmonary embolism: results of a multicenter registry. Circulation 96:882–888
16. Konstantinides S, Geibel A, Heusel G, Heinrich F, Kasper W (2002) Heparin plus alteplase compared with heparin alone in patients with submassive pulmonary embolism. N Engl J Med 347:1143–1150
17. (1973) The urokinase pulmonary embolism trial. A national cooperative study. Circulation 47:II1–II108
18. Tibbutt DA, Davies JA, Anderson JA et al (1974) Comparison by controlled clinical trial of streptokinase and heparin in treatment of life-threatening pulmonary embolism. Br Med J 1:343–347
19. Ly B, Arnesen H, Eie H, Hol R (1978) A controlled clinical trial of streptokinase and heparin in the treatment of major pulmonary embolism. Acta Med Scand 203:465–470
20. Marini C, Di Ricco G, Rossi G, Rindi M, Palla R, Giuntini C (1988) Fibrinolytic effects of urokinase and heparin in acute pulmonary embolism: a randomized clinical trial. Respiration 54:162–173
21. Levine M, Hirsh J, Weitz J et al (1990) A randomized trial of a single bolus dosage regimen of recombinant tissue plasminogen activator in patients with acute pulmonary embolism. Chest 98:1473–1479
22. (1990) Tissue plasminogen activator for the treatment of acute pulmonary embolism. A collaborative study by the PIOPED Investigators. Chest 97:528–533
23. Dalla-Volta S, Palla A, Santolicandro A et al (1992) PAIMS 2: alteplase combined with heparin versus heparin in the treatment of acute pulmonary embolism. Plasminogen activator Italian multicenter study 2. J Am Coll Cardiol 20:520–526
24. Goldhaber SZ, Haire WD, Feldstein ML et al (1993) Alteplase versus heparin in acute pulmonary embolism: randomised trial assessing right-ventricular function and pulmonary perfusion. Lancet 341:507–511
25. Meneveau N, Seronde MF, Blonde MC et al (2006) Management of unsuccessful thrombolysis in acute massive pulmonary embolism. Chest 129:1043–1050
26. Daniels LB, Parker JA, Patel SR, Grodstein F, Goldhaber SZ (1997) Relation of duration of symptoms with response to thrombolytic therapy in pulmonary embolism. Am J Cardiol 80:184–188
27. Dalen JE, Banas JS Jr, Brooks HL, Evans GL, Paraskos JA, Dexter L (1969) Resolution rate of acute pulmonary embolism in man. N Engl J Med 280:1194–1199

28. Konstantinides S, Tiede N, Geibel A, Olschewski M, Just H, Kasper W (1998) Comparison of alteplase versus heparin for resolution of major pulmonary embolism. Am J Cardiol 82:966–970

29. (1974) Urokinase-streptokinase embolism trial. Phase 2 results. A cooperative study. JAMA 229:1606–1613

30. Meyer G, Sors H, Charbonnier B et al (1992) Effects of intravenous urokinase versus alteplase on total pulmonary resistance in acute massive pulmonary embolism: a European multicenter double-blind trial. The European Cooperative Study Group for Pulmonary Embolism [see comments]. J Am Coll Cardiol 19:239–245

31. Goldhaber SZ, Kessler CM, Heit J et al (1988) Randomised controlled trial of recombinant tissue plasminogen activator versus urokinase in the treatment of acute pulmonary embolism. Lancet 2:293–298

32. Meneveau N, Schiele F, Metz D et al (1998) Comparative efficacy of a two-hour regimen of streptokinase versus alteplase in acute massive pulmonary embolism: immediate clinical and hemodynamic outcome and one-year follow-up. J Am Coll Cardiol 31:1057–1063

33. Meneveau N, Schiele F, Vuillemenot A et al (1997) Streptokinase vs alteplase in massive pulmonary embolism. A randomized trial assessing right heart haemodynamics and pulmonary vascular obstruction. Eur Heart J 18:1141–1148

34. Goldhaber SZ, Agnelli G, Levine MN (1994) Reduced dose bolus alteplase vs conventional alteplase infusion for pulmonary embolism thrombolysis. An international multicenter randomized trial. The Bolus Alteplase Pulmonary Embolism Group. Chest 106:718–724

35. Sors H, Pacouret G, Azarian R, Meyer G, Charbonnier B, Simonneau G (1994) Hemodynamic effects of bolus vs 2-h infusion of alteplase in acute massive pulmonary embolism. A randomized controlled multicenter trial. Chest 106:712–717

36. Tebbe U, Graf A, Kamke W et al (1999) Hemodynamic effects of double bolus reteplase versus alteplase infusion in massive pulmonary embolism. Am Heart J 138:39–44

37. Kline JA, Hernandez-Nino J, Jones AE (2007) Tenecteplase to treat pulmonary embolism in the emergency department. J Thromb Thrombolysis 23(2):101–105

38. Verstraete M, Miller GA, Bounameaux H et al (1988) Intravenous and intrapulmonary recombinant tissue-type plasminogen activator in the treatment of acute massive pulmonary embolism. Circulation 77:353–360

39. Kanter DS, Mikkola KM, Patel SR, Parker JA, Goldhaber SZ (1997) Thrombolytic therapy for pulmonary embolism. Frequency of intracranial hemorrhage and associated risk factors. Chest 111:1241–1245

40. Goldhaber SZ, Kessler CM, Heit JA et al (1992) Recombinant tissue-type plasminogen activator versus a novel dosing regimen of urokinase in acute pulmonary embolism: a randomized controlled multicenter trial. J Am Coll Cardiol 20:24–30

41. Konstantinides S, Marder VJ (2006) Thrombolysis in venous thromboembolism. In: Colman RW, Marder VJ, Clowes AW, George JN, Goldhaber SZ (eds) Hemostasis and Thrombosis. Lippincott Williams and Wilkins, Philadelphia, pp 1317–1329

42. Stein PD, Hull RD, Raskob G (1994) Risks for major bleeding from thrombolytic therapy in patients with acute pulmonary embolism. Consideration of noninvasive management [see comments]. Ann Intern Med 121:313–317

43. Hamel E, Pacouret G, Vincentelli D et al (2001) Thrombolysis or heparin therapy in massive pulmonary embolism with right ventricular dilation: results from a 128-patient monocenter registry. Chest 120:120–125

44. Meyer G, Gisselbrecht M, Diehl JL, Journois D, Sors H (1998) Incidence and predictors of major hemorrhagic complications from thrombolytic therapy in patients with massive pulmonary embolism. Am J Med 105:472–477

45. Kucher N, Rossi E, De Rosa M, Goldhaber SZ (2006) Massive pulmonary embolism. Circulation 113:577–582

46. Stein PD, Henry JW (1995) Prevalence of acute pulmonary embolism among patients in a general hospital and at autopsy. Chest 108:978–981

47. Jerjes-Sanchez C, Ramírez-Rivera A, de Lourdes G et al (1995) Streptokinase and Heparin versus Heparin Alone in Massive Pulmonary Embolism: A Randomized Controlled Trial. J Thromb Thrombolysis 2:227–229

48. Wan S, Quinlan DJ, Agnelli G, Eikelboom JW (2004) Thrombolysis compared with heparin for the initial treatment of pulmonary embolism: a meta-analysis of the randomized controlled trials. Circulation 110:744–749

49. Torbicki A, Perrier A, Konstantinides SV et al. Guidelines on the diagnosis and management of acute pulmonary embolism: The Task Force for the Diagnosis and Management of Acute Pulmonary Embolism of the European Society of Cardiology (ESC). Eur Heart J 2008; 29:2276–2315

50. Kearon C, Kahn SR, Agenlli G, Goldhaber S, Raskob GE, Comerota AJ. Antithrombotoc therapy for venous thromboembolic disease: American College of Chest Physicians Evidence-Based Clinical Practice Guidelines (8th Edition). Chest 2008; 133(6 Suppl):454S–545S

51. Rose PS, Punjabi NM, Pearse DB (2002) Treatment of right heart thromboemboli. Chest 121:806–814

52. Chartier L, Bera J, Delomez M et al (1999) Free-floating thrombi in the right heart: diagnosis, management, and prognostic indexes in 38 consecutive patients. Circulation 99:2779–2783

53. Vieillard-Baron A, Page B, Augarde R et al (2001) Acute cor pulmonale in massive pulmonary embolism: incidence, echocardiographic pattern, clinical implications and recovery rate. Intensive Care Med 27:1481–1486

54. Grifoni S, Olivotto I, Cecchini P et al (2000) Short-term clinical outcome of patients with acute pulmonary embolism, normal blood pressure, and echocardiographic right ventricular dysfunction. Circulation 101:2817–2822

55. Ribeiro A, Lindmarker P, Johnsson H, Juhlin-Dannfelt A, Jorfeldt L (1999) Pulmonary embolism: one-year follow-up with echocardiography Doppler and five-year survival analysis [see comments]. Circulation 99:1325–1330

56. ten Wolde M, Sohne M, Quak E, Mac Gillavry MR, Buller HR (2004) Prognostic value of echocardiographically assessed right ventricular dysfunction in patients with pulmonary embolism. Arch Intern Med 164:1685–1689

57. Sanchez O, Trinquart L, Colombet I et al (2008) Prognostic value of right ventricular dysfunction in patients with haemodynamically stable pulmonary embolism: a systematic review. Eur Heart J 29(12):1569–1577

58. Kasper W, Geibel A, Tiede N et al (1993) Distinguishing between acute and subacute massive pulmonary embolism by conventional and Doppler echocardiography. Br Heart J 70:352–356

59. Schoepf UJ, Kucher N, Kipfmueller F, Quiroz R, Costello P, Goldhaber SZ (2004) Right ventricular enlargement on chest computed tomography: a predictor of early death in acute pulmonary embolism. Circulation 110:3276–3280

60. van der Meer RW, Pattynama PM, van Strijen MJ et al (2005) Right ventricular dysfunction and pulmonary obstruction index at helical CT: prediction of clinical outcome during 3-month follow-up in patients with acute pulmonary embolism. Radiology 235:798–803

61. Becattini C, Vedovati MC, Agnelli G (2007) Prognostic value of troponins in acute pulmonary embolism: a meta-analysis. Circulation 116:427–433

62. Klok FA, Mos IC, Huisman MV. Brain-type natriuretic peptide levels in the prediction of adverse outcome in patients with pulmonary embolism: a systematic review and meta-analysis. Am J Respir Crit Care Med 2008; 178(4):425–430

63. Puls M, Dellas C, Lankeit M et al (2007) Heart-type fatty acid-binding protein permits early risk stratification of pulmonary embolism. Eur Heart J 28:224–229

64. Lankeit M, Kempf T, Dellas C et al (2008) Growth differentiation factor-15 for prognostic assessment of patients with acute pulmonary embolism. Am J Respir Crit Care Med 177:1018–1025

65. Binder L, Pieske B, Olschewski M et al (2005) N-terminal pro-brain natriuretic peptide or troponin testing followed by echocardiography for risk stratification of acute pulmonary embolism. Circulation 112:1573–1579

66. Scridon T, Scridon C, Skali H, Alvarez A, Goldhaber SZ, Solomon SD (2005) Prognostic significance of troponin elevation and right ventricular enlargement in acute pulmonary embolism. Am J Cardiol 96:303–305

67. Van De WF, Ardissino D, Betriu A et al (2003) Management of acute myocardial infarction in patients presenting with ST-segment elevation. The Task Force on the Management of Acute Myocardial Infarction of the European Society of Cardiology. Eur Heart J 24:28–66

68. Meyer G (2007) Thrombolysis. In: Konstantinides SV (ed) Management of acute pulmonary embolism. Humana, Totowa, pp 125–136

69. Konstantinides SV (2008) Acute pulmonary embolism revisited: thromboembolic venous disease. Heart 94:795–802

19 Duration of Anticoagulant Therapy After Venous Thromboembolism

Clive Kearon

CONTENTS

ABSTRACT Long-term treatment of venous thromboembolism (VTE) primarily focuses on the duration of anticoagulant therapy, usually with vitamin K antagonists (VKA). The duration of therapy should be individualized based on the risk of recurrent VTE if treatment is stopped and the risk of bleeding if treatment is continued. The risk of recurrence is low if thrombosis was provoked by a reversible risk factor such as surgery; 3 months of treatment is usually adequate for such patients. The risk of recurrence is high if thrombosis was associated active cancer; indefinite anticoagulant therapy, with low-molecular-weight heparin for at least the first 3 months, is often indicated for such patients. Risk of recurrence is intermediate if thrombosis was an unprovoked proximal deep vein thrombosis or pulmonary embolism; indefinite anticoagulant therapy is often appropriate for such patients. Among patients with unprovoked proximal deep vein thrombosis or pulmonary embolism, more than one previous episode of VTE, presentation as pulmonary embolism, male sex, and a positive D-dimer test 1 month after stopping anticoagulant therapy, particularly favor indefinite anticoagulant therapy. High risk of bleeding and patient preference favor treatment for only 3 months. New anticoagulants, that may improve the risk: benefit ratio of anticoagulant therapy and should reduce the burden of therapy, are expected to be available soon.

Key words: Deep vein thrombosis; Pulmonary embolism; Anticoagulation; Warfarin; INR; Monitoring

Long-term treatment of venous thromboembolism (VTE) is usually with a vitamin K antagonist (VKA) and less commonly with a low-molecular weight heparin (LMWH). Long-term therapy has two goals that overlap in timing: (1) to complete treatment of the acute episode of VTE (predominantly in the first 3 months); and (2) to prevent new episodes of VTE that are not directly related to the acute event (predominantly after the first 3 months).

The need for long-term therapy of VTE after an initial 5–10 day course of therapeutic-dose heparin has been established by trials that have shown that long-term therapy with VKA markedly reduced recurrent VTE in patients with: (1) symptomatic isolated distal deep vein thrombosis (DVT) com-

From: *Contemporary Cardiology: Antithrombotic Drug Therapy in Cardiovascular Disease*
Edited by: A.T. Askari and A.M. Lincoff (eds.), DOI 10.1007/978-1-60327-235-3_19
© Humana Press, a part of Springer Science+Business Media, LLC 2010

pared with controls who did not receive long-term therapy (0/23 vs. 8/28 [29%] at 3 months; $p<0.01$) *(1)*; and *(2)* proximal DVT compared with low dose (5,000 U twice daily) subcutaneous heparin (0/17 vs. 9/19 [47%] at 3 months; $p<0.001$) *(2)*. High rates of recurrent VTE in patients who are only treated for 4 or 6 weeks with VKA compared to those treated for 3 or 6 months further supports the need for long-term therapy (see below) *(3–5)*.

MANAGEMENT OF VITAMIN K ANTAGONIST THERAPY
Initiation of VKA

Studies have shown that about 5 days of heparin therapy (VKA started on first or second day) was as effective as 10–14 days of heparin therapy (VKA started after about 5 days), and thus, established that VKA could be started the same day as heparin *(6,7)*. Two trials in hospitalized patients showed that starting warfarin at a dose of 5 mg, compared with 10 mg, is associated with less excessive anticoagulation and does not meaningfully delay onset of anticoagulation *(8,9)*. However, a similar study in outpatients with acute VTE found that starting with 10 mg of warfarin was superior to starting with 5 mg *(10)*. Observational studies have shown that lower VKA maintenance doses are required in older patients, women, and those with impaired nutrition and vitamin K deficiency *(11,12)*. Thus, these data suggest that warfarin can usually be started at a first dose of 10 mg in younger (e.g., less than 60 years) and healthy outpatients, and at a first dose of 5 mg in older and hospitalized patients. Nomograms, to guide the first days of warfarin dosing, were published from previous studies *(9,10)*.

Long-Term Monitoring and Adjustment of VKA

Many factors modify the anticoagulant response to VKA therapy and, therefore, there are marked differences in VKA dosing required to achieve an International Normalized Ratio (INR) of 2.0–3.0, both among patients and in the same patient over time *(11)*. Consequently, VKA dosing needs to be adjusted in response to ongoing INR measurements in order to maximize the time a patient is in the target INR range. Good anticoagulant control is important as: (1) subtherapeutic anticoagulation (particularly below INR 1.5) increases recurrent VTE, (2) supratherapeutic anticoagulation (particularly over INR 5.0) increases bleeding, and (3) poor anticoagulant control increases the burden of anticoagulant therapy and discourages patients and healthcare providers from continuing VKA therapy when it is indicated *(11)*. Principles and management strategies that facilitate optimal long-term anticoagulation are summarized in Table 1.

Optimal Intensity of Vitamin K Antagonist Therapy

VKA inhibits two enzymes (vitamin K epoxide reductase and vitamin K reductase) that convert vitamin K epoxide, via vitamin K, to hydroquinone (vitamin KH_2). Subsequently, hydroquinone deficiency results in defective carboxylation, and reduced functional levels of coagulation factors II, VII, IX, and X, thereby achieving anticoagulation. The degree, or intensity, of resultant anticoagulation is measured as a prothrombin time ratio, usually expressed in a standardized form as the INR *(11)*. Hull and colleagues established that acute treatment of VTE (i.e., first 3 months) with a target INR of 2.5 (range 2.0–3.0) was as effective but caused less bleeding than treatment with a target INR of 3.5 (range 3.0–4.0) *(13)*. In patients with an antiphospholipid antibody and mostly VTE, two studies have shown that targeting an INR of 2.5 is as effective as targeting an INR of 3.5 *(14,15)*.

The observation in two trials *(3,16)* that there were no episodes of recurrent VTE among patients who remained on extended-duration VKA targeted an INR of ~2.5 *(3,16)* (Table 3) suggesting that

Table 1
Principles and recommendations for maintenance of vitamin K antagonist therapy

Interval between INR measurements
- Gradually increase interval from every 2–3 days in the first week to every 2–4 weeks (e.g., after 6 weeks) *(11)*.
- Decrease interval between testing if the patient becomes ill or if a medication is added or stopped *(11,116)*.
- Decrease interval if INR results become unstable.

Dosing of warfarin
- Average daily warfarin dose is about 6 mg at age 50 and about 3.5 mg at age 80 *(12)*.
- If warfarin maintenance dose needs to be increased or decreased, steps of 10% are usually suitable. This can be done by calculating the total dose of warfarin given in the preceding week, and adjusting the next week(s) total dose by 10%; this often translates into a change in the total week's dose of 2.5–5.0 mg of warfarin *(11)*.
- If INR >5.0, 1 or 2 doses of warfarin should be withheld in addition to reducing the maintenance of warfarin dose. If INR >5.0, the patient has a risk of bleeding, or INR >10.0, 1–2.5 mg of oral vitamin K should also be given *(11,117,118)*.

Method of anticoagulant monitoring
- A systematic process for monitoring VKA should be used that includes patient education, and explicit patient and healthcare provider responsibility for each stage of the process (e.g., patient attends a designated laboratory for INR testing; INR results are communicated to healthcare providers at pre-specified time (e.g., same or following day); INR results are recorded in the patient's anticoagulation record; VKA dose is selected; VKA dose and timing of next INR measurement are communicated to the patient) *(11)*.
- Use of a dedicated anticoagulant service can improve delivery of VKA therapy *(11)*.
- Self-testing, or self-dosing, is appropriate in selected well educated and motivated patients *(11,119)*.
- Computer programs can facilitate selection of warfarin dose, tracking of INR and VKA dosing, and communication of VKA dosing to patients (e.g., via mail) *(11)*.

Interruption of VKA
- After 1 month, and particularly after 3 months, of VKA therapy for VTE, short interruptions of VKA (e.g., ≤5 days) are well tolerated (i.e., associated with a low risk of recurrence) provided patients have not undergone a procedure that is associated with VTE *(11,62)*.
- Patients who have had a procedure that is associated with VTE (e.g., surgery with general anesthetic) should receive supplemental VTE prophylaxis (e.g., a heparin preparation) until their INR increases, or is expected to have increased (e.g., ~3 days), to above INR 1.5 *(11,120)*.

lowering the intensity of anticoagulation to a target INR of ~1.75 after the first 3 months of conventional intensity therapy might reduce bleeding without loss of efficacy. When this hypothesis was subsequently tested in a double-blind trial of patients with unprovoked VTE, the lower intensity of anticoagulation was less effective in preventing recurrent VTE (intention-to-treat analysis: 1.9% vs. 0.7% per patient-year; hazard ratio 2.8 [95% CI 1.1–7.0]) and was associated with the same frequency of major bleeding (1.1% vs. 0.9% per patient-year; hazard ratio 1.2 [95% CI 0.4–3.0]) as conventional intensity therapy (Table 3) *(17)*. As discussed later in this chapter, after the first 3 months of conventional intensity VKA therapy, low intensity anticoagulation (target INR of 1.75) has been shown to reduce the risk of recurrent VTE by about two-thirds and is compatible with a less frequent INR testing (e.g., about 2 months) than is usual with conventional intensity anticoagulation (Table 3) *(18)*.

Based on these studies, a target INR of 2.5 (range 2.0–3.0) is recommended as the optimal intensity of anticoagulation for both acute and long-term treatment of VTE.

Duration of Anticoagulant Therapy

Anticoagulant therapy for VTE should be continued until: (1) its benefits (reduction of recurrent VTE) no longer clearly outweigh its risks (increase in bleeding); or (2) the patient prefers to stop treatment even if continuing treatment is beneficial. In patients with an average risk of bleeding while on anticoagulant therapy, therefore, the decision to stop or continue therapy is dominated by the risk of recurrent VTE if treatment is stopped. Current evidence suggests that the risk of recurrence after stopping therapy is largely determined by two factors: (1) whether the acute episode of VTE has been effectively treated, and (2) the patient's intrinsic risk of having a new episode of VTE (i.e., not arising directly from the episode of thrombosis for which patients have been receiving treatment). If therapy is stopped before the acute episode of thrombosis is adequately treated, the risk of recurrent VTE will be higher than if treatment was stopped after a longer course of anticoagulation. If patients have a persistently high intrinsic risk for thrombosis, even if the acute episode of thrombosis has effectively been treated, they will have a high risk of recurrence once anticoagulant therapy is stopped; if this risk is high enough relative to the patient's increased risk of bleeding on anticoagulants, indefinite therapy will be indicated. As patients' intrinsic risk of recurrent VTE has influenced the enrolling of patients in trials that have compared durations of anticoagulant therapy and needs to be considered in the interpretation of these studies, risk factors for recurrent VTE in individual patients will be considered before reviewing the studies that have compared different durations of VKA in patients with VTE.

Patient Related Risk Factors for Recurrent VTE After Stopping Anticoagulant Therapy

CANCER

Cancer is associated with about a threefold increased risk of recurrent VTE both during (19–23) and after (22,24–26) anticoagulant therapy, and among patients with cancer, the risk of recurrence is about threefold higher in those with metastatic disease (23) (Table 2). The risk of recurrent VTE after stopping anticoagulant therapy is expected to be high (i.e., 10–20% in the first year) in cancer patients, particularly if there is progressive or metastatic disease, poor mobility, or ongoing chemotherapy (25–27). The risk of recurrence is uncertain, and likely to be lower, if the cancer has responded to therapy, or if the initial VTE was provoked by an additional reversible risk factor, such as surgery or chemotherapy (see below). Because cancer is considered to be such a strong risk factor for recurrent VTE, there is widespread agreement that most patients with VTE and cancer require long-term anticoagulant therapy and these patients have been excluded from the randomized trials that have compared different durations of anticoagulant therapy.

REVERSIBILITY OF RISK FACTORS FOR VTE

It has become clear that patients with VTE provoked by a major reversible risk factor, such as surgery, have a low risk of recurrence (i.e., about 3% in the first year) after 3 or more months of anticoagulant therapy, whereas the risk is high (i.e., about 10% in the first year) in patients with an unprovoked (also termed "idiopathic") VTE and in those with a persistent risk for thrombosis (Table 2) (4,5,18,26–31). If VTE was provoked by a minor reversible risk factor, such as leg trauma, estrogen therapy, or prolonged air travel (e.g., a flight of over 8 h), there is an intermediate risk of recurrent VTE after stopping anticoagulant therapy (i.e., approximately 5% in the first year) (25,31,32). Because of this difference in the risk of recurrence, many recent trials selectively enrolled patients with unprovoked VTE and compared longer durations of therapy (16–18,33–35), or enrolled patients

Table 2
Risk factors for recurrent VTE after stopping anticoagulant therapy

Variable	Relative risk
Transient risk factor *(4,5,24,26,28,29,31,42,58)*	≤0.5
Persistent risk factor *(4,5,24,26,28,29,42)*	≥2
Unprovoked VTE *(4,5,16,26,28,31)*	≥2
Protein C, protein S and antithrombin deficiencies *(24,31,52,58)*	~1.5
Heterozygous for factor V Leiden or the G20210A prothrombin gene *(16,18,42,55)*	~1.5
Homozygous for factor V Leiden *(42,56–58)*	1.5–2
Heterozygous for both factor V Leiden and G20210A prothrombin gene *(56,58,121–123)*	1.5–2
Factor VIII level >150 IU/dL *(54,58,65)*	~1.4
Antiphospholipid antibodies *(16,36,42,59)*	1.5–2
Mild hyperhomocysteinemia *(69,124)*	1.5–2.5
D-dimer elevation after stopping therapy *(35,52–54)*	~2.5
Family history of VTE *(28,56,73)*	~1
Cancer *(23–26)*	~3
Metastatic vs. non-metastatic *(23)*	~3
Chemotherapy *(25)*	~2
Discontinuation of estrogen *(25,58,125–131)*	~0.5
Proximal DVT vs. PE *(16,28,38)*	~1
Distal DVT vs. proximal DVT or PE *(28,30)*	~0.5
Residual thrombosis *(4,16,22,28,34,62,132)*	1–2
Vena caval filter *(38,63,64,132)*	1–1.5
Second vs. first episode of VTE *(3,18,38,39)*	1.5–2
Age *(16,25,38,56)*	~1
Gender *(60)*	~1.5
Asian *(38)*	~0.8

with VTE that was provoked by a reversible risk factor and compared shorter durations of therapy *(36)* (Table 3).

ISOLATED CALF DVT VS. PROXIMAL DVT

Patients with DVT that is confined to the distal veins (often called "isolated calf" DVT) have about half the risk of recurrence than patients with DVT that involves the proximal veins (i.e., popliteal or more proximal veins) *(28,30,37)*. If ultrasound rather than venography is used to diagnose distal DVT, the risk of recurrence after distal DVT may be even lower as a higher proportion of such patients may have false-positive findings or may have thrombosis of the muscular rather than of the deep veins. Many studies that compared durations of anticoagulation excluded patients with isolated distal DVT *(4,20,34,35)*.

SECOND VS. FIRST EPISODE OF VTE

After a second or subsequent episode of VTE, the risk of recurrence appears to be about 1.5-fold higher than that after a first episode *(18,38,39)*. Many studies that compared durations of anticoagulation excluded patients if their VTE was not a first episode *(28,30,33–35)*.

PULMONARY EMBOLISM VS. DEEP VEIN THROMBOSIS

Patients with pulmonary embolism (PE) appear to have the same risk of recurrent VTE as those with proximal DVT *(25,28,38,40)*. However, after a PE, about 60% of recurrent episodes of VTE are

Table 3
Comparisons of Durations and Intensities of Anticoagulant Therapy for DVT and PE

First author/ year (acronym)	Intervention	Blinding	# pts analyzed	Length follow-up	Recurrent DVT or PE	Major bleeding	Total mortality	Comments
Short (4 or 6 weeks) vs. Intermediate (3 or 6 months) durations of anticoagulation								
Kearon 2004 (36) (SOFAST)	VKA stopped (Placebo) VKA (INR 2.0–3.0) For 2 more month	Allocation: yes Patients: yes Caregivers: yes Adjudications: yes Data analysts: yes	84/84 81/81	11 month 11 month	5/84 (6%) 3/81 (4%) RR 0.6 (0.1, 2.5)	0/84 0/81 RR 1.0 (0.0, 51.6)	0/84 1/81 (1%) RR 3.1 (0.1,)	Population: first DVT or PE. Treated for 1 month VTE was asymptomatic in 9%, and isolated calf DVT in 18%. One VTE occurred while on warfarin.
Pinede 2001 (30) (DOT AVK)	VKA (INR 2.0–3.0) for 1.5 month VKA (INR 2.0–3.0) for 3 month	Allocation: yes Patients: no Caregivers: no Adjudications: yes Data analysts: unlikely	105/105 92/92	15 month	2/105 (2%) 3/92 RR 1.7 (0.3, 10.0)	1/105 (1%) 3/92 RR 3.4 (0.4, 33.4)	Not specified	Population: first isolated calf DVT.
Schulman 1995 (28) (DURAC 1)	VKA (INR 2.0–2.85) for 1.5 month VKA (INR 2.0–2.85) for 6 month	Allocation: yes Patients: no Caregivers: no Adjudications: VTE, yes Other, unlikely Data analysts: unlikely	443/443 454/454	2 years	80/443 (18%) 43/454 (9%) RR 0.5 (0.4, 0.7)	1/443 5/454 (1%) RR 4.9 (0.6, 41.6)	22/443 (5%) 17/454 (4%) RR (0.7, 1.4)	First VTE: DVT (distal or proximal) or PE. Only asked about bleeding while on VKAs.
Levine 1995 (4)	VKA stopped (Placebo) VKA (INR 2.0 –3.0) for 2 more month	Allocation: yes Patients: no Caregivers: no Adjudications: VTE, yes Data analysts: unlikely	105/107 109/113	9 month	12/105 (11%) 7/109 (6%) RR 0.6 (0.2, 1.4)	0/105 1/109 (1%) RR 2.9 (0.1, 70.2) (within 2 month of randomization)	9/105 (9%) 9/109 (8%) RR 1.0 (0.4, 2.5)	Proximal DVT (first episode in 91%). Cancer in 21%

Study	Intervention	N	Duration	Recurrent VTE	Major bleeding	Death	Comments
British Thoracic Society (5)	VKA (INR 2.0–3.0) For 1 month; VKA (INR 2.0–3.0) for 3 months	358/358; 354/354	1 year; 1 year	28/358 (11%); 14/354 (4%); RR 0.5 (0.3, 0.9)	5/358 (1%); 4/354 (1%); RR 0.8 (0.2, 3.0)	26/358 (7%); 28/354 (8%); RR 1.1 (0.6, 1.8)	Population: DVT or PE; only 71% objectively diagnosed; proportion with a previous VTE not known. All bleeds were on VKA. Only 1 recurrent VTE among 116 pts with post operative VTE.
Summary		2,198		RR 0.53 (0.40, 0.70)	RR 1.84 (0.76, 4.50)	RR 1.04 (0.74, 1.48)	For all analyses, $p \geq 0.1$ for heterogeneity. SOFAST (36) not included in estimate for major bleeding as no events in either group.

Different intermediate durations (6 or 12 months vs. 3 months) of anticoagulation

Study	Intervention	N	Duration	Recurrent VTE	Major bleeding	Death	Comments
Campbell 2004 (75)	VKA (INR 2.0–3.5) for 3 months; VKA (INR 2.0–3.5) for 6 months	369/396; 380/414	1 year; 1 year	31/369 (8%); 29/380 (8%); RR 0.9 (0.6, 1.5)	0/369 (during 3 month treatment); 8/380 (2%) (during 6 month treatment); RR 16.5 (1.0, 285)	15/369 (4%); 19/369 (5%); RR 1.3 (0.6, 2.5)	Population: DVT or PE; proportion with calf DVT not known; Only bleeding during treatment is reported. 20% of VTE outcomes were not objectively verified.

(continued)

Table 3
(continued)

First author/year (acronym)	Intervention	Blinding	# pts analyzed	Length follow-up	Recurrent DVT or PE	Major bleeding	Total mortality	Comments
Agnelli 2003 (34) (WODIT-PE)	VKA stopped / VKA (INR 2.0–3.0) for 9 more month	Allocation: yes, Patients: no, Caregivers: no, Adjudications: yes, Data analysts: unlikely	91/91, 90/90	2.6 years (mean), 2.9 years (mean)	11/91 (12%), 11.90 (12%), RR 1.0 (0.5, 2.2)	1/91 (1%), 2/90 (2%), RR 2.0 (0.5, 21.9)	7/91 (8%), 8/90 (9%), RR 1.16 (0.4, 3.0)	Population: first unprovoked PE. Treated for ≥3 month. Among the 4 groups, only 1 recurrent VTE while on VKA.
	VKA stopped / VKA (INR 2.0–3.0) for 3 more month		70/70, 75/75	2.8 years (mean), 2.9 years (mean)	7/70 (10%), 4/75 (5%), RR 0.5 (0.2, 1.7)	0/70 (0%), 1/75 (1%), RR 1.9 (0.1, 56)	0/70 (0%), 4/75 (5%), RR 8.4 (0.5, 153)	Population: first provoked PE. Treated for ≥3 month (see above)
Agnelli 2001 (33) (WODIT-DVT)	VKA stopped / VKA (INR 2.0–3.0) for 9 month	Allocation: yes, Patients: no, Caregivers: no, Adjudications: yes, Data analysts: unlikely	133/133, 134/134	3.2 years (mean), 3.1 years (mean)	21/133 (16%), 21/134 (16%), RR 1.0 (0.6, 1.7)	2/133 (2%), 4/134 (3%), RR 2.0 (0.4, 10.7)	7/133 (5%), 7/134 (5%), RR 1.0 (0.4, 2.8)	Population: first unprovoked proximal DVT treated for 3 month. One patient had recurrent VTE on VKA. Bleeding in the intervention group was while on VKA.
Pinede 2001 (30)(DOT AVK)	VKA (INR 2.0–3.0) for 3 month & VKA (INR 1.0–3.0) for 6 month	Allocation: yes, Patients: no, Caregivers: no, Adjudications: yes, Data analysts: unlikely	270/270, 269/269	15 month	21/270 (8%), 23/269 (9%), RR 1.1 (0.6, 1.9)	5/270 (2%), 7/269 (3%), RR 1.4 (0.4, 4.4)	not specified	Population: first proximal DVT or PE. Recurrent VTE occurred after VKA in 26/28 of the short duration groups and 21/27 of the long duration groups.
Summary			1881		RR 0.95 (0.72, 1.26)	RR 2.53 (1.18, 5.46)	RR 1.3 (0.82, 2.08)	For all analyses, p≥0.1 for heterogeneity.

Indefinite vs. intermediate durations of anticoagulation (INR ~20–3.0)

Study	Remain aff (stop)	Methods	N	Duration				Population / Comments
Palereti 2006 (35) (PROLONG)	VKA Restart Indefinitely VKA (INR 2.0-3.0) (not blinded)	Allocation: yes Patients: no Caregivers: no Adjudications: yes Data analysts: unlikely	103/105 120/122	1.4 years (mean) (max 1.5 years)	18/103 (17%) 2/120 (2%) RR 0.1 (0.0, 0.4)	0/103 1/120 (1%) RR 2.6 (0.1, 62.6)	1/103 (1%) 1/120 (1%) RR 0.9 (0.1, 13.6)	Population: first unprovoked proximal DVT or PE. Treated for ≥3 month. VKA stopped & D-dimer positive 1 month later. Eight control pts. Restarted VKA, some after superficial phlebitis. 1 recurrent VTE in VKA group after VKA stopped.
Kearon 1999 (16) (LAFIT)	VKA stopped (Placebo) VKA (INR 2.0-3.0) for 2 more years	Allocation: yes Patients: yes Caregivers: yes Adjudications: yes Data analysts: yes	83/83 79/79	10 month (mean) (max 2 years)	17/83 (20%)1/79 (1%) RR 0.1 (C.0, 0.5)	0/83 3/79 (4%) RR 7.4 (0.4, 140)	3/83 (4%) 1/79 (1%) RR 0.3 (0.0, 3.3)	Population: first unprovoked proximal DVT or PE (5%) had previous provoked VTE). The recurrent VTE in the VKA patient was after stopping VKA.
Schulman 1997 (3) (DURAC 2)	VKA (INR 2.0-2.85) for 6 month VKA (INR 2.0-2.85) indefinitely.	Allocation: yes Patients: no Caregivers: no Adjudications: VTE, yes Other, unlikely Data analysts: unlikely	111/111 116/116	4 years	23/111 (2%) 3/116 (3%) RR 0.1 (0.0, 0.4)	3/111 (3%) 10/116 (9%) RR 3.2 (0.9, 11.3)	16/111 (14%) 10/116 (9%) RR 0.6 (0.3, 1.3)	Second VTE: DVT (distal or proximal) or PE. All recurrent VTE in the indefinite VKA group were after stopping VKAs. Bleeding during the first 6 month of VKA in 1 of 6 month group and 6 of indefinite group. (Only asked about bleeding while on VKAs.
Summary					RR 0.1 (0.04, 0.22)	RR 3.61 (1.22, 10.7)	RR 0.58 (0.29, 1.14)	For all analyses, $p \geq 0.1$ for heterogeneity.

(continued)

Table 3
(continued)

First author/year (acronym)	Intervention	Blinding	# pts analyzed	Length follow-up	Recurrent DVT or PE	Major bleeding	Total mortality	Comments
Indefinite vs. intermediate durations of anticoagulation (INR ~1.5–2.0 after initial INR 2.0–3.0 in both groups)								
Ridker 2003 (18) (PREVENT)	VKA stopped or not restarted (Placebo) VKA INR 1.5–2.0	Allocation: yes Patients: yes Caregivers: yes Adjudications: yes Data analysts: yes	253/253 255/255	2.1 years (mean (max 4.3 years)	37/253 (15%) 14/255 (5%) RR 0.4 (0.2, 0.7)	2/253 (1%) 5/255 (2%) RR 2.5 (0.5, 12.7)	8/253 (3%) 4/255 (2%) RR 0.5 (0.1, 1.6)	Population: unprovoked DVT (distal or proximal) or PE (first episode in 38%) 8 recurrent VTE in the VKA group after stopping VKAs.
Low intensity (INR 1.5–1.9) vs. conventional intensity (INR 2.0–3.0)								
Kearon 2003 (17) (ELATE)	VKA INR 1.5–1.9 VKA INR 2.0–3.0 (blinded)	Allocation: yes Patients: yes Caregivers: yes Adjudications: yes Data analysts: yes	369/369 369/369	2.4 years (mean)	16/369 (4%) 6/369 (2%) RR 0.4 (0.1, 0.9)	9/369 (2%) 8/369 (2%) RR 0.9 (0.3, 2.3)	16/369 (4%) 8/369 (2%) RR 0.5 (0.2, 1.2)	Population: unprovoked proximal DVT or PE (first episode in 31%). Treated for ≥3 month VKA (INR 2.0–3.0) (mean 12 month) 5 recurrent VTE in INR 1.5–1.9 and 3 in the INR 2.0–3.0 group after stopping VKAs.

also PE, whereas only about 20% of recurrent episodes of VTE are a PE after an initial DVT *(33,34,38,40–42)*. This pattern of recurrence, with about a three-fold higher risk of PE after an initial PE than after an initial DVT, appears to persist long-term *(38,41,42)*. About 10% of symptomatic PE are considered to be rapidly fatal *(43–45)* and another 5% of patients whose PE is diagnosed and treated also die from PE *(38,41,46–50)*. Thus, after 3 or more months of treatment for DVT or PE, recurrent VTE that presents as PE probably has a case-fatality of about 15%. The risk of dying from acute DVT, because of early subsequent PE or other complications (e.g., bleeding, precipitation of myocardial infarction), appears to be 2% or less *(24,38,41,47,50,51)*. Based on these estimates, the case-fatality associated with late recurrent VTE after a preceding PE is expected to be about 10%, whereas that after a preceding DVT is expected to be about 5%. Consistent with the latter estimate, an overview of randomized trials calculated a 5.1% case-fatality for recurrent VTE in patients with DVT who had completed 3 months of treatment *(40)*. Therefore, although the risk of a recurrence is the same after PE and proximal DVT, the case-fatality for a recurrence is expected to be two-fold higher after PE than after DVT.

D-DIMER LEVEL AFTER WITHDRAWAL OF TREATMENT

A negative D-dimer test 1 month after withdrawal of VKA appears to identify patients with a substantially reduced risk of recurrent VTE (relative risk ~0.4) *(35,52–54)*.

HEREDITARY THROMBOPHILIAS

A recent meta-analysis estimated that the risk of recurrent VTE associated with heterozygous factor V Leiden was 1.4 (95% CI 1.1–1.8) and that associated with prothrombin G20210A was 1.7 (1.3–2.3), with heterogeneity of these estimates among studies *(55)*. Among the five large prospective studies that included a total of 2,691 patients with a first episode of VTE (provoked and unprovoked), and of whom 117 (4.3%) had homozygous factor V Leiden, homozygous prothrombin gene G20210A, double heterozygous states for these two mutations, or deficiency of protein C, protein S or antithrombin, the overall odds ratio for recurrent VTE associated with these major thrombophilias was 1.5 (95% CI 0.9–2.4) *(31,52,56–58)*.

ANTIPHOSPHOLIPID ANTIBODIES

Schulman et al. found that an anticardiolipin antibody was associated with recurrent VTE in the first 4 years after the first VTE *(59)*, but at the end of 10 years of follow-up it was no longer predictive *(42)*. Kearon found that an anticardiolipin antibody or lupus anticoagulant was associated with recurrent VTE after an unprovoked VTE (hazard ratio 4.0, 95% CI 1.2–13) *(16)*, but not after a provoked VTE (hazard ratio 1.3, 95% CI 0.2–11) *(36)*.

SEX

A recent meta-analysis estimated that the risk of recurrent VTE is higher in males than in females (RR 1.6, 95% CI 1.2–2.0), with heterogeneity of this association among studies *(60)*.

RESIDUAL DEEP VEIN THROMBOSIS

A relation between the presence of residual DVT on ultrasound and the risk of recurrent VTE has been reported *(22,61)*. However, a number of other studies have not found the residual DVT to be an independent predictor of recurrence *(16,34,36,62)*, and why residual DVT would be associated with DVT in the contralateral leg remains unexplained *(61)*.

VENA CAVAL FILTER

In patients who have had a vena caval filter inserted, followed by standard anticoagulant therapy, a trend to a higher risk of a new episode of DVT (RR 1.3; 95% CI 0.9–1.8), a lower risk of PE (RR 0.4; 95%

CI 0.2–0.9), and no difference in the risk of VTE (DVT and/or PE; RR 1.0; 95% CI 0.7–1.4) was observed after 8 years of follow-up *(63,64)*.

OTHER MARKERS FOR RECURRENCE

Factor VIII *(54,58,65,66)*, factor IX *(58)*, factor XI *(58,67)*, homocysteine *(58,68,69)*, thrombin generation *(70)*, activated partial thromboplastin time *(71)*, family history of VTE *(72)*, and age at diagnosis *(25,38)* have been evaluated, but the evidence that they are clinically important risk factors for recurrent VTE is generally weak.

Comparisons of Different Durations of Anticoagulation Therapy for Venous Thromboembolism

Trials that have evaluated different durations of anticoagulant therapy in patients with VTE can be divided into three categories, according to the durations of the therapy that were compared: (1) short vs. intermediate durations, (2) different intermediate durations, and (3) indefinite therapy vs. intermediate durations. Within each of these categories, studies that included heterogeneous (i.e., less selected) patients with VTE will be considered first, followed by studies that enrolled subgroups of (i.e., selected) patients who were expected to have either a lower (e.g., associated with reversible risk factors) or a higher (e.g., unprovoked, or second episodes of VTE) risk of recurrence.

SHORT (4 OR 6 WEEKS) VS. INTERMEDIATE (3 OR 6 MONTHS) DURATIONS OF THERAPY

Five trials have evaluated shortening the duration of oral anticoagulant therapy from 3 or 6 months to 4 or 6 weeks in patients with mostly first episodes of VTE (Table 3) *(4,5,28,30)*. The first three studies (British Thoracic Society, Levine, DURAC 1; Table 3), which mainly enrolled unselected patients with proximal DVT or PE, found that shortening the duration of anticoagulation was associated with about double the frequency of recurrent VTE during follow-up of 1 to 2 years (an absolute risk increase of ~5%) *(4,5,28)*. Major bleeding was uncommon during the incremental period of anticoagulation in these three studies (estimated as seven episodes among 1,009 patients during 259-patient years of additional treatment [2.7% per year]) *(4,5,28)*. Therefore, the main finding of these studies was that anticoagulant therapy should not be shortened to 4 or 6 weeks in patients with VTE.

Subgroup analyses of one of the above studies (DURAC 1) suggest that isolated distal DVT provoked by a major transient risk factor can safely be treated with only 6 weeks of therapy *(28)*. A subsequent study (component of DOTVAK), which compared 6 vs. 12 weeks of therapy in patients with isolated calf DVT (unprovoked or provoked; mostly diagnosed by ultrasound), found no evidence to suggest that shortening therapy increased the risk of recurrence (RR 0.6; 95% CI 0.01–3.4) and, in general, observed a low frequency of recurrent VTE with isolated calf DVT (~2% in the first year) compared to proximal DVT or PE (~6% in the first year) *(30)*. These findings suggest that if anticoagulants need to be stopped after 6 weeks of therapy in patients with isolated distal DVT, the subsequent risk of recurrence is not expected to be excessive. The fifth of these studies enrolled only patients with VTE that was associated with a major reversible risk factor (SOFAST; Table 3); however, because only 165 patients were enrolled, its findings were not definitive *(36)*. A meta-analysis of five studies (retrospective identification of the patient's subgroup in four studies *(4,5,28,73)*; prospective enrollment of patients in one study *(36)*) that compared 4 or 6 weeks with 3 or 6 months of treatment among 725 patients with VTE provoked by a reversible risk factor found that the shorter durations of therapy were associated with more than double the risk of recurrent VTE during the subsequent year (odds ratio 2.9; 95% CI 1.2–6.9; absolute increase of ~3.4%) *(36)*.

DIFFERENT INTERMEDIATE DURATIONS OF THERAPY (6 OR 12 MONTHS VS. 3 MONTHS)

Two studies have compared 6 vs. 3 months of anticoagulant therapy in patients with predominantly first episodes of DVT or PE (unprovoked, or provoked by a reversible risk factor) (DOTAVK, Campbell; Table 3) (30,74). There was no difference in the risk of recurrence during follow-up in both studies, and one study (74) reported a lower risk of bleeding in the 3-month group (Campbell; Table 3).

Agnelli and colleagues compared stopping anticoagulant therapy at 3 months with continuing it for another 9 months after a first episode of unprovoked proximal DVT (WODIT-DVT; Table 3) (33). At the end of the first year, recurrent VTE was less frequent in the group that continued on anticoagulant therapy (3.0% vs. 8.3%) but this benefit was no longer present after 2 years of follow-up (RR 1.0; 95% CI 0.6–1.7). The same investigators obtained similar results in a comparable study of patients with unprovoked PE (WODIT PE and Table 3) (34).

Based on the findings of these five studies (including the two components of WODIT-PE) (30,33,34,74), anticoagulants are found to be very effective in preventing recurrence when patients are receiving therapy but, at the end of extended follow-up after stopping treatment, a similar risk of recurrence is expected if anticoagulants are stopped at 6 or 12 months compared to at 3 months (RR for the five studies 0.95; 95% CI 0.72–1.26; Table 3) (30,33,34,74), including among patients with unprovoked proximal DVT or PE.

INDEFINITE THERAPY VS. INTERMEDIATE DURATIONS OF ANTICOAGULANT THERAPY

Four trials have compared indefinite (i.e., extended therapy without scheduled stopping of treatment and subsequent follow-up) anticoagulation (target INR of 2.0–2.85 (3), 2.0–3.0 (16,35), 1.5–2.0 (18)) with stopping therapy in patients with VTE who were believed to have a high risk of recurrence because thrombosis was a second episode (3), unprovoked (16,18), or was unprovoked and had a positive D-dimer result 1 month after stopping therapy (35) (DURAC 2, LAFIT, PREVENT, PROLONG; Table 3). The results indicate that randomization to indefinite treatment with conventional-intensity VKA (target INR 2.5) reduces recurrent VTE by about 90% (RR for the three studies 0.10; 95% CI 0.04–0.22; Table 3) (3,16,35), and randomization to low-intensity therapy (target INR 1.75) reduces VTE by 64% (95% CI for HR, 23–81%) (18) (Table 3; both risk reductions are appreciably greater among patients who remain on VKA therapy).

Bleeding During Long-Term Anticoagulant Therapy

A meta-analysis of seven studies (4,16,18,33,39,75,76) that compared durations of conventional-intensity anticoagulant therapy for VTE (not all patients had unprovoked VTE) estimated the rate of major bleeding to be 1.1% per patient-year (18 episodes in 1,571 years) during the extended phase of anticoagulation compared with 0.6% per patient-year (9 episodes during 1,497 years) without anticoagulation (RR of 1.80; 95% CI 0.72–4.51) (77). Similar low rates on major bleeding were observed during long-term treatment of unprovoked VTE in the more recent ELATE and PROLONG studies (Table 3) (17,74).

Of factors that have been evaluated as risk factors for major bleeding during anticoagulant therapy, the following appear to have the greatest potential to be clinically useful markers of increased risk: old age, particularly after 75 years; previous gastrointestinal bleeding, particularly if not associated with a reversible cause; previous non-cardioembolic stroke; chronic renal or hepatic disease; concomitant antiplatelet therapy (to be avoided if possible); other serious acute or chronic illness; poor anticoagulant control; and suboptimal monitoring of anticoagulant therapy (17,78–85).

Balancing Reduction of VTE with Increase of Bleeding During Long-Term Therapy

As noted previously, the likelihood of dying from recurrent VTE depends on whether the recurrence is a PE or a DVT, with PE being much more common after an initial PE than after an initial DVT. After completing 3 or more months of initial anticoagulant therapy, case-fatality for recurrent VTE is expected to be about 10% after an initial PE and 5% after an initial DVT (see above). Case-fatality with major bleeding during long-term anticoagulant therapy for VTE is about 10% (86). Comparison of associated case-fatalities suggests that the consequence of major bleeding during long-term anticoagulation is similar to that of a recurrent episode of VTE that occurs after a PE, and is about twice as severe as the consequences of a recurrent episode of VTE that occurs after a DVT. Therefore, given a relative risk reduction for recurrent VTE of over 90%, and a relative risk for bleeding of 2.5, with long-term anticoagulation, if the annual rate of major bleeding on anticoagulant therapy is 2%, the annual risk of recurrent VTE needs to exceed 1.2% after a PE, and 2.4% after a DVT just to offset the increased fatal bleeding.

As the average rate of recurrence is about 6% per year in the first 5 years after stopping anticoagulant therapy in patients with a first episode of unprovoked proximal DVT or PE (4,5,16,18,27,28,30,31,33,34), indefinite anticoagulant therapy is expected to be beneficial in a majority of such patients (see also Table 3). Consistent with this risk:benefit analysis, the combined results of the five randomized trials that have compared long-term conventional-intensity (3,16,35) or low-intensity (18) therapy with stopping therapy, and conventional-intensity with low-intensity therapy (17), in patients with mostly unprovoked VTE suggests that long-term therapy reduces all-cause mortality (risk ratio 0.53; 95% CI 0.33–0.87 (87) [see Baglin (88) for the argument against long-term anticoagulation for a first unprovoked VTE]).

Patient Preferences and the Burden of Anticoagulation

The perceived burden associated with being on VKA therapy differs markedly among patients. For example, Locadia and colleagues identified that being on VKA was associated with a median utility of 0.92 (where 0 is equivalent to death and 1.0 is equivalent to perfect health) by 124 patients who had a recent or remote VTE; however, the associated utility was 0.77 or lower for a quarter of patients, and was 0.98 or higher for another quarter of patients (i.e., rated more highly that the median utility of 0.96 associated with not being on VKA). Consistent with these large differences in patients' perception of the burden of VKA therapy, irrespective of whether the risk of recurrence was assumed to be high or low after stopping therapy, 25% of surveyed patients always opted to stop therapy and 23% always opted to continue with the therapy. There were also marked difference in how negatively (i.e., "bad") patients consider it would be to have an episode of bleeding or VTE (90).

Alternatives to Vitamin K Antagonists

SUBCUTANEOUS UNFRACTIONATED HEPARIN

Adjusted-dose subcutaneous UFH is an effective approach for the long-term treatment of DVT (91), whereas low-dose UFH (5,000 U twice daily) is inadequate for this purpose (2,92). In a study of 80 patients with DVT, contraindications to VKA therapy that compared 10,000 U UFH with 5,000 IU dalteparin, each administered subcutaneously twice daily for 3 months, there was a similar low frequency of recurrent VTE and bleeding in both groups, and a less frequent spinal fracture in the LMWH group (93).

SUBCUTANEOUS LOW-MOLECULAR-WEIGHT-HEPARIN

Fourteen randomized trials have compared VKA (INR of 2.0–3.0) with widely differing regimens of five LMWH preparations (dalteparin (94–96), enoxaparin (29,97–101), nadroparin (102,103), tinzaparin *(104,105)*, bemiparin *(106))*. In these studies, the daily LMWH dose was as low as 4,000 IU *(29,97)* to as high as 200 IU/kg *(96,103)*; approximately a 3.5-fold difference. Two meta-analyses of studies that compared LMWH with VKA, each given for 3 months after initial heparin therapy, have been performed *(107,108)*. In the analysis by Iorio and colleagues, which includes seven studies *(29,94,97,98,102–104)* and a total of 1,379 patients, there were trends towards less recurrent VTE (odds ratio 0.66; 95% CI 0.41–1.07) and less major bleeding (odds ratio 0.45; 95% CI 0.18–1.11) with 3 months of LMWH compared with VKA *(108)*. Compared with outcomes in patients who received VKA therapy, between study differences of mean daily dose of LMWH had little effect on efficacy but did appear to influence the risk of major bleeding (odds ratio of about 0.2 with ~4,000 IU/day to about 0.7 with 12,000 IU/day, relative to the VKA groups [$p=0.03$]) *(108)*. Three subsequent studies that selectively enrolled a total of 1,019 patients with VTE in association with active cancer found that, compared to VKA therapy, 3 *(99,109)* or 6 *(96)* months of therapeutic-dose LMWH was associated with less recurrent VTE in one study *(96)* and less bleeding in another *(99)* (Table 4) (RR for the three studies: recurrent VTE 0.56 [95% CI 0.38–0.82]; major bleeding 1.01 [95% CI 0.62–1.64]; mortality 0.92 [95% CI 0.78–1.10] Table 4) *(99,108,109)*. Randomized trials have not evaluated approaches to anticoagulant therapy after the first 6 months of VKA or LMWH therapy in patients with VTE and cancer, either to assess the duration of therapy or to compare VKA with LMWH for extended therapy. Observational studies suggest that the risk of recurrent VTE is unacceptably high in patients with active cancer who terminate anticoagulant therapy *(24–26,38)*.

NEW ANTICOAGULANTS

Ximelagatran, an oral direct thrombin inhibitor, has been shown to be effective for the initial and long-term treatment of VTE but has been withdrawn because of hepatic toxicity *(39,110)*. Idraparinux, the synthetic long-acting pentasaccharide, was recently reported to be as effective (recurrent VTE at 3 months: 2.9% vs. 3.0%) and as safe as VKA for the first 3 or 6 months of treatment of DVT but less effective than VKA (recurrent VTE at 3 months: 3.4% vs. 1.6%; $p<0.05$) in patients with PE *(111)*. After 6 months of treatment of VTE with idraparinux or VKA, compared with placebo, 6 months of further treatment with idraparinux reduced their recurrence (1.0% vs. 3.7%; $p=0.002$) but was associated with increased major bleeding (1.9% vs 0%; $p<0.001$) *(112)*. New Anticoagulants including dabigatran etexilate, rivaroxaban and apizaban, are at an advanced of development.

ANTIPLATELET THERAPY FOR TREATMENT OF VTE

Antiplatelet therapy, usually with aspirin, reduces the risk of postoperative VTE by about 40% (i.e., primary prophylaxis) *(113,114)*. This has led to the hypothesis that aspirin may also reduce the risk of recurrent VTE if it is started after anticoagulant therapy, which is being tested in two ongoing placebo-controlled trials in patients with unprovoked VTE *(114)*. If patients were on long-term antiplatelet therapy before starting treatment for VTE, it is usually appropriate to restart this therapy if anticoagulants are stopped. Currently, there is insufficient evidence to support use of aspirin in patients with unprovoked VTE who are not candidates for indefinite anticoagulant therapy.

RECOMMENDED DURATION OF ANTICOAGULATION IN INDIVIDUAL PATIENTS

Based largely on the preceding analysis of risk factors for recurrent thrombosis and bleeding, and on the findings of studies that compared different durations and intensities of anticoagulation, an approach to selection of duration of anticoagulation for individual patients with VTE is outlined in

Table 4
LMWH vs. VKA for long-term treatment of VTE in patients with active cancer

First author (acronym)	Interventions	Blinding	# pts analyzed	Length of follow-up	Recurrent DVT or PE	Major bleeding	Total mortality	Comments
Meyer 2002 (99)	VKA (INR 2.0–3.0) for 3 months after Initial enoxaparin; Enoxaparin 1.5 mg/kg OD for 3 months	Allocation: likely; Patients: no; Caregivers: no; Adjudications: yes; Data analysts: unlikely	75/75; 71/71	3 month; 3 month	3/75 (4%); 2/71 (3%); RR 0.7 (0.1, 4.1)	12/75 (16%); 5/71 (7%); RR 0.4 (0.2, 1.2)	17/75 (23%); 8/71 (11%); RR 0.5 (0.2, 1.1)	Population: DVT (proportion with calf DVT not known) or PE and active cancer. All fatal bleeding (n=6) were in VKA group.
Lee 2003 (96) (CLOT)	VKA (INR 2.0–3.0) for 6 months after initial dalteparin-Dalteparin 200 U/kg OD for 1 month followed by 150 U/kg for 5 months	Allocation: yes; Patients: no; Caregivers: no; Adjudications: yes; Data analysts: likely	336/338; 336/338	6 month; 6 month	53/336 (16%); 27/336 (8%); RR 0.5 (0.3, 0.8)	12/335 (4%); 19/338 (6%); RR 1.6 (0.8, 3.2)	136/336 (40%); 130/336 (37%); RR 1.0 (0.8, 1.2)	Population: proximal DVT or PE and active cancer. Difference in efficacy mainly due to recurrent DVT (14 vs. 37 episodes)
Hull 2006 (109) (Main LITE-cancer)	VKA (INR 2.0–3.0) for 3 months after initial IV UFH; Tinzaparin 175 mg/kg OD for 3 months.	Allocation: likely; Patients: no; Caregivers: no; Adjudications: yes; Data analysts: likely	100/100; 100/100	3 month; 3 month	10/100 (10%); 6/100 (6%); RR 0.6 (0.2, 1.6)	7/100 (7%); 7/100 (7%); RR 1.0 (0.4, 2.8)	19/100 (19%); 20/100 (20%); RR 1.0 (0.6, 1.9)	Population: proximal DVT and active cancer. Pre-specified, stratification, subgroup within a larger trial. Outcomes at 12 months were also reported.
Summary			1019		RR 0.7 (0.4, 0.8)v	RR 1.0 (0.6, 1.6)	RR 0.9 (0.8, 1.1)	Heterogeneity $p < 0.1$ for all estimates

Table 5
Recommendations for duration of anticoagulant therapy for VTE

Risk factor for VTE	Durations of treatment (Target INR 2.5, range 2.0–3.0)
Transient risk factor[a]	3 months
UnprovokedIf also:	Indefinite[b]3 months
isolated distal DVT; or a first proximal DVT or PE and a moderate or higher risk of bleeding[c]; or an informed patient's preference to stop therapy	
Uncontrolled malignancyIf also:	Indefinite(preferably with LMWH for at least
a very high risk of bleeding[c]; isolated distal DVT; or an additional major reversible provoking risk factor for VTE[a]	the first 3 months)
	consider stopping therapy at 3 or when cancer becomes inactive

[a]Transient risk factors include: major factors, such as surgery with general anesthesia, plaster cast immobilization of a leg, or hospitalization, all within the past month; and minor factors, such as estrogen therapy, pregnancy, prolonged travel (e.g., longer than 8 h), less marked leg injury, or the previously noted "major factors" when they occur 1–3 months before diagnosis of VTE

[b]Decision should be reviewed annually to consider if the patient's risk of bleeding has increased, or if patient preference has changed. Additional factors favoring indefinite therapy include: more than one episode of unprovoked VTE; PE vs. proximal DVT at presentation; male sex; antiphospholipid antibodies; hereditary thrombophilia

[c]Risk factors for bleeding include: age 65 years or older, particularly after 75 years; previous non-cardioembolic stroke; previous bleeding (e.g., gastrointestinal), particularly if there was not a reversible cause; active peptic ulcer disease; renal impairment; anemia; thrombocytopenia; liver disease; diabetes mellitus; use of antiplatelet therapy (to be avoided); poor patient compliance; poor control of anticoagulation; structural lesion (including tumor) expected to be associated with bleeding. One or two risk factors suggests moderate risk, and three or more risk factors suggests high risk, of bleeding

Table 5. Because the presence of a reversible risk factor for VTE, lack of a provoking factor, or cancer, at the time of thrombosis has the greatest prognostic influence on the risk of recurrence, this assessment carries most weight.

For patients whose VTE is associated with a major reversible risk factor, such as recent surgery, stopping anticoagulant therapy after 3 months of treatment is expected to be associated with a subsequent risk of recurrent VTE of about 3% in the first year and about 10% over 5 years (4,5,18,24,26,29,30,34,39). For patients whose VTE is associated with a lesser reversible risk factor, such as a soft tissue injury to the leg or a prolonged flight, stopping anticoagulant therapy after 3 months of treatment is expected to be associated with a subsequent risk of recurrent VTE of about 5% in the first year and about 15% over 5 years (31). These rates of VTE are not high enough to justify treatment for longer than 3 months.

For patients with unprovoked VTE, stopping anticoagulant therapy after 3 or more months of treatment is expected to be associated with a subsequent risk of recurrent VTE of about 10% in the first year and about 30% over 5 years (26,28,30,33). This rate is high enough to justify long-term anticoagulation in the majority of patients. The argument favoring long-term therapy is stronger if the unprovoked episode of VTE was a second or subsequent episode of unprovoked VTE, a PE, occurred in a male, or was associated with an antiphospholipid antibody or a hereditary thrombophilia. A low D-dimer level (e.g., corresponding to a "negative test" result using a D-dimer assay that has a high sensitivity for diagnosing acute VTE) 1 month after stopping anticoagulant therapy may identify patients with unprovoked proximal but or be who have a low risk of recurrence, and do not require long-term anticoagulant therapy (35,52,54,115). However, this author suggests that the use of D-dimer testing to identify patients with unprovoked proximal DVT or PE who can safely discontinue anticoagulant therapy requires further prospective validation before this can be recommended in usual clinical practice (the author is currently involved in such a study).

Patients with active cancer should generally remain on long-term anticoagulant therapy (LMWH or VKA) because the risk of recurrent VTE is expected to be higher than 10% within a year of stopping treatment.

If anticoagulant therapy is expected to be associated with a high risk of bleeding because of risk factors for bleeding or lack of access to appropriate anticoagulant monitoring, longer than 3 months of treatment generally should be avoided in patients with a first unprovoked VTE. Annual review is recommended for patients on long-term therapy to ensure that the benefits of continuing therapy are likely to exceed the risks (e.g., that contraindications have not developed).

REFERENCES

1. Lagerstedt CI, Olsson CG, Fagher BO, Oqvist BW, Albrechtsson U (1985) Need for long-term anticoagulant treatment in symptomatic calf-vein thrombosis. Lancet 2(8454):515–518
2. Hull R, Delmore T, Genton E, Hirsh J, Gent M, Sackett D et al (1979) Warfarin sodium versus low-dose heparin in the long-term treatment of venous thrombosis. N Engl J Med 301:855–858
3. Schulman S, Granqvist S, Holmstrom M, Carlsson A, Lindmarker P, Nicol P et al (1997) The duration of oral anticoagulant therapy after a second episode of venous thromboembolism. N Engl J Med 336:393–398
4. Levine MN, Hirsh J, Gent M, Turpie AG, Weitz J, Ginsberg J et al (1995) Optimal duration of oral anticoagulant therapy: a randomized trial comparing four weeks with three months of warfarin in patients with proximal deep vein thrombosis. Thromb Haemost 74:606–611
5. Research Committee of the British Thoracic Society (1992) Optimum duration of anticoagulation for deep-vein thrombosis and pulmonary embolism. Lancet 340:873–876
6. Gallus AS, Jackaman J, Tillett J, Mills W, Sycherley A (1986) Safety and efficacy of warfarin started early after submassive venous thrombosis or pulmonary embolism. Lancet 2:1293–1296
7. Hull RD, Raskob GE, Rosenbloom D, Panju AA, Brill-Edwards P, Ginsberg JS et al (1990) Heparin for 5 days as compared with 10 days in the initial treatment of proximal venous thrombosis. N Engl J Med 322:1260–1264
8. Harrison L, Johnston M, Massicotte MP, Crowther M, Moffat K, Hirsh J (1997) Comparison of 5-mg and 10-mg loading doses in initiation of warfarin therapy. Ann Intern Med 126:133–136
9. Crowther MA, Ginsberg JS, Kearon C, Harrison L, Johnson J, Massicotte P et al (1999) A randomized trial comparing 5 mg and 10 mg warfarin loading doses. Arch Intern Med 159:46–48
10. Kovacs MJ, Rodger M, Anderson DR, Morrow B, Kells G, Kovacs J et al (2003) Comparison of 10-mg and 5-mg warfarin initiation nomograms together with low-molecular-weight heparin for outpatient treatment of acute venous thromboembolism. A randomized, double-blind, controlled trial. Ann Intern Med 138:714–719
11. Ansell J, Hirsh J, Poller L, Bussey H, Jacobson A, Hylek E (2004) The pharmacology and management of the vitamin K antagonists: the Seventh ACCP Conference on Antithrombotic and Thrombolytic Therapy. Chest 126:204S–233S
12. Garcia D, Regan S, Crowther M, Hughes RA, Hylek EM (2005) Warfarin maintenance dosing patterns in clinical practice: implications for safer anticoagulation in the elderly population. Chest 127:2049–2056
13. Hull R, Hirsh J, Jay R, Carter C, England C, Gent M et al (1982) Different intensities of oral anticoagulant therapy in the treatment of proximal-vein thrombosis. N Engl J Med 307:1676–1681
14. Crowther MA, Ginsberg JS, Julian J, Denburg J, Hirsh J, Douketis J et al (2003) A comparison of two intensities of warfarin for prevention of recurrent thrombosis in patients with antiphospholipid antibody syndrome. N Eng J Med 349:1133–1138
15. Finazzi G, Marchioli R, Brancaccio V, Schinco P, Wisloff F, Musial J et al (2005) A randomized clinical trial of high-intensity warfarin vs. conventional antithrombotic therapy for the prevention of recurrent thrombosis in patients with the antiphospholipid syndrome (WAPS). J Thromb Haemost 3:848–853
16. Kearon C, Gent M, Hirsh J, Weitz J, Kovacs MJ, Anderson DR et al (1999) A comparison of three months of anticoagulation with extended anticoagulation for a first episode of idiopathic venous thromboembolism. N Engl J Med 340:901–907
17. Kearon C, Ginsberg JS, Kovacs MJ, Anderson DR, Wells PS, Julian JA et al (2003) Comparison of low-intensity warfarin therapy with conventional-intensity warfarin therapy for long-term prevention of recurrent venous thromboembolism. N Eng J Med 349:631–639

18. Ridker PM, Goldhaber SZ, Danielson E, Rosenberg Y, Eby CS, Deitcher SR et al (2003) Long-term, low-intensity warfarin therapy for prevention of recurrent venous thromboembolism. N Eng J Med 348:1425–1434

19. Hutten BA, Prins M, Gent M, Ginsberg J, Tijssen J, Buller H (2000) Incidence of recurrent thromboembolic and bleeding complications among patients with venous thromboembolism in relation to both malignancy and achieved international normalized ratio: a retrospective analysis. J Clin Oncol 18:3078–3083

20. Merli G, Spiro TE, Olsson CG, Abildgaard U, Davidson BL, Eldor A et al (2001) Subcutaneous enoxaparin once or twice daily compared with intravenous unfractionated heparin for treatment of venous thromboembolic disease. Ann Intern Med 134:191–202

21. Palareti G, Legnani C, Lee A, Manotti C, Hirsh J, D'Angelo A et al (2000) A comparison of the safety and efficacy of oral anticoagulation for the treatment of venous thromboembolic disease in patients with or without malignancy. Thromb Haemost 84:805–810

22. Piovella F, Crippa L, Barone M, Vigano DS, Serafini S, Galli L et al (2002) Normalization rates of compression ultrasonography in patients with a first episode of deep vein thrombosis of the lower limbs: association with recurrence and new thrombosis. Haematologica 87:515–522

23. Prandoni P, Lensing AW, Piccioli A, Bernardi E, Simioni P, Girolami B et al (2002) Recurrent venous thromboembolism and bleeding complications during anticoagulant treatment in patients with cancer and venous thrombosis. Blood 100:3484–3488

24. Prandoni P, Lensing AWA, Cogo A, Cuppini S, Villalta S, Carta M et al (1996) The long-term clinical course of acute deep venous thrombosis. Ann Intern Med 125:1–7

25. Heit JA, Mohr DN, Silverstein MD, Petterson TM, O'Fallon WM, Melton LJ III (2000) Predictors of recurrence after deep vein thrombosis and pulmonary embolism: a population-based cohort study. Arch Intern Med 160:761–768

26. Palareti G, Legnani C, Cosmi B, Guazzaloca G, Pancani C, Coccheri S (2002) Risk of venous thromboembolism recurrence: high negative predictive value of D-dimer performed after oral anticoagulation is stopped. Thromb Haemost 87:7–12

27. Prandoni P, Lensing AWA, Buller HR, Cogo A, Prins MH, Cattelan AM et al (1992) Deep-vein thrombosis and the incidence of subsequent symptomatic cancer. N Engl J Med 327:1128–1133

28. Schulman S, Rhedin A-S, Lindmarker P, Carlsson A, Lärfars G, Nicol P et al (1995) A comparison of six weeks with six months of oral anticoagulant therapy after a first episode of venous thromboembolism. N Engl J Med 332:1661–1665

29. Pini M, Aiello S, Manotti C, Pattacini C, Quintavalla R, Poli T et al (1994) Low molecular weight heparin versus warfarin the prevention of recurrence after deep vein thrombosis. Thromb Haemost 72(2):191–197

30. Pinede L, Ninet J, Duhaut P, Chabaud S, Demolombe-Ragué S, Duricu I et al (2001) Comparison of 3 and 6 months of oral anticoagulant therapy after a first episode of proximal deep vein thrombosis or pulmonary embolism and comparison of 6 and 12 weeks of therapy after isolated calf deep vein thrombosis. Circulation 103:2453–2460

31. Baglin T, Luddington R, Brown K, Baglin C (2003) Incidence of recurrent venous thromboembolism in relation to clinical and thrombophilic risk factors: prospective cohort study. Lancet 362:523–526

32. Spiezia L, Bernardi E, Tormene D, Simioni P, Girolami A, Prandoni P (2003) Recurrent thromboembolism in fertile women with venous thrombosis: incidence and risk factors. Thromb Haemost 90:964–966

33. Agnelli G, Prandoni P, Santamaria MG, Bagatella P, Iorio A, Bazzan M et al (2001) Three months versus one year of oral anticoagulant therapy for idiopathic deep vein thrombosis. N Engl J Med 345:165–169

34. Agnelli G, Prandoni P, Becattini C, Silingardi M, Taliani MR, Miccio M et al (2003) Extended oral anticoagulant therapy after a first episode of pulmonary embolism. Ann Intern Med 139:19–25

35. Palareti G, Cosmi B, Legnani C, Tosetto A, Brusi C, Iorio A et al (2006) D-dimer testing to determine the duration of anticoagulation therapy. N Engl J Med 355:1780–1789

36. Kearon C, Ginsberg JS, Anderson DR, Kovacs MJ, Wells P, Julian JA et al (2004) Comparison of 1 month with 3 months of anticoagulation for a first episode of venous thromboembolism associated with a transient risk factor. J Thromb Haemost 2:743–749

37. Hansson PO, Sorbo J, Eriksson H (2000) Recurrent venous thromboembolism after deep vein thrombosis: incidence and risk factors. Arch Intern Med 160:769–774

38. Murin S, Romano PS, White RH (2002) Comparison of outcomes after hospitalization for deep vein thrombosis or pulmonary embolism. Thromb Haemost 88:407–414

39. Schulman S, Wahlander K, Lundström T, Clason SB, Eriksson H (2003) for the THRIVE III Investigators. Secondary prevention of venous thromboembolism with the oral direct thrombin inhibitor ximelagatran. N Engl J Med 349:1713–1721

40. Douketis JD, Kearon C, Bates S, Duku EK, Ginsberg JS (1998) Risk of fatal pulmonary embolism in patients with treated venous thromboembolism. JAMA 279:458–462

41. Kniffin WD Jr, Baron JA, Barrett J, Birkmeyer JD, Anderson FA (1994) The epidemiology of diagnosed pulmonary embolism and deep venous thrombosis in the elderly. Arch Intern Med 154:861–866

42. Schulman S, Lindmarker P, Holmstrom M, Larfars G, Carlsson A, Nicol P et al (2006) Post-thrombotic syndrome, recurrence, and death 10 years after the first episode of venous thromboembolism treated with warfarin for 6 weeks or 6 months. J Thromb Haemost 4:734–742

43. Bell WR, Simon TL (1982) Current status of pulmonary embolic disease: pathophysiology, diagnosis, prevention, and treatment. Am Heart J 103:239–261

44. Stein PD, Henry JW (1995) Prevalence of acute pulmonary embolism among patients in a general hospital and at autopsy. Chest 108:978–981

45. Kearon C (2003) Natural history of venous thromboembolism. Circulation 107(Suppl 1):I22–I30

46. Goldhaber SZ, Visni L, De Rosa M (1999) Acute pulmonary embolism: clinical outcomes in the International Cooperative Pulmonary Embolism Registry (ICOPER). Lancet 353:1386–1389

47. Heit JA, Silverstein MD, Mohr DN, Petterson TM, O'Fallon WM, Melton LJ III (1999) Predictors of survival after deep vein thrombosis and pulmonary embolism: a population-based, cohort study. Arch Intern Med 159:445–453

48. Ribeiro A, Lindmarker P, Juhlin-Dannfelt A, Johnsson H, Jorfeldt L (1997) Echocardiography Doppler in pulmonary embolism: right ventricular dysfunction as a predictor of mortality rate. Am Heart J 134:479–487

49. Bell CM, Redelmeier DA (2002) Mortality among patients admitted to hospitals on weekends as compared with weekdays. N Engl J Med 345:663–668

50. Naess IA, Christiansen SC, Romundstad P, Cannegieter SC, Rosendaal FR, Hammerstrom J (2007) Incidence and mortality of venous thrombosis: a population-based study. J Thromb Haemost 5:692–699

51. Beyth RJ, Cohen AM, Landefeld CS (1995) Long-term outcomes of deep-vein thrombosis. Arch Intern Med 155:1031–1037

52. Palareti G, Legnani C, Cosmi B, Valdre L, Lunghi B, Bernardi F et al (2003) Predictive value of D-dimer test for recurrent venous thromboembolism after anticoagulation withdrawal in subjects with a previous idiopathic event and in carriers of congenital thrombophilia. Circulation 108:313–318

53. Eichinger S, Minar E, Bialonczyk C, Hirschl M, Quehenberger P, Schneider B et al (2003) D-dimer levels and risk of recurrent venous thromboembolism. JAMA 290:1071–1074

54. Shrivastava S, Ridker PM, Glynn RJ, Goldhaber SZ, Moll S, Bounameaux H et al (2006) D-dimer, factor VIII coagulant activity, low-intensity warfarin and the risk of recurrent venous thromboembolism. J Thromb Haemost 4:1208–1214

55. Ho WK, Hankey GJ, Quinlan DJ, Eikelboom JW (2006) Risk of recurrent venous thromboembolism in patients with common thrombophilia: a systematic review. Arch Intern Med 166:729–736

56. Lindmarker P, Schulman S, Sten-Linder M, Wiman B, Egberg N, Johnsson H (1999) The risk of recurrent venous thromboembolism in carriers and non-carriers of the G1691A Allele in the coagulation factor V gene and the G20210A Allele in the prothrombin gene. Thromb Haemost 81:684–689

57. Eichinger S, Pabinger I, Stumpflen A, Hirschl M, Bialonczyk C, Schneider B et al (1997) The risk of recurrent venous thromboembolism in patients with and without Factor V Leiden. Thromb Haemost 77(4):624–628

58. Christiansen SC, Cannegieter SC, Koster T, Vandenbroucke JP, Rosendaal FR (2005) Thrombophilia, clinical factors, and recurrent venous thrombotic events. JAMA 293:2352–2361

59. Schulman S, Svenungsson E, Granqvist S (1998) Anticardiolipin antibodies predict early recurrence of thromboembolism and death among patients with venous thromboembolism following anticoagulant therapy. Am J Med 104:332–338

60. McRae S, Tran H, Schulman S, Ginsberg J, Kearon C (2006) Effect of patient's sex on risk of recurrent venous thromboembolism: a meta-analysis. Lancet 368:371–378

61. Prandoni P, Lensing AW, Prins MH, Bernardi E, Marchiori A, Bagatella P et al (2002) Residual venous thrombosis as a predictive factor of recurrent venous thromboembolism. Ann Intern Med 137:955–960

62. Cosmi B, Legnani C, Cini M, Guazzaloca G, Palareti G (2005) D-dimer levels in combination with residual venous obstruction and the risk of recurrence after anticoagulation withdrawal for a first idiopathic deep vein thrombosis. Thromb Haemost 94:969–974

63. Decousus H, Leizorovicz A, Parent F, Page Y, Tardy B, Girard P et al (1998) A clinical trial of vena caval filters in the prevention of pulmonary embolism in patients with proximal deep-vein thrombosis. N Engl J Med 338:409–415

64. PREPIC Study Group (2005) Eight-year follow-up of patients with permanent vena cava filters in the prevention of pulmonary embolism: the PREPIC (Prevention du Risque d'Embolie Pulmonaire par Interruption Cave) randomized study. Circulation 112:416–422

65. Kryle P, Minar E, Hirschl M, Bialonczyk C, Stain M, Schneider B et al (2000) High plasma levels of factor VIII and the risk of recurrent venous thromboembolism. N Engl J Med 343:457–462

66. Kraaijenhagen RA, in't Anker PS, Koopman MM, Reitsma PH, Prins MH, van den Ende A et al (2000) High plasma concentration of factor VIIIc is a major risk factor for venous thromboembolism [see comments]. Thromb Haemost 83:5–9

67. Weltermann A, Eichinger S, Bialonczyk C, Minar E, Hirschl M, Quehenberger P et al (2003) The risk of recurrent venous thromboembolism among patients with high factor IX levels. J Thromb Haemost 1:28–32

68. Eichinger S, Stumpflen A, Hirschl M, Bialonczyk C, Herkner K, Stain M et al (1998) Hyperhomocysteinemia is a risk factor of recurrent venous thromboembolism. Thromb Haemost 80:566–569

69. Den Heijer M, Willems HP, Blom HJ, Gerrits WBJ, Cattaneo M, Eichinger S et al (2003) Homocysteine lowering by B vitamins and the prevention of secondary deep vein thrombosis and pulmonary embolism: a randomized, placebo-controlled, double-blind trial. J Thromb Haemost (Suppl 1 July 2003):OC161

70. Hron G, Kollars M, Binder BR, Eichinger S, Kyrle PA (2006) Identification of patients at low risk for recurrent venous thromboembolism by measuring thrombin generation. JAMA 296:397–402

71. Hron G, Eichinger S, Weltermann A, Quehenberger P, Halbmayer WM, Kyrle PA (2006) Prediction of recurrent venous thromboembolism by the activated partial thromboplastin time. J Thromb Haemost 4:752–756

72. Hron G, Eichinger S, Weltermann A, Minar E, Bialonczyk C, Hirschl M et al (2006) Family history for venous thromboembolism and the risk for recurrence. Am J Med 119:50–53

73. Schulman S, Lockner D, Juhlin-Dannfelt A (1985) The duration of oral anticoagulation after deep vein thrombosis. Acta Med Scand 217:547–552

74. Campbell IA, Bentley DP, Prescott RJ, Routledge PA, Shetty HG, Williamson IJ (2007) Anticoagulation for three versus six months in patients with deep vein thrombosis or pulmonary embolism, or both: randomised trial. BMJ 334(7595):674

75. Schweizer J, Elix H, Altmann E, Hellner G, Forkmann L (1998) Comparative results of thrombolysis treatment with rt-PA and urokinase: a pilot study. VASA 27:167–171

76. Holmgren K, Andersson G, Fagrell B, Johnsson H, Ljungberg B, Nilsson E et al (1985) One-month versus six-month therapy with oral anticoagulants after symptomatic deep vein thrombosis. Acta Med Scand 218:279–284

77. Ost D, Tepper J, Mihara H, Lander O, Heinzer R, Fein A (2005) Duration of anticoagulation following venous thromboembolism: a meta-analysis. JAMA 294:706–715

78. Palareti G, Leali N, Coccheri S, Poggi M, Manotti C, D'Angelo A et al (1996) Bleeding complications of oral anticoagulant treatment: An inception-cohort, prospective collaborative study (ISCOAT). Lancet 348:423–428

79. Beyth RJ, Quinn LM, Landefeld S (1998) Prospective evaluation of an index for predicting the risk of major bleeding in outpatients treated with warfarin. Am J Med 105:91–99

80. Kuijer PMM, Hutten BA, Prins MH, Buller HR (1999) Prediction of the risk of bleeding during anticoagulant treatment for venous thromboembolism. Arch Intern Med 159:457–460

81. Pengo V, Legnani C, Noventa F, Palareti G (2001) Oral anticoagulant therapy in patients with nonrheumatic atrial fibrillation and risk of bleeding. A Multicenter Inception Cohort Study. Thromb Haemost 85:418–422

82. Beyth RJ, Quinn L, Landefeld CS (2000) A multicomponent intervention to prevent major bleeding complications in older patients receiving warfarin. A randomized, controlled trial. Ann Intern Med 133:687–695

83. Dentali F, Douketis JD, Lim W, Crowther M (2007) Combined aspirin–oral anticoagulant therapy compared with oral anticoagulant therapy alone among patients at risk for cardiovascular disease: a meta-analysis of randomized trials. Arch Intern Med 167:117–124

84. Schulman S, Beyth RJ, Kearon C, Levine MN (2008) Hemorrhagic complications of anticoagulant and thrombolytic treatment. Chest 2008;133:257S–298S

85. Gage BF, Yan Y, Milligan PE, Waterman AD, Culverhouse R, Rich MW et al (2006) Clinical classification schemes for predicting hemorrhage: results from the National Registry of Atrial Fibrillation (NRAF). Am Heart J 151:713–719

86. Linkins LA, Choi PT, Douketis JD. Clinical impact of bleeding in patients taking oral anticoagulant therapy for venous thromboembolism: a meta-analysis. Am Intern Med. 2003;139:893–900

87. Kearon C (2007) Indefinite anticoagulation after a first episode of unprovoked venous thromboembolism: yes. J Thromb Haemost 5:2330–2335

88. Baglin T (2007) Unprovoked deep vein thrombosis should be treated with long-term anticoagulation – no. J Thromb Haemost 5:2336–2339

89. Locadia M, Bossuyt PM, Stalmeier PF, Sprangers MA, van Dongen CJ, Middeldorp S et al (2004) Treatment of venous thromboembolism with vitamin K antagonists: patients' health state valuations and treatment preferences. Thromb Haemost 92:1336–1341

90. Hull R, Delmore T, Carter C, Hirsh J, Genton E, Gent M et al (1982) Adjusted subcutaneous heparin versus warfarin sodium in the long-term treatment of venous thrombosis. N Engl J Med 306:189–194

91. Bynum LJ, Wilson Je (1979) Low-dose heparin therapy in the long-term management of venous thromboembolism. Am J Med 67:553–556

92. Monreal M, Lafoz E, Olive A, del Rio L, Vedia C (1994) Comparison of subcutaneous unfractionated heparin with a low molecular weight heparin (fragmin) in patients with venous thromboembolism and contraindications to coumarin. Thromb Haemost 71(1):7–11

93. Das SK, Cohen AT, Edmondson RA, Melissari E, Kakkar VV (1996) Low-molecular-weight heparin versus warfarin for prevention of recurrent venous thromboembolism: a randomized trial. World J Surg 20:521–527

94. Hamann H (1998) Rezidivprophylaxe nach phlebothrombose – orale antikoagulation oder niedermolelulares heparin subkutan. Vasomed 10:133–136

95. Lee AY, Levine MN, Baker RI, Bowden C, Kakkar AK, Prins M et al (2003) Low-molecular-weight heparin versus a coumarin for the prevention of recurrent venous thromboembolism in patients with cancer. N Engl J Med 349:146–153

96. Gonzalez-Fajardo JA, Arreba E, Castrodeza J, Perez JL, Fernandez L, Agundez I et al (1999) Venographic comparison of subcutaneous low-molecular weight heparin with oral anticoagulant therapy in the long-term treatment of deep venous thrombosis. J Vasc Surg 30:283–292

97. Veiga F, Escriba A, Maluenda MP, Lopez RM, Margalet I, Lezana A et al (2000) Low molecular weight heparin (enoxaparin) versus oral anticoagulant therapy (acenocoumarol) in the long-term treatment of deep venous thrombosis in the elderly: a randomized trial. Thromb Haemost 84:559–564

98. Meyer G, Marjanovic Z, Valcke J, Lorcerie B, Gruel Y, Solal-Celigny P et al (2002) Comparison of low-molecular-weight heparin and warfarin for the secondary prevention of venous thromboembolism in patients with cancer: a randomized controlled study. Arch Intern Med 162:1729–1735

99. Beckman JA, Dunn K, Sasahara AA, Goldhaber SZ (2003) Enoxaparin monotherapy without oral anticoagulation to treat acute symptomatic pulmonary embolism. Thromb Haemost 89:953–958

100. Kucher N, Quiroz R, McKean S, Sasahara AA, Goldhaber SZ (2005) Extended enoxaparin monotherapy for acute symptomatic pulmonary embolism. Vasc Med 10:251–256

101. Lopaciuk S, Bielska-Falda H, Noszczyk W, Bielawiec M, Witkiewicz W, Filipecki S et al (1999) Low molecular weight heparin versus acenocoumarol in the secondary prophylaxis of deep vein thrombosis. Thromb Haemost 81:26–31

102. Lopez-Beret P, Orgaz A, Fontcuberta J, Doblas M, Martinez A, Lozano G et al (2001) Low molecular weight heparin versus oral anticoagulants in the long- term treatment of deep venous thrombosis. J Vasc Surg 33:77–90

103. Hull R, Pineo G, Mah A, Brant R, for the LITE Investigators (2000) Long-term low molecular weight heparin treatment versus oral anticoagulant therapy for proximal deep vein thrombosis. Blood 96:449a

104. Hull RD, Pineo GF, Brant RF, Mah AF, Burke N, Dear R et al (2007) Self-managed long-term low-molecular-weight heparin therapy: the balance of benefits and harms. Am J Med 120:72–82

105. Kakkar V, Gebska M, Kadziola Z, Saba N, Carrasco P (2003) Low-molecular-weight heparin in the acute and long-term treatment of deep vein thrombosis. Thromb Haemost 89:674–680

106. van der Heijden JF, Hutten BA, Buller HR, Prins MH (2002) Vitamin K antagonists or low molecular weight heparin for the long term treatment of symptomatic venous thromboembolism (Cochrane Review), Issue 4. The Cochrane Library, Update Software, Oxford

107. Iorio A, Guercini F, Pini M (2003) Low-molecular-weight heparin for the long-term treatment of symptomatic venous thromboembolism: meta-analysis of the randomized comparisons with oral anticoagulants. J Thromb Haemost 1:1906–1913

108. Hull RD, Pineo GF, Brant RF, Mah AF, Burke N, Dear R et al (2006) Long-term low-molecular-weight heparin versus usual care in proximal-vein thrombosis patients with cancer. Am J Med 119:1062–1072

109. Fiessinger JN, Huisman MV, Davidson BL, Bounameaux H, Francis CW, Eriksson H et al (2005) Ximelagatran vs low-molecular-weight heparin and warfarin for the treatment of deep vein thrombosis: a randomized trial. JAMA 293:681–689

110. Buller HR, Cohen AT, Davidson B, Decousus H, Gallus AS, Gent M et al (2007) Extended prophylaxis of venous thromboembolism with idraparinux. N Engl J Med 357:1105–1112

111. Buller HR, Cohen AT, Davidson B, Decousus H, Gallus AS, Gent M et al (2007) Idraparinux versus standard therapy for venous thromboembolic disease. N Engl J Med 357:1094–1104

112. (2000) Prevention of pulmonary embolism and deep vein thrombosis with low dose aspirin: Pulmonary Embolism Prevention (PEP) trial [see comments]. Lancet 355:1295–1302

113. Hovens MM, Snoep JD, Tamsma JT, Huisman MV (2006) Aspirin in the prevention and treatment of venous thromboembolism. J Thromb Haemost 4:1470–1475

114. Buller HR, Agnelli G, Hull RD, Hyers TM, Prins MH, Raskob GE (2004) Antithrombotic therapy for venous thromboembolic disease: the Seventh ACCP Conference on Antithrombotic and Thrombolytic Therapy. Chest 126:401S–428S

115. Holbrook AM, Pereira JA, Labiris R, McDonald H, Douketis JD, Crowther M et al (2005) Systematic overview of warfarin and its drug and food interactions. Arch Intern Med 165:1095–1106

116. Dentali F, Ageno W, Crowther M (2006) Treatment of coumarin-associated coagulopathy: a systematic review and proposed treatment algorithms. J Thromb Haemost 4:1853–1863

117. Dezee KJ, Shimeall WT, Douglas KM, Shumway NM, O'malley PG (2006) Treatment of excessive anticoagulation with phytonadione (vitamin K): a meta-analysis. Arch Intern Med 166:391–397

118. Heneghan C, Alonso-Coello P, Garcia-Alamino JM, Perera R, Meats E, Glasziou P (2006) Self-monitoring of oral anticoagulation: a systematic review and meta-analysis. Lancet 367:404–411

119. O'Donnell M, Kearon C (2006) Perioperative management of oral anticoagulation. Clin Geriatr Med 22:199–213 p xi

120. Margaglione M, Brancaccio V, Giuliani N, D'Andrea G, Cappucci G, Iannaccone L, Vecchione G, Grandone E, Di Minno G (1998) Increased risk for venous thrombosis in carriers of the prothrombin G – a 20210 gene variant. Annals of Internal Medicine 129:89–93

121. DeStefano V, Martinelli I, Mannucci PM, Paciaroni K, Chiusolo P, Casorelli I et al (1999) The risk of recurrent deep venous thrombosis among heterozygous carriers of both factor V Leiden and the G20210A prothrombin mutation [see comments]. N Engl J Med 341:801–806

122. Miles JS, Miletich JP, Goldhaber SZ, Hennekens CH, Ridker PM (2001) G20210A mutation in the prothrombin gene and the risk of recurrent venous thromboembolism. J Am Coll Cardiol 37:215–218

123. Den Heijer M, Willems HP, Blom HJ, Gerrits WB, Cattaneo M, Eichinger S et al (2007) Homocysteine lowering by B vitamins and the secondary prevention of deep vein thrombosis and pulmonary embolism: a randomized, placebo-controlled, double-blind trial. Blood 109:139–144

124. Grady D, Wenger NK, Herrington D, Khan S, Furberg C, Hunninghake D et al (2000) Postmenopausal hormone therapy increases risk for venous thromboembolic disease. The Heart and Estrogen/progestin Replacement Study. Ann Intern Med 132:689–696

125. Hoibraaten E, Qvigstad E, Arnesen H, Larsen S, Wickstrom E, Sandset PM (2000) Increased risk of recurrent venous thromboembolism during hormone replacement therapy – results of the randomized, double-blind, placebo- controlled estrogen in venous thromboembolism trial (EVTET). Thromb Haemost 84:961–967

126. Rossouw JE, Anderson GL, Prentice RL, LaCroix AZ, Kooperberg C, Stefanick ML et al (2002) Risks and benefits of estrogen plus progestin in healthy postmenopausal women: principal results From the Women's Health Initiative randomized controlled trial. JAMA 288:321–333

127. Hulley S, Furberg C, Barrett-Connor E, Cauley J, Grady D, Haskell W et al (2002) Noncardiovascular disease outcomes during 6.8 years of hormone therapy: Heart and Estrogen/progestin Replacement Study follow-up (HERS II). JAMA 288:58–66

128. Baglin T, Luddington R, Brown K, Baglin C (2004) High risk of recurrent venous thromboembolism in men. J Thromb Haemost 2:2152–2155

129. Cushman M, Glynn RJ, Goldhaber SZ, Moll S, Bauer KA, Deitcher S et al (2006) Hormonal factors and risk of recurrent venous thrombosis: the prevention of recurrent venous thromboembolism trial. J Thromb Haemost 4:2199–2203

130. Kyrle PA, Minar E, Bialonczyk C, Hirschl M, Weltermann A, Eichinger S (2004) The risk of recurrent venous thromboembolism in men and women. N Engl J Med 350:2558–2563

131. Lindmarker P, Schulman S (2000) The risk of ipsilateral versus contralateral recurrent deep vein thrombosis in the leg. The DURAC Trial Study Group. J Intern Med 247:601–606

132. White RH, Zhou H, Kim J, Romano PS (2000) A population-based study of the effectiveness of inferior vena cava filter use among patients with venous thromboembolism. Arch Intern Med 160:2033–2041

Part VII
Clinical Consideration

20

Antithrombotic Therapy for Atrial Fibrillation and Cardioversion

Carmel M. Halley and Allan L. Klein

CONTENTS

ABSTRACT Thromboembolism, especially the cerebrovascular events, due to atrial fibrillation leads to significant morbidity and mortality. A fundamental part of the management of any patient with atrial fibrillation is stratification of this risk, and deciding upon suitable antithrombotic therapy. Currently, the cornerstone of anticoagulation in high risk patients is the warfarin therapy. However, despite its efficacy, warfarin has many practical limitations, and is known to be underused even when identified as the best therapy. This has led to the search for a safe and effective alternative to warfarin which, if discovered, would revolutionize anticoagulation in atrial fibrillation.

Key words: Atrial fibrillation • Thromboembolism • Stroke • Warfarin • Heparin • Cardioversion

INTRODUCTION

Atrial fibrillation is the most common cardiac arrhythmia, with an estimated prevalence of 2.3 million people in North America and 4.5 million people in the European Union *(1)*. Atrial fibrillation (AF) is characterized by chaotic uncoordinated atrial activity, resulting in deterioration of mechanical function. This predisposes to thrombus formation, especially in the left atrial appendage, due to a combination of factors including blood stasis, endothelial dysfunction, and systemic hypercoagulability *(2)*.

Thromboembolism due to AF leads to significant morbidity and mortality. Therefore, the stratification of risk and anticoagulation therapies to reduce the risk are essential aspects of the clinical management of all patients with AF, irrespective of other management strategies such as rate or rhythm control.

From: *Contemporary Cardiology: Antithrombotic Drug Therapy in Cardiovascular Disease*
Edited by: A.T. Askari and A.M. Lincoff (eds.), DOI 10.1007/978-1-60327-235-3_20
© Humana Press, a part of Springer Science+Business Media, LLC 2010

RISK OF THROMBOEMBOLISM IN ATRIAL FIBRILLATION

The risk of stroke and thromboembolism is increased up to fivefold in non-valvular AF and up to 17-fold in valvular AF. The risk of embolic events does not depend on whether AF is paroxysmal or permanent, or on the treatment strategy chosen *(3,4)*. Overall, AF is responsible for up to 25% of all ischemic cerebrovascular events. Patients with AF who have suffered a stroke have a higher mortality, greater disability, and longer hospital admissions compared to patients without AF *(5–9)*. However, it should be noted that the pathogenesis of thromboembolism in AF is complex and not solely related to embolism of thrombus generated in the left atrial appendage, with up to 25% of the events resulting from intrinsic cerebrovascular disease, other cardiac source of embolism, and atherosclerosis of the aorta *(10,11)*.

Several clinical and echocardiographic characteristics have been identified that serve as predictors of thromboembolic events in patients with AF. Clinical risk factors include a history of a prior embolic event, hypertension, diabetes mellitus, old age, coronary artery disease, and heart failure *(1)*. Echocardiographic risk factors, often more accurately identified with transesophageal echocardiography (TEE) *(12)* (Fig. 1), include increased left atrial size, impaired left ventricular systolic function, left atrial thrombus, spontaneous echocardiographic contrast (SEC), complex aortic atheroma, and evidence of left atrial mechanical dysfunction. Reduced left atrial appendage emptying velocity

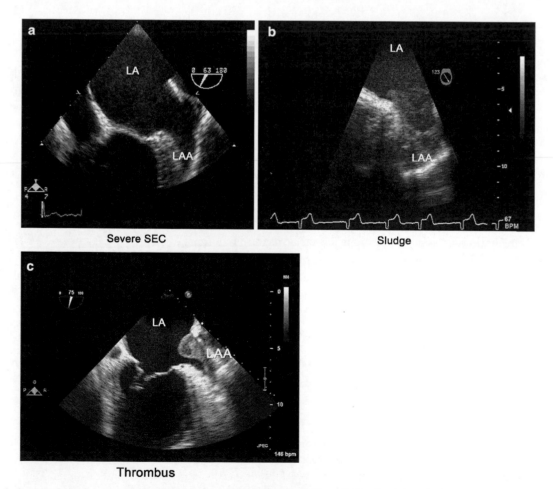

Fig. 1. Spectrum of left atrial appendage (*LAA*) thrombogenic milieu within the left atrium (*LA*) identified by transesophageal echocardiography (TEE) with (**a**) severe spontaneous contrast (SEC) (**b**) sludge and (**c**) thrombus.

(<20 cm/s) results from the loss of organized mechanical function in AF, and is associated with an increased risk of thromboembolism *(13)*. In addition, the dynamic mechanical dysfunction that occurs following cardioversion is also associated with an increased risk of thromboembolic events *(14)*. SEC attributes the smoke-like swirling echocardiographic appearance to the presence of a low flow state and red blood cell–protein interactions (rouleau formation) *(13)*. The presence of SEC has been associated with an increased risk of thromboembolism. In one study of 302 patients undergoing TEE prior to cardioversion or catheter ablation or as part of a clinical evaluation for cardiac source of embolism, the presence of a viscid layered SEC or "sludge" in the left atrial appendage is an independent predictor of all-cause mortality or thromboembolism *(15)*. The incorporation of these risk factors into predictive risk models has become an integral component of clinical decision-making.

Several risk stratification schemes for anticoagulation in AF have evolved, incorporating data from clinical trials and expert opinion (Table 1). However, a recent comparison of five different risk stratification schemes had a comparable but limited ability to predict thromboembolism. Clearly, better methods are needed to select patients for anticoagulation.

The role of other imaging modalities, including cardiac CT, continues to evolve. Despite being able to distinguish severe left atrial appendage SEC or thrombus from lesser grades of SEC *(16,17)*, a high interobserver variability and modest diagnostic accuracy for detecting left atrial thrombus in patients undergoing catheter ablation *(18)* have precluded the use of cardiac CT for the purpose of predicting events following cardioversion.

The annual stroke rate in patients with AF ranges between 3 and 8% depending on the presence of risk factors *(19)*. The lowest risk is in the so-called "lone" AF (defined as a patient younger than 60 years with no clinical history or echocardiographic features of cardiopulmonary disease) at 0.5%/year *(20)*. In patients with non-valvular AF, prior embolic event and age are the two most powerful predictors of risk. The incremental relative risk, associated with prior embolic event, is estimated at approximately 3.0 *(1,19,21)*. The annual risk of embolic events in AF is 1.5% in those younger than 60 years but increases to 23.5% in octogenarians *(19)*. It should be emphasized that based on the available data, the type of AF (paroxsysmal versus permanent) and the treatment strategy chosen (rate versus rhythm control) should not be considered as major factors in the anticoagulant decision-making process *(22–27)*.

MANAGEMENT OPTIONS

Oral anticoagulant therapy is the basis on which thromboembolism is prevented in patients with AF with over 24 published trials in patients with non-valvular AF including 20,012 patients and an average follow-up time of 1.6 years *(1,28)*. Alternative strategies such as surgical removal of the left atrial appendage have not been proven to reduce thromboembolic risk *(28)*. Ongoing clinical trials will examine the long-term safety and efficacy of surgical ligation and percutaneous occluder devices of the left atrial appendage *(29–32)*. Recently presented data from the Embolic Protection in Patients with Atrial Fibrillation (PROTECT-AF) trial have demonstrated showed that device closure using the Watchman device (Atritech, Plymouth, MN) was associated with a reduction in hemorrhagic stroke risk versus warfarin and all cause stroke was non inferior to warfarin. Further data is awaited in this developing area.

Warfarin

Warfarin, a synthetic derivative of coumarin, inhibits the vitamin K γ-carboxylation of coagulation factors II, VII, IX, and X, resulting in the synthesis of inactive coagulation proteins of the prothrombin complex *(33)*. After rapid and complete absorption, it is almost completely bound to plasma albumin with a half-life of 37 h. Clinically, there is a delay of 2–7 days in the onset of action. It is metabolized in the liver, and therefore is subject to many (up to 80) drug and food interactions.

Table 1

Risk stratification schemes for anticoagulation in atrial fibrillation

Scheme	High risk	Intermediate risk	Low risk	Management
ACC/AHA/ESC guidelines 2006	Prior thromboembolism, mitral stenosis, prosthetic heart valve	Age ≥75 years, Hypertension, heart failure, EF <35% or less, diabetes mellitus	Age 65–74 years, coronary artery disease, female gender, thyrotoxicosis (these are considered less validated or weaker risk factors)	No risk factor → Aspirin One moderate risk factor → Aspirin or Warfarin Any high risk factor or >1 moderate risk factor → Warfarin
CHADS2 2001	Score 3–6 (Score 1 for each of the recent heart failure, hypertension, diabetes; score 2 for prior stroke or TIA)	Score 1–2	Score 0	Score 0 → Aspirin Score 1–2 → Aspirin or Warfarin Score 3–6 → Warfarin
Framingham 2003	14–31 points (old age – max score <10, sex – women=6, men=0, hypertension <4, diabetes=6)	8–13 points	0–7 points	Total score corresponds to predicted 5-year stroke risk
ACCP 2004	Previous stroke or TIA or systemic thromboembolism, age >75 years, moderately or severely impaired LV function with or without heart failure, hypertension, diabetes	Age 65–75 without other risk factors	Age <65 years with no risk factors	Low risk → Aspirin Moderate risk → Aspirin or Warfarin High risk → Warfarin
Atrial Fibrillation Investigators (AFI) 1994	Age >65 years, hypertension, coronary artery disease or diabetes	Hypertension, no high risk features	Age <65, no high risk features	
SPAF Investigators trial 1995	Women >75 years, systolic blood pressure >160 mmHg, left ventricular dysfunction clinically or on echocardiogram	Hypertension, no high risk features	No history of hypertension, no high risk features	

Five large randomized trials (AFSAK 1, SPAF 1, BAATAF, CAFA and SPINAF) *(34–38)* have evaluated warfarin compared with either placebo or control in the primary prevention of thromboembolism in patients with non-valvular AF (Fig. 2) *(39)*. The European Atrial Fibrillation Trial compared phenprocoumon or acenocoumarol (other synthetic derivatives of coumarin with the same action mechanism but with different half-life compared to warfarin) and placebo in the secondary prevention of stroke among patients with non-valvular AF *(40)*. In a meta-analysis of these six trials, adjusted-dose warfarin reduced the relative risk of stroke (both ischemic and hemorrhagic) by 61% *(95% CI 47–71%)* compared to placebo *(41)*. When only ischemic strokes are considered, treatment with adjusted-dose warfarin was associated with a 65% *(95% CI 52–74)* relative risk reduction, and was equally effective in preventing disabling and non-disabling strokes *(41)*. The absolute risk reduction for all strokes is far greater for secondary stroke prevention (8.4% per year; number needed to treat for 1 year to prevent one stroke, 12) than for primary stroke prevention (2.7% per year; number needed to treat for 1 year to prevent one stroke, 37 *(41)*). In addition, adjusted-dose warfarin significantly reduced the all-cause mortality compared to placebo *(RR 0.69, 95% CI 0.53–0.89; p = 0.005) (42)*.

The main risk associated with warfarin therapy is major bleeding. Patient age and intensity of anticoagulation are the most powerful predictors of major bleeding *(43–46)*. Other factors, besides intensity of anticoagulation, associated with an increased risk of bleeding include hypertension (systolic blood pressure >180 mmHg or diastolic blood pressure >100 mmHg), alcoholism or liver disease, poor drug adherence, presence of bleeding lesions (e.g., peptic ulcer disease, intracranial hemorrhage, bleeding diatheses), and concomitant use of non-steroidal antiinflammatory drugs or specific antibiotics.

The optimum intensity of anticoagulation balances the prevention of ischemic stroke with the risk of hemorrhagic complications *(45)*. Patients with an INR of 1.7 have twice the odds of stroke *(95% CI 1.6–2.4)*, and those with an INR of 1.5 have 3.3 times the odds of stroke *(95% CI 2.4–4.6 times)* compared with those achieving an INR of 2.0 *(47)*. An INR above 3.0 increases the risk of major bleeding threefold *(OR 3.21, 95% CI 1.24–8.28) (48,49)*. Therefore, the optimum target intensity in protection against ischemic stroke is probably achieved at an INR range 2.0–3.0 *(1)*.

Clinical practice differs from the carefully selected and closely monitored population of clinical trials. Warfarin, with an unpredictable dose–response relationship, delayed the onset and offset of action and significant drug–drug and drug–food interactions requires careful monitoring with blood tests and dose adjustments. However, even with careful monitoring, initiation of warfarin dosing is associated with highly variable responses between individuals, possibly related to genetic variation. Variants of two genes, CYP2C9 and VKORC1, account for 30–50% of the variability in warfarin dosing. Recent data suggest that initial variability in the INR response to warfarin is more strongly associated with VKORC1 than with CYP2C9 *(50)*. Although the routine use of warfarin genotyping is not recommended at this time, in certain situations, CYP2C9 and VKORC1 testing may be useful and warranted in determining the cause of unusual therapeutic responses to warfarin therapy *(51)*.

These factors may help to explain the under-utilization of warfarin for anticoagulation in AF in clinical practice. A number of observational studies have confirmed that under half of all patients eligible for warfarin for AF, actually receive it *(52)*. Even among patients who have been prescribed warfarin for AF, therapeutic anticoagulation is achieved in only about 30–50% of the time *(53,54)*.

Aspirin

Aspirin offers a modest protection against stroke for patients with AF, but is inferior to warfarin in this regard and should not be considered an adequate substitute in high-risk patients. A recent large meta-analysis of 29 trials (*n* = 28,044, mean age 71 years, mean follow-up 1.5 years) concluded that

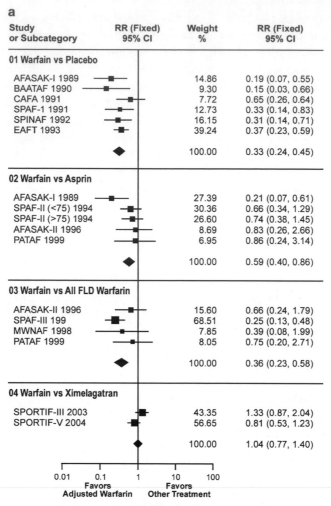

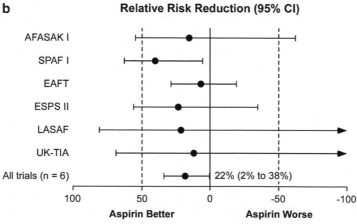

Fig. 2. (**a**) Meta-analysis of ischemic stroke or systemic embolism for adjusted-dose warfarin compared with placebo, aspirin, fixed low-dose warfarin (with or without aspirin), and ximelagatran in patients with non-valvular atrial fibrillation (*AFASAK* Copenhagen atrial fibrillation, aspirin, and anticoagulation study, *BAATAF* Boston Area Anticoagulation Trial for Atrial Fibrillation, *CAFA* Canadian Atrial Fibrillation Anticoagulation study, *CI* confidence interval, *EAFT* European Atrial Fibrillation Trial, *MWNAF* Minidose Warfarin in Non-rheumatic Atrial Fibrillation, *PATAF* Primary Prevention of Arterial Thromboembolism in Non-rheumatic Atrial Fibrillation, *RR* relative risk, *SPAF*

compared with controls, adjusted-dose warfarin (six trials, $n=2{,}900$) and antiplatelet agents (eight trials, $n=4{,}876$) reduced stroke by 64% *(95% CI 49–74)* and 22% *(95% CI 22–52)*, respectively *(55)*. Adjusted-dose warfarin was substantially more efficacious than antiplatelet therapy (RR reduction 39% *[95% CI 22–52%])* *(55)*. However, there did not appear to be an increased hemorrhagic stroke risk with warfarin as compared with aspirin *(55)*. The combination of antiplatelet therapy and low-dose warfarin is not as effective as the adjusted-dose warfarin *(56,57)*.

Meta-analysis of six randomized clinical trials ($n=3{,}119$ participants) showed a stroke reduction of 22% *(CI 2–38%)* with aspirin compared to placebo; absolute risk reductions were 1.5% per year for primary prevention and 2.5% per year for secondary prevention *(39,41)* (Fig. 2). This level of stroke reduction is similar to the effect of antiplatelet treatment in patients without AF who are at high risk for vascular disease *(58)*. Aspirin has been shown to be more effective for non-cardioembolic strokes that tend to be less disabling *(41,59)*. Therefore, the greater the risk of disabling cardioembolic stroke in a population of patients with AF, the lesser is the protection provided by aspirin *(59)*.

There is differing opinion regarding the optimum dose of aspirin in patients with AF. Based on the Antithrombotic Trialists' Collaboration, trials with a higher daily dose of aspirin did not result in statistically different proportional reductions in vascular events – 19% with 500–1,500 mg/day, 26% with 160–325 mg/day, and 32% with 75–150 mg/day compared with placebo *(58)*. The current ACC/AHA/ACC guidelines recommend aspirin use at 81–325 mg/day, while the current ACCP guidelines recommend a dose of 75–325 mg/day *(1,60)*.

Antiplatelet Therapy

Given the practical limitations associated with warfarin use and the proven effectiveness of combination antiplatelet therapy in cardiovascular disease, the ACTIVE W study was designed to test the effectiveness and safety of dual antiplatelet therapy instead of warfarin in AF *(61)*. In this study, 6,706 patients with AF were randomly assigned aspirin and clopidogrel or warfarin. However, this study was discontinued prematurely because of a lack of efficacy relative to warfarin. The ACTIVE A a randomized trial of aspirin plus clopidogrel versus aspirin alone in patients with AF unwilling or incapable of using oral anticoagulants, has found that the addition of clopidogrel to aspirin reduced the risk of stroke (2.4 % per year in clopidrogrel group vs 3.3 % in placebo, RR 0.72; 95% CI, 0.62 to 0.83; P<0.001) and increased the risk of major bleeding (2% per year occurred in 251 patients receiving clopidogrel (2.0% per year in clopidrogrel group vs 1.3% per year in placebo, RR 1.57; 95% CI, 1.29 to 1.92; P<0.001).

Low Weight Molecular Heparins

Low weight molecular heparins (LWMHs) were discovered accidentally in the late 1970s, and are prepared by depolymerization of unfractionated heparin (UFH) *(62)*. LWMHs have many pharmacological and biological advantages over UFH and have replaced it in many clinical scenarios in cardiology. These include predictable bioavailability and anticoagulant response, and fixed or weight-adjusted doses in most clinical scenarios *(63)*. Like UFH, LWMHs produce an anticoagulant effect by activating antithrombin and accelerating the rate at which it inhibits factor Xa and thrombin *(63)*.

Stroke Prevention in Atrial Fibrillation study, *SPINAF* Stroke Prevention in Non-rheumatic Atrial Fibrillation, *SPORTIF* Stroke Prevention Using the Oral Thrombin Inhibitor in Patients with Non-valvular Atrial Fibrillation). (**b**) Meta-analysis of trials comparing aspirin with placebo in reducing risk of thromboembolism in patients with atrial fibrillation (*ESPS* European Stroke Prevention Study, *LASAF* Low-Dose Aspirin, Stroke, and Atrial Fibrillation pilot study, *UK-TIA* United Kingdom Transient Ischemic Attack). Reproduced with permission from *(39)*.

There have been limited randomized controlled trials to assess the efficacy of LWMH for the prevention of thromboembolism in AF. The Anticoagulation for Cardioversion using Enoxaparin (ACE) trial demonstrated that enoxaparin was not inferior to heparin and phenprocoumon, an oral vitamin K antagonist with a serum half-life longer than warfarin *(64)*. The ACUTE II randomized trial compared the safety and efficacy of enoxaparin with UFH as antithrombotic bridging therapy in patients with AF of >48 h duration undergoing TEE-guided cardioversion *(65)*. No differences in safety outcomes were observed between the two strategies; however, the enoxaparin group was associated with a shorter hospital stay *(65)*. Further analysis with regard to resource uses and cost effectiveness demonstrated that costs of initial and subsequent hospitalizations, outpatient procedures, and emergency room visits were lower in the enoxaparin group as were average total costs *(66)*. Therefore, the use of enoxaparin as a bridging therapy for patients with AF undergoing TEE-guided cardioversion can be considered a cost-saving strategy with similar clinical outcomes and lower costs *(66)*.

NEW ANTITHROMBOTIC THERAPY FOR ATRIAL FIBRILLATION

Given the practical limitations, there has been much interest in finding agents that could replace warfarin. In the search for an alternative, two key targets in the coagulation cascade have been identified – factor Xa and thrombin (factor IIa) (Table 2). If a safe and effective alternative is discovered, it will revolutionize anticoagulation in AF.

Direct Thrombin Inhibitors

Direct thrombin inhibitors bind to thrombin (fibrin bound and fluid-phase) and block its interaction with substrates *(67)*. Three parenteral direct thrombin inhibitors are licensed in the United States for limited clinical indications – hirudin for the treatment of heparin-induced thrombocytopenia (HIT); argatroban for the treatment of HIT and for patients with or at risk of HIT who are undergoing percutaneous intervention; and bivalirudin as an alternative to UFH in patients undergoing percutaneous intervention *(62)*.

Ximelagatran is the first orally active direct thrombin inhibitor and is a prodrug of the active site-directed thrombin inhibitor, melagatran, which is eliminated via the kidneys *(67)*. Ximelagatran has a plasma half-life of 4–5 h and is administered orally twice daily without dosage adjustments or monitoring compared to warfarin *(67)*. The Stroke Prevention using an Oral Thrombin Inhibitor in AF (SPORTIF) III and V trials randomized more than 7,000 patients with non-valvular AF to adjusted-dose warfarin (INR 2–3) or fixed-dose ximelagatran *(68,69)*. These trials concluded that ximelagatran was not inferior to warfarin for the prevention of stroke and systemic embolic events. Rates of major bleeding were similar in the two groups but minor bleeding was lower in the ximelagatran group. The drug was not approved by the FDA and was removed from the European market due to hepatotoxicity, an idiosyncratic event which led to the death of three patients in preclinical testing.

Dabigatran etexilate, a prodrug of dabigatran, is an orally active, specific, competitive and reversible inhibitor of thrombin. A phase 3 trial (Randomized Evaluation of Long-term anticoagulant therapY – the RELY trial) with 14,000 patients is currently underway using dabigatran administered twice daily for the prevention of stroke or thromboembolism in patients with AF.

Factor Xa Inhibitors

Factor Xa inhibitors block factor Xa either directly by binding to the active site of factor Xa or indirectly via antithrombin *(67)*. These agents have not yet been systematically evaluated in patients with AF and cannot be recommended as a therapeutic option at this point in time.

Table 2
Possible alternatives to warfarin for anticoagulation in atrial fibrillation

Drug	Pharmacological target	Parenteral	Oral	Indications	Ongoing trials
Direct thrombin inhibitors	Bind to thrombin and block its interaction with substrates	Hirudin		Treatment of HIT	
		Argatroban		Treatment of HIT or for patient with or at high risk of HIT undergoing PCI	
		Bivalirudin		Alternative to UFH in PCI	
			Ximelagatran	Not approved by FDA	Non-inferior to warfarin in SPORTIF III and V but concerns over effects on liver enzymes
			Dabigatran	Undergoing clinical trials	RELY trial with 14,000 patients ongoing for prevention of stroke/thromboembolism in AF
Factor Xa inhibitors	Direct inhibitors act by binding to the active site of Xa		Rivaroxaban	Undergoing clinical trials	Ongoing phase 3 non-inferiority trial in patients with AF and high risk of stroke
			Apixaban	Undergoing clinical trials	Ongoing phase 3 non-inferiority trial in patients with AF for prevention of stroke and phase 3 superiority trial with aspirin
	Indirect Factor Xa inhibitors act via antithrombin	Fondaparinux (subcutaneous injection)		Treatment of ACS and DVT	
		Idraparinux (subcutaneous injection)			Excess bleeding when evaluated for stroke prevention in AF

DIRECT XA (ANTI-XA) INHIBITORS

Direct inhibitors of factor Xa inactivate both free factor Xa and factor Xa incorporated within the prothrombinase complex (70). Rivaroxaban and apixaban are oral anti-Xa inhibitors with similar properties except for the pathway of excretion – renal for rivaroxaban and biliary/fecal for apixaban. The clinical development of rivaroxaban is more advanced than apixaban with phase 2 trials in patients with deep vein thrombosis, providing proof of principle for efficacy and safety. Rivaroxaban is being compared with warfarin in a phase 3 non-inferiority, randomized, controlled trial in patients with AF at a high risk of stroke (previous ischemic stroke or at least two vascular risk factors) (62). Apixaban is being compared with warfarin for the prevention of stroke or thromboembolism in patients with AF in a phase 3 non-inferiority trial, and is being compared with aspirin in patients with AF not treated with warfarin in a phase 3 superiority trial (62).

INDIRECT FACTOR XA INHIBITORS

Fondaparinux is the only commercially available agent in this class and has been extensively evaluated in patients with acute coronary syndrome and deep vein thrombosis. It is administered once daily by subcutaneous injection. Idraparinux is a longer acting subcutaneous agent which only requires once weekly administration; however, when evaluated for prevention of stroke in patients with AF, it caused excess bleeding and is no longer being developed for this indication (62).

ANTICOAGULATION IN PATIENTS WITH ATRIAL FIBRILLATION IN CLINICAL PRACTICE

Cardioversion

Up to 50% of patients with new onset of AF spontaneously convert back to sinus rhythm within 24 h (71). If this does not occur in the stable patient, pharmacological or electrical cardioversion can be attempted. The guidelines of anticoagulation are the same irrespective of the approach undertaken--electrical or chemical. However, if the patient is hemodynamically unstable (hypotension, cardiac failure, or ischemia related to arrhythmia) at the time of presentation, immediate cardioversion may be required without further delay of achieving therapeutic anticoagulation, although heparin--either intravenous or subcutaneous--should be initiated before cardioversion (1).

Cardioversion without anticoagulation has a risk of thromboembolism that can be as high as 5.6% and usually occurs within the first week after the procedure (72). There is no significant difference in this embolic risk between electrical and chemical cardioversions (72). TEE studies have demonstrated that left atrial mechanical function declines or SEC increases after cardioversion reflecting transient left atrial mechanical dysfunction or "stunning" (14). It has also been demonstrated that transmitral atrial wave does not return to normal until 3–4 weeks after cardioversion (73). These form the basis for the current recommendations that regardless of the approach to anticoagulation pre-cardioversion and the method of cardioversion, anticoagulation should be continued empirically for 4 weeks afterwards (1).

Generally, in stable patients without high risk features and with duration of AF <48 h, cardioversion can be performed after the initiation of anticoagulation with heparin (1). In patients with AF >48 h in duration or AF of uncertain duration, there are two approaches to pre-cardioversion anticoagulation – either empirical anticoagulation for 3 weeks prior to cardioversion or a TEE-guided strategy (1). With a TEE-guided strategy, TEE is used to exclude atrial thrombi and allow immediate cardioversion with concomitant heparin (intravenous or subcutaneous). The ACUTE study was a randomized multi-center clinical trial in which 1,222 patients with either AF persisting longer than 48 h or atrial flutter were randomized to a TEE-guided strategy or a conventional strategy (74). There was no difference in the rate of stroke or thromboembolism between the two groups (0.81% vs. 0.5%,

$p = 0.5)$ but there was a significant difference in the composite end-point of major and minor bleeding $(2.9\%$ vs. 5.5%, $p = 0.02)$ (74). These results helped to establish a TEE-guided strategy to cardioversion as a safe and clinically-effective alternative to conventional management. The ACUTE II trial established that enoxaparin as a bridging therapy for patients with AF undergoing TEE-guided cardioversion is a safe and efficacious alternative to UFH and is more cost-effective $(65,66)$.

Anticoagulation and Catheter Ablation

There are two main interventional approaches for the management and potential cure of AF – percutaneous catheter-based ablation and surgical approaches (Maze procedure with associated left atrial appendage ligation or removal). Radiofrequency catheter ablation of AF with pulmonary vein isolation, although not a first-line therapy for AF, is continuing to grow as a common procedure in major hospitals throughout the world (75). Thromboembolism is recognized as one of the potential major complications of this procedure. In addition to the inherent risk of the patient population in AF, the procedure itself involves catheter manipulation in the left atrium and ablation of the left atrial endothelium can be a potential nidus for thrombus. In patients who are in AF at the time of the procedure, AF termination may be achieved at the time of the procedure by either catheter ablation or cardioversion. It is important to remember that guidelines regarding anticoagulation at the time of cardioversion apply in this circumstance. On the other hand, peri-procedural anticoagulation can contribute to complications such as hemopericardium, cardiac tamponade and vascular complications (76). Therefore, as emphasized by the recent HRS/EHRA/ECAS expert Consensus Statement, careful attention must be paid to peri-procedural anticoagulation (75).

It is recommended that in patients with persistent AF, who are in AF at the time of the procedure, a TEE be performed to screen for thrombus whether or not they have been anticoagulated prior to the procedure (75). Most operators discontinue warfarin prior to the procedure with some advocating the use of LWMH until the evening prior to the procedure. A small number of operators chose to continue anticoagulation with warfarin in a therapeutic range before, during and after the procedure. The main concern with this approach is the difficulty of managing potential bleeding complications, although it has been reported as a safe strategy (77). After the procedure if warfarin has been discontinued, anticoagulation with intravenous heparin or LWMH should be started until therapeutic anticoagulation with warfarin has been re-established. The HRS/EHRA/ECAS expert Consensus Statement advises that warfarin be continued in all patients for at least 2 months post procedure. Decisions about continuing use after 2 months should be made on the basis of risk factors for stroke and not on the presence of AF. Discontinuation of warfarin therapy is not advised in patients who have a CHADS2 score ≥2 (Table 1).

Anticoagulation and Percutaneous Coronary Intervention

For the majority of patients with stable coronary artery disease and AF, warfarin therapy alone should be a sufficient antithrombotic therapy (1). A common clinical scenario is the management of patients with AF undergoing percutaneous intervention or presenting with an acute coronary syndrome where aspirin and clopidogrel have become standard antiplatelet therapy. The combination of these therapies with warfarin increases the risk of intracranial bleeding, especially in the elderly. There have been no clinical trials to date specifically addressing this issue. The recent ACC/AHA/ESC guidelines advise that the use of dual antiplatelet therapy with 81 mg of aspirin daily and clopidogrel is pivotal in maintaining stent and coronary patency, and that these agents should be used in combination with ongoing warfarin therapy $(78,79)$. While warfarin may need to be temporarily discontinued around the time of any percutaneous procedure, it should be recommenced as soon as it is safe to do so. The intensity of anticoagulation should be carefully monitored when these agents are combined with warfarin.

Anticoagulation and Acute Stroke

There have been limited trials involving anticoagulation in patients with AF presenting with acute ischemic stroke. The presence of intracranial hemorrhage on computed tomography or magnetic resonance imaging is a contraindication to the immediate and possibly the long-term use of warfarin. If a large infarct is revealed, the initiation of anticoagulation should be delayed for 2–4 weeks because of the potential risk of hemorrhagic transformation. Randomized trials comparing aspirin with heparin during the first 2 weeks of acute ischemic stroke among patients in AF show no benefit from early anticoagulation because any net gains from reduction in ischemic strokes are offset by the excess hazards of hemorrhagic stroke *(80,81)*.

Anticoagulation and Elective Diagnostic and Therapeutic Procedures

When a need to stop anticoagulant therapy in patients with AF undergoing elective procedures arises, there is a need to balance the risk of stroke against the risk of bleeding complications if bridging short-acting anticoagulant therapy is used. In high risk patients (prosthetic heart valves, prior stroke or embolic event), it is appropriate to substitute unfractionated or LMWH once INR falls below 2.0 *(1,60)*. In patients with low risk of thromboembolism, it is reasonable to stop warfarin for a period up to 1 week for procedures that carry a risk of bleeding without substituting heparin *(1,60)*. This is based on extrapolation from the annual rate of thromboembolism in patients with non-valvular AF.

REFERENCES

1. Go AS, Hylek EM, Phillips KA et al (2001) Prevalence of diagnosed atrial fibrillation in adults: national implications for rhythm management and stroke prevention: the AnTicoagulation and Risk Factors in Atrial Fibrillation (ATRIA) Study. JAMA 285(18):2370–2375
2. Fuster V, Ryden LE, Cannom DS et al (2006) ACC/AHA/ESC 2006 Guidelines for the Management of Patients with Atrial Fibrillation: a report of the American College of Cardiology/American Heart Association Task Force on Practice Guidelines and the European Society of Cardiology Committee for Practice Guidelines (Writing Committee to Revise the 2001 Guidelines for the Management of Patients With Atrial Fibrillation): developed in collaboration with the European Heart Rhythm Association and the Heart Rhythm Society. Circulation 114(7):e257–e354
3. Kannel WB, Abbott RD, Savage DD, McNamara PM (1982) Epidemiologic features of chronic atrial fibrillation: the Framingham study. N Engl J Med 306(17):1018–1022
4. Wolf PA, Dawber TR, Thomas HE Jr, Kannel WB (1978) Epidemiologic assessment of chronic atrial fibrillation and risk of stroke: the Framingham study. Neurology 28(10):973–977
5. Saxena R, Lewis S, Berge E, Sandercock PA, Koudstaal PJ (2001) Risk of early death and recurrent stroke and effect of heparin in 3169 patients with acute ischemic stroke and atrial fibrillation in the International Stroke Trial. Stroke 32(10):2333–2337
6. Lin HJ, Wolf PA, Kelly-Hayes M et al (1996) Stroke severity in atrial fibrillation. The Framingham Study. Stroke 27(10):1760–1764
7. Marini C, De Santis F, Sacco S et al (2005) Contribution of atrial fibrillation to incidence and outcome of ischemic stroke: results from a population-based study. Stroke 36(6):1115–1119
8. Kimura K, Minematsu K, Yamaguchi T (2005) Atrial fibrillation as a predictive factor for severe stroke and early death in 15,831 patients with acute ischaemic stroke. J Neurol Neurosurg Psychiatr 76(5):679–683
9. Steger C, Pratter A, Martinek-Bregel M et al (2004) Stroke patients with atrial fibrillation have a worse prognosis than patients without: data from the Austrian Stroke registry. Eur Heart J 25(19):1734–1740

10. Bogousslavsky J, Van Melle G, Regli F, Kappenberger L (1990) Pathogenesis of anterior circulation stroke in patients with nonvalvular atrial fibrillation: the Lausanne Stroke Registry. Neurology 40(7):1046–1050

11. Miller VT, Rothrock JF, Pearce LA, Feinberg WM, Hart RG, Anderson DC (1993) Ischemic stroke in patients with atrial fibrillation: effect of aspirin according to stroke mechanism. Stroke Prevention in Atrial Fibrillation Investigators. Neurology 43(1):32–36

12. Mugge A, Kuhn H, Nikutta P, Grote J, Lopez JA, Daniel WG (1994) Assessment of left atrial appendage function by biplane transesophageal echocardiography in patients with nonrheumatic atrial fibrillation: identification of a subgroup of patients at increased embolic risk. J Am Coll Cardiol 23(3):599–607

13. Feigenbaum H, Armstrong W, Ryan T (2005) Feigenbaum's Echocardiography, 6th edn. Lippincott, William and Wilkins, Philadelphia, PA

14. Grimm RA, Stewart WJ, Maloney JD et al (1993) Impact of electrical cardioversion for atrial fibrillation on left atrial appendage function and spontaneous echo contrast: characterization by simultaneous transesophageal echocardiography. J Am Coll Cardiol 22(5):1359–1366

15. Lowe B, Varr B, Shrestha K, Whitman C, Klein AL (2007) Prognostic significance of left atrial appendage "sludge" in patients with atrial fibrillation: a new transesophageal echocardiographic thromboembolic risk factor. Circulation 116:II_687

16. Jaber WA, White RD, Kuzmiak SA et al (2004) Comparison of ability to identify left atrial thrombus by three-dimensional tomography versus transesophageal echocardiography in patients with atrial fibrillation. Am J Cardiol 93(4):486–489

17. Kim YY, Klein AL, Halliburton SS et al (2007) Left atrial appendage filling defects identified by multidetector computed tomography in patients undergoing radiofrequency pulmonary vein antral isolation: a comparison with transesophageal echocardiography. Am Heart J 154(6):1199–1205

18. Gottlieb I, Pinheiro A, Brinker JA, Lima JA, Abraham TP, Henrikson CA (2008) Resolution of left atrial appendage thrombus by 64-detector CT scan. J Cardiovasc Electrophysiol 19(1):103

19. Wolf PA, Abbott RD, Kannel WB (1991) Atrial fibrillation as an independent risk factor for stroke: the Framingham Study. Stroke 22(8):983–988

20. Kopecky SL, Gersh BJ, McGoon MD et al (1987) The natural history of lone atrial fibrillation. A population-based study over three decades. N Engl J Med 317(11):669–674

21. Stewart S, Hart CL, Hole DJ, McMurray JJ (2002) A population-based study of the long-term risks associated with atrial fibrillation: 20-year follow-up of the Renfrew/Paisley study. Am J Med 113(5):359–364

22. Carlsson J, Miketic S, Windeler J et al (2003) Randomized trial of rate-control versus rhythm-control in persistent atrial fibrillation: the Strategies of Treatment of Atrial Fibrillation (STAF) study. J Am Coll Cardiol 41(10):1690–1696

23. Hohnloser SH, Kuck KH, Lilienthal J (2000) Rhythm or rate control in atrial fibrillation – Pharmacological Intervention in Atrial Fibrillation (PIAF): a randomised trial. Lancet 356(9244):1789–1794

24. Opolski G, Torbicki A, Kosior DA et al (2004) Rate control vs rhythm control in patients with nonvalvular persistent atrial fibrillation: the results of the Polish How to Treat Chronic Atrial Fibrillation (HOT CAFE) Study. Chest 126(2):476–486

25. Van Gelder IC, Hagens VE, Bosker HA et al (2002) A comparison of rate control and rhythm control in patients with recurrent persistent atrial fibrillation. N Engl J Med 347(23):1834–1840

26. Wyse DG, Waldo AL, DiMarco JP et al (2002) A comparison of rate control and rhythm control in patients with atrial fibrillation. N Engl J Med 347(23):1825–1833

27. Fang MC, Go AS, Chang Y, Borowsky L, Pomernacki NK, Singer DE (2008) Comparison of risk stratification schemes to predict thromboembolism in people with nonvalvular atrial fibrillation. J Am Coll Cardiol 51(8):810–815

28. Healey JS, Crystal E, Lamy A et al (2005) Left Atrial Appendage Occlusion Study (LAAOS): results of a randomized controlled pilot study of left atrial appendage occlusion during coronary bypass surgery in patients at risk for stroke. Am Heart J 150(2):288–293

29. Sick PB, Schuler G, Hauptmann KE et al (2007) Initial worldwide experience with the WATCHMAN left atrial appendage system for stroke prevention in atrial fibrillation. J Am Coll Cardiol 49(13):1490–1495

30. Mobius-Winkler S, Schuler GC, Sick PB (2008) Interventional treatments for stroke prevention in atrial fibrillation with emphasis upon the WATCHMAN device. Curr Opin Neurol 21(1):64–69

31. Halperin JL, Gomberg-Maitland M (2003) Obliteration of the left atrial appendage for prevention of thromboembolism. J Am Coll Cardiol 42(7):1259–1261

32. Ostermayer SH, Reisman M, Kramer PH et al (2005) Percutaneous left atrial appendage transcatheter occlusion (PLAATO system) to prevent stroke in high-risk patients with non-rheumatic atrial fibrillation: results from the international multi-center feasibility trials. J Am Coll Cardiol 46(1):9–14

33. Holmes DR et al, 2009 .Protect AF :Randomized Prospective Trial of Percutaneous LAA Closure vs Warfarin for Stroke Prevention in AF. J Am Coll Cardiol.2009;53:A100-A143

34. (1990) The effect of low-dose warfarin on the risk of stroke in patients with nonrheumatic atrial fibrillation. The Boston Area Anticoagulation Trial for Atrial Fibrillation Investigators. N Engl J Med 323(22):1505–1511.

35. (1991) Stroke prevention in atrial fibrillation study. Final results. Circulation 84(2):527–539

36. Connolly SJ, Laupacis A, Gent M, Roberts RS, Cairns JA, Joyner C (1991) Canadian Atrial Fibrillation Anticoagulation (CAFA) Study. J Am Coll Cardiol 18(2):349–355

37. Ezekowitz MD, Bridgers SL, James KE et al (1992) Warfarin in the prevention of stroke associated with nonrheumatic atrial fibrillation. Veterans Affairs Stroke Prevention in Nonrheumatic Atrial Fibrillation Investigators. N Engl J Med 327(20):1406–1412

38. Petersen P, Boysen G, Godtfredsen J, Andersen ED, Andersen B (1989) Placebo-controlled, randomised trial of warfarin and aspirin for prevention of thromboembolic complications in chronic atrial fibrillation. The Copenhagen AFASAK study. Lancet 1(8631):175–179

39. Lip GY, Boos CJ (2006) Antithrombotic treatment in atrial fibrillation. Heart 92(2):155–161

40. (1993) Secondary prevention in non-rheumatic atrial fibrillation after transient ischaemic attack or minor stroke. EAFT (European Atrial Fibrillation Trial) Study Group. Lancet 342(8882):1255–1262.

41. Hart RG, Benavente O, McBride R, Pearce LA (1999) Antithrombotic therapy to prevent stroke in patients with atrial fibrillation: a meta-analysis. Ann Intern Med 131(7):492–501

42. Lip GY, Edwards SJ (2006) Stroke prevention with aspirin, warfarin and ximelagatran in patients with non-valvular atrial fibrillation: a systematic review and meta-analysis. Thromb Res 118(3):321–333

43. Fang MC, Chang Y, Hylek EM et al (2004) Advanced age, anticoagulation intensity, and risk for intracranial hemorrhage among patients taking warfarin for atrial fibrillation. Ann Intern Med 141(10):745–752

44. Fihn SD, Callahan CM, Martin DC, McDonell MB, Henikoff JG, White RH (1996) The risk for and severity of bleeding complications in elderly patients treated with warfarin. The National Consortium of Anticoagulation Clinics. Ann Intern Med 124(11):970–979

45. Hylek EM, Singer DE (1994) Risk factors for intracranial hemorrhage in outpatients taking warfarin. Ann Intern Med 120(11):897–902

46. Oden A, Fahlen M, Hart RG (2006) Optimal INR for prevention of stroke and death in atrial fibrillation: a critical appraisal. Thromb Res 117(5):493–499

47. Hylek EM, Skates SJ, Sheehan MA, Singer DE (1996) An analysis of the lowest effective intensity of prophylactic anticoagulation for patients with nonrheumatic atrial fibrillation. N Engl J Med 335(8):540–546

48. Hylek EM, Go AS, Chang Y et al (2003) Effect of intensity of oral anticoagulation on stroke severity and mortality in atrial fibrillation. N Engl J Med 349(11):1019–1026

49. Reynolds MW, Fahrbach K, Hauch O et al (2004) Warfarin anticoagulation and outcomes in patients with atrial fibrillation: a systematic review and metaanalysis. Chest 126(6):1938–1945

50. Schwarz UI, Ritchie MD, Bradford Y et al (2008) Genetic determinants of response to warfarin during initial anticoagulation. N Engl J Med 358(10):999–1008

51. Flockhart DA, O'Kane D, Williams MS et al (2008) Pharmacogenetic testing of CYP2C9 and VKORC1 alleles for warfarin. Genet Med 10(2):139–150

52. Sudlow M, Thomson R, Thwaites B, Rodgers H, Kenny RA (1998) Prevalence of atrial fibrillation and eligibility for anticoagulants in the community. Lancet 352(9135):1167–1171

53. Bungard TJ, Ackman ML, Ho G, Tsuyuki RT (2000) Adequacy of anticoagulation in patients with atrial fibrillation coming to a hospital. Pharmacotherapy 20(9):1060–1065

54. Jones M, McEwan P, Morgan CL, Peters JR, Goodfellow J, Currie CJ (2005) Evaluation of the pattern of treatment, level of anticoagulation control, and outcome of treatment with warfarin in patients with non-valvar atrial fibrillation: a record linkage study in a large British population. Heart 91(4):472–477

55. Hart RG, Pearce LA, Aguilar MI (2007) Meta-analysis: antithrombotic therapy to prevent stroke in patients who have nonvalvular atrial fibrillation. Ann Intern Med 146(12):857–867

56. Cowburn P, Cleland JG (1996) SPAF-III results. Eur Heart J 17(7):1129

57. Gullov AL, Koefoed BG, Petersen P et al (1998) Fixed minidose warfarin and aspirin alone and in combination vs adjusted-dose warfarin for stroke prevention in atrial fibrillation: Second Copenhagen Atrial Fibrillation, Aspirin, and Anticoagulation Study. Arch Intern Med 158(14):1513–1521

58. Antithrombotic Trialists' Collaboration (2002) Collaborative meta-analysis of randomised trials of antiplatelet therapy for prevention of death, myocardial infarction, and stroke in high risk patients. BMJ 324(7329):71–86

59. Hart RG, Pearce LA, Miller VT et al (2000) Cardioembolic vs. noncardioembolic strokes in atrial fibrillation: frequency and effect of antithrombotic agents in the stroke prevention in atrial fibrillation studies. Cerebrovasc Dis 10(1):39–43

60. Singer DE, Albers GW, Dalen JE, Fang MC, Go AS, Halperin JL, Lip G, Manning WJ (2008) Antithrombotic therapy in atrial fibrillation: the Eighth ACCP Conference on Antithrombotic and Thrombolytic Therapy. Chest 133:546S–592S

61. Connolly S, Yusuf S, Budaj A et al (2006) Rationale and design of ACTIVE: the atrial fibrillation clopidogrel trial with irbesartan for prevention of vascular events. Am Heart J 151(6):1187–1193
62. ACTIVE A investigators. (2009) Effect of clopidogrel added to aspirin in patients with atrial fibrillation. NEJM 14;360(20):2066–2078
63. De Caterina R, Husted S, Wallentin L et al (2007) Anticoagulants in heart disease: current status and perspectives. Eur Heart J 28(7):880–913
64. Stellbrink C, Nixdorff U, Hofmann T et al (2004) Safety and efficacy of enoxaparin compared with unfractionated heparin and oral anticoagulants for prevention of thromboembolic complications in cardioversion of nonvalvular atrial fibrillation: the Anticoagulation in Cardioversion using Enoxaparin (ACE) trial. Circulation 109(8):997–1003
65. Klein AL, Jasper SE, Katz WE et al (2006) The use of enoxaparin compared with unfractionated heparin for short-term antithrombotic therapy in atrial fibrillation patients undergoing transoesophageal echocardiography-guided cardioversion: assessment of Cardioversion Using Transoesophageal Echocardiography (ACUTE) II randomized multicentre study. Eur Heart J 27(23):2858–2865
66. Zhao L, Zhang Z, Kolm P et al (2008) Cost in the use of Enoxaparin compared with unfractionated heparin in patients with atrial fibrillation undergoing a transesophageal echocardiography-guided cardioversion (from assessment of cardioversion using transesophageal echocardiography [ACUTE] II randomized multicenter study). Am J Cardiol 101(3):338–342
67. Hirsh J, O'Donnell M, Weitz JI (2005) New anticoagulants. Blood 105(2):453–463
68. Olsson SB (2003) Stroke prevention with the oral direct thrombin inhibitor ximelagatran compared with warfarin in patients with non-valvular atrial fibrillation (SPORTIF III): randomised controlled trial. Lancet 362(9397):1691–1698
69. Albers GW, Diener HC, Frison L et al (2005) Ximelagatran vs warfarin for stroke prevention in patients with nonvalvular atrial fibrillation: a randomized trial. JAMA 293(6):690–698
70. Eikelboom JW, Weitz JI (2007) A replacement for warfarin: the search continues. Circulation 116(2):131–133
71. Naccarelli GV, Wolbrette DL, Khan M et al (2003) Old and new antiarrhythmic drugs for converting and maintaining sinus rhythm in atrial fibrillation: comparative efficacy and results of trials. Am J Cardiol 91(6A):15D–26D
72. Klein AL, Murray RD, Grimm RA (2001) Role of transesophageal echocardiography-guided cardioversion of patients with atrial fibrillation. J Am Coll Cardiol 37(3):691–704
73. Prystowsky EN, Benson DW Jr, Fuster V et al (1996) Management of patients with atrial fibrillation. A Statement for Healthcare Professionals. From the Subcommittee on Electrocardiography and Electrophysiology, American Heart Association. Circulation 93(6):1262–1277
74. Klein AL, Grimm RA, Murray RD et al (2001) Use of transesophageal echocardiography to guide cardioversion in patients with atrial fibrillation. N Engl J Med 344(19):1411–1420
75. Calkins H, Brugada J, Packer DL et al (2007) HRS/EHRA/ECAS expert Consensus Statement on catheter and surgical ablation of atrial fibrillation: recommendations for personnel, policy, procedures and follow-up. A report of the Heart Rhythm Society (HRS) Task Force on catheter and surgical ablation of atrial fibrillation. Heart Rhythm 4(6):816–861
76. Cappato R, Calkins H, Chen SA et al (2005) Worldwide survey on the methods, efficacy, and safety of catheter ablation for human atrial fibrillation. Circulation 111(9):1100–1105
77. Wazni OM, Beheiry S, Fahmy T et al (2007) Atrial fibrillation ablation in patients with therapeutic international normalized ratio: comparison of strategies of anticoagulation management in the periprocedural period. Circulation 116(22):2531–2534
78. Lip GY, Karpha M (2006) Anticoagulant and antiplatelet therapy use in patients with atrial fibrillation undergoing percutaneous coronary intervention: the need for consensus and a management guideline. Chest 130(6):1823–1827
79. Lip GY, Tse HF (2007) Management of atrial fibrillation. Lancet 370(9587):604–618
80. (1997) The International Stroke Trial (IST): a randomised trial of aspirin, subcutaneous heparin, both, or neither among 19435 patients with acute ischaemic stroke. International Stroke Trial Collaborative Group. Lancet 349(9065):1569–1581
81. Berge E, Abdelnoor M, Nakstad PH, Sandset PM (2000) Low molecular-weight heparin versus aspirin in patients with acute ischaemic stroke and atrial fibrillation: a double-blind randomised study. HAEST Study Group. Heparin in Acute Embolic Stroke Trial. Lancet 355(9211):1205–1210

21

Antithrombotic Therapy for Valvular Heart Disease

Noah Rosenthal and Brian D. Hoit

CONTENTS

ABSTRACT Certain native valvular diseases and prosthetic valves require anticoagulation in order to prevent catastrophic thrombotic consequences. Anticoagulation strategies and the treatment of complications are areas under constant reevaluation and study. There are multiple sources of recommendations, and three major societies have produced guidelines (ACCP, AHA/ACC, ESC) which make up the bulk of commonly accepted practice. This is a review and evaluation of the guidelines and a counterpoint of current study and opinions

Key words: Anticoagulation; Antithrombotic therapy; Atrial fibrillation; Mitral annular calcification; Mitral stenosis; Mitral valve prolapse; Pregnancy; Prosthetic valve; Prosthetic valve thrombosis; Fibrinolysis

Although the elegant design of cardiac valves provides reduced shear surfaces for linear flow and efficient function, the interruption of this blueprint by aging, disease, or prosthesis and the resulting imbalance of anti- and pro-coagulant forces that comprise Virchow's triad (injury, turbulent flow, and stasis) create the milieu for thromboembolism (TE). Because of the potentially devastating effects that may follow, optimization of anti-thrombotic regimens has been an intense area of refinement and exploration. The present chapter summarizes the most recent publications and recommendations from the three major guideline documents from the 7th American College of Chest Physicians conference on antithrombotic and thrombolytic therapy (ACCP, 2004), the American Heart Association/American College of Cardiology (AHA/ACC, 2006), and the European Society of Cardiology which published their guidelines in 2005 and 2007 *(1–4)*. This body of work comprises the contemporary foundation for the management of antithrombotic therapy in valvular heart disease.

From: *Contemporary Cardiology: Antithrombotic Drug Therapy in Cardiovascular Disease*
Edited by: A.T. Askari and A.M. Lincoff (eds.), DOI 10.1007/978-1-60327-235-3_21
© Humana Press, a part of Springer Science+Business Media, LLC 2010

NATIVE VALVE DISEASE

Risk Factors

In accordance with all currently published guidelines for patients in normal sinus rhythm with native valvular disease, primary prophylaxis against thromboembolic events is indicated only for mitral stenosis, and then, only when additional risk factors are present (antithrombotic therapy is recommended for mitral valve prolapse and mitral annular calcification after an embolic episode, see below). Mitral stenosis creates a milieu of stasis in the left atrium upon which additional risk factors greatly increase the risk of a subsequent thrombotic event. Factors currently recognized as imparting the greatest risk are atrial fibrillation (AF), left ventricular dysfunction, prior thromboembolic events, and perturbations of the coagulation cascade.

From a pathophysiological perspective, hypertension and its cardiovascular complications – AF, heart failure, and left ventricular hypertrophy – produce a prothrombotic state *(5)*. Although heart failure and left ventricular dysfunction are known prothrombotic states imparting an increased risk of thromboembolic events, prophylactic anticoagulation with warfarin has not been shown to improve outcomes *(6,7)*.

The risk factor of thrombophilias (e.g., antiphospholipid antibodies, resistance to activated protein C, factor V Leiden, prothrombin gene polymorphisms, protein C deficiency, protein S deficiency, Antithrombin III deficiency) are themselves sufficient grounds for anticoagulation.

Atrial fibrillation is increasingly common as the population ages. It conveys an increased risk of thromboembolism with advancing age, hypertension, heart failure, diabetes, and prior thrombotic event, in turn elevating the relative risk of an embolic event in men by 2.4 and in women by 3 compared to matched controls *(8,9)*. While the rate of stroke is higher in selected patient populations with an increasing number of risk factors (greater than 10 strokes per 100 patient-years in those most at risk) *(10)*, the use of warfarin in an unselected group of individuals with atrial fibrillation will reduce the incidence of stroke by approximately 65% *(9)*. As alluded to earlier, atrial fibrillation may itself impart a prothrombotic state beyond simple flow-related effects. Investigators found increased levels of plasma von Willebrand factor, vascular endothelial growth factor, and angiopoietin-2 in 59 chronic AF patients compared to healthy controls and postulated that these changes altered tissue factor expression and endothelial integrity, consistent with earlier, preliminary observations *(11,12)*.

It is no surprise that patients with the highest incidence of stroke are those with previous thromboembolic events, having already demonstrated a substrate prone to generating thrombi. A recent meta-analysis showed that in the absence of antithrombotic therapy among patients with prior strokes, the yearly average stroke rate is approximately 13% compared to 4.1% in those without a prior stroke *(13)*. This trend holds true in patients with mitral stenosis as well.

Mitral Stenosis

The presumptive mechanism of increased thrombogenicity in mitral stenosis (MS) is the remodeling of the left atrium and appendage that occurs due to pressure and volume overload. Slow and non-linear flow in the enlarged atrium leads to further atrial dysfunction and increased spontaneous echo contrast associated with an increased risk of atrial thrombus *(14)*. In addition, the expression of immunoreactive von Willebrand factor is increased in the endothelium of the left atrial appendage in patients with mitral valve disease (with and without atrial fibrillation) and may be a predisposing factor for atrial thrombus *(15)*. Compounding the risk of thrombus is the common presence of superimposed atrial fibrillation which imparts a sevenfold increase in the risk of TE events *(16)*.

While non-anticoagulated mitral stenosis is uncommon in countries with intensive health care surveillance, older studies cited in the 7th ACCP review reported an associated incidence of TE events in up to 27% in these patients, with a future risk of detectable TE event in a patient with unrepaired rheumatic mitral valve disease of approximately one in five *(1)*, making MS the highest risk valvular lesion for TE. Guidelines support anticoagulation with vitamin K antagonists (VKA) for mitral stenosis patients in normal sinus rhythm only when additional risk factors are present. These risk factors are: prior thromboembolism, dense spontaneous echocardiographic contrast on TEE, and a moderately enlarged left atrial size – a reflection of the functional impact of stenosis and harbinger of further dysfunction. If atrial fibrillation develops [a frequency of 30–40% in the MS population *(17)*], then anticoagulation is recommended. As mentioned earlier, the highest incidence of embolus occurs in those who have already had emboli, and these patients should have rigorously monitored anticoagulation therapy.

There has been debate regarding the optimal degree of anticoagulation. A sub-analysis of the multicenter randomized NASPEAF (National Study for Prevention of Embolism in Atrial Fibrillation) trial compared 184 high-embolic-risk patients with atrial fibrillation to 311 patients with atrial fibrillation and mitral stenosis (including bioprosthetic valve replacements). Patients were randomized to achieve an INR 2–3 or a more moderate dose anticoagulation (INR 1.4–2.4) plus 600 mg triflusal (antiplatelet agent equivalent to 300 mg aspirin). The combined antiplatelet/moderate anticoagulant therapy compared to anticoagulant alone significantly reduced the number of vascular events (14 vs. 29 in an intention to treat analysis and 6 vs. 28 for "on-therapy" analysis). The study concluded that a combined regimen of moderate intensity anticoagulation and antiplatelet agent is effective in mitral stenosis *(18)*.

Mitral Valvuloplasty

The 7th ACCP guidelines recommend a limited period of anticoagulation both before and after mitral valvuloplasty to reduce the theoretical risk of periprocedural stroke. However, there are no randomized control trials (RCT) to support this premise, and the data is extrapolated from prior atrial fibrillation studies and "good sense."

Mitral Valve Prolapse

Mitral valve prolapse (MVP) is a frequently identified form of valvular disease in adults. Once thought to be the most common form of valvular heart disease, Freed et al. showed that the true prevalence of MVP in an unselected, community-based sample of ambulatory subjects (2.4%) is lower than previously reported (up to 15%) *(19)*. The association of MVP and ischemic stroke has been controversial, in part due to this overdiagnosis. Revision of the diagnostic criteria in the 1980s led to a reduced incidence of MVP, casting doubt on the validity of earlier studies linking MVP to stroke. Supporting this, Gilon et al. showed that MVP was no more common among young patients with unexplained cerebral embolic events than among control subjects *(20)*. In contrast, Avierinos showed a small but significant independent risk of stroke associated with MVP, conferring a lifetime excess rate of events twice that of a comparable population; in patients without other risk factors for TE, age, and increased valve thickness conferred higher risk *(21)*. However, the incidence of overall TE in this population remains low and the guidelines do not endorse antithrombotic therapy in asymptomatic patients.

In the event of a transient ischemic attack (TIA), the institution of long-term aspirin (50–162 mg/day) therapy should be initiated. Patients with subsequent TIA on aspirin or documented systemic embolism should progress to full anticoagulation with VKA (goal INR 2.0–3.0).

Mitral Annular Calcification

Population-based studies have shown both an increased relative risk of stroke *(22)* and a reduced time to first TE event *(23)* in patients with mitral annular calcification compared to those without MAC. Interestingly, although associated with all the same atherosclerotic risk factors, aortic valve sclerosis has not been shown to confer an increased risk of stroke *(23)*. Patients with MAC have a higher incidence of AF, diffuse atherosclerotic disease, left atrial enlargement, and disruption of laminar flow across the valve, all of which increase the risk of TE *(24)*. Importantly, embolism from this type of lesion may also be calcific, for which anticoagulation is not therapeutic. Therefore for patients with a demonstrated TE lesion that is not calcific, the ACCP recommends anticoagulation (INR 2–3). For the asymptomatic patient with MAC, optimal management is uncertain. Although there is an empiric rationale for prophylactic anticoagulation, MAC is typically a degenerative process more common in elderly patients, and the ACCP encourages careful consideration of risk/benefits in this population without severe disease. They offer the "uncertain compromise" of antiplatelet therapy with aspirin or clopidogrel, although there are no data to support this strategy. Table 1 is a composite of the guideline recommendations for the management of native valve disease and antithrombotic therapy.

PROSTHETIC HEART VALVES

By current guidelines, anticoagulation is indicated for all mechanical valves, for bioprosthetic valves in patients with high-risk features for TE, and for the first 3 months after the implantation of a bioprosthetic heart valve, as this time period has the highest incidence of thromboembolic risk (i.e., before endothelialization of implanted hardware). The benefit of a bioprosthetic valve is the reduced need for life-long anticoagulation and thus freedom from the added morbidity of vitamin K antagonists (VKA) in patients who (1) otherwise do not need anticoagulation, (2) are at high risk for bleeding complications, or (3) cannot take VKA.

Mechanical Valves

It is well known that all current mechanical heart valves require anticoagulation with warfarin or a VKA in order to prevent TE. However, the degree of anticoagulation necessary to prevent TE has been a topic of considerable debate, and since 2004 three major writing groups (ACCP, ACC/AHA, ESC) have formalized the management of these patients *(1,2,4)*. Their recommendations are similar, with occasional divergence reserved for specialized situations. Table 2 shows current recommendations for the ACCP and ACC/AHA, and Fig. 1 shows a scheme from the ESC.

While VKAs and heparin have been well studied in the PHV population, newer agents like low molecular weight heparins have been a source of some controversy in selected populations (pregnant women specifically) and will be addressed in the section on pregnant patients. LMWH is generally considered an acceptable alternative to heparin for temporary or bridging therapy in non-pregnant patients *(1–4)*. It has been studied in multiple trials and shown to be efficacious and potentially cost saving. Routine checking of anti-factor Xa levels (therapeutic range defined as 0.5–1.0 IU/ml) is not typically required, with the exception of pregnant patients in whom variable plasma volumes and renal clearance require surveillance*(25)* (for details, see section on pregnancy and PHV). A well-known limitation to the use of LMWH is the lack of easy reversibility in the setting of a bleed (although enoxaparin is described as being up to 60% reversible with 1 mg protamine per 1 mg enoxaparin) *(26)*.

Current studies report a yearly incidence of TE around 4% in patients with prosthetic valves, whereas older analyses range up to a high of 22% annual incidence in patients without anticoagulation *(27–32)*. The ranges in reported incidence of stroke rates differ depending on the method of data collection and patient-related factors *(2)*. It is certain that the likelihood of stroke is dependent on the type of valve (mechanical vs. bioprosthetic), the type of design (e.g., caged ball, tilting disk, bileaflet), the material used (newer valves are less thrombogenic), the number of valves and their position (e.g., aortic vs. mitral). The variability in incidence is also due in part to the evolving population of

Table 1
Succinct guidelines for native valve disease and anticoagulation

	Mitral stenosis and NSR Only if:	Mitral stenosis and atrial fib or previous history of embolism	Mitral stenosis on anticoagulation with additional thromboembolic event or TIA	Mitral valve prolapse Only if:	Mitral valve valvulotomy	MAC	Mobile aortic atheromas
ACCP 2004 (1)	LA≥55 mm: INR 2–3	INR 2–3	INR 2–3+ASA 75–100 mg or Dipyridamole 400 mg/day or Clopidogrel 75 mg/day	TIA:ASA 50–162 mg/day Systemic embolism on ASA: INR 2–3	2–3 for 3 weeks prior and 4 weeks after procedure	If systemic non-calcific embolism: INR 2–3	>4 mm by TEE: INR 2–3
ESC 2007 (3)	Prior embolism LA>50 mm TEE with dense spontaneous contrast INR 2–3	INR 2–3	INR 2–3	NR	NR	NR	NR
ACC/AHA 2006 (4)	Severe MS and LA≥55 mm or LA thrombus	Indicated[a]	Indicated[a]	TIA or prior CVA without risk factors[b]:ASA 75–325 mg/day Stroke and/or MR, AF, atrial thrombus: INR 2–3 Prior stroke + Thickened/redundant valve leaflets >5 mm recurrent TIA on aspirin: INR 2–3	NR	NR	NR

NR No Recommendation provided in guidelines

[a] ACC/AHA guidelines do not specify a range for anticoagulation

[b] Risk factors: evidence of MR, atrial fibrillation, left atrial thrombus, echocardiographic evidence of valvular thickening > 5 mm

Table 2
Summary of guideline recommendations for antithrombotic therapy for prosthetic

ACCP guidelines (1): recommendations for prosthetic heart valves – mechanical

Use warfarin or other vitamin K antagonist bridged with UFH or LMWH until the INR is stable and at goal for 2 days. When VKA must be discontinued, use LMWH for bridging

Goal INR 2.5 (range 2.0–3.0)	*Goal INR 3.0 (range 2.5–3.5)*	*Goal INR 3.0 (range 2.5–3.5)+ASA 75–100 mg/day*
Aortic position St. Jude Medical or CarboMedics bileaflet mechanical valves without other risk factors	Mitral position tilting disk and bileaflet mechanical valves	Mechanical valves in the setting of additional risk factors[a] Systemic embolism despite a therapeutic INR
		Caged ball or caged disk valves

ACCP guidelines (1): recommendations for prosthetic heart valves – bioprosthetic

Warfarin or other vitamin K antagonist with UFH or LMWH bridging until the INR is stable and at goal for 2 days

Goal INR 2.5 (range 2.0–3.0)for a limited time period	*Goal INR 2.5 (range 2.0–3.0)*	*ASA 75–100 mg/day*
Bioprosthetic MV for the first 3 months after valve implant	Bioprosthetic valves with: Left atrial thrombus at surgery	Bioprosthetic valve, sinus rhythm without a history of atrial fibrillation
Bioprosthetic AV for the first 3 months after valve insertion OR aspirin 80–100 mg/day	Atrial fibrillation	Bioprosthetic AV for the first 3 months after valve insertion (or VKA with a goal INR 2–3)
Bioprosthetic valves and a history of systemic embolism, for 3–12 months		

ACC/AHA guidelines (4): prosthetic heart valves – mechanical and bioprosthetic

INR 2.0–3.0	*ASA 75–100 mg/day*	*Warfarin+ASA 75–100 mg/day*
Aortic position mechanical valve: bileaflet or Medtronic HallBioprosthetic AVR+risk factors[a]	Aortic or mitral bioprosthesis and no risk factors	Mechanical or bioprosthetic heart valves+risk factors[a]
Aortic or mitral bioprosthetic valve: For 3 months after implant and no risk factors	*ASA 75–325 mg/day*	*INR 3.5–4.5OR Clopidogrel 75 mg/day*
INR 2.5–3.5		High-risk[a] patients with prosthetic heart valves when aspirin cannot be used
Aortic position mechanical valve: For 3 months after implant	Patients who are unable to take VKA after MV replacement or AVR	
Bileaflet or Medtronic Hall+risk factors[a] (with option of ASA)		
Starr-Edwards or disc valves (other than Medtronic Hall)		
Mechanical MV (any type)		
Bioprosthetic MV+risk factors[a]		

INR international normalized ratio, *AVR* aortic valve replacement, *MV* mitral valve, *VKA* vitamin K antagonist

[a]Risk factors include: AF, myocardial infarction, left atrial enlargement, endocardial damage, or low ejection fraction, prior thromboembolism, left ventricular dysfunction, and a hypercoagulable state

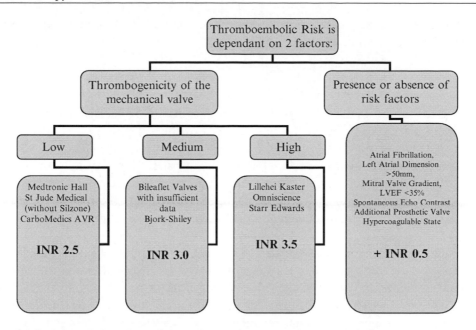

Fig. 1. General principles of thromboembolic risk according to the ESC. [Adapted from ESC Guidelines *(2,3)*.] Optimal INR is determined by inherent valve thrombogenicity and addition of applicable risk factors.

implanted valves (i.e., TE incidence has decreased as older generations of more thrombogenic valves are replaced or their hosts die).

Further confounding the definition of an optimal INR is the variability of INR levels in a single patient over time. The value of a recommended INR goal is based on the expectation that patients are actually at goal. Kulik et al. show subtherapeutic INRs are recorded in up to 50% of patients followed in large studies *(33)*. Further, Kulik showed that TE events occurring early (but after the first 6 months of anticoagulation to permit time for endothelialization) are up to seven times greater than those occurring later. They go on to suggest that this trend is due to improved compliance and familiarity with VKA. Ultimately, all the guidelines recommend that tailoring therapy to the individual patient with their particular set of risk factors is necessary to attain the most appropriate level of anticoagulation.

While the likelihood of TE can be reduced by increasing the level of anticoagulation, this benefit is counterbalanced by an increased risk of both major and minor bleeding. A similar dilemma exists for aspirin, particularly if the median INR is >3.0 *(1)*, and so the ACCP limits their recommendation of adding aspirin only to certain patient subsets felt to pose a higher risk. In contrast, a best evidence review of all published data from 1966 to 2004 concluded that low-dose aspirin (80–100 mg daily) in addition to warfarin reduces all cause long-term mortality (NNT = 19), with significant reductions in thromboembolism, and the increased bleeding was significant only for minor bleeds *(34)*.

GUIDELINES AND RECOMMENDATIONS

Although there are a few specific items of discrepancy, the three major guideline formats are similar *(1,3,4)*. The recommendations can be found in Table 2. The degree of anticoagulation for aortic valves is generally accepted as an INR of 2–3. Mitral valves are recommended to have a higher INR goal of 2.5–3.5, and aspirin can be added for additional risk factors or embolus in the setting of therapeutic anticoagulation. The ESC guidelines for anticoagulation with PHV can be thought of as stepwise levels of anticoagulation based on the inherent valve thrombogenicity and superimposed risk factors (see Fig. 1). Specific circumstances are discussed below.

Bioprosthetic Valves

The advantage of bioprosthetic valves is their decreased thrombogenicity, making lifelong anticoagulation unnecessary in the absence of TE risk factors. Low-dose aspirin (75–100 mg) is universally recommended, with increased doses (up to 325 mg) appropriate for compelling reasons (status post percutaneous intervention or stroke), or in the event that a patient has the indication for VKA, but cannot take warfarin. Warfarin is endorsed in the setting of TE risk factors (atrial fibrillation, prior TE, LV dysfunction, hypercoagulable state). If warfarin is used, then the patient should be bridged with unfractionated heparin or low molecular weight heparin until therapeutic INRs are established for 2 days.

While all three guidelines support the use of routine anticoagulation after bioprosthetic valve implantation for the first 90 days with at least aspirin or warfarin if possible, the data supporting this practice are conflicting. After 3 months, the valve is considered to be endothelialized and treated as a native valve early postoperatively with the addition of lifelong low-dose aspirin. However, recent reviews highlight that no study has shown anticoagulation with VKA leads to a reduction or increase in adverse outcomes (35,36); the authors conclude that with more research, aspirin alone may suffice for TE prophylaxis in the first 90 days after implantation, effectively removing the indication for warfarin in this setting (36).

PREGNANCY AND ANTICOAGULATION

In patients with prosthetic valves, persistent high-grade reliable anticoagulation is necessary to reduce the incidence of valve thrombosis and thromboembolism. Pregnancy itself is not only a procoagulant state, but is associated with an asymmetric risk/benefit; that is, the benefits associated with anticoagulation must be weighed against the risks attendant to both the fetus and mother. Bleeding (both fetal and maternal) as well as the teratogenic effect of the anticoagulant lie on one end of the spectrum with strokes and valve thrombosis at the other. While warfarin and other coumarin derivatives cross the placenta with demonstrated potential for teratogenic and hemorrhagic side effects, unfractionated and low molecular weight heparins do not cross and are safer for the fetus. However, retrospective cohorts have shown that this protection to the fetus comes at the expense of a higher incidence of maternal complications. Coumadin use for the entirety of pregnancy is associated with lowest all-cause maternal mortality and TE (1.8 and 3.9%, respectively), but a high rate of embryopathy (>6.4%) (37). Exchange of VKA for heparin at or prior to week 6 and continuing through the first trimester reduced the incidence of embryopathy to 0%, but increases the risk of valve thrombosis (9.2%) (37). However, none of the anticoagulation regimens markedly impacts the incidence of spontaneous abortion or fetal demise (ranges of 23.8–24.8% and 26.5–42.9%, respectively) (37).

It should be noted that recommendations are hampered by a paucity of data in this area, with a notable lack of randomized controlled trials evaluating the various methods of anticoagulation for these patients. Therefore data are based on literature reviews of case series and retrospective cohorts with consensus agreements. With no well-defined optimal method of anticoagulation, warfarin, unfractionated heparin, and most controversially low molecular weight heparin are the available options.

Warfarin has not been shown to cause an anticoagulant effect in breast milk fed infants, and may be resumed after delivery. Provided the mother is hemodynamically stable, the ACC recommends resumption of unfractionated heparin to therapeutic levels 4–6 h after delivery as a bridge *(4)* until INR returns to goal.

Subcutaneous BID dosing of UFH derived to keep the PTT at least twice normal (i.e., in the therapeutic range) 6 h after administration for the duration of the pregnancy is an option. However, long-term exposure to UFH yields an increased risk of heparin-induced thrombocytopenia (HIT) and heparin-induced osteoporosis(HIO), as well as evidence of variable anticoagulation: as adjusted dose heparin alone has the highest incidence of TE complications (29% in one study)*(38)*. Two leading reviews offer similar recommendations suggesting if UFH is used, high doses (35,000–40,000 units split BID) should be given and titrated to keep the PTT therapeutic in a range of 2–2.5× normal *(37,39)*.

Given its convenient ease of administration, presumed lack of teratogenicity, reduced incidence of HIT and HIO, and typically weight-based formulation, LMWH is one of the more appealing anticoagulation agents for the pregnant population. However, the degree of anticoagulation turns out to be less certain for weight-based dosing in pregnant women, and the vital necessity to assure adequate levels of anticoagulation has made for controversy regarding its use. In a study comparing enoxaparin to warfarin and UFH in pregnant women with prosthetic valves, two deaths (out of seven) from acute valve thrombosis led to the early termination of the study and a labeling change from the makers of Lovenox. Ultimately revised, according to Sanofi-Aventis and the package insert "the use of Lovenox has not been adequately studied for thromboprophylaxis in patients with mechanical prosthetic heart valves and has not been adequately studied for long-term use in this patient population" *(26)*. However, anti-factor Xa levels were subtherapeutic in one patient, were unclear in the other *(40)*, and further reviews of all available data suggest LMWH compared to UFH may be a safe and effective option in patients with mechanical prosthetic heart valves but require vigilant dosing to account for changes in clearance *(40)*. A scheme proposed by Elkayam *(39)* is shown compared to the recommendations of the ACC/AHA and ACCP in Table 3. Endorsing a monitored regimen, a review of 51 pregnancies with monitored anti-factor Xa levels had only one reported thromboembolic complication *(41)*. As such, recommendations have been made to monitor weekly anti-factor Xa levels in the first trimester as plasma volume and creatinine clearance fluctuate. Thereafter it is left to the discretion of the treating physician *(40)*.

A recent study evaluating nadroparin (available in Europe) substitution from weeks 6–12 and at delivery compared to coumarin derivative and aspirin throughout the pregnancy in 25 women over 31 pregnancies, showed less fetopathy and markedly more live and healthy births in the former group. Although this benefit was balanced by an increase in maternal death and valve thrombosis, the incidence was too small to be significant *(42)*.

The 7th ACCP Conference on Anticoagulation and Thrombolytic Therapy concluded that a definitive recommendation was not possible due to the lack of studies and data, but recommendations based on what evidence is available are shown in Table 3. In sum, there is no ideal plan as all carry varied risk either to the mother or to the fetus. However, of utmost importance is a detailed discussion and therapeutic plan in conjunction with the patient, cardiologist, and high-risk obstetrician, being sure that all parties are aware of the risks of bleeding, fetal wastage, teratogenesis, and mortality. Ideally, this discussion happens prior to conception, so that frequent pregnancy testing and UFH or LMWH substitution can occur when pregnancy is achieved. However, any of the three regimens are possible: (1) Warfarin with initiation of UFH or LMWH from conception until week 13 and late into the third trimester or at delivery (to avoid an anticoagulated fetus) with a goal INR 3.0 (range 2.5–3.5). For bileaflet aortic valves without concurrent atrial fibrillation or impaired ventricular function, a goal of 2.0–3.0 is acceptable. (2) Aggressive dose-adjusted UFH throughout the pregnancy. (3) Dose-adjusted LMWH throughout the pregnancy.

Table 3
A comparison of anticoagulation schemes for pregnant women with PHV

	6–12 weeks	13–35 weeks	36 weeks–delivery
7th ACCP (1)3 methods (1)	LMWH q 12 h (4 h anti-Xa 1.0–1.2) or SC UFH BID (35,000–40,000 U/day) Q 6 h aPTT "therapeutic"	Warfarin (INR 2.5–3.5) (2.0–3.0 for bileaflet AV)	LMWH or SC UFH
(2)	Aggressive dose-adjusted UFH		
(3)	Aggressive dose-adjusted LMWH "Some women at high risk" should have 75–162 mg aspirin daily added to the regimen throughout		
ACC/AHA (4)	Avoid warfarin Continuous(IV)/Dose-adjusted (SC) UFH (goal q 6 h aPTT 2× control) or Dose-adjusted LMWH BID (4 h anti-Xa 0.7–1.2)	Warfarin (INR 3.0) or Continuous/Dose-adjusted UFH or Dose-adjusted LMWH Aspirin 75–100 mg daily starting in second trimester	Continuous/Dose-adjusted UFH (2–3 week prior to planned delivery) Resume 4–6 h after delivery is completed
Elkayam et al. (39) High Risk[a]	Warfarin (INR 2.5–3.5) SC UFH (aPTT >2.5×) or LMWH (predose anti-Xa ~0.7)	Warfarin (INR 3.0)	IV UFH (aPTT 2.5–3.5×)+ aspirin 80–100 mg daily or LMWH+aspirin 80–100 mg daily
Low Risk[b]	SC UFH (aPTT 2.0–3.0×) or LMWH (4 h anti-Xa ~0.6)		
Low Risk[b]	SC UFH (aPTT 2.0–3.0×) or LMWH (predose anti-Xa ~0.6)	Warfarin (INR 2.5–3.0)	SC UFH or LMWH

[a]High-risk valves are older generation mechanical prosthetic valves, those in mitral position, atrial fibrillation, and a history of thromboembolism on anticoagulation
[b]Low-risk valves are newer generation or those in aortic position

All guidelines agree that VKA should be changed to UFH or LMWH in the middle of the third trimester prior to delivery in order to reduce bleeding complications at time of delivery, with UFH carrying the additional ease of brisk reversibility.

PROSTHETIC VALVE THROMBOSIS

Thrombotic and bleeding calamities comprise the majority of complications in patients with prosthetic valves. Prosthetic valve thrombosis (PVT) occurs most often with mechanical prostheses and to a lesser extent, early after implantation of bioprosthetic valves (i.e., before endothelialization of the suture zone); it is more common in right-sided prostheses compared to left sided, and more common in the mitral than aortic position. The incidence of obstructive PVT is estimated at 0.3–1.3% patient-years. Thromboemboli occur more commonly (0.7–6% patient-years), and small, non-obstructing thrombi are surprisingly common (an incidence as high as 24% in the first postoperative year) *(43,44)*. Thus, PVT should be considered in any patient with a prosthetic valve presenting with an embolic event, shortness of breath, or fatigue. The clinical presentation is variable, depending to a large extent on the presence and degree of prosthetic obstruction. The duration of symptoms is not particularly helpful, as valve dysfunction can evolve slowly, permitting cardiac compensation with mounting thrombus or pannus burden and progressive impairment, or abrupt valvular failure leading to sudden cardiac compromise. PVT can be due to outflow obstruction by the mass of the thrombus or pannus or by impairing leaflet mobility (Figs. 2 and 3). Inadequate anticoagulation has been shown to be the most potent factor in the pathogenesis of valve thrombosis *(45)*; therefore non-compliance or planned interruption of anticoagulation in particular as well as a new prothrombotic environment or low-flow state should further raise suspicion. Although rare, native valve thrombosis has been described, typically in the aortic position and associated with valvular abnormalities or a hypercoagulable state *(46–51)*. Valvular dysfunction can be due to thrombus, pannus (an excessive cicatrical inflammatory response to the foreign valve surface usually seen in proximity to the suture site), or frequently, a combination of the two. Even in the presence of distinct clinical clues (e.g., inadequate anticoagulation, recent implantation, prothrombotic milieu), it is important to try and differentiate between the two, as pannus ingrowth is not treatable with fibrinolytics. One small study of 24

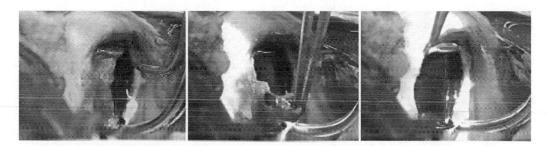

Fig. 2. Thrombosed mechanical valve intraoperative view of a bileaflet mechanical mitral valve with obstructive thrombus before *(left panel)*, during *(middle panel)*, and after *(right panel)* thrombectomy (Courtesy of Dr. A. Cobanoglu, University Hospitals Case Medical Center).

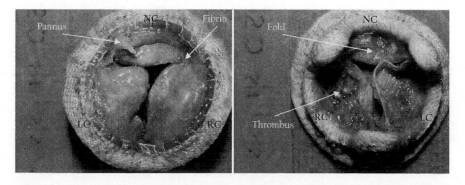

Fig. 3. Thrombosed bioprosthetic homograft with frozen leaflets due to thrombus. (Courtesy of Dr. A. Markowitz, University Hospitals Case Medical Center.) *RC* right coronary cusp; *NC* non-coronary cusp; *LC* left coronary cusp.

patients evaluated clinical and echocardiographic parameters (TEE) to distinguish between pannus and thrombus: 92% of thrombi were soft masses, pannus tended to be smaller and denser, and a videointensity ratio (videointensity of the mass compared to that of the prosthetic valve) was lower in thrombi: a ratio < 0.70 had a positive predictive value of 87% and a negative predictive value of 89% for thrombus *(52)*.

Diagnosis

The physical examination as well as imaging modalities are employed to assist diagnosis. A change in heart sounds, muffled prosthetic clicks, new murmurs, and signs of heart failure or embolism should heighten concern and further imaging should be pursued without delay. A subtherapeutic INR, inflammatory markers, and elevated D-dimer may be seen. While transthoracic and transesophageal echocardiography are the mainstay of bedside evaluation, fluoroscopy can confirm the diagnosis with mechanical prostheses by showing restricted leaflet movement, or with contrast injection to demonstrate valvular reflux. However, cinefluoroscopy is less valuable in cases of non-obstructive PVT. If thrombosis is the cause of valve dysfunction, it is important to investigate the etiology, as merely blaming the valve, patient, or medical compliance and intensifying the antithrombotic regimen may hide another diagnosis such as malignancy, endocarditis, or paroxysmal or asymptomatic atrial fibrillation.

Echocardiography allows direct visualization of the prosthesis and estimation of valvular gradients, flows, and effective orifice areas. For a mitral prosthesis, a mean gradient (measured by planimetry of diastolic mitral inflow) greater than 8 mmHg and an effective orifice area less than 1.4 cm^2 (measured by pressure half-time) suggest PVT. Values for aortic PVT include a mean transaortic gradient greater than 45 mmHg and an obstructive index (the ratio of LV outflow tract to peak aortic velocity) less than 0.25 *(53)*. However, prosthesis size in conjunction with underlying hemodynamics must be taken into account; although reference tables are available for the different prostheses, the most valuable reference is a patient's baseline postoperative echocardiogram (e.g., at the first postoperative office visit). A transesophageal echocardiogram should be performed if any clinical suspicion persists after a transthoracic examination. Thrombi may be sized (see below) and to a certain extent, differentiated from pannus, sutures, vegetations, and fibrous strands. Because of acoustic shadowing from the esophageal window, the ventricular surface of prosthesis is often poorly visualized; for this reason, the transthoracic and transesophageal approaches should be considered complimentary.

Treatment

Treatment consists of anticoagulation with heparin, fibrinolysis, thrombectomy, or valve replacement in both pregnant and non-pregnant patients *(54)*. Lysis and surgery carry both morbidity and mortality rates proportional to NYHA class *(55)*. Streptokinase, urokinase, and recombinant tissue plasminogen activator have all been used successfully for lysis. Traditionally, surgery has been considered first line therapy with left-sided PVT, given the risk of TE with lysis. Though carrying the added morbidity and mortality of reoperation, surgery has a reduced risk of thromboembolism, stroke, and hemorrhage. For those too unstable or decompensated for surgery, fibrinolysis is considered a feasible alternative. However, there is debate endorsing the use of fibrinolytics, and optimal management is unclear beyond the recognition that rational decision-making and therapy should be tailored to the set of circumstances particular to each patient (location of the valve, hemodynamic stability, degree of obstruction, size of thrombus, comorbidities, and services available at the institution).

The ACC/AHA guidelines (Fig. 4) endorse surgery as a "reasonable" (Class IIa) first line management with fibrinolysis reserved for specific situations. However, the lack of Class I therapeutic recommendations reflect the sources of data from small cohorts and case studies. The ACC/AHA document deems

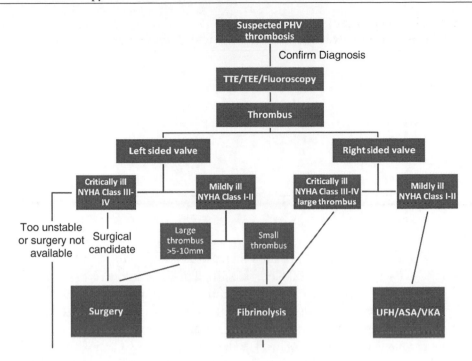

Fig. 4. Management of prosthetic valve thrombosis according to the ACC/AHA *(4)*.

Table 4
Indications for surgical management of PVT

Obstruction from endocarditis
Abscess
Large thrombus
Mobile mass
Thrombolytic therapy failure

Adapted from Lengyel et al. *(56)*

fibrinolysis reasonable for right-sided valves with NYHA class III-IV symptoms. Citing ineffectiveness and a 12–15% incidence of cerebral emboli, the ACC/AHA reserve lysis with left-sided thromboses to patients with small clot burden and minor symptoms (NYHA class I-II) or with severe failure (NYHA III-IV) if they are high surgical risk or if surgery is unavailable *(4)*. The ESCs recommendations are congruent but more aggressive than the ACC/AHA. Acknowledging that any therapy is high risk, surgery for critically ill patients without serious comorbidities is given a Class I indication. Fibrinolysis is recommended only for patients not likely to survive surgery or with right-sided prostheses.

In marked distinction, supporting fibrinolysis since 1997 *(56)* Lengyel et al. writing for the Society for Heart Valve Disease in 2005 published recommendations reiterating support for fibrinolysis as the first line therapy independent of position, NYHA class, or thrombus size *(57)*. A meta-analysis from the same author reported improved outcomes over the last 30 years with a lower overall lower embolic rate than cited by the AHA guidelines (4%), improved success (90%), and low mortality (2.5%) *(58)*. Further, if lytic therapy fails to improve valve hemodynamics, the patient can still be taken to surgery. Serial TEEs are strongly recommended during lytic therapy to monitor hemodynamics and cardiac response to lytic intervention *(57)*. The embolic risk of lytic use is directly proportional to the size of

Table 5
Patients at risk for adverse outcomes from fibrinolytic therapy

Active internal bleeding
History of hemorrhagic stroke
Recent cranial trauma or neoplasm
Hemorrhagic retinopathy
Large thrombi
Mobile thrombi
Hypertension (>200/120)
Hypotension or shock
NYHA Class III–IV

Adapted from Bonow et al. *(4)*

the clot. Tong et al. showed the odds of a complication increase as a linear function by 2.41 for every 1 cm^2 of thrombus, but that a thrombus area of <0.8 cm^2 identified patients at low risk for complications independent of NYHA class *(59)*. These data can help to define a group of patients that would benefit from fibrinolytics regardless of their degree of illness. Clearly not all patients are candidates for lytic therapy, and the surgical indications and lytic contraindications are shown in Tables 4 and 5.

Valve thrombosis in pregnant patients is not well addressed in the ACCP, ACC/AHA, or ESC guidelines. In recent publications, the prevailing opinion proposes lytic therapy as first line treatment (in the absence of contraindications) due to the attendant risks of anesthesia and surgery to the mother and fetus *(54,59,60)*.

While anticoagulation alone may be used for smaller thrombi, especially if lytics are contraindicated, this strategy is inadequate for thrombi greater than 5 mm *(57)*.

Prevention

Following a TE event, attention should be focused on ameliorating or reversing the potential risk factors and optimizing the consistency of anticoagulation. A regimen can be enhanced by adding ASA or increasing goal INR by 0.5 to a maximum of 3.5–4.5. If ASA is added, it should be low dose (<100 mg/day) and used with INR<2.5–3.5 *(2)*. While 20% of PVT treated with lytics will recur, more than 90% of those can be treated successfully with repeated fibrinolysis *(61)*.

MISCELLANEOUS TOPICS: WITHOLDING ANTICOAGULATION, BRIDGING THERAPY, OVER-ANTICOAGULATION, BLEEDING EMERGENCIES

Withholding Anticoagulation

The theoretical risk of withholding chronic anticoagulation on a daily basis is low. For a patient at the highest risk with a normal INR (an estimated yearly risk of TE=20%) the additive daily risk is 0.20/365=.055%. Thus, the risk of TE while holding anticoagulation for 1 week would be 0.055%×7=0.38%. A small retrospective study examining bleeding events in patients with PHVs found no thrombotic complications in patients with anticoagulation held for up to 3 weeks *(62)*. Those patients on chronic anticoagulation presenting for surgery with a low risk of bleeding can ideally have surgery without reversal (often cited examples are dermatologic and ophthalmologic procedures or dental extractions). If therapy must be suspended then a decision regarding thromboembolic risk and whether to bridge the patient with a parenteral anticoagulant must be made. Usually at least 81 mg of aspirin can be tolerated during the surgery to provide a margin of protection, but if aspirin or ADP antagonists need to be stopped, 5 to 7 days provide adequate washout. Oral anticoagulation is usually stopped 48 to 72 h prior to surgery and the patient is either admitted for continuous infusion UFH or allowed to remain at home for self-administrated LMWH (BID UFH is less commonly used). However, not all PHVs require an anticoagulant bridge, and as per the ACC/AHA: for low-risk patients (bi-leaflet AVR with no risk factors) a heparin bridge is usually unnecessary; and warfarin can then be restarted 24 h following surgery. For all other situations, bridging should begin when the INR drops below 2, and resumed 4–6 h after surgery is completed as hemodynamic stability permits. Heparin is discontinued once the INR is therapeutic again.

Bridging Therapy

There are two scenarios that classically invoke the issue of "bridging therapy," that is, the use of a "bridging" anticoagulant to provide seamless anticoagulation therapy during times of stoppage or initiation of oral VKA: (1) initiation of anticoagulation after new prosthetic valve implantation, and (2) the stoppage of anticoagulation in anticipation of a surgery with high bleeding risk that requires normalization of INR. The issue of initiation of anticoagulation with UFH or LMWH is still a subject of continued debate, given the large risk of hemorrhagic complications after valve surgery compared to the thromboembolic risks of a foreign surface, turbulent prosthetic flow, and a postoperative pro-thrombotic state (see section regarding new valve implantation for details).

In general, there are two options for parenteral anticoagulant: UFH or LMWH (enoxaparin and dalteparin in most studies). Continuous intravenous UFH has traditionally been the agent of choice. However, the use of LMWH has been increasingly frequent despite the relatively limited data available for its use compared to heparin. The justification for LMWH advantage over UFH includes the daily or q 12 h dosing (reducing the patient tethering to intravenous infusions), the simplicity of sub-cutaneous injections, ease of self-administration, fewer dosing errors, less underdosing with a weight-based algorithm (thus faster therapeutic levels), reduced incidence of heparin-induced thrombocytopenia, and during long-term administration, less osteoporosis. A major advantage of UFH over LMWH is its straightforward and rapid reversibility. Although the unit cost of LMWH is seven times more expensive than UFH, when the associated cost of administration, lab testing, nursing assistance, and extra hospital days are factored into the equation, LMWH often ends up being a more cost-effective option *(25,40,63,64).*

When patients with prosthetic valves need to have their oral anticoagulation interrupted for invasive procedures, the simplicity and reduced patient discomfort from fewer blood draws makes LMWH desirable. This has been shown to be an effective method of bridging anticoagulation in 116 patients (31 with mitral valve replacements, 76 aortic valve replacements, 9 double valve replacements). There was one major bleeding complication, no valve thrombosis, and minor bleeding occurred in 10 patients *(65).* Routine monitoring of anti-Xa levels in the absence of renal failure (serum creatinine >1.5 or creatinine clearance <30 ml/min) or pregnancy is not warranted. When checked, then levels should be 0.5–1.0 IU/ml, checked pre-dose as well as 3–4 h after administration, and the goal should be maintained at high levels (~0.7 IU/ml) *(40).* However, in counterpoint to the recommendations of Seshadri et al., the ESC endorses the use of UFH over LMWH. They acknowledge that LMWH can be used, but has limited data and is best tailored with anti-Xa levels if possible.

One of the expected complications of VKA therapy is over-anticoagulation. Management can usually be conservative, with simple holding or reduction of further doses of warfarin until the INR trend returns to therapeutic range. The risk of hemorrhage increases markedly for INR>6 (up to 4% of patients treated with simple withholding of warfarin) *(66),* and so at this level caution and further recommendations have been proposed, although there are no formal guidelines, and therapeutic intervention (or lack thereof) should be directed to the particular patient situation. Reversal of anticoagulation and abrupt changes in INR poses a theoretical risk of increased thrombogenicity. However, this is not well demonstrated in clinical data, and so reversal, if deemed necessary, should not be withheld for fear of thrombosis. To this end, the ACC/AHA discourage the use of high-dose vitamin K in emergencies, preferring the use of FFP (class IIa), and make routine administration for non-emergent situations a class III indication.

The optimal method of reversal remains poorly defined. The understood goal for the over-anticoagulated patient who is not actively bleeding is to return to appropriate levels of INR without leaving the patient subtherapeutic and thus at risk of thrombosis. Vitamin K in all forms: IV, oral, and subcutaneous have been used and are effective. Vitamin K is usually given in low dose (1 mg) and is comparable to 1 unit of fresh frozen plasma (FFP) at 6 h *(67)*. One milligram of oral vitamin K compared to watchful waiting for patients with INRs 6–12 showed faster correction into therapeutic range in 24 h, with 10% of patients' INR less than 1.8; however, no thrombotic complications occurred *(68)*. When an anticoagulated patient presents with a life-threatening bleed, complete reversal is necessary. Oral vitamin K has been shown to have a slower onset, but equal effectiveness in reversing supra-therapeutic INR compared to IV formulations *(69)*. The recognized drawback of intravenous administration is a small risk of anaphylactoid reactions which can be minimized by slow administration of vitamin K over 60 min diluted in 50 cc of normal saline. FFP, though only transiently providing complete reversal, is as effective an option as IV vitamin K *(67)*. For patients on ADP receptor antagonists, platelet transfusion is usually unnecessary, but can be used to provide functional platelets in a crisis.

REFERENCES

1. Salem DN, Stein PD, Al-Ahmad A et al (2004) Antithrombotic therapy in valvular heart disease – native and prosthetic: the Seventh ACCP Conference on Antithrombotic and Thrombolytic Therapy. Chest 126(3 Suppl):457S–482S
2. Butchart EG, Gohlke-Bärwolf C, Antunes MJ et al (2005) Working groups on valvular heart disease, thrombosis, and cardiac rehabilitation and exercise physiology, European Society of Cardiology. Recommendations for the management of patients after heart valve surgery. Eur Heart J 26(22):2463–71
3. Vahanian A, Baumgartner H, Bax J et al (2007) Guidelines on the management of valvular heart disease: the task force on the management of valvular heart disease of the European Society of Cardiology. Eur Heart J 28:230–268
4. Bonow RO, Carabello BA, Chatterjee K et al (2006) ACC/AHA 2006 guidelines for the management of patients with valvular heart disease: a report of the American College of Cardiology/American Heart Association Task Force on Practice Guidelines (writing committee to revise the 1998 Guidelines for the Management of Patients with Valvular Heart Disease): developed in collaboration with the Society of Cardiovascular Anesthesiologists: endorsed by the Society for Cardiovascular Angiography and Interventions and the Society of Thoracic Surgeons. Circulation 114:e84–e231
5. Varughese GI, Lip GY (2005) Is hypertension a prothrombotic state? Curr Hypertens Rep 7(3):168–73
6. Cleland JG, Findlay I, Jafri S et al (2004) The Warfarin/Aspirin Study in Heart Failure (WASH): a randomized trial comparing antithrombotic strategies for patients with heart failure. Am. Heart J 148(1):157–64
7. Massie BM, Krol WF, Ammon SE et al (2004) The Warfarin and Antiplatelet Therapy in Heart Failure trial (WATCH): rationale, design, and baseline patient characteristics. J Card Fail 10(2):101–12
8. Wolf PA, Abott RD, Kannel WB (1991) Atrial fibrillation as an independent risk factor for stroke: the Framingham Study. Stroke 22((8):983–8
9. Hart RG, Halperin JL, Pearce LA et al (2003) Stroke prevention in atrial fibrillation investigators. Lessons from the stroke prevention in atrial fibrillation trials. Ann Intern Med 138:831–838
10. Gage BF, van Walraven C, Pearce L et al (2004) Selecting patients with atrial fibrillation for anticoagulation: stroke risk stratification in patients taking aspirin. Circulation 110(16):2287–2292
11. Freestone B, Chong AY, Lim HS, Blann A, Lip GY (2005) Angiogenic factors in atrial fibrillation: a possible role in thrombogenesis? Ann Med 37(5):365–72

12. Nakamura Y, Nakamura K, Fukushima-Kusano K et al (2003) Tissue factor expression in atrial endothelia associated with nonvalvular atrial fibrillation: possible involvement in intracardiac thrombogenesis. Thromb Res 111(3):137–42

13. Hart RG, Pearce LA, Aguilar MI (2007) Meta-analysis: antithrombotic therapy to prevent stroke in patients who have nonvalvular atrial fibrillation. Ann Intern Med 146(12):857–67

14. Fatkin D, Kelly RP, Feneley MP (1994) Relations between left atrial appendage blood flow velocity, spontaneous echocardiographic contrast and thromboembolic risk in vivo. J Am Coll Cardiol 23(4):961–9

15. Fukuchi M, Watanabe J, Kumagai K et al (2001) Increased von Willebrand factor in the endocardium as a local predisposing factor for thrombogenesis in overloaded human atrial appendage. J Am Coll Cardiol 37(5):1436–42

16. Szekely P (1964) Systemic embolization and anticoagulant prophylaxis in rheumatic heart disease. BMJ 1:209–212

17. Rowe JC, Bland EF, Sprague HB, White PD (1960) The course of mitral stenosis without surgery: ten- and twenty-year perspectives. Ann Intern Med 52:741–9

18. Perez-Gomez F, Salvador A, Zumalde F, for the National Study for Prevention of Embolism in Atrial Fibrillation Investigators et al (2006) Effect of antithrombotic therapy in patients with mitral stenosis and atrial fibrillation: a subanalysis of NASPEAF randomized trial. European Heart Journal 27:960–967

19. Freed LA, Levy D, Levine RA et al (1999) Prevalence and clinical outcome of mitral-valve prolapse. N Engl J Med 341:1–7

20. Gilon D, Buonanno FS, Joffe M (1999) Lack of evidence of an association between mitral-valve prolapse and stroke in young patients. N Engl J Med 341:8–13

21. Avierinos JF, Brown RD, Foley DA et al (2003) Cerebral ischemic events after diagnosis of mitral valve prolapse: a community-based study of incidence and predictive factors. Stroke 34:1339–1344

22. Benjamin EJ, Plehn JF, D'Agostino RB et al (1992) Mitral annular calcification and the risk of stroke in an elderly cohort. N Engl J Med 327(24):1761–2

23. Kizer JR, Wiebers DO, Whisnant JP et al (2005) Mitral annular calcification, aortic valve sclerosis, and incident stroke in adults free of clinical cardiovascular disease: the strong heart study. Stroke 36(12):2533–2537

24. Fox CS, Parise H, Vasan RS et al (2004) Mitral annular calcification is a predictor for incident atrial fibrillation. Atherosclerosis 173(2):291–4

25. Goldhaber SZ (2006) "Bridging" and mechanical heart valves: perils, promises, and predictions. Circulation 113:470–472

26. Lovenox package insert; Sanofi-Adventis U.S. LLC Bridgewater, NJ 08807

27. Cannegieter SC, Rosendaal FR, Wintzen AR et al (1995) Optimal oral anticoagulant therapy in patients with mechanical heart valves. N Engl J Med 333.11

28. Cannegieter SC, Rosendaal FR, Brlet E (1994) Thromboembolic and bleeding complications in patients with mechanical heart valve prostheses. Circulation 89:635

29. Kontozis L, Skudicky D, Hopley MJ et al (1998) Long-term follow-up of St. Jude medical prosthesis in a young rheumatic population using low-level warfarin anticoagulation: an analysis of the temporal distribution of cause of death. Am J Cardiol 81.736

30. Hammermeister KE, Sethi GK, Henderson WG et al (2000) Outcomes 15 years after valve replacement with a mechanical versus bioprosthetic valve. J Am Coll Cardiol 36:1152–1158

31. Baudet EM, Puel V, McBride JT et al (1995) Long-term results of valve replacement with the St. Jude Medical prosthesis. J Thorac Cardiovasc Surg 109:858–870

32. Bjork VO, Henze A (1975) Management of thrombo-embolism after aortic valve replacement with the Bjork-Shiley tilting disc valve: medicamental prevention with dicumarol in comparison with dipyridamole-acetylsalicylic acid; surgical treatment of prosthetic thrombosis. Scand J Thorac Cardiovasc Surg 9:183–191

33. Kulik A, Rubens FD, Wells PS et al (2006) Early postoperative anticoagulation after mechanical valve replacement: a systematic review. Ann Thorac Surg 81(2):770–81

34. Nagarajan DV, Lewis PS, Botha P, Dunning J (2004) Is addition of anti-platelet therapy to warfarin beneficial to patients with prosthetic heart valves? Interact CardioVasc Thorac Surg 3:450–455

35. Nowell J, Wilton E, Markus H, Jahangiri M (2007) Antithrombotic therapy following bioprosthetic aortic valve replacement. Eur J Cardiothorac Surg 31(4):578–85

36. Colli A, Verhoye JP, Leguerrier A, Gherli T (2007) Anticoagulation or antiplatelet therapy of bioprosthetic heart valves recipients: an unresolved issue. Eur J Cardiothorac Surg 31(4):573–7

37. Chan WS, Anand S, Ginsberg JS (2000) Anticoagulation of pregnant women with mechanical heart valves: a systematic review of the literature. Arch Intern Med 160(2):191–196

38. Sadler L, McCowan L, White H, Stewart A, Bracken M, North R (2000) Pregnancy outcomes and cardiac complications in women with mechanical, bioprosthetic and homograft valves. BJOG 2:245–53

39. Elkayam U, Singh H, Irani A, Akhter MW (2004) Anticoagulation in pregnant women with prosthetic heart valves. J Cardiovasc Pharmacol Ther 9(2):107–15

40. Seshadri N, Goldhaber SZ, Elkayam U et al (2005) The clinical challenge of bridging anticoagulation with low-molecular-weight heparin in patients with mechanical prosthetic heart valves: an evidence-based comparative review focusing on anticoagulation options in pregnant and nonpregnant patients. Am Heart J 150:27–34
41. Oran B, Lee-Parritz A, Ansell J (2004) Low molecular weight heparin for the prophylaxis of thromboembolism in women with prosthetic mechanical heart valves during pregnancy. Thromb Haemost 92(4):747–51
42. Lee JH, Park NH, Keum DY, Choi SY, Kwon KY, Cho CH (2007) Low molecular weight heparin treatment in pregnant women with a mechanical heart valve prosthesis. J Korean Med Sci 22(2):258–261
43. Laplace G, Lafitte S, Labeque JN et al (2004) Clinical significance of early thrombosis after prosthetic mitral valve replacement: a postoperative monocentric study of 680 patients. J Am Coll Cardiol 43(7):1283–90
44. Deviri E, Sareli P, Wisenbaugh T, Cronje SL (1991) Obstruction of mechanical heart valve prostheses: clinical aspects and surgical management. J Am Coll Cardiol 17(3):646–50
45. Dürrleman N, Pellerin M, Bouchard D et al (2004) Prosthetic valve thrombosis: twenty-year experience at the Montreal Heart Institute. J Thorac Cardiovasc Surg 127(5):1388–92
46. Jobic Y, Provost K, Larlet JM et al (1999) Intermittent left coronary occlusion caused by native aortic valve thrombosis in a patient with protein S deficiency. J Am Soc Echocardiogr 12:1114–6
47. Massetti M, Babatasi G, Saloux E, Bhoyroo S, Grollier G, Khayat A (1999) Spontaneous native aortic valve thrombosis. J Heart Valve Dis 8:157–9
48. Unger P, Plein D, Pradier O, LeClerc JL (2004) Thrombosis of aortic valve homograft associated with lupus anticoagulant antibodies. Ann Thorac Surg 77:312–4
49. Wan S, DeSmet JM, Vincent JL, LeClerc JL (1997) Thrombus formation on a calcific and severely stenotic bicuspid aortic valve. Ann Thorac Surg 64:535–6
50. Yasaka M, Tsuchiya T, Yamaguchi T (1993) Mobile string-like thrombus on the calcified aortic valve in cardioembolic stroke – a case report. Angiology 44:655–9
51. Barandon L, Clerc P, Chauvel C, Plagnol P (2004) Native aortic valve thrombosis: a rare cause of acute ischemia of the lower limb. Interact Cardiovasc Thorac Surg 3(4):675–7
52. Barbetseas J, Nagueh SF, Pitsavos C, Toutouzas PK, Quinones MA, Zoghbi WA (1998) Differentiating thrombus from pannus formation in obstructed mechanical prosthetic valves: an evaluation of clinical, transthoracic and transesophageal echocardiographic parameters. J Am Coll Cardiol 32(5):1410–7
53. Roudaut R, Serri K, Lafitte S (2007) Thrombosis of prosthetic heart valves: diagnosis and therapeutic considerations. Heart 93(1):137–42
54. Koller PT, Arom KV (1995) Thrombolytic therapy of left-sided prosthetic valve thrombosis. Chest 108(6):1683–9
55. Elkayam U, Bitar F (2005) Valvular heart disease and pregnancy: part II: prosthetic valves. J Am Coll Cardiol 46(3):403–10
56. Lengyel M, Fuster V, Keltai M et al (1997) Guidelines for management of left-sided prosthetic valve thrombosis: a role for thrombolytic therapy. Consensus Conference on Prosthetic Valve Thrombosis. J Am Coll Cardiol 30(6):1521–6
57. Lengyel M, Horstkotte D, Völler H, Mistiaen WP (2005) Working Group Infection, Thrombosis, Embolism and Bleeding of the Society for Heart Valve Disease. Recommendations for the management of prosthetic valve thrombosis. J Heart Valve Dis 14(5):567–75
58. Lengyel M (2005) Thrombolysis should be regarded as first-line therapy for prosthetic valve thrombosis in the absence of contraindications. J Am Coll Cardiol 45(2):325 author reply 326
59. Tong AT, Roudaut R, Ozkan M et al (2004) Prosthetic Valve Thrombolysis-Role of Transesophageal Echocardiography (PRO-TEE) Registry Investigators. Transesophageal echocardiography improves risk assessment of thrombolysis of prosthetic valve thrombosis: results of the international PRO-TEE registry. J Am Coll Cardiol 43(1):77–84
60. Choi C, Midwall S, Chaille P, Conti CR (2007) Treatment of mechanical valve thrombosis during pregnancy. Clin Cardiol 30(6):271–6
61. Cáceres-Lóriga FM, Pérez-López H, Morlans-Hernández K et al (2006) Thrombolysis as first choice therapy in prosthetic heart valve thrombosis. A study of 68 patients. J Thromb Thrombolysis 21(2):185–90
62. Ananthasubramaniam K, Beattie JN, Rosman HS, Jayam V, Borzak S (2001) How safely and for how long can warfarin therapy be withheld in prosthetic heart valve patients hospitalized with a major hemorrhage? Chest 119(2):478–84
63. Amorosi SL, Tsilimingras K, Thompson D, Fanikos J, Weinstein MC, Goldhaber SZ (2004) Cost analysis of "bridging therapy" with low-molecular weight heparin versus unfractionated heparin during temporary interruption of chronic anticoagulation. Am J Cardiol 93:509–511
64. Spyropoulos AC, Frost FJ, Hurley JS, Roberts M (2004) Costs and clinical outcomes associated with low-molecular-weight heparin vs. unfractionated heparin for perioperative bridging in patients receiving long-term oral anticoagulant therapy. Chest 125:1642–1650

65. Hammerstingl C et al (2007) Periprocedural bridging therapy with low-molecular-weight heparin in chronically anticoagulated patients with prosthetic mechanical heart valves: experience in 116 patients from the prospective BRAVE registry. J Heart Valve Dis 16(3):285–92

66. Hylek EM, Chang YC, Skates SJ, Hughes RA, Singer DE (2000) Prospective study of the outcomes of ambulatory patients with excessive warfarin anticoagulation. Arch Intern Med 160(11):1612–7

67. Yiu KH, Siu CW, Jim MH, Tse HF, Fan K, Chau MC, Chow WH (2006) Comparison of the efficacy and safety profiles of intravenous vitamin K and fresh frozen plasma as treatment of warfarin-related over-anticoagulation in patients with mechanical heart valves. Am J Cardiol 97(3):409–11

68. Ageno W, Garcia D, Silingardi M, Galli M, Crowther M (2005) A randomized trial comparing 1 mg of oral vitamin K with no treatment in the management of warfarin-associated coagulopathy in patients with mechanical heart valves. J Am Coll Cardiol 46(4):732–3

69. Lubetsky A, Yonath H, Olchovsky D, Loebstein R, Halkin H, Ezra D (2003) Comparison of oral versus intravenous phytonadionc (Vitamin K1) in patients with excessive anticoagulation: a prospective randomized controlled study. Arch Intern Med 163(20):2469–73

22 Antithrombotic Therapy in Heart Failure and Cardiomyopathy

Zuheir Abrahams, George Sokos, and W. H. Wilson Tang

Contents

Abstract Patients with heart failure and cardiomyopathy often present with risk factors that may warrant anti-thrombotic therapy, such as atrial fibrillation, left ventricular thrombus, and the presence of a hyper-coagulable state. Decades of clinical studies have provided a wealth of information and speculations, but the current role of prophylactic antiplatelet and anticoagulant therapies remained controversial. Post hoc analyses from large heart failure trials provided evidence that warfarin use was associated with improved clinical outcomes despite the lack of a significant reduction in thromboembolic risks. However, prospective randomized trials have identified an unexpected benefit of reduced heart failure hospitalizations in those treated with warfarin, which may also be interpreted as potential risk with *routine* administration of aspirin therapy. Ongoing clinical trials may provide the necessary clinical evidence to guide future recommendations.

Key words: Anticoagulation; Aspirin; Cardiomyopathy; Heart failure; Thrombosis

INTRODUCTION

Heart failure and cardiomyopathy remain highly morbid and costly diseases, accounting for approximately 250,000 deaths per year in the United States and a mortality approaching 50% at 5 years *(1)*. Among these patients, the risk of stroke is increased by an estimated 3.5% per year and more than doubles the risk of death even in the setting of sinus rhythm *(2–4)*. However, the long-term cumulative risk of thromboembolism, the benefits and risks of treatment, and the relationship of

From: *Contemporary Cardiology: Antithrombotic Drug Therapy in Cardiovascular Disease*
Edited by: A.T. Askari and A.M. Lincoff (eds.), DOI 10.1007/978-1-60327-235-3_22
© Humana Press, a part of Springer Science+Business Media, LLC 2010

425

thromboembolic risk to other clinical parameters in patients with heart failure remain largely unclear.

This chapter will focus on anti-thrombotic therapy for chronic heart failure and cardiomyopathy (specifically those in sinus rhythm). The role of anti-thrombotic therapy in conditions frequently found in patients with heart failure (including venous thromboembotic disease, pulmonary embolism, and atrial fibrillation) is covered in detail in other chapters of this book.

EPIDEMIOLOGY OF THROMBOEMBOLISM IN HEART FAILURE

The primary goal of anti-thrombotic therapy is to reduce the risk of thromboembolic events. Therefore, justification for their use requires a heightened risk of thromboembolism in the heart failure population. Early autopsy studies reported a very high frequency of thromboembolic events in patients with heart failure *(5)* with an estimated prevalence of vascular events ranging from 3% to 50% in the published literature *(6)*, an overall estimated incidence of systemic and cerebral thromboembolism of 2.7 and 1.7 per 100 patient-years, respectively *(7,8)*, and an incidence of arterial embolic events in an advanced heart failure population of 3.2 per 100 patient-years *(9)*. It is important to emphasize, however, that much of these data were collected decades ago. Advancing age and improved survival may result in significant differences in contemporary patients with heart failure.

In the Studies of Left Ventricular Dysfunction (SOLVD), the annual incidence of vascular thrombotic events (including strokes, pulmonary emboli, and peripheral emboli) in patients with left ventricular dysfunction and sinus rhythm was 2.4% in women and 1.8% in men *(2)*. These figures were similar to that reported from the Vasodilators in Heart Failure Trials (V-HeFT) I and II studies (2.7 and 2.1 per 100 patient-years, respectively) *(10)*. In contrast to patients with underlying atrial fibrillation, more current data suggest an overall incidence of up to 4% of fatal and non-fatal stroke rate in patients with heart failure followed for a mean of 37.7 months (approximately 2.5% per year) irrespective of ejection fraction (EF) *(11)*. In a non-atrial fibrillation cohort of the Sudden Cardiac Death in Heart Failure Trial (SCD-HeFT), the annual thromboembolic rate for moderately symptomatic systolic heart failure was 1.7% per year without anti-arrhythmic therapy *(12)* and the four-year rate of thromboembolism was highest in patients with an EF≤20% (4.6% vs. 3.5% 3.5% in patients with an EF between 20% and 35%).

RATIONALE FOR ANTI-THROMBOTIC THERAPY

Patients with advanced heart failure frequently have all three components of Virchow's triad (blood stasis, endothelial dysfunction, hypercoagulable state). Epidemiologic observations suggested that the risk of thromboembolic events can be related to the patients' functional capacity, the degree of left ventricular dysfunction, or the presence of co-morbid conditions *(10,13)*. More recent data have suggested that the presence of heart failure itself rather than the degree of cardiac dysfunction may impact thromboembolic risks *(11,12)*. Patients with heart failure are more prone to thromboembolic events if they have concomitant risk factors such as atrial fibrillation, poor myocardial contractility, or low cardiac output. Dilated cardiac chambers and decreased cardiac output also interfere with the efficient forward movement of circulating blood resulting in stasis.

The other two components of Virchow's triad, hypercoagulability and endothelial dysfunction, seem to be integrally related. Endothelial dysfunction is manifest by elevated levels of von Willebrand factor and increased markers of thrombin production and platelet activation *(14)*. Furthermore, decreased nitric oxide (NO) production may provide additional explanation for hypercoagulability. Decreased levels of NO result in reduced antiplatelet activity and an increased release of prothrombotic mediators *(15)*.

Hypercoagulability is also related to the compensatory mechanisms activated in patients with heart failure. Activation of the renin angiotensin aldosterone system (RAAS) contributes to the hypercoagulable state through elevated levels of angiotensin II that stimulate the expression of plasminogen activator inhibitor-1 in endothelial and smooth muscle cells as well as through increased degradation of bradykinin, both of which adversely alter the fibrinolytic equilibrium (16).

TREATING THROMBOEMBOLISM IN HEART FAILURE

Potential cardiac sources of embolism requiring anticoagulation include left atrial appendage thrombi, left ventricular thrombi, and mural thrombi. Cardiac sources of embolism account for ≥15% of ischemic strokes. Left ventricular thrombus formation is a frequent complication of ischemic heart disease or low-output heart failure, occurring in at least 5% of patients after acute transmural myocardial infarction that may result in systemic embolization. In addition, left atrial appendage is a common source of cardiac thrombus formation associated with systemic embolism, primarily in association with atrial fibrillation and/or rheumatic mitral valve disease. Despite the varied locales for cardiac sources of embolism, the potential devastation is uniform, prompting the need for both preventive and therapeutic measure.

Anticoagulation therapy may significantly decrease the incidence of embolic events by 33% compared to untreated patients (17). According to the Heart Failure Society of America (HFSA) guidelines, the presence of left ventricular thrombus in cardiomyopathies should be considered for chronic anticoagulation, depending on the characteristics of the thrombus, such as its size, mobility, and degree of calcification (18). The Canadian Cardiovascular Society (CCS) guidelines further recommended that anticoagulation should be considered for patients with demonstrated intracardiac thrombus, spontaneous echocardiographic contrast, or severe reduction in left ventricular systolic function when intraventricular thrombus cannot be excluded (19).

It was previously believed that chronic laminated mural thrombi have a low incidence of embolization and do not necessarily need anticoagulation. However, a recent study of 361 patients with ischemic heart disease undergoing evaluation of surgical left ventricular reconstruction with infarct exclusion and eventual surgical or pathological evaluation of the left ventricle reported a 29% prevalence of left ventricular thrombus (20). In this study, patients with left ventricular thrombus were not significantly different compared to patients without thrombus, except in incidence of recent systemic embolic events. This study also reported a 6.1% risk of recent systemic embolization in patients with confirmed left ventricular thrombus compared to only 0.8% risk in patients without LV thrombus (20). Another interesting finding of this study was that in patients with confirmed left ventricular thrombus and recent systemic embolic events, pathologic evaluation identified chronic organized mural thrombus (67%) as opposed to recent thrombus (33%) (20) as the major source of embolism. Chronic mural thrombi represent a significant risk factor for systemic embolization either from increased incidence of embolization of mural thrombus or new clot formation on its surface is reinforced.

Many thrombotic events in patients with heart failure can be associated with interventions. For example, an increasingly common source of thrombosis emerged with the broad adoption of device therapy in heart failure, particularly implantable cardioverter defibrillator (ICD) and biventricular devices (21). Venous thrombosis, especially at the subclavian vein, has been reported on average in 12% (range 2–22%) of patients, from several days to years post-implantation (22). Early detection of clinical presentation of venous thrombosis is crucial, and treatment approach largely follows standard anticoagulation therapy for venous thrombosis (see Chaps. 17 and 19).

PROPHYLATIC ANTI-THROMBOTIC THERAPY IN HEART FAILURE

Aspirin Monotherapy

The anti-thrombotic effects of aspirin monotherapy have been well established in ischemic heart disease. Aspirin also reduces the incidence of stroke and death in patients with a history of transient ischemic attacks and reduces the rate of stroke and systemic embolism in patients with atrial fibrillation. However, it is also important to point out that in only two of the many studies supporting the use of aspirin in preventing serious vascular events were patients with heart failure (totaling 134) included *(23)*. When assessed in heart failure trials, the use of aspirin was not randomized, but likely related to underlying indications. Nevertheless, the incidence of thromboembolism in patients receiving aspirin was reduced from 2.1–2.7 to 0.5–1.6 events/100 patient-years in the two V-HeFT studies *(10)*. Among all patients enrolled in the SAVE trial, aspirin use significantly reduced the risk of stroke by 56% *(13)*. Importantly, the protective effect of aspirin was most pronounced in patients with an LVEF ≤ 28%, with a reduction in risk of stroke of 66% ($p < 0.001$) *(13)*. Similarly, the SOLVD trial showed a beneficial effect of aspirin monotherapy, with a 23% reduction in the risk of thromboembolism in men, a 53% reduction in risk in women *(24)*, and a 24% reduction in the risk of sudden death in all patients enrolled *(25)*.

However, concerns regarding the concomitant use of aspirin and angiotensin-converting enzyme (ACE) inhibition have also been raised *(25,26)*. The most common pathophysiologic explanation is their combined adverse effects on the production of vasodilating prostaglandins. Nevertheless, this has not been observed in other post hoc analyses *(27)*, and a recent observational study of over 7,000 patients demonstrated that aspirin use was not associated with an increase in mortality or heart failure readmission rates and aspirin did not affect the benefits of ACE inhibitors *(28)*. This has been further demonstrated in an elderly population with underlying heart failure and atrial fibrillation *(29)*.

Current national and international guidelines differ slightly about use of aspirin in patients with heart failure. The European Society of Cardiology (ESC) guidelines recommend against aspirin: "Aspirin should be avoided in patients with recurrent hospitalization with worsening heart failure (Class of recommendation IIb, level of evidence B)" *(30)*. This is in contrast with the guidelines of the American College of Cardiology/American Heart Association (ACC/AHA), stating "there may be an important interaction between aspirin and ACE inhibitors, but there is controversy regarding this point, and it requires further study" *(31)*. The HFSA guidelines recommend aspirin for certain patients only: "Aspirin is recommended in most patients [with ischemic cardiomyopathy] for whom anticoagulation is not specifically indicated. However, routine use of aspirin is not recommended in patients with heart failure from non-ischemic cardiomyopathy and without other evidence of atherosclerotic vascular disease. Aspirin and an ACE inhibitor in combination may be considered for patients with heart failure where an indication for both drugs exists" *(18)*. The Canadian guidelines recommended a similar approach *(19)*.

Anticoagulant Therapy (Warfarin)

Data regarding the use of warfarin following myocardial infarction came from the WARIS (Warfarin, aspirin, reinfarction study) *(32)* and the ASPECT (Anticoagulants in the secondary prevention of events in coronary thrombosis) *(33)*. Both studies demonstrated significant benefit (relative risk 0.45 and 0.58, respectively) with warfarin targeted at INR of 2.8–4.8. However, they were all-inclusive of myocardial infarction patients without specifying LV ejection fraction; these data are 2–3 decades old; and subsequent studies have failed to demonstrate mortality benefits with warfarin over standard anti-platelet therapy. Therefore, the latest ST elevation myocardial infarction guidelines advocate warfarin use primarily in the presence of left ventricular thrombus for the initial 3 months after myocardial infarction, in patients with persistent or paroxysmal atrial fibrillation, or in those unable to take antiplatelet agents *(18,34)*.

For patients with chronic heart failure treated with anticoagulant agents, concerns have been raised regarding the balance between risks and benefits. In V-HeFT I, the thromboembolic event rate in patients treated with anticoagulant agents was similar to that in patients not receiving anticoagulation (2.9 vs. 2.7/100 patient-years, respectively) *(10)*. However, the rates of thromboembolism were higher in the anticoagulant group than in the non-anticoagulant group in V-HeFT II (4.9 vs. 2.1/100 patient-years, $p = 0.01$) *(10)*. Because neither the decision to initiate anticoagulation nor the intensity of anticoagulation was controlled, it is likely that patients judged to be at highest risk for thromboembolism (i.e., those with atrial fibrillation or known LV thrombus or even patients with mechanical valve replacement) were treated with warfarin. As for post hoc analyses from clinical trials, the use of anticoagulants did not confer lower thromboembolic risks in patients with chronic systolic heart failure with sinus rhythm in SOLVD (relative risk 1.14 in men, 1.51 in women, both statistically non-significant). Also in SCD-HeFT, there was no significant risk reduction in thromboembolism with the use of aspirin or warfarin *(12)*. These neutral results in the chronic heart failure setting were in contrast with the association of anticoagulant therapy with significant reduction in stroke rates in the post-infarction setting *(24)*.

Significant reductions in sudden cardiac deaths and long-term prognosis have been observed with anticoagulant use in specific populations of patients with heart failure *(35,36)*. In the EPICAL study (Epidémiologie de l'Insuffisance Cardiaque Avancée en Lorraine), a total of 417 consecutive patients surviving at hospital discharge were followed for up to 5 years. The investigators found better 5-year survival in patients on anti-thrombotic therapy (40% vs. 31%), with no interaction between aspirin and ACE inhibitor use on survival *(37)*. These are the first suggestions that there may be discordance between the potential benefits of warfarin therapy with the lack of reduction in thromboembolic risks.

Such discrepancies have prompted the need for prospective clinical trials to better define the risks and benefits of anti-thrombotic therapy in patients with heart failure and, in particular, those in sinus rhythm. Three trials have been completed to date, although they all had crucial limitations. Nevertheless, the three trials demonstrate consistent findings: (1) Neither aspirin nor warfarin therapy decreases the risk of subsequent death, MI, or stroke, (2) patients with heart failure receiving aspirin may experience increased hospitalization rates, and (3) in no way are these data conclusive.

The Warfarin/Aspirin Study in Heart Failure (WASH) trial was an open-label pilot study that randomized 279 patients with chronic systolic heart failure (6% with atrial fibrillation, and 70% NYHA Class II with LV ejection fraction ≤ 35%) to receive aspirin (300 mg/day), warfarin (INR target at 2.5), or no anti-thrombotic therapy for a mean of 27 ± 1 months. There were no statistically significant differences in the composite endpoint of death, myocardial infarction, and stroke, but in the first 12 months patients randomized to aspirin were twice as likely to be hospitalized for cardiovascular reasons compared to warfarin, particularly related to worsening heart failure ($p = 0.044$) *(38)*.

The Warfarin and Anti-platelet Therapy in Chronic Heart failure (WATCH) trial assumed that patients with heart failure needed anti-thrombotic therapy, did not provide a placebo group. It was a multicenter study sponsored by the Department of Veterans' Affairs designed to compare open-label warfarin (target INR 2.5–3) vs. double-blind aspirin (162 mg/day), vs. double-blind clopidogrel (75 mg/day) in 1,587 subjects with chronic systolic heart failure (NYHA II–IV, LV ejection fraction ≤35%, 70% beta-blocker use) in sinus rhythm over a follow-up period of 23 months (originally targeted for 4,500 subjects) *(39)*. Again, there was no statistically significant difference between the three treatment groups on the primary outcome of death, myocardial infarction, or stroke (20.5% vs.

Table 1
Meta-analysis of prospective studies evaluating warfarin versus aspirin *(39)*

	Odds ratio		
	WATCH	WASH	*Pooled*
Mortality, myocardial infarction, and stroke	0.96 (0.70–1.31)	0.75 (0.37–1.50)	0.92 (0.69–1.22)
All-cause mortality	0.94 (0.67–1.30)	0.78 (0.38–1.58)	0.91 (0.67–1.22)
Heart failure hospitalization	0.67 (0.49–0.93)*	0.49 (0.23–1.01)	0.64 (0.48–0.85)*

*$p < 0.05$. 95% confidence interval is given within parentheses

19.8% vs. 21.8%, statistically non-significant). However, there was once again a 28% relative risk reduction in heart failure hospitalizations comparing the warfarin and aspirin groups (16.1% vs. 22.2%, $p = 0.01$).

A recent meta-analysis including the previous two trials further supported that warfarin use may favorably impact heart failure hospitalization rates when compared with aspirin (OR 0.64, 95% confidence interval 0.48–0.85) (Table 1). The underlying explanation is unclear, although it is conceivable that high doses of aspirin may share the same risks as non-steroidal anti-inflammatory drugs and may aggravate fluid retention in patients with heart failure, especially in those with concomitant risk factors for decompensation.

Recently, investigators from the Heart failure long-term anti-thrombotic study (HELAS) reported their results on 197 patients (NYHA II–IV, LVEF < 35%, no atrial fibrillation) who were randomized to either aspirin (325 mg/day) vs. warfarin (INR 2–3) in ischemic cardiomyopathy, or warfarin vs. placebo in dilated cardiomyopathy *(40)*. There were no significant differences in composite event rates among the groups, although the absolute number of events was small (a total of only 5 embolic events).

The use of anticoagulant therapy was more consistent across the various guidelines, however as stated in the latest ACC/AHA guidelines, "in the absence of definitive trials, it is not clear how anticoagulation should be prescribed in patients with heart failure" *(31)*. At present, the use of anticoagulation medication is recommended in patients with heart failure and atrial fibrillation, presence of left ventricular thrombus, or a prior embolic event (such as pulmonary embolism, including stroke and transient ischemic attack) unless contraindicated *(18,30,31)*. Aspirin use should be reserved for patients in whom secondary prevention of atherosclerotic disease is the goal.

Considerations of Bleeding Risks

The incidence of major hemorrhage in patients receiving anticoagulant therapy ranges from 2.3 to 6.8/100 patient-years, and the rate of intracranial bleeding approximates 0.62/100 patient-years, with each 10-year increase in age after 40 years imparting a 46% increase in the relative risk of major bleeding *(41)*. In the Stroke Prevention in Atrial Fibrillation (SPAF) II study, the rate of intracranial bleed was calculated to be 0.9/100 patient-years, and an increased risk of both thromboembolism as well as major bleeding in patients with heart failure aged ≥75 years was observed *(42)*. Even when adjustments were made for the intensity of anticoagulation, patients ≥80 year old may still present with a fourfold greater risk of life-threatening or fatal bleeding *(43)*. Bleeding complications occur far less frequently with antiplatelet therapy than with anticoagulant agents. Although low-dose aspirin carries a risk of gastrointestinal hemorrhage, review of the various placebo-controlled aspirin trials suggests that the risk is especially increased only when higher doses (>1,000 mg) are used. As expected, across all randomized studies there were more bleeding episodes for warfarin compared to aspirin.

CLINICAL PERSPECTIVES

The role of anti-thrombotic therapy in patients with heart failure and cardiomyopathy remains contentious. Despite data suggesting a benefit with warfarin compared to aspirin therapy, important limitations preclude widespread implementation in this patient population. It will be of interest to see if newer anticoagulants such as anti-factor Xa or anti-factor IIa agents can provide similar efficacy as warfarin without the monitoring hassles in the setting of heart failure.

Nevertheless, it is important to point out that the risk of thromboembolic events in patients with heart failure in sinus rhythm is low (1–3% per year), thus, prophylactic use of warfarin is controversial and has not been widely accepted. The ongoing Warfarin vs. Aspirin in Reduced Cardiac Ejection Fraction (WARCEF) trial is a National Institutes of Health funded, randomized, double-blind, placebo-controlled trial designed to test the hypothesis that there is no difference between warfarin (INR 2.5–3.0) and aspirin (325 mg daily) in three- to five-year event-free survival for the composite endpoint of death or stroke (ischemic or hemorrhagic) among patients with cardiac ejection fraction ≤ 35% who do not have atrial fibrillation or mechanical valves *(44)*. However, at present, warfarin should be considered in patients with heart failure with persistent or paroxysmal atrial fibrillation, evidence of left ventricular thrombi (especially mobile) or left ventricular aneurysms, known hypercoagulable states, history of thromboembolism, and patent foramen ovale. Aspirin is primarily indicated in patients with ischemic heart diseases as secondary prevention, and although there is a lack of evidence to indicate an adverse interaction with ACE inhibitors, routine use of aspirin in patients with non-ischemic cardiomyopathy has yet to be supported.

REFERENCES

1. Rosamond W, Flegal K, Friday G et al (2009) Heart disease and stroke statistics 2009 update: a report from the American Heart Association Statistics Committee and Stroke Statistics Subcommittee. Circulation 119(3):480–406
2. Dries DL, Domanski MJ, Waclawiw MA, Gersh BJ (1997) Effect of antithrombotic therapy on risk of sudden coronary death in patients with congestive heart failure. Am J Cardiol 79(7):909–913
3. Dunkman WB (1995) Thromboembolism and antithrombotic therapy in congestive heart failure. J Cardiovasc Risk 2(2):107–117
4. Fuster V, Gersh BJ, Giuliani ER, Tajik AJ, Brandenburg RO, Frye RL (1981) The natural history of idiopathic dilated cardiomyopathy. Am J Cardiol 47(3):525–531
5. Spodick DH, Littmann D (1958) Idiopathic myocardial hypertrophy. Am J Cardiol 1(5):610–623
6. Sirajuddin RA, Miller AB, Geraci SA (2002) Anticoagulation in patients with dilated cardiomyopathy and sinus rhythm: a critical literature review. J Card Fail 8(1):48–53
7. Cioffi G, Pozzoli M, Forni G et al (1996) Systemic thromboembolism in chronic heart failure. A prospective study in 406 patients. Eur Heart J 17(9):1381–1389
8. Katz SD, Marantz PR, Biasucci L et al (1993) Low incidence of stroke in ambulatory patients with heart failure: a prospective study. Am Heart J 126(1):141–146
9. Natterson PD, Stevenson WG, Saxon LA, Middlekauff HR, Stevenson LW (1995) Risk of arterial embolization in 224 patients awaiting cardiac transplantation. Am Heart J 129(3):564–570
10. Dunkman WB, Johnson GR, Carson PE, Bhat G, Farrell L, Cohn JN (1993) Incidence of thromboembolic events in congestive heart failure. The V-HeFT VA Cooperative Studies Group. Circulation 87(6 Suppl):VI94–VI101
11. Olsson LG, Swedberg K, Ducharme A et al (2006) Atrial fibrillation and risk of clinical events in chronic heart failure with and without left ventricular systolic dysfunction: results from the Candesartan in Heart failure-Assessment of Reduction in Mortality and morbidity (CHARM) program. J Am Coll Cardiol 47(10):1997–2004
12. Freudenberger RS, Hellkamp AS, Halperin JL et al (2007) Risk of thromboembolism in heart failure: an analysis from the sudden cardiac death in heart failure trial (SCD-HeFT). Circulation 115(20):2637–2641

13. Loh E, Sutton MS, Wun CC et al (1997) Ventricular dysfunction and the risk of stroke after myocardial infarction. N Engl J Med 336(4):251–257
14. Dotsenko O, Kakkar VV (2007) Antithrombotic therapy in patients with chronic heart failure: rationale, clinical evidence and practical implications. J Thromb Haemost 5(2):224–231
15. Jafri SM, Ozawa T, Mammen E, Levine TB, Johnson C, Goldstein S (1993) Platelet function, thrombin and fibrinolytic activity in patients with heart failure. Eur Heart J 14(2):205–212
16. Smith D, Gilbert M, Owen WG (1985) Tissue plasminogen activator release in vivo in response to vasoactive agents. Blood 66(4):835–839
17. Vaitkus PT, Barnathan ES (1993) Embolic potential, prevention and management of mural thrombus complicating anterior myocardial infarction: a meta-analysis. J Am Coll Cardiol 22(4):1004–1009
18. Heart Failure Society of America (2006) Executive summary: HFSA 2006 Comprehensive Heart Failure Practice Guideline. J Card Fail 12:10–38
19. Arnold JM, Liu P, Demers C et al (2006) Canadian Cardiovascular Society consensus conference recommendations on heart failure 2006: diagnosis and management. Can J Cardiol 22(1):23–45
20. Srichai MB, Junor C, Rodriguez LL et al (2006) Clinical, imaging, and pathological characteristics of left ventricular thrombus: a comparison of contrast-enhanced magnetic resonance imaging, transthoracic echocardiography, and trans-esophageal echocardiography with surgical or pathological validation. Am Heart J 152(1):75–84
21. Rozmus G, Daubert JP, Huang DT, Rosero S, Hall B, Francis C (2005) Venous thrombosis and stenosis after implantation of pacemakers and defibrillators. J Interv Card Electrophysiol 13(1):9–19
22. Bracke F, Meijer A, Van Gelder B (2003) Venous occlusion of the access vein in patients referred for lead extraction: influence of patient and lead characteristics. Pacing Clin Electrophysiol 26(8):1649–1652
23. Antiplatelet Trialists' Collaboration (1994) Collaborative overview of randomised trials of antiplatelet therapy–I: prevention of death, myocardial infarction, and stroke by prolonged antiplatelet therapy in various categories of patients. BMJ 308(6921):81–106
24. Dries DL, Rosenberg YD, Waclawiw MA, Domanski MJ (1997) Ejection fraction and risk of thromboembolic events in patients with systolic dysfunction and sinus rhythm: evidence for gender differences in the studies of left ventricular dysfunction trials. J Am Coll Cardiol 29(5):1074–1080
25. Al-Khadra AS, Salem DN, Rand WM, Udelson JE, Smith JJ, Konstam MA (1998) Antiplatelet agents and survival: a cohort analysis from the Studies of Left Ventricular Dysfunction (SOLVD) trial. J Am Coll Cardiol 31(2):419–425
26. Nguyen KN, Aursnes I, Kjekshus J (1997) Interaction between enalapril and aspirin on mortality after acute myocardial infarction: subgroup analysis of the Cooperative New Scandinavian Enalapril Survival Study II (CONSENSUS II). Am J Cardiol 79(2):115–119
27. Leor J, Reicher-Reiss H, Goldbourt U et al (1999) Aspirin and mortality in patients treated with angiotensin-converting enzyme inhibitors: a cohort study of 11, 575 patients with coronary artery disease. J Am Coll Cardiol 33(7):1920–1925
28. McAlister FA, Ghali WA, Gong Y, Fang J, Armstrong PW, Tu JV (2006) Aspirin use and outcomes in a community-based cohort of 7352 patients discharged after first hospitalization for heart failure. Circulation 113(22):2572–2578
29. Desai A, Healey J, Pfeffer M (2006) Aspirin and the risk of heart failure hospitalization in patients with atrial fibrillation and a prior history of heart failure: an ACTIVE-W analysis. Presented at the 10th annual scientific meeting of the Heart Failure Society of America; September 10–13, 2006
30. Swedberg K, Cleland J, Dargie H et al (2005) Guidelines for the diagnosis and treatment of chronic heart failure: executive summary (update 2005): the task force for the Diagnosis and Treatment of Chronic Heart Failure of the European Society of Cardiology. Eur Heart J 26(11):1115–1140
31. Hunt SA, Abraham WT, Chin MH et al (2009) Focused update incorporated into the ACC/AHA 2005 Guidelines for the Diagnosis and Management of Heart Failure in Adults A Report of the American College of Cardiology Foundation/American Heart Association Task Force on Practice Guidelines Developed in Collaboration With the International Society for Heart and Lung Transplantation. Circulation 119(14):e391–479
32. Smith P, Arnesen H, Holme I (1990) The effect of warfarin on mortality and reinfarction after myocardial infarction. N Engl J Med 323(3):147–152
33. Warfarin versus aspirin for prevention of thromboembolism in atrial fibrillation (1994) Stroke prevention in atrial fibrillation II study. Lancet 343(8899):687–691
34. Antman EM, Anbe DT, Armstrong PW et al (2008) 2007 Focused Update of the ACC/AHA 2004 Guidelines for the Management of Patients With ST-Elevation Myocardial Infarction: a report of the American College of Cardiology/American Heart Association Task Force on Practice Guidelines: developed in collaboration With the Canadian Cardiovascular Society endorsed by the American Academy of Family Physicians: 2007 Writing Group to Review New

Evidence and Update the ACC/AHA 2004 Guidelines for the Management of Patients With ST-Elevation Myocardial Infarction, Writing on Behalf of the 2004 Writing Committee. Circulation 117(2):296–329

35. Al-Khadra AS, Salem DN, Rand WM, Udelson JE, Smith JJ, Konstam MA (1998) Warfarin anticoagulation and survival: a cohort analysis from the Studies of Left Ventricular Dysfunction. J Am Coll Cardiol 31(4):749–753

36. de Boer RA, Hillege HL, Tjeerdsma G, Verheugt FW, van Veldhuisen DJ (2005) Both antiplatelet and anticoagulant therapy may favorably affect outcome in patients with advanced heart failure. A retrospective analysis of the PRIME-II trial. Thromb Res 116(4):279–285

37. Echemann M, Alla F, Briancon S et al (2002) Antithrombotic therapy is associated with better survival in patients with severe heart failure and left ventricular systolic dysfunction (EPICAL study). Eur J Heart Fail 4(5):647–654

38. Cleland JG, Findlay I, Jafri S et al (2004) The warfarin/aspirin study in heart failure (WASH): a randomized trial comparing antithrombotic strategies for patients with heart failure. Am Heart J 148(1):157–164

39. Massie BM, Collins JF, Ammon SE, et al. (2009) Randomized trial of warfarin, aspirin, and clopidogrel in patients with chronic heart failure: the Warfarin and Antiplatelet Therapy in Chronic Heart Failure (WATCH) trial. Circulation 119(12):1616–1624.

40. Cokkinos DV, Haralabopoulos GC, Kostis JB, Toutouzas PK (2006) Efficacy of antithrombotic therapy in chronic heart failure: the HELAS study. Eur J Heart Fail 8(4):428–432

41. van der Meer FJ, Rosendaal FR, Vandenbroucke JP, Briet E (1993) Bleeding complications in oral anticoagulant therapy. An analysis of risk factors. Arch Intern Med 153(13):1557–1562

42. The Stroke Prevention in Atrial Fibrillation Investigators (1996) Bleeding during antithrombotic therapy in patients with atrial fibrillation. Arch Intern Med 156(4):409–416

43. Fihn SD, Callahan CM, Martin DC, McDonell MB, Henikoff JG, White RH (1996) The risk for and severity of bleeding complications in elderly patients treated with warfarin. The national consortium of anticoagulation clinics. Ann Intern Med 124(11):970–979

44. Pullicino P, Thompson JL, Barton B, Levin B, Graham S, Freudenberger RS (2006) Warfarin versus aspirin in patients with reduced cardiac ejection fraction (WARCEF): rationale, objectives, and design. J Card Fail 12(1):39–46

23   Heparin-Induced Thrombocytopenia

John R. Bartholomew

CONTENTS

ABSTRACT Heparin-induced thrombocytopenia (HIT) is a transient, prothrombotic, immune-mediated complication of unfractionated heparin (UFH) or any of the low molecular weight heparin (LMWH) preparations that can result in venous or arterial thrombosis, amputation or death. It classically develops within 5–14 days of administration of either agent, although it may occur more rapidly if there has been recent exposure; or delayed days to weeks after either preparation has been discontinued. Thrombocytopenia, once considered necessary for the diagnosis is no longer essential, whereas a 50% reduction from the patients baseline count is considered a more specific finding. Immediate cessation of UFH or LMWH is recommended once the diagnosis is suspected, and therapy initiated with a non-heparin anticoagulant to prevent and/or treat the potentially devastating complications.

Key words: Heparin; Low molecular weight heparin; Heparin-induced thrombocytopenia; Isolated heparin-induced thrombocytopenia; Heparin antibodies; Direct thrombin inhibitors; Fondaparinux; Warfarin; Percutaneous coronary transluminal angioplasty; Percutaneous coronary intervention; Coronary artery bypass surgery

From: *Contemporary Cardiology: Antithrombotic Drug Therapy in Cardiovascular Disease*
Edited by: A.T. Askari and A.M. Lincoff (eds.), DOI 10.1007/978-1-60327-235-3_23
© Humana Press, a part of Springer Science+Business Media, LLC 2010

INTRODUCTION

Heparin induced thrombocytopenia is a common, transient, iatrogenic disorder that can occur in any patient population exposed to UFH or LMWH. Cardiovascular patients are at increased risk according to data from the Complication After Thrombocytopenia Caused by Heparin (CATCH) registry. Approximately 25,000–50,000 of these patients will develop this complication annually in the US with health care costs approaching $300 million (1). Patients undergoing endovascular procedures percutaneous transluminal angioplasty (PTA), percutaneous coronary artery angioplasty (PTCA), percutaneous coronary intervention (PCI), and coronary artery bypass (CABG) or vascular surgery appear particularly vulnerable. The cause for its increased incidence in the cardiovascular patient population is not known. However, it is speculated that it may be the result of an increase in the percentage of this population exposed to UFH or LWMH, greater use of UFH or LMWH during treatment for the acute coronary syndromes (ACS), and an increase in the number of individuals who have repeated exposures or undergo repeat coronary procedures (2).

INCIDENCE

The incidence of HIT varies depending on the type of heparin preparation- (bovine lung>porcine intestine) and (UFH>LMWH), patient population (surgical>medical), gender (women>men), dose (treatment>prophylaxis), and the definition of thrombocytopenia used (a>50% decline in the platelet count is more sensitive than an absolute count ≤150,000 mm³) (3)

The American College of Chest Physicians (ACCP) estimate the risk of HIT as 1–5% in patients receiving UFH, but less than 1% in individuals exposed to LMWH (4,5). The incidence is lower in patients receiving thromboprophylaxis approaching 2.6% for UFH and 0.2% for LMWH (6,7).

PATHOGENESIS

Heparin-induced thrombocytopenia is an immune-mediated disorder that develops following exposure to UFH or LMWH. It is less common with LMWH, believed to be due to the smaller size of the molecule, but both agents are capable of triggering the release of platelet factor 4 (PF4), a heparin-neutralizing protein found in the alpha granules of platelets (6). An immune response can develop in susceptible individuals, forming IgG platelet activating antibodies. These "HIT antibodies" bind to heparin-PF4 on the FcγIIa receptors of platelet surfaces forming immune complexes that are capable of platelet activation and the release of procoagulant microparticles that promote thrombin generation. These immune complexes can also bind to heparan sulfate on endothelial cells and monocytes where they have the potential to initiate the release of tissue factor (TF) and contribute further to the hypercoagulable state (8–11) (Fig. 1).

CLINICAL FEATURES

Thrombocytopenia, defined as a platelet count less than 150,000 mm³ is the most common clinical finding of HIT, although most patients will have platelet counts well under this number. In a review of 142 serologically confirmed cases, Warkentin et al reported the median figure as 59,000 mm³ but counts as low as 15,000 mm³ were reported (12). Thrombocytopenia can occur in the absence of thrombosis and is referred to as isolated HIT. Not all patients develop thrombocytopenia and a 50% or greater drop in the platelet count from baseline in patients receiving UFH or LMWH is a more sensitive marker (3,5,12–14).

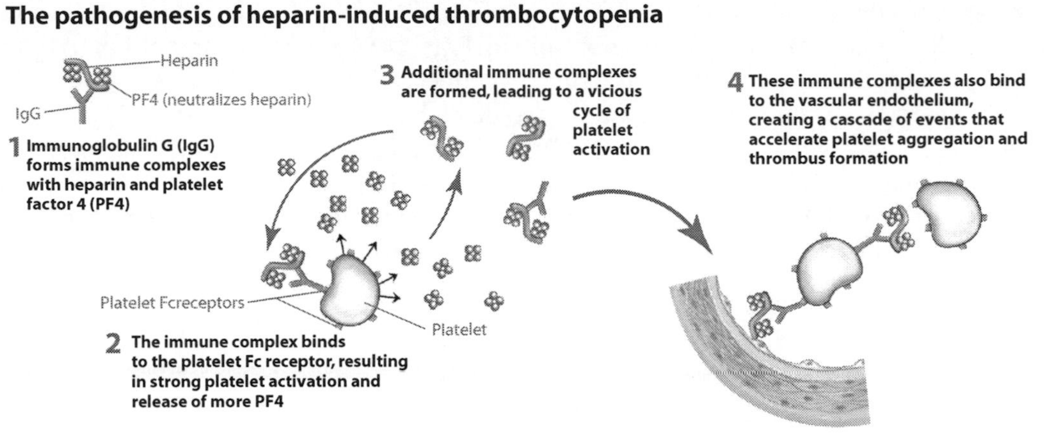

The pathogenesis of heparin-induced thrombocytopenia

Fig. 1. The pathogenesis of heparin-induced thrombocytopenia *(11,56).*

Patients are also at an increased risk of thrombosis. Approximately 30–75% develop a thrombotic event (depending on the patient population) and four out of five events are venous. Deep vein thrombosis (DVT) of the lower extremity occurs in approximately 50% of patients and pulmonary embolism (PE) is found in nearly 25% of individuals *(3,5).* Deep vein thrombosis is also seen in the upper extremity, more often associated with a central venous catheter or pacemaker wire. Other less commonly reported events include mesenteric venous thrombosis, adrenal hemorrhagic infarction, and cerebral venous (dural sinus) thrombosis.

Acute limb occlusion is the most common arterial event usually developing in areas of arteriosclerosis, at the site of a recent endovascular or surgical procedure, or following vascular trauma, and as many as 10% of these patients will require amputation. HIT may also present as an acute thrombotic stroke, myocardial infarction (MI), intracardiac thrombus, and thrombosis of an extracorporeal circuit, or rarely mesenteric or renal arteries. Occlusion of bypass conduits (saphenous veins more likely than arterial grafts) may also result following open heart surgery *(15).* Despite recent advances in the diagnosis and treatment of HIT, mortality rates approach 10–20% *(3,14,16).*

There are a number of atypical manifestations of HIT including coumarin-induced venous limb gangrene (VLG), coumarin-induced skin necrosis, heparin-induced skin necrosis, acute systemic reaction following intravenous bolus of UFH or subcutaneous injection of UFH, or LMWH, and disseminated intravascular coagulation (DIC) *(17).*

Coumarin-induced VLG is characterized by distal extremity necrosis, an ipsilateral limb DVT, and a supratherapeutic international normalized ratio (INR). It differs from coumarin-induced skin necrosis, which develops in areas of fatty tissue including breasts, buttocks, and thighs *(17,18).* Either condition can develop when the vitamin K antagonist (VKA) warfarin is initiated during acute HIT prior to the patient's platelet count recovery. This depletes the vitamin-K dependent natural anticoagulant protein C, and results in an additional prothrombotic condition. Both forms of coumarin-induced necrosis can also occur if a VKA is administered unopposed (without a direct thrombin inhibitor (DTI) or given despite the initiating of a DTI in the setting of persistent thrombocytopenia *(17,18).* Coumarin-induced skin necrosis is 100 times more frequent in patients with HIT (5–10%) compared to the skin necrosis seen in patients receiving a VKA in non-HIT conditions (0.001%) *(19).*

Heparin-induced Necrotizing skin lesions are found at the site of subcutaneous injections of UFH or LMWH and erythematous plaques, nodules, or skin necrosis have also been reported. Necrotizing lesions are characterized by an area of central ischemia surrounded by erythema and are characteristically extremely painful *(20).*

Acute systemic reactions develop anywhere from 5 to 30 min following an intravenous bolus of UFH or up to 2 h after subcutaneous injections of UFH or LMWH *(21)*. An abrupt fall in the platelet count is observed followed by fever, tachycardia, hypertension, dyspnea, chest pain, or transient global amnesia. Sudden cardiorespiratory collapse and death have also been reported *(5)*.

Disseminated intravascular coagulation (DIC) is characterized by hypofibrinogenemia, a transient acquired deficiency of antithrombin and protein C, and a prolonged international normalized ratio (INR) and activated partial thromboplastin time (aPTT). Schistocytes, livedo reticularis, renal failure, and other signs of microvascular thrombosis may be observed.

TEMPORAL PATTERNS OF HIT

Three distinct temporal patterns of HIT are described - typical-onset, rapid-onset, and delaye-donset *(5,22)*. Approximately two thirds of HIT patients develop the typical-onset form that develops within 4–14 days after an initial exposure to either anticoagulant, but may occur several days later with the LMWH preparations *(5,20,22)*.

Rapid-onset HIT develops in 25–30% of all patients and occurs within hours to days after either anticoagulant is initiated. In 243 serologically confirmed HIT cases, 30% of the individuals had this type with a median time to onset of thrombocytopenia of 10.5 h. All patients had recent exposure, commonly within the previous 30 days *(5,22)*. Rapid-onset HIT is due to residual heparin-platelet factor 4 (PF4) antibodies that developed during a previous exposure.

Delayed-onset HIT is the least common pattern developing in 3–5% of all HIT patients. It usually occurs within 7–40 days after either UFH or LMWH is discontinued, and often after discharge *(5)*. Patients have very high titers of HIT IgG antibodies and are often readmitted with a new thrombosis. Thrombocytopenia may not be initially observed, but develops soon after UFH or LMWH is administered, if this pattern is not recognized.

LABORATORY TESTING FOR HIT

Thrombocytopenia is a common finding in the hospital setting and possibilities other than HIT must be considered in the differential diagnosis including: pseudothrombocytopenia, sepsis, thrombotic thrombocytopenic purpura (TTP), idiopathic thrombocytopenic purpura (ITP), alcohol, aplastic anemia, hypersplenism, DIC, drug-related (glycoprotein IIb/IIIa inhibitors and thienopyridines), mechanically induced (intra-aortic balloon pump) or hemodilution from blood transfusions.

HIT should also be considered in the differential diagnosis of a new thrombosis or extension of an existing thrombus in a patient receiving either anticoagulant and in patients resistant to UFH, defined as individuals who require unusually high doses to attain a therapeutic aPTT.

The diagnosis of HIT is based on clinical presentation and laboratory testing. Warkentin et al developed a scoring system to assess the pretest probability of HIT, known as the 4 T's. This system is based on four criteria - thrombocytopenia, timing of the platelet count fall, thrombosis, and exclusion of other causes of thrombocytopenia. It appears to be most helpful in deciding which patient needs laboratory testing as noted in Table 1 *(3,5,23)*.

Two types of laboratory tests are available - functional tests that detect heparin-dependent platelet activation in the presence of the patient's sera and UFH or LMWH and immunoassays that measure IgG, IgM, or IgA antibodies that bind PF4 to either anticoagulant. To avoid over diagnosis, laboratory testing should only be ordered when there is a moderate to high clinical suspicion of HIT. Both tests have high negative predictive values but only moderate positive predictive values *(5,9,24)*.

Table 1
Estimating pretest probability of HIT: The four T's. *(3,5)*

	2 points	*1 point*	*0 points*
Thrombocytopenia	>50% fall or platelet nadir 20–100 mm³	30–50% fall or platelet nadir 10–19 mm³	<30% fall or platelet nadir <10 mm³
Timing of platelet drop or other sequelae	Onset between day 5 and 10 or < 1 day if recent exposure	Onset after day 10 or not clear (missing counts)	Falls too early without heparin exposure
Thrombosis or other sequelae	New thrombosis; skin necrosis; acute systemic reaction	Progressive or recurrent thrombosis; erythematous skin lesions; suspected thrombosis	None
Other causes of thrombocytopenia	None evident	Possible other causes	Definite other causes

Pretest probability: 6–8 = high, 4–5 = intermediate, 0–3 = low

Several functional tests are available of which two are heparin induced platelet aggregation assay (HIPA) and serotonin release assay (SRA). These assays have greater specificity but less sensitivity. The HIPA uses platelet-rich plasma mixed with the patient's plasma plus UFH, whereas the SRA uses donor platelets labeled with radioactive ¹⁴C serotonin. Although the latter is more sensitive and specific and the standard by which other tests are judged, it is not readily available at all hospitals because it requires radioisotopes. It is also technically more demanding to perform *(23)*.

Immunoassays have higher sensitivity but lower specificity and are technically easier to perform than functional tests. Results are reported as optical density (OD) values, with results ≥0.40 considered positive. Titers are generally higher in clinically confirmed cases as demonstrated by Zwicker and colleagues in a retrospective review. They found that values (>1.0) were more likely to be associated with thrombosis *(25)*. False positive results are more likely with the immunoassays because they detect all three immunoglobulin classes, whereas only a minority of these anti-PF4 heparin antibodies (generally 1%) is pathogenic *(9,24)*.

According to Arepally and Ortel, there are several approaches the clinician should take using the pretest probability screening tool (4Ts), once HIT is suspected. If the clinical suspicion is low, no laboratory testing should be performed. If the clinical suspicion is intermediate or high however, an immunoassay should be performed. If the results are positive with an indeterminate pretest probability, a functional assay should be obtained. If this test is positive, HIT is likely. If the functional test is negative, however, HIT is considered indeterminate. If the pretest probability is high and the immunoassay positive, HIT is confirmed. If the pretest is high and the immunoassay negative, HIT is considered to be indeterminate and repeating the test may be helpful *(14)*. It must be remembered that HIT remains a clinical diagnosis and results of laboratory testing may not always coincide with the clinical picture.

Management of HIT

Heparin and LMWH must be discontinued immediately once HIT is suspected and a thorough search performed to identify either of these agents in unsuspected locations like; bound to UFH coated-catheters, arterial line flushes, added to intravenous solutions for angiographic procedures, administered during dialysis or added to total parenteral nutrition solutions. Low molecular weight heparin should not be substituted for UFH because of the cross-reactivity of the HIT antibodies *(5)*.

Table 2
Treatment guidelines for HIT

1. Discontinue heparin or low molecular weight heparin immediately once HIT is suspected
2. Remove any hidden source(s) of heparin or LMWH
3. Do not wait for laboratory confirmation to begin treatment
4. Initiate an alternative anticoagulant using a direct thrombin inhibitor
5. Do not start warfarin until the platelet count has recovered to 100,000 mm^3 and preferably to 150,000 mm^3
6. Begin with low doses of warfarin and overlap a DTI for a minimum of 5 days and until the INR is ≥2.0 for two consecutive days
7. Avoid placement of inferior vena cava filters
8. Avoid platelet transfusions unless the patient is actively bleeding

Numerous studies have demonstrated that discontinuing UFH or LMWH is inadequate treatment even if there is no evidence of acute thrombosis like isolated HIT, because of the potential risk of new thrombosis, amputation or death (5,26–29). Treatment should not be delayed while waiting for laboratory confirmation as this delay only increases the risk of complications (26,27). Physicians should avoid platelet transfusions unless there is active bleeding; defer administration of a VKA until the platelet count has recovered to ≥100,000 mm^3 and preferably 150,000 mm^3; and avoid placement of an inferior vena cava filter (Table 2) (3).

DIRECT THROMBIN INHIBITORS

Currently, the Food and Drug Administration (FDA) has approved two DTI's for treating HIT (argatroban and lepirudin; one agent for the treatment of isolated HIT (argatroban) and two agents for patients with HIT requiring PCI (argatroban and bivalirudin).

LEPIRUDIN

Lepirudin is a recombinant form of hirudin, the natural anticoagulant derived from the medicinal leech, Hirudo Medicinalis. It irreversibly binds thrombin, has a half-life of approximately 1.3 h, and is eliminated by the kidneys. It is given by intravenous infusion.

Three prospective trials (designated heparin-associated thrombocytopenia or HAT-1, 2, 3) compared 403 patients treated with lepirudin to 120 historical controls - the latter group treated with the best available therapy at the time (26,27). The reported combined outcome of new thrombosis, amputation, and death was lower among patients receiving lepirudin, although after further analysis, only a statistical difference in new thrombotic events was reached. Bleeding was significantly higher in the lepirudin population (14,26,27).

In the initial HAT trials, patients with normal renal function received a weight-based bolus of 0.4 mg/kg followed by an infusion of 0.15 mg/kg/h. Based on data from the HAT trials however, the manufacturer no longer recommends a bolus dose (unless there is life threatening thrombosis) and advises lowering the initial infusion rate to between 0.05 and 0.10 mg/kg/h (26,27).

The aPTT (targeted to 1.5–2.5 times the baseline level) is used to monitor lepirudin. It should be checked 4 h after initiating therapy, with necessary dose adjustments and daily, once a therapeutic level is reached.

Lepirudin does not cross-react with UFH or LMWH, but anti-hirudin antibodies develop in as many as 60% of patients *(3,5,30)*. Although these antibodies are not associated with an increased risk of thrombosis, they may extend lepirudin's half-life and will require more frequent dose adjustments. Anaphylaxis and death in patients re-exposed to lepirudin have been reported; therefore caution is recommended when using it inpatients with a previous exposure *(14,31)*.

ARGATROBAN

Argatroban is a small synthetic molecule derived from L-arginine. It binds in a reversible fashion to the catalytic site of thrombin, is eliminated via hepatobiliary excretion, and has a half-life of 39–51 min. Argatroban lacks cross reactivity with UFH and is currently approved for the prevention (isolated HIT) and treatment of HIT, as well as for patients undergoing PCI.

Argatroban was used in two prospective trials (Arg 911 and Arg 915) involving 772 patients with HIT or suspected HIT and compared to historical controls. The combined outcomes of death, amputation, and new thrombosis were lower in individuals receiving argatroban when compared to historical controls (34% vs.43%) *(28,29,32)*. As in the HAT trials, fewer new thromboembolic events were reported, but no differences in amputations or death rates were noted. Unlike the lepirudin trials however, there was no increase in bleeding rates compared to the historical controls.

Argatroban does not require a loading dose for the treatment or prevention of HIT. It is given by continuous infusion at a rate of 0.2 µg/kg/min. Lower doses of 0.05 µg/kg/min are recommended for patients with moderate to severe liver disease or multisystem organ failure *(33)*. Argatroban is monitored using the aPTT targeted to 1.5–3.0 times the baseline level. The aPTT should be evaluated 2 h after initiating therapy and once daily after therapeutic levels have been attained.

A bolus dose of 350 µg/kg is required for patients who undergo PCI followed by an infusion rate of 25 µg/kg/min adjusted to achieve an activated clotting time (ACT) of 300–450 s. Argatroban does not produce antibodies.

BIVALIRUDIN

Bivalirudin is a small synthetic 20-amino-acid peptide, which is a specific and reversible inhibitor of thrombin. Currently, the major indications for bivalirudin are for use in patients with unstable angina undergoing PTCA and or with provisional glycoprotein IIb/IIIa receptor inhibitor treatment to reduce acute ischemic events in select patients undergoing PCI.

The FDA has approved bivalirudin for PCI in patients who have, or are at risk of HIT *(34)*. A bolus of 0.75 mg/kg/intravenously should be followed by a 1.75 mg/kg/h infusion for 4 h to attain a target ACT of >300 s. It has also been used in several trials as an alternative anticoagulant to UFH in on-pump or off-pump cardiac surgery in patients with HIT who require an alternative anticoagulant *(35,36)*. Bivalirudin has been used "off label" for the treatment of HIT patients in a number of small studies, where the dose is much lower (0.1–0.2 mg/kg/h *(37–39)*. Patients with moderate to severe renal insufficiency may require dose adjustments.

Bivalirudin has several advantages including a shorter half-life (25 min), enzymic (80%) and renal (20%) metabolism, low immunogenicity and a minimal effect on the INR *(39)*. It shares an 11-amino acid sequence with hirudin; therefore, it is possible that patients with antilepirudin antibodies resulting from treatment with lepirudin could cross react with bivalirudin. For that reason caution extreme should be exercised *(39)*, if bivalirudin is used in patients previously treated with lepirudin.

Alternative Therapies

FONDAPARINUX

Fondaparinux is a synthetic pentasaccharide metabolized in the kidneys. It has a half-life of 17–21 h and is administered subcutaneously with 100% bioavailability. Its elimination is prolonged in patients with renal impairment and is not advised in patients with a creatinine clearance of less than 30 ml/min. Fondaparinux is a selective indirect factor Xa inhibitor that binds specifically to antithrombin. It inhibits thrombin generation, does not prolong the prothrombin time (PT), INR, or aPTT, and no laboratory monitoring is usually needed.

Fondaparinux is currently approved for the prophylaxis of DVT and PE for orthopedic and abdominal surgery as well as for treatment of DVT and PE. It has also been used "off-label" in a number of patients with HIT *(40)*. Warkentin et al reported similar immunogenicity between fondaparinux and LMWH in a study of 2,726 patients; however, PF4/fondaparinux was poorly recognized by the HIT antibodies leading the authors to rationalize that the risk of HIT was very low *(41)*. Recently, Warkentin and colleagues published the first reported case of HIT associated with fondaparinux in a patient with no previous UFH or LWMH exposure and advised that it can cause a disorder resembling HIT on rare occasions *(40–42)*.

DANAPAROID

Danaparoid is a non-heparin low molecular weight glycosaminoglycan derived from porcine intestinal mucosa. It is approved for the treatment and prevention of HIT-associated thrombosis outside the United States. However,it is no longer available in this country.

None of the currently available alternative anticoagulants used in the US have an antidote. If clinically significant bleeding occurs, the agent should be discontinued immediately and supportive therapy initiated. A comparison of the current alternative anticoagulants available for the treatment of HIT is found in Table 3.

Warfarin

Warfarin should be avoided in patients with acute HIT to avoid coumarin-induced-VLG or coumarin-induced skin necrosis. Current ACCP guidelines advise that warfarin only be initiated in lower doses

Table 3
Comparison of available agents used in the treatment of HIT

	Argatroban	Bivalirudin	Fondaparinux	Lepirudin
Monitoring	aPTT, ACT	aPTT, ACT, ECT	Anti-Xa level	aPTT, ACT, ECT
Half-life	39–51 min	25 min	17 h	80 min
Clearance	Hepatic	Enzymic and renal	Renal	Renal
Dose adjustment	Hepatic insufficiency	Moderate to severe renal insufficiency	Renal insufficiency	Renal insufficiency
Cross-reaction with HIT antibodies	No	No	Yes	No
Antibody development	No	May cross-react with anti-hirudin antibodies	No	Anti-hirudin antibodies in up to 60% of patients

(≤5 mg); overlapped concurrently with a DTI for a minimum of 5 days, only started once the patient has improved clinically and the platelets have recovered to ≥100,000 mm^3 and preferably 150,000 mm^3; and the DTI discontinued only when the INR is ≥2 for two consecutive days *(5,17,18)*. Reversal with oral or intravenous vitamin K is advised to prevent VLG or coumarin-induced skin necrosis if warfarin has already been started before HIT is recognized *(3)*.

All DTIs prolong the INR because of differences in their molar concentrations required to achieve the desired inhibition of thrombin *(43)*. Argatroban causes the most pronounced increase in the INR and the manufacturer recommends a INR ≥4.0 during cotherapy. The INR is least affected by lepirudin *(44)*.

Once the INR is within the targeted range (and only after a minimum 5-day overlap), the INR and aPTT should be checked after holding the DTI 4–6 h. If the INR is between 2 and 3 (or) and the aPTT is at baseline, the DTI can be safely discontinued *(44)*. The recommended length of therapy with warfarin following acute HIT is 3–6 months.

Reducing the Incidence of HIT

Low molecular weight heparin or fondaparinux are alternatives to UFH for prophylaxis and/or treatment of DVT and PE and should reduce the incidence of HIT as they are less likely to trigger this condition. Early transition to warfarin (before HIT has a chance to develop) in patients receiving UFH or LMWH for acute DVT or PE is also recommended. Porcine UFH preparation should be used rather than bovine products, and all patients receiving UFH should have their platelet count monitored regularly. Current ACCP guidelines recommend monitoring platelet counts at baseline and every other day from days 4 to 14. If there is no recent exposure however, patients with exposure within the previous 100 days must be monitored within 24 h of administration *(5,45)*. The ACCP guidelines do not recommend routine platelet count monitoring for LMWH. This is however recommended by the British Committee for Standards in Haematology *(46)*.

Special Conditions

ISOLATED HIT

Isolated HIT was previously treated by just discontinuing UFH or LMWH. However, this approach places patients at an increased risk of new thromboembolic rates of 20–50% *(5,16,32,46)*. Current ACCP guidelines recommend treatment with a DTI followed by a short course of warfarin and performing a venous duplex ultrasound of the lower extremities due to the high frequency of asymptomatic DVT's in this situation *(5)*.

HIT AND PCI

Argatroban and bivalirudin are the only agents currently approved by the FDA for PCI and HIT, although there is limited experience with lepirudin, and all three agents have been used successfully in previous trials *(32,47)*. The Anticoagulant Therapy with Bivalirudin to Assist in the performance of PCI in patients with heparin-induced Thrombocytopenia trial (ATBAT) used bivalirudin in 52 patients *(34)*. Clinical success was defined as procedural success without death, emergency bypass surgery, or q wave MI, and procedural and clinical successes were achieved in 98 and 96% of patients. Only one death was reported - a cardiac arrest 46 h after a successful PCI *(34)*.

Lewis and colleagues analyzed 91 patients who underwent 112 PCIs in three prospective randomized trials (ARG-261, ARG-310, and ARG-311) using Argatroban *(48)*. Satisfactory outcomes of the procedure and adequate anticoagulation were primary efficacy endpoints and were achieved in

94.5 and 97.8% of patients respectively. There was only one major bleeding event, four MIs, and revascularization was necessary in seven patients. Results were comparable to historical heparin controls *(48)*.

Percutaneous coronary intervention was also performed using lepirudin in 25 HIT patients by Cochran et al. Many of their patients received GPIIb/IIIa inhibitors and clinical success - defined as freedom from death, MI, stroke, or revascularization -was achieved in 92% of the patients *(47)*.

According to Jolicoeur et al ,who recommend bivalirudin, experience with PCI and HIT is limited (to only 228 patients) *(49)*. The ACCP guidelines recommend using any of the three DTIs for patients with acute or previous HIT who require cardiac catheterization or PCI *(5)*.

Fondaparinux has also been used in PCI, but not in patients with HIT *(50)*. In the recently published Sixth Organization to Assess Strategies in Acute Ischemic Syndromes trial or OASIS, an increase in catheter-related thromboses was reported. Based on this finding, the authors recommended adjunctive therapy with UFH to prevent this complication, thereby eliminating fondaparinux as a suitable alternative for HIT patients *(50)*.

HIT AND CARDIAC SURGERY

Several issues confront the cardiac surgical patient with HIT, including difficulty in making the postoperative diagnosis of HIT and how best to manage the patient with acute HIT who requires urgent CABG.

The incidence of HIT approaches 2–3% following CABG; however, antibody formation is much higher approaching 50% by 1 week postoperatively. If routine HIT testing is done after surgery (because of thrombocytopenia), there is often a potential to over diagnose HIT based on laboratory results alone *(14)*.There are several clues helpful in making the diagnosis of "postoperative HIT." One, it classically presents as a biphasic pattern of platelet recovery; with an initial postoperative decline followed by recovery and then a second decline *(14)*. Other clues may include unusual or unexpected thromboembolic events, prolonged thrombocytopenia, and immunoassay values >1.0 or positive functional testing *(51)*.

Anticoagulation for the acute HIT patient who requires urgent CABG presents a difficult problem because currently available alternative anticoagulants are limited by their lack of an antidote and their need for special intraoperative monitoring using the ecarin clotting time (ECT). Several recent trials using bivalirudin in both "on-pump" and "off-pump" cardiac surgery have been described however *(35,36)*. The *C*ABG*HIT/TS* *O*n and *O*ff Pump *S*afety and *E*fficacy (CHOOSE-ON and CHOOSE-OFF) trials reported satisfactory procedural success and an acceptable incidence of bleeding *(35,36)*. If surgery cannot wait, recent data appears to favor bivalirudin in this setting, although lepirudin has been successfully used as well *(5,35,36)*.

Reexposure to UFH in patients with HIT is an area of controversy, although this approach has been used successfully for CABG and vascular surgery, when the surgeon feels alternative anticoagulants are not acceptable. Current strategies advise waiting approximately 100 days after the last UFH or LMWH exposure, thus allowing time for transient HIT antibodies to disappear. If testing confirms their absence, re-administration of UFH (during the procedure) appears to be safe *(22,45,52)*. A DTI should be considered postoperatively if the clinical situation warrants it.

The ACCP and the task force of the British Committee for Standards in Haematology guidelines recommend delaying surgery if possible, until the HIT antibody disappears., If however surgery is urgently needed, options include bivalirudin and lepirudin using the ECT for monitoring, or UFH plus the antiplatelet agents tirofiban (not recommended by the manufacturer) or epoprostenol *(5,45)*.

PLATELET FACTOR 4 HEPARIN ANTIBODIES IN PATIENTS WITHOUT HIT

Several recently published studies have suggested that the mere presence of "heparin antibodies" (without evidence for thrombocytopenia or overt HIT) may lead to adverse outcomes for cardiovascular patients *(53,54)*. Mattioli and colleagues reviewed the composite end point of death, MI, recurrent angina, and need for revascularization in 124 patients presenting with unstable angina who received at least 5 days of UFH *(53)*. The combined incidence of new thrombotic events including death, MI, recurrent angina, urgent revascularization, and stroke was more common (66% in patients with positive HIT antibodies and 44% in those without) at one year follow up *(53)*. Williams et al also reported adverse outcomes in 109 patients from the GUSTO IV-ACS trial who also received UFH exposure. They found that patients with PF4/heparin antibodies (without thrombocytopenia and no evidence for HIT) had a significantly higher rate of 30-day MI compared to those without antibodies *(54)*. Arnold and Kelton suggested that although these patients likely have what should be considered "false positive HIT", these antibodies, in certain populations may result in thrombosis *(55)*. Although these and other reports are intriguing, their significance is unknown and will need further research.

CONCLUSION

Heparin-induced thrombocytopenia is a serious complication of UFH or LMWH preparations that affects both the venous and arterial circulation. Although thrombocytopenia is the most common presentation, bleeding is an unusual complication. Thrombosis develops in over one half of all patients and lower extremity DVT and PE are the most common events, while acute limb occlusion involving the arterial circulation occurs more often than stroke or myocardial infarction.

HIT is an immune-mediated process that requires both clinical and laboratory findings to confirm the diagnosis. It is commonly referred to as a clinicopathologic syndrome. A high clinical suspicion, a pre-test probability score using the 4T's (thrombocytopenia, timing of the platelet count drop, thrombosis, and exclusion of other diagnostic possibilities) and positive laboratory testing will help confirm the diagnosis. Immediate discontinuation of UFH or LMWH,and the initiation of a DTI followed by warfarin therapy once the platelet count has recovered, is recommended.

Prevention is best achieved by close monitoring of the platelet count while the patient is receiving UFH. The use of alternatives to UFH (LMWH or fondaparinux) as primary prevention or treatment agents should be considered given their lower incidence of HIT.

REFERENCES

1. Oliveira GB, Anstrom KJ, Honeycutt EF et al (2004) Days on intravenous heparin predicts thrombocytopenia and drop in platelet count on heparin predicts mortality; findings from the Complications After Thrombocytopenia Caused by Heparin (CATCH) registry [abstract]. Circulation 110(Suppl):2604
2. Foo SY, Everett BM, Yeh RW et al (2006) Prevalence of heparin-induced thrombocytopenia in patients undergoing cardiac catheterization. Am Heart J 152(290):e1–e7
3. Warkentin TE (2003) Heparin induced thrombocytopenia: pathogenesis and management. Br J Haematol 123:373–374
4. Warkentin TE, Levine MN, Hirsh J et al (1995) Heparin-induced thrombocytopenia in patients treated with low-molecular weight heparin or unfractionated heparin. N Engl J Med 332:1330–1335
5. Warkentin TE, Greinacher A (2004) Heparin induced thrombocytopenia: recognition, treatment, and prevention the Seventh ACCP Conference on Antithrombotic and Thrombolytic Therapy. Chest 126(suppl 4):311S–337S

6. Martel N, Lee J, Wells PS (2005) Risk for heparin-induced thrombocytopenia with unfractionated and low-molecular-weight heparin thromboprophylaxis: a meta-analysis. Blood 106:2710–2715

7. Prandoni P, Siragusa S, Girolami B, Fabris F (2005) The incidence of heparin-induced thrombocytopenia in medical patients treated with low molecular weight heparin: a prospective cohort study. Blood 106:3049–3054

8. Cines DB, Rauova L, Arepally G et al (2007) Heparin-induced thrombocytopenia: an autoimmune disorder regulated through dynamic autoantigen assembly/disassembly. J Clin Apher 22:31–36

9. Warkentin TE, Sheppard JAI (2006) Testing from heparin-induced thrombocytopenia antibodies. Transfus Med Rev 20:254–272

10. Kelton JG (2005) The pathophysiology of heparin-induced thrombocytopenia: biological basis for treatment. Chest 127:9S–20S

11. Bartholomew JR, Begelman SM, AlMahameed A (2005) Heparin-induced thrombocytopenia: principles for early recognition and management. Cleve Clin J Med 72(Suppl 1):S31–S36

12. Warkentin TE (1998) Clinical presentation of heparin-induced thrombocytopenia. Semin Hematol 35(Suppl):9–16

13. Warkentin TE, Roberts RS, Hirsh J et al (2003) An improved definition of immune heparin-induced thrombocytopenia in postoperative orthopedic patients. Arch Intern Med 163:2518–2524

14. Arepally GM, Ortel TL (2006) Heparin-induced thrombocytopenia. N Engl J Med 355:809–817

15. Liu JC, Lewis BE, Steen LH et al (2002) Patency of coronary artery bypass grafts in patients with heparin-induced thrombocytopenia. Am J Cardiol 89:979–981

16. Warkentin TE, Kelton JG (1996) A 14 year study of heparin-induced thrombocytopenia. Am J Med 101:502–507

17. Warkentin TE, Elavathil LJ, Hayward CPM et al (1997) The pathogenesis of venous limb gangrene associated with heparin-induced thrombocytopenia. Ann Intern Med 127:804–812

18. Srinivasan AF, Rice L, Bartholomew JR et al (2004) Warfarin-induced skin necrosis and venous limb gangrene in the setting of heparin-induced thrombocytopenia. Arch Intern Med 164:66–70

19. Warkentin TE (2006) Coumarin-induced skin necrosis and venous limb gangrene. In: Colman RW, Marder VJ, Clowes AW, George JN, Goldhaber SZ (eds) Hemostasis and thrombosis: basic principles and clinical practice, 5th edn. Lippincott Williams & Wilkins, Philadelphia, pp 1663–1671

20. Warkentin TE (2007) Clinical picture of heparin-induced thrombocytopenia. In: Warkentin TE, Greinacher A (eds) Heparin-induced thrombocytopenia, 4th edn. Marcel Dekker, New York, pp 21–66

21. Mims MP, Manian P, Rice L (2004) Acute cardiorespiratory collapse from heparin: a consequence of heparin-induced thrombocytopenia. Eur J Haematol 72:366–369

22. Warkentin TE, Kelton JG (2001) Temporal aspects of heparin-induced thrombocytopenia. N Engl J Med 344:1286–1292

23. Warkentin TE, Heddle NM (2003) Laboratory diagnosis of immune heparin-induced thrombocytopenia. Curr Hematol Rep 2:148–157

24. Warkentin TE, Sheppard JI, Moore JC et al (2005) Laboratory testing for the antibodies that cause heparin-induced thrombocytopenia: how much class do we need. J Lab Clin Med 146:341–346

25. Zwicker JI, Uhl L, Huang WY, Shaz BH, Bauer KA (2004) Thrombosis and ELISA optical density values in hospitalized patients with heparin-induced thrombocytopenia. J Thromb Haemost 2:2133–2137

26. Greinacher A, Eichler P, Lubenow N, Kwasny H, Luz M (2000) Heparin-induced thrombocytopenia with thromboembolic complications; meta-analysis of 2 prospective trials to assess the value of parenteral treatment with lepirudin and its therapeutic aPTT range. Blood 96:846–851

27. Lubenow N, Eichler P, Lietz T, Greinacher A (2005) HIT investigators Group. Lepirudin in patients with heparin-induced thrombocytopenia-results of the third prospective study (HAT-3) and a combined analysis of HAT-1, HAT-2 and HAT-3. J Thromb Haemost 3:2428–2436

28. Lewis BE, Wallis DE, Berkowitz SD et al (2001) Argatroban anticoagulant therapy in patients with heparin-induced thrombocytopenia. Circulation 103:1838–1843

29. Hirsh J, Heddle N, Kelton JG (2004) Treatment of heparin-induced thrombocytopenia: a critical review. Arch Intern Med 164:361–369

30. Song X, Huhle G, Wang L, Hoffman U, Harenberg J (1999) Generation of anti-hirudin antibodies in heparin-induced thrombocytopenic patients treated with r-hirudin. Circulation 100:1528–1532

31. Greinacher A, Lubenow N, Eichler P (2003) Anaphylactic and anaphylactoid reactions associated with lepirudin in patients with heparin-induced thrombocytopenia. Circulation 108:2062–2065

32. Lewis BE, Wallis DE, Leya F, Hursting MJ, Kelton JG (2003) Argatroban anticoagulation in patients with heparin-induced thrombocytopenia. Arch Intern Med 163:1849–1856

33. Baghdasarian S, Singh I, Militello MA et al (2004) Argatroban dosage in critically ill patients with HIT. Blood 104:1179 (abstract)

34. Mahaffey KW, Lewis BE, Wilderman NM et al (2003) ATBAT investigators. The anticoagulant therapy with bivalirudin to assist in the performance of percutaneous coronary intervention in patients with heparin-induced thrombocytopenia (ATBAT) study: main results. J Invasive Cardiol 15:611–616

35. Dyke CM, Aldea G, Koster A et al (2007) Off pump coronary artery bypass with bivalirudin for patients with heparin-induced thrombocytopenia or anti-platelet factor 4/heparin antibodies. Ann Thorac Surg 84:836–839

36. Koster A, Dyke CM, Aldea G et al (2007) Bivalirudin during cardiopulmonary bypass in patients with previous or acute heparin-induced thrombocytopenia and heparin antibodies: results of the CHOOSE-ON trial. Ann Thorac Surg 83:572–577

37. Chamberlin JR, Lewis B, Leya F et al (1995) Successful treatment of heparin-associated thrombocytopenia and thrombosis using Hirulog. Can J Cardiol 11:511–514

38. Ramirez L, Carman T, Begelman SM, Bartholomew JR (2005) Bivalirudin in patients with HIT or clinically suspected HIT. Blood 106:269a abstract 918

39. Bartholomew JR (2007) Bivalirudin for the treatment of heparin-induced thrombocytopenia. In: Warkentin TE, Greinacher A (eds) Heparin-induced thrombocytopenia, 4th edn. Marcel Dekker, New York

40. Efird LE, Kockler DR (2006) Fondaparinux for thromboembolic treatment and prophylaxis of heparin-induced thrombocytopenia. Ann Pharmacother 40:1383–1387

41. Warkentin TE, Cook RJ, Marder VJ, Sheppard JA, Moore JC, Eriksson BI et al (2005) Anti-platelet factor 4/heparin antibodies in orthopedic surgery patients receiving antithrombotic prophylaxis with fondaparinux or enoxaparin. Blood 106(12):3791–3796

42. Warkentin TE, Maurer BT, Aster RH (2007) Heparin-induced thrombocytopenia associated with fondaparinux. N Engl J Med 356:2653–2655

43. Warkentin TE, Greinacher A, Craven S et al (2005) Differences in the clinically effective molar concentrations of four direct thrombin inhibitors explaining their variable prothrombin time prolongation. Thromb Haemost 94:958–964

44. Kearon C, Johnston M, Moffat K, McGinnis J, Ginsberg JS (1998) Effect of warfarin on activated partial thromboplastin time in patients receiving heparin. Arch Intern Med 158:1140–1143

45. Keeling D, Davidson S, Watson H (2006) On behalf of the Haemostasis and Thrombosis Task Force of the British Committee for Standards in Haematology. The management of heparin-induced thrombocytopenia. Br J Haematol 133:259–269

46. Wallis DE, Workman KL, Lewis BE et al (1999) Failure of early heparin cessation as treatment for heparin-induced thrombocytopenia. Am J Med 106:629–635

47. Cochran K, Demartini TJ, Lewis BE et al (2003) Use of lepirudin during percutaneous vascular interventions in patients with heparin-induced thrombocytopenia. J Invasive Cardiol 15:617–621

48. Lewis BE, Matthai WH, Cohen M et al (2002) Argatroban anticoagulation during percutaneous coronary intervention in patients with heparin-induced thrombocytopenia. Catheter Cardiovasc Interv 57:177–184

49. Jolicoeur EM, Wang T, Lopes RD et al (2007) Percutaneous coronary interventions in patients with heparin-induced thrombocytopenia. Curr Cardiol Rep 9:396–405

50. Yusuf S, Mehta SR, Chrolavicius S, OASIS-6 Trial Group et al (2006) Effects of fondaparinux on mortality and reinfarction in patients with acute ST-segment elevation myocardial infarction: the OASIS-6 randomized trial. JAMA 295(13):1519–1530

51. Das P, Ziada K, Steinhubl SR et al (2006) Heparin-induced thrombocytopenia and cardiovascular diseases. Am Heart J 152:19–26

52. Potzsch B, Klovekorn WP, Madlener K (2000) Use of heparin during cardiopulmonary bypass in patients with a history of heparin-induced thrombocytopenia (letter). N Engl J Med 343:515

53. Mattioli AV, Bonetti L, Sternieri S, Mattioli G (2000) Heparin-induced thrombocytopenia in patients treated with unfractionated heparin: prevalence of thrombosis in a 1 year follow-up. Ital Heart J 1:39–42

54. Williams RT, Damaraju LV, Mascelli MA et al (2003) Anti-platelet factor 4/heparin antibodies: an independent predictor of 30-day myocardial infarction after acute coronary ischemic syndromes. Circulation 107:2307–2312

55. Arnold DM, Kelton JG (2005) Heparin-induced thrombocytopenia: an iceberg rising. Mayo Clin Proc 80:988–990

56. Caiola E (2000) Heparin-induced thrombocytopenia: how to manage it, how to avoid it. Cleve Clin J Med 67:621–624

24 Resistance to Antiplatelet Drugs

Gerald C. Koenig and Hitinder S. Gurm

Contents

ABSTRACT Platelet activation and aggregation are central events in arterial thrombosis underlying acute coronary syndromes and progression of atherosclerotic vascular disease, and constitute complex processes involving multiple interdependent pathways. Aspirin remains the most well-studied antiplatelet agent and the backbone of therapy for patients with atherothrombosis. The thienopyridines (i.e., clopidogrel) have emerged as important additions for the management of patients with atherothrombotic diseases including those with acute coronary syndromes, those undergoing percutaneous coronary intervention, and selected patients with known vascular disease. Despite the use of these agents alone or in combination, a proportion of patients will continue to experience recurrent events. Some of these patients may be considered "resistant" to the currently available antiplatelet agents. Once thought of as simply a laboratory phenomenon, antiplatelet resistance has more recently been associated with adverse clinical events. Therefore, an understanding of the mechanism(s) behind treatment failure and therapeutic regimens needed to remedy them remain an area of essential research and of significant clinical importance.

Key words: Clopidogrel; Aspirin; Resistance; Outcomes; Assessment; Platelet function

From: *Contemporary Cardiology: Antithrombotic Drug Therapy in Cardiovascular Disease*
Edited by: A.T. Askari and A.M. Lincoff (eds.), DOI 10.1007/978-1-60327-235-3_24
© Humana Press, a part of Springer Science+Business Media, LLC 2010

INTRODUCTION

Platelets play an integral role in the pathogenesis of atherothrombotic disorders. While the clinical benefits of antiplatelet drugs are well recognized, there has been growing awareness of resistance to these agents. This chapter aims to highlight the definitions, mechanisms, and significance of resistance to antiplatelet drugs.

BACKGROUND

Platelet activation and aggregation are central events in arterial thrombosis underlying acute coronary syndromes and progression of atherosclerotic vascular disease, and constitute complex processes involving multiple interdependent pathways. In the acute coronary syndromes, atherosclerotic plaque rupture exposes collagen, von Willebrand factor, and other adhesive proteins within the subendothelium and intima to circulating platelets. Adhered platelets undergo conformational changes via the action of extrinsic activators, such as collagen, thrombin, and epinephrine. Upon activation platelets then release additional factors from their dense- and alpha-granules, including thromboxane A_2, adenosine diphosphate (ADP), and pro-inflammatory and pro-thrombotic factors. The activated and degranulated platelets expose glycoprotein IIb/IIIa receptors on their surface resulting in fibrinogen binding and platelet aggregation.

Aspirin, or acetylsalicylic acid, was first developed in 1897 by Felix Hoffman of Friedrich Bayer & Company in a stable, commercially available form *(1)*. However, the potential benefits of salicin, or salicylic acid, an extract of willow bark, had been known centuries prior and can be dated back to the Egyptians for its analgesic and anti-inflammatory activity *(2)*. Aspirin has now become essential therapy in cardiovascular medicine based on several clinical trials documenting primary and secondary prevention of myocardial infarction, stroke, and cardiovascular mortality. Aspirin serves as an irreversible inhibitor of platelet cyclooxygenase and platelet thromboxane A_2 production. However, aspirin does not prevent platelet aggregation due to thrombin, epinephrine, or serotonin, which are alternative pathways of platelet activation and aggregation.

Clopidogrel and ticlopidine are thienopyridine derivatives which exert their antiplatelet effects by inhibiting adenosine diphosphate (ADP)-mediated platelet activation. Use of clopidogrel, in combination with aspirin therapy, has shown significant risk reduction in myocardial infarction, stroke, and cardiovascular mortality in patients with both stable and unstable coronary artery disease [(CAPRIE *(3)*, CURE *(4)*, CREDO *(5)*, CLARITY-TIMI-28 *(6)*, COMMIT *(7)*] (Fig. 1).

However, despite millions of patients worldwide taking monotherapy or combination antiplatelet therapy, many continue to have cardiovascular events. Further laboratory evaluation of platelet function has revealed widespread variation in the degree of platelet inhibition in response to these agents. The understanding of the mechanism(s) behind treatment failure and therapeutic regimens needed to remedy them remain an area of essential research and of significant clinical importance.

DEFINITION

A true definition of aspirin and clopidogrel resistance has yet to be established. In the literature, it has been defined in both clinical and pharmacodynamic terms. Predicting clinical events has been difficult, and there exists a significant inter-assay discordance. Additionally, resistance may be more of a continuum than a binary determination and the occurrence of thrombotic events is a culmination of multiple signaling pathways encompassing complex platelet biology and function (Fig. 2).

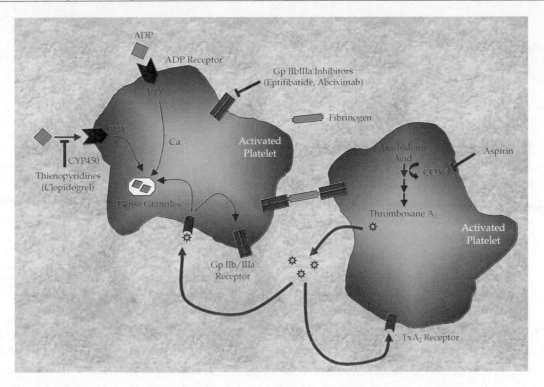

Fig. 1. Mechanism of platelet activation and regulation by aspirin and clopidogrel.

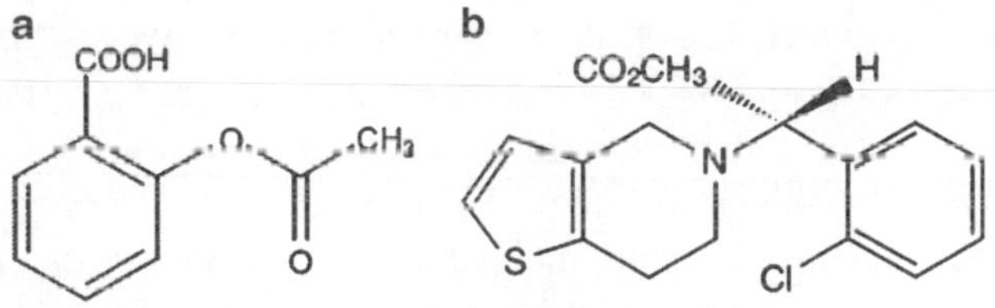

Fig. 2. Chemical structure of aspirin (**a**) and clopidogrel (**b**).

Clinical Failure

By strictest terms, the clinical definition of aspirin or clopidogrel failure is the occurrence of a vascular event despite treatment with aspirin and clopidogrel for thromboprophylaxis. Per the Antithrombotic Trialists' Collaboration (8), the frequency of aspirin failure can be estimated to range from 10.9% to 17.3%, depending on the aspirin dose. There has been no clear relationship between dosage and clinical failure rate, but several studies have suggested a dose response and time-dependent variability to both aspirin and clopidogrel treatment. However, because of the complex pathophysiology of ischemic heart disease, multiple factors potentially contribute to these events including inflammation, vascular biology, thrombosis, and hemodynamics. Recurrent events may also be mediated by non-platelet factors. Therefore, treatment failure is not synonymous with pharmacodynamic resistance and should not be used interchangeably.

Pharmacodynamic or Laboratory Resistance

The pharmacodynamic definition is the inability of antiplatelet therapy to inhibit the target of its action, that is, reduce platelet aggregation, using various assay systems. The frequency of aspirin resistance can be estimated to range from 5.5% to 60%, depending on the assay used.

PREVALENCE

Aspirin resistance has been reported in patients with coronary artery disease, cerebrovascular disease, peripheral artery disease, chronic heart failure, and atrial fibrillation. The frequency of reported cases has ranged from 5.5% in patients with stable cardiovascular disease and abnormal pharmacodynamics to 60% in patients with claudication symptoms on aspirin therapy *(8–19)*.

Clopidogrel resistance has been reported to have a prevalence between 4% and 30% 24 h after administration, depending on the assay utilized and baseline platelet reactivity *(20–24)*.

MECHANISMS

Aspirin

The action of acetylsalicylic acid, or aspirin, on platelet activity has been previously well characterized *(25)*. Aspirin acts by irreversibly acetylating platelet cyclooxygenase (COX)-1 at serine residue 530 to exert its anti-platelet effect *(26–28)*. The enzyme COX-1 is then permanently inhibited from converting arachadonic acid to several eicosanoids, such as leukotrienes, prostaglandins, thromboxane A_2 (TXA_2), and prostacyclin (PGI_2). Thromboxane A_2 is a potent vasoconstrictor and platelet agonist found in the alpha-granules of platelets. Prostacyclin is a vasodilator and platelet inhibitor produced by platelets and vascular endothelium. When COX-1 is inhibited by aspirin, platelet thromboxane A_2 production is eliminated for the life span of the anucleated platelet, but prostacyclin synthesis continues via the vascular endothelium which is able to replenish enzyme levels *(28,29)*. In addition, PGI_2 is produced by the enzymatic activity of COX-2 which is dramatically less affected by aspirin binding *(30)*.

Despite this well-characterized and clearly defined mechanism of action, the antiplatelet effects of aspirin are not uniform in all patients and the inhibition of platelet aggregation is highly variable. Several theories have been postulated on its mechanism of action and can be generally categorized into clinical, cellular, and genetic factors. Among the more evaluated mechanisms are platelet hypersensitivity to collagen *(31)*, increased COX-2 activity or over-expression *(30)*, and platelet alloantigen 2 (PLA2) polymorphism of platelet glycoprotein IIIa *(32,33)*. Additional mechanisms include poor patient compliance *(34)*, poor gastrointestinal absorption *(35)*, interactions with other medications *(36–38)*, tachyphylaxis *(39)*, increased isoprostane activity *(40)*, CD40–CD40 ligand interaction *(41)*, thromboxane production by non-platelet cells *(42)*, exercise and catecholamine levels *(43)*, and COX-1 polymorphism *(44)*. While the theories all appear plausible, the complex nature of platelet physiology and redundancy of multiple platelet agonists argue for numerous factors being involved.

Clopidogrel

Unlike aspirin, clopidogrel is a prodrug that effects platelet activation and aggregation by a secondary active hepatic metabolite converted by cytochrome P450 3A4 (CYP3A4) *(45)*. The thiol metabolite, in turn, acts by blocking adenosine diphosphate (ADP)-mediated platelet activation via irreversible inhibition of one of three platelet ADP receptors ($P2Y_{12}$) via disulfide bond bridging *(46,47)*. $P2Y_{12}$ receptor binding liberates G_i protein subunits, which leads to the inhibition of cAMP-mediated phosphorylation of vasodilator-stimulated phosphoprotein (VASP), a known inhibitor of glycoprotein IIb/IIIa receptor activation *(48)*. This prevents upregulation of the glycoprotein IIb/IIIa receptor which is involved in the final common pathway for platelet activation. Shear stress-induced platelet activation is largely dependent on ADP and is resistant to aspirin, as is ADP-induced platelet activation in vivo in the presence of physiologic calcium concentrations. The effects of clopidogrel on platelet activity are both time and dose dependent. Inhibition of platelet aggregation appears limited to 50–60% secondary to either incomplete $P2Y_{12}$ receptor occupancy or effects of the $P2Y_1$ receptor binding sites *(49)*. Steady-state levels are achieved by 4–24 h following loading doses (300–600 mg) and 4–7 days following daily maintenance dosing (75 mg) *(21,22,50,51)*. Also, it has been reported that nearly half of initially reported non-responders at 24 h post-loading doses of clopidogrel prior to PCI became responders by 30 days, a finding postulated to arise as a result of delayed post-stent platelet activation *(52)*.

Similar to aspirin resistance, the mechanism of clopidogrel resistance may also be generally categorized into clinical, cellular, and genetic factors. These mechanisms include poor patient compliance, variable gastrointestinal absorption and conversion to active metabolite *(53,54)*, inappropriate dosing, drug–drug interactions *(45,55)*, body mass index *(56)*, upregulation of other platelet activation pathways, greater baseline platelet reactivity *(57)*, and variable expression and polymorphism of ADP receptors *(53,58–60)*.

TESTING

To date there is no clinically accepted and validated method to specifically determine the effect of aspirin or other anti-platelet agents on platelet aggregation. Several methods of measuring platelet function and activity have been developed over the years, including aggregation, receptor expression, intracellular signaling, point-of-care and platelet-released factors. The more commonly accepted method and historical "gold standard" is that of Born *(61)* which extrapolates aspirin sensitivity by platelet function in an in vitro measurement of light transmittance aggregometry (LTA). Basically, platelet-rich plasma prepared from citrated whole blood samples is induced to aggregate by the addition of an agonist (e.g., ADP, arachidonic acid, collagen, epinephrine, and thrombin) and the turbidity of the solution is measured by optical light transmission *(62,63)*. Aspirin almost completely inhibits platelet aggregation induced by arachidonic acid and collagen. Modifications to the assay have also been widely used to monitor the effects of other antiplatelet agents, such as clopidogrel, other $P2Y_{12}$ inhibitors, and platelet glycoprotein IIb/IIIa inhibitors *(64)*. The aggregation assay, however, is sensitive to changes in temperature and pH, necessitating sample assessment within hours of collection, and is labor intensive.

Additional methods using immunoassay and flow cytometry techniques include measurement of platelet-released factors and receptor expression, including plasma-soluble CD40 ligand, platelet-derived microparticles, platelet surface P-selectin (CD62p) and GP IIb/IIIa, and serum thromboxane B_2 *(64)*. The stable urinary TXA_2 metabolite 11-dehydro-TXB_2 has been used to predict outcomes along with aspirin responsiveness using radioimmunoassay and enzyme immunoassay (AspirinWorks, Creative Clinical Concepts Inc., Denver, CO) systems *(10,65)*. This assay is non-invasive and normalized with standard controls given COX-1 dependency, but is based on a retro-spective case-control study for its abnormal range determination, an indirect measure, and depends on renal function.

Intracellular signaling pathway activation has further been measured using flow cytometry techniques in combination with platelet membrane permeabilizing agents. By quantifying the amount of phosphorylated vasodilator-stimulated phosphoprotein (VASP) using monoclonal antibodies, increased specificity for the $P2Y_{12}$ signaling pathway activation by the thienopyridines can be determined *(48)*.

Also, two automated, point-of-care assays have been studied, the Platelet Function Analyzer (PFA)-100 (Dade Behring Inc., Deerfield, IL) and the VerifyNow Rapid Platelet Function Assay (Accumetrics Inc., San Diego, CA) *(66,67)*. The PFA-100 functions by aspirating a blood sample through a capillary tube and passing through a small slit aperture that is cut into a membrane coated with either collagen-epinephrine (CEPI) or collagen-ADP (CADP) serving as a platelet aggregation agonist. The time for the aggregate to occlude the slit aperture is inversely related to platelet activity, with closure times of <193 s considered normal. However, the time point of aspirin sensitivity by CEPI (aspirin has little effect on CADP measurements) remains ill-defined, is weakly correlated with increased risk of clinical events in a selected cohort study, and depends on vWF and hematocrit levels.

The VerifyNow assay is designed to only detect platelet dysfunction when exposed to antiplatelet agents, such as aspirin, clopidogrel, and glycoprotein IIb–IIIa inhibitors, using arachadonic acid (AA) for aspirin agonist and combination ADP and prostaglandin E1 for clopidogrel agonist. The agglutination of platelets on fibrinogen-coated beads is detected by an optical turbidimetric method. Platelet responsiveness to aspirin is expressed in aspirin response units (ARU), with the cutoff at >550 ARU, and has shown good correlation with measurements performed by the PFA-100 and traditional optical platelet aggregation techniques. Platelet responsiveness to clopidogrel is expressed in $P2Y_{12}$ reaction units (PRU), but has no consensually defined cutoff value to identify non-responders. In consideration of the factors affecting platelet aggregation, relative measures of reactivity compared to baseline measures are considered more appropriate rather than arbitrary cutoff values. Empirically defined cutoff values have ranged between <10 and <40% *(22,23)*.

More recently consideration has been placed on assessing the platelet–fibrin interaction, kinetics of thrombin generation, and platelet-fibrin clot strength as possible important mediators in predicting cardiovascular events in those patients on antiplatelet therapy *(68,69)*. These thromboelastography measurements may potentially yield better predictive tools independently or in combination with isolated platelet function assays.

CLINICAL CONFOUNDERS

The action of aspirin and clopidogrel therapy on platelet responsiveness is additionally confounded by other cyclooxygenase inhibitors, lipid levels, BMI, diabetes, smoking status, gender, and other drug interactions, such as statin medications. Diabetic patients with stable CAD have been found to exhibit higher aspirin resistance at 81 mg/day compared to non-diabetic patients with stable CAD (27% vs. 4% with collagen-induced LTA) using several different platelet function assays, and increasing the aspirin dosing resulted in similar rates of resistance and platelet function *(70)*. Similar rates of aspirin resistance have been identified in both type I and type II diabetic patients *(71)*. Compared with clopidogrel-resistant patients, patients with effective clopidogrel inhibition have significantly lower BMI (26.1 vs. 28.8 kg/m^2, $p < 0.05$), even after adjustment for other risk factors and medications *(72)*. Smoking has also been shown to induce platelet hyper-reactivity and correlated with increased aspirin resistance, potentially limiting or negating the therapeutic effect of antiplatelet agents in these patients *(73,74)*. Gender difference has been correlated with aspirin resistance or semi-responder status in patients with stable CAD with women having greater propensity for resistance (25.3% vs. 46.1% and 17.3% vs. 34.4%, respectively) *(75,76)*. Poor responsiveness to aspirin therapy in patients with known CAD, or at least two risk factors for CAD, has been shown to correlate with higher mean concentrations of total cholesterol and LDL cholesterol (6.2% vs. 4.8% and 4.0% vs. 3.0%, respectively), but not with HDL cholesterol and triglycerides *(77)*. Among medication interactions, several studies have revealed a decreased clinical benefit of aspirin with concomitant administration of ibuprofen, but not significantly with diclofenac or rofecoxib, correlating with in vitro analysis of ibuprofen's action of interfering with the ability of aspirin to irreversibly inhibit COX-1 enzyme *(36,37,78)*. In addition, the ability of clopidogrel to inhibit platelet function has been demonstrated to be attenuated by some HMG CoA reductase inhibitors, such as atorvastatin, likely via inhibition of the CYP 3A4 enzyme *(45,79,80)*. However, post hoc analysis has revealed no difference in clinical outcomes between patients taking clopidogrel and a variety of HMG-CoA reductase inhibitors, suggesting the interaction observed appears to be only significant in vitro *(81–83)*.

CLINICAL SIGNIFICANCE

An estimated 26 million patients in the United States currently take aspirin for cardiovascular thromboprophylaxis. Given the reported prevalence of aspirin resistance of 5–60% and clopidogrel resistance from 4% to 30%, there exist a substantial number of patients who are likely resistant to these medications and potentially at risk for breakthrough events. Definitive data to support a clinically relevant impact of antiplatelet therapy, however, are lacking. Establishing the clinical significance of antiplatelet resistance has been hindered by lack of reliable measurement of aspirin and clopidogrel effect and poses the biggest challenge to the current research.

Aspirin Resistance

Despite evidence in using biochemical measures to determine aspirin responsiveness, the causal association with cardiovascular disease and the magnitude of associated risk holds the greatest implications for clinical importance and relevance.

Initial studies by Grotemeyer and colleagues *(84)* prospectively evaluated the effects of aspirin resistance in 180 acute stroke patients. Aspirin non-responders made up 30% of post-stroke patients who were all treated with 500 mg of aspirin and were 89% more likely to have recurrent cerebrovascular events within 2 years compared to aspirin responders. Mueller et al. *(16)* followed with a study of patients with intermittent claudication presenting for peripheral vascular angioplasty and found a 40% incidence of aspirin resistance. After 18 months of follow-up, aspirin non-response was associated with an 87% increase in the risk of arterial reocclusion. Eikelboom and colleagues *(10)* performed a case-control study from the Heart Outcomes Prevention Evaluation (HOPE) trial that found patients with the highest levels of urinary 11-dehydro thromboxane B_2, implying incomplete platelet inhibition, had a 3.5-fold increase in cardiovascular mortality, and a twofold increase in myocardial infarction. Gum et al. *(9)* prospectively studied 326 patients with stable cardiovascular disease on 325 mg of daily aspirin and found 5–9% to be aspirin resistant (optical aggregation vs. PFA-100 assay, respectively). Women and non-smokers were more likely to be ASA non-responders, along with a trend toward those with increased age. A threefold increase in risk of death, MI, or CVA was found in those patients with aspirin resistance [4 of 17 (24%) vs. 30 of 309 (10%), $p=0.03$]. More recently, Chen et al. *(14)* studied 151 patients with stable CAD presenting for elective percutaneous coronary intervention and found a 19.2% incidence of aspirin resistance, as measured by the Ultegra Rapid Platelet Function Assay-ASA (Accumetrics Inc., San Diego, CA), that was associated with a nearly threefold increased risk of post-PCI creatinine kinase-MB elevation, defined as any elevation above the upper limit of normal of ≥ 16 U/L.

SIGNIFICANCE OF ANTI-PLATELET FAILURE

Observational studies from larger randomized clinical trials involving patients with known CAD have further lent support to aspirin failure as a potential mechanism for atherothrombotic events in individuals on aspirin therapy. Antman and colleagues *(85)* have reported that prior aspirin use in those patients presenting with acute coronary syndromes is an independent predictor of increased cardiovascular risk. However, Barnes and colleagues (86) found no significant difference in 6-month stroke, death, or major adverse cardiac events (MACEs) in patients on no prior antiplatelet therapy, aspirin only, or aspirin and clopidogrel. These findings suggest a possible role for confounding in the earlier studies and that prior antiplatelet therapy may well be a marker of cardiovascular disease and not of worse outcomes.

Clopidogrel Resistance

A limited number of studies exist in the literature assessing the clinical relevance of platelet response to clopidogrel therapy. The studies have used dissimilar assay systems for measuring platelet reactivity and have compared small populations of patients. Additionally, the potential benefit of clopidogrel therapy beyond that of platelet aggregation inhibition, namely the anti-inflammatory properties, has not been assessed.

Barragan et al. (87) performed an initial small, prospective evaluation using a vasodilator-stimulated phosphoprotein (VASP) phosphorylation assay on 36 patients with subacute stent thrombosis and found significantly higher platelet reactivity compared to controls receiving similar therapies. However, the results were limited given the high inter-individual variability and lack of baseline platelet aggregation levels for assessment of relative changes. Müller and colleagues (22) followed with a study of 105 patients with stable coronary artery disease undergoing elective PCI and found 5–11% (ADP 5 μmol/L vs. ADP 20 μmol/L) were non-responders to clopidogrel therapy. Of two patients who developed subacute stent thrombosis following intracoronary stent placement, both were non-responders. Gurbel et al. (21) studied 96 patients undergoing elective coronary stenting and measured platelet aggregation at baseline and at multiple times after a standard 300 mg loading dose and 75 mg daily maintenance dose. Resistance to clopidogrel was defined as <10% reduction in platelet aggregation to 5 μmol/L ADP compared to pretreatment values. The findings showed clopidogrel resistance in 63% of patients at 2 h, 31% at 24 h, 31% at 5 days, and 15% at 30 days. Significant interindividual variability was noted in the platelet inhibitory response, and those with high baseline reactivity were least protected. Mobley et al. (23) published a small prospective study of 50 patients with stable coronary artery disease undergoing elective PCI for which platelet function was analyzed by three separate instruments. Using a similar definition of <10% reduction in platelet aggregation, 30% of patients were found to be non-responders, but no correlation was found with clinical pretreatment variables, including major adverse coronary events at 1 and 6 months. Matetzky and colleagues (88) followed with a study of 60 patients undergoing primary PCI with stenting and ten patients undergoing primary angioplasty for acute ST elevation myocardial infarction. Patients received 300 mg aspirin loading dose, along with eptifibatide and heparin during PCI. Turbidimetric analysis was used to measure platelet aggregation to 5 μmol/L ADP and 10 μmol/L epinephrine. Patients were divided into quartiles based on the level of platelet inhibition at 6 days compared to baseline: first quartile with aggregation 103% (non-responders), second quartile 69%, third quartile 58%, and fourth quartile 33%. At 6-month follow-up, 40% of non-responders, 7% of patients in the second quartile, and none in the remaining quartiles had recurrent cardiovascular events, including stent thrombosis, MI, and recurrent ACS. This was the first study to show that clopidogrel resistance may be a marker for increased secondary cardiovascular events. More recently, Serebruany et al. (24) analyzed the response to clopidogrel treatment on 544 heterogeneous patients, consisting of volunteers ($n=94$), patients after coronary stenting ($n=405$), with heart failure ($n=25$), and after stroke ($n=20$). The findings showed a wide variability in response with a normal, bell-shaped distribution, for which 4.2 and 4.8% of patients were deemed hypo-responsive and hyper-responsive, respectively, based on being greater or less than two standard deviations from the mean. The clinical implications, however, are unknown. Further, Cuisset et al. *(89)* studied post-treatment platelet reactivity rather than antiplatelet responsiveness in 106 patients and showed an increased risk of recurrent cardiovascular events after stenting for acute coronary syndrome by comparing the upper quartile group to the lower quartiles (12 total events, OR 22.4). Similarly, Lev et al. *(90)* found aspirin-resistant patients ($n=19$) had more than a twofold increase in the incidence of myonecrosis (CK-MB > 5 ng/ml) following PCI (38.9% vs. 18.3%), and clopidogrel-resistant patients ($n=36$) had slightly less than a twofold increase in myonecrosis following PCI (32.4% vs. 17.3%) compared to aspirin and clopidogrel responders, respectively. Finally, Angiolillo et al. *(91)* studied 173 diabetic patients with coronary artery disease on standard chronic treatment with clopidogrel and aspirin over 2 years and found high platelet reactivity, defined as upper quartile of maximal platelet aggregation, was associated with a higher major adverse cardiovascular events (15.2, 12.2, 12.2, and 37.7%, respectively).

TREATMENT

Aspirin

Several placebo-controlled trials and a number of meta-analyses to confirm the benefit of aspirin in the primary and secondary prevention of atherosclerotic disease complications in various clinical settings have used doses ranging from 30 to 1,300 mg/d *(8,92)*. Universally, a significant benefit favoring higher doses of aspirin has not been demonstrated, and in most trials the low-dose groups achieved the lowest event rates and improved outcomes. Retrospective analyses of large-scale clinical trials have also consistently shown the lack of increased benefit with higher aspirin doses *(93,94)*.

Despite the population-based evidence, individual variability in the response to aspirin exists using ex vivo diagnostic measures has been correlated to clinical outcomes *(95)*. Higher doses of maintenance aspirin have been proposed that may accordingly be of clinical benefit in those specific sub groups. In support of such a tactic, a comprehensive comparison of studies that have examined aspirin resistance in users of aspirin at ≥300 mg daily versus ≤100 mg daily showed a significantly lower prevalence rate *(96)*. An increase in the aspirin dose has been shown to alleviate aspirin resistance in 44–92% of the individuals in small, selected populations *(97,98)*. However, this benefit has yet to be correlated with a reduction in clinical events. In addition, the potential benefit of higher aspirin doses in reducing the prevalence of aspirin resistance may be offset by the more profound suppression of the vasculoprotective effects of prostacyclin and the higher incidence of bleeding complications *(99–101)*.

Clopidogrel

The standard dosing regimen of clopidogrel was derived mainly from studies involving healthy volunteers and stable patients with coronary artery disease *(51,102,103)*. Clinical benefit on improving cardiovascular outcomes was further corroborated in the observational PCI-CURE (Percutaneous Coronary Intervention – Clopidogrel in Unstable Angina to Prevent Recurrent Events) trial and randomized CREDO (Clopidogrel for the Reduction of Events During Observation) trial *(5,104)*. However, platelet reactivity in patients with coronary atherosclerosis undergoing PCI may be significantly elevated due to several factors, including increased platelet reactivity induced by stenting *(21,105)*, primed platelets *(106)*, genetic polymorphisms *(59,60)*, and drug–drug interactions *(79,107,108)*.

Observational studies have shown that higher loading doses of clopidogrel, such as 600 mg versus 300 mg, provide a more rapid and greater inhibition of platelet aggregation, reducing the incidence of clopidogrel non-responders and high post-procedural platelet aggregation, for a distinct set of platelet activation assays (106,109–112). Furthermore, the higher loading dose regimen of clopidogrel has also been shown to potentially improve 30-day clinical outcomes with significantly reduced periprocedural MI and overall cardiovascular events in patients undergoing percutaneous coronary intervention (113,114). However, a significant interindividual variability of platelet inhibition still persisted, and postulated to be as a result of the high number of factors contributing to the modulation of platelet function. Despite the limitations, the current ACC/AHA guidelines for PCI have given a Class IIa recommendation to using a greater than 300 mg loading dose of clopidogrel to achieve a higher, more rapid level of antiplatelet activity (115).

In addition to the short-term effects, patients may sustain a heightened level of platelet reactivity during the maintenance phase of therapy (116). Supporting this hypothesis is the fact that a more pronounced inhibition has been observed with clopidogrel re-loading in patients on chronic therapy, suggesting higher clopidogrel doses might be needed for maintenance therapy (110). In addition, a higher maintenance dose of clopidogrel (150 mg vs. 75 mg daily) was shown to reduce platelet reactivity in a high-risk group of diabetics with coronary artery disease who demonstrated suboptimal baseline platelet inhibition, but clinical outcomes were not assessed (117). Based on this level of evidence, the current ACC/AHA guidelines for PCI have given a Class IIb recommendation to using a platelet aggregation study in certain high-risk individuals and an increased maintenance clopidogrel dose of 150 mg if less than 50% platelet aggregation inhibition can be demonstrated (115).

Additionally, the relative potential pleiotropic properties of clopidogrel, namely that of anti-inflammatory characteristics and reductions in serum C-reactive protein level (110), have not been evaluated with respect to its anti-platelet effect. Therefore, whether patients deemed unresponsive to clopidogrel via platelet reactivity still receive benefit through other avenues remains to be determined.

Alternative or other antithrombotic strategies, such as newly designed thienopyridines (118,119), non-thienopyridine P2Y inhibitors (120,121), and antagonists of other platelet targets (53), have been proposed for those patients who continue to show high platelet aggregation levels despite increased loading and maintenance doses of clopidogrel in combination with aspirin. Recently, the TRITON-TIMI 38 phase 3 clinical trial results were released comparing prasugrel, a novel thienopyridine, to standard-dosing regimen of clopidogrel in 13,608 patients with acute coronary syndromes with scheduled PCI (119). Prasugrel therapy was associated with significantly reduced rates of the primary endpoints of death from cardiovascular causes, nonfatal myocardial infarction, or non-fatal stroke (9.9% vs. 12.1%, $p < 0.001$), with nonfatal myocardial infarction being the major driving component (7.3% vs. 9.5%, $p < 0.001$), along with urgent target-vessel revascularization (2.5% vs. 3.7%, $p < 0.001$) and stent thrombosis (1.1% vs. 2.4%, $p < 0.001$). However, unlike the JUMBO-TIMI-26 trial findings (122), these results were accompanied by higher rates of bleeding endpoints (32% increase in TIMI major hemorrhage), including life-threatening and fatal hemorrhage.

Additional clinical studies remain to be performed to validate these hypotheses, identify safety margins for increased bleeding complications, and determine the need for individualized antithrombotic regimens to optimally inhibit platelet activity.

CONCLUSIONS

The inability of aspirin or clopidogrel to prevent clinical atherothrombotic ischemic events has been termed clinical aspirin or clopidogrel failure, respectively. Several mechanisms have been proposed and most likely are a combination of clinical, biological, and genetic properties on platelet function. Numerous laboratory assays have been established to measure platelet reactivity and aggregation in an effort to establish a causal relationship between aspirin and clopidogrel resistance and clinical outcomes for cardiovascular risk. There is a growing body of literature suggesting that laboratory measures of aspirin and clopidogrel non-responsiveness are clinically correlated to outcomes, and that biologic aspirin reactivity can be altered by dose adjustments.

However, significant speculation and uncertainty remain as to whether the laboratory measurement of platelet activity and aggregation fully encompasses the biological effect of antiplatelet therapy. Additionally, the antiplatelet effects of aspirin and clopidogrel remain highly variable and follow a continuous distribution of values. In this context, antiplatelet resistance remains poorly defined and without a standardized definition. Further research is still required to both establish a valid, specific, reliable, and reproducible standard measurement, and appropriately correlate the findings with ischemic or other cardiovascular events using adequately powered, long-term clinical trials. Only at that point will it then be possible to adequately and accurately determine the specific population at risk, evaluate the effectiveness of treatment, and assess the utility and cost-effectiveness of laboratory testing for resistance.

In the interim, it remains to be determined whether we should be regularly measuring platelet activity in patients with known cardiovascular disease or presenting with acute coronary syndromes, and what if any therapeutic strategies should be employed to potentially improve clinical outcomes. However, given the significant implications for thromboprophylaxis on cardiovascular outcomes, the intuitive notion of measuring the biochemical activity of antiplatelet therapy in targeting treatment, much like that performed for cholesterol and blood pressure, is likely to yield further significant understanding of treatment failure, to improve individualized antiplatelet therapy, and to develop new antithrombotic agents.

REFERENCES

1. Schadewaldt H (1990) Historical aspects of pharmacologic research at Bayer. 1890-1990. Stroke 21:IV5–IV8
2. Jack DB (1997) One hundred years of aspirin. Lancet 350:437–439
3. CAPRIE Steering Committee (1996) A randomised, blinded, trial of clopidogrel versus aspirin in patients at risk of ischaemic events (CAPRIE). CAPRIE Steering Committee. Lancet 348:1329–1339
4. Mehta SR (2003) Aspirin and clopidogrel in patients with ACS undergoing PCI: CURE and PCI-CURE. J Invasive Cardiol 15(Suppl B):17B–20B discussion 20B–21B
5. Steinhubl SR, Berger PB, Mann JT 3 rd, Fry ET, DeLago A, Wilmer C, Topol EJ (2002) Early and sustained dual oral antiplatelet therapy following percutaneous coronary intervention: a randomized controlled trial. JAMA 288:2411–2420
6. Sabatine MS, Cannon CP, Gibson CM, Lopez-Sendon JL, Montalescot G, Theroux P, Claeys MJ, Cools F, Hill KA, Skene AM, McCabe CH, Braunwald E (2005) Addition of clopidogrel to aspirin and fibrinolytic therapy for myocardial infarction with ST-segment elevation. N Engl J Med 352:1179–1189
7. Chen ZM, Jiang LX, Chen YP, Xie JX, Pan HC, Peto R, Collins R, Liu LS (2005) Addition of clopidogrel to aspirin in 45, 852 patients with acute myocardial infarction: randomised placebo-controlled trial. Lancet 366:1607–1621
8. Antithrombotic Trialists' Collaboration (2002) Collaborative meta-analysis of randomised trials of antiplatelet therapy for prevention of death, myocardial infarction, and stroke in high risk patients. BMJ 324:71–86
9. Gum PA, Kottke-Marchant K, Welsh PA, White J, Topol EJ (2003) A prospective, blinded determination of the natural history of aspirin resistance among stable patients with cardiovascular disease. J Am Coll Cardiol 41:961–965
10. Eikelboom JW, Hirsh J, Weitz JI, Johnston M, Yi Q, Yusuf S (2002) Aspirin-resistant thromboxane biosynthesis and the risk of myocardial infarction, stroke, or cardiovascular death in patients at high risk for cardiovascular events. Circulation 105:1650–1655
11. Harrison P, Segal H, Blasbery K, Furtado C, Silver L, Rothwell PM (2005) Screening for aspirin responsiveness after transient ischemic attack and stroke: comparison of 2 point-of-care platelet function tests with optical aggregometry. Stroke 36:1001–1005
12. Helgason CM, Bolin KM, Hoff JA, Winkler SR, Mangat A, Tortorice KL, Brace LD (1994) Development of aspirin resistance in persons with previous ischemic stroke. Stroke 25:2331–2336

13. Alberts MJ, Bergman DL, Molner E, Jovanovic BD, Ushiwata I, Teruya J (2004) Antiplatelet effect of aspirin in patients with cerebrovascular disease. Stroke 35:175–178

14. Chen WH, Lee PY, Ng W, Tse HF, Lau CP (2004) Aspirin resistance is associated with a high incidence of myonecrosis after non-urgent percutaneous coronary intervention despite clopidogrel pretreatment. J Am Coll Cardiol 43:1122–1126

15. Andersen K, Hurlen M, Arnesen H, Seljeflot I (2002) Aspirin non-responsiveness as measured by PFA-100 in patients with coronary artery disease. Thromb Res 108:37–42

16. Mueller MR, Salat A, Stangl P, Murabito M, Pulaki S, Boehm D, Koppensteiner R, Ergun E, Mittlboeck M, Schreiner W, Losert U, Wolner E (1997) Variable platelet response to low-dose ASA and the risk of limb deterioration in patients submitted to peripheral arterial angioplasty. Thromb Haemost 78:1003–1007

17. Coma-Canella I, Velasco A, Castano S (2005) Prevalence of aspirin resistance measured by PFA-100. Int J Cardiol 101:71–76

18. Fateh-Moghadam S, Plockinger U, Cabeza N, Htun P, Reuter T, Ersel S, Gawaz M, Dietz R, Bocksch W (2005) Prevalence of aspirin resistance in patients with type 2 diabetes. Acta Diabetol 42:99–103

19. Malinin A, Spergling M, Muhlestein B, Steinhubl S, Serebruany V (2004) Assessing aspirin responsiveness in subjects with multiple risk factors for vascular disease with a rapid platelet function analyzer. Blood Coagul Fibrinolysis 15:295–301

20. Jaremo P, Lindahl TL, Fransson SG, Richter A (2002) Individual variations of platelet inhibition after loading doses of clopidogrel. J Intern Med 252:233–238

21. Gurbel PA, Bliden KP, Hiatt BL, O'Connor CM (2003) Clopidogrel for coronary stenting: response variability, drug resistance, and the effect of pretreatment platelet reactivity. Circulation 107:2908–2913

22. Muller I, Besta F, Schulz C, Massberg S, Schonig A, Gawaz M (2003) Prevalence of clopidogrel non-responders among patients with stable angina pectoris scheduled for elective coronary stent placement. Thromb Haemost 89:783–787

23. Mobley JE, Bresee SJ, Wortham DC, Craft RM, Snider CC, Carroll RC (2004) Frequency of nonresponse antiplatelet activity of clopidogrel during pretreatment for cardiac catheterization. Am J Cardiol 93:456–458

24. Serebruany VL, Steinhubl SR, Berger PB, Malinin AI, Bhatt DL, Topol EJ (2005) Variability in platelet responsiveness to clopidogrel among 544 individuals. J Am Coll Cardiol 45:246–251

25. Vane JR (1971) Inhibition of prostaglandin synthesis as a mechanism of action for aspirin-like drugs. Nat New Biol 231:232–235

26. Roth GJ, Calverley DC (1994) Aspirin, platelets, and thrombosis: theory and practice. Blood 83:885–898

27. Roth GJ, Majerus PW (1975) The mechanism of the effect of aspirin on human platelets. I. Acetylation of a particulate fraction protein. J Clin Invest 56:624–632

28. Burch JW, Stanford N, Majerus PW (1978) Inhibition of platelet prostaglandin synthetase by oral aspirin. J Clin Invest 61:314–319

29. Patrignani P, Filabozzi P, Patrono C (1982) Selective cumulative inhibition of platelet thromboxane production by low-dose aspirin in healthy subjects. J Clin Invest 69:1366–1372

30. Cipollone F, Rocca B, Patrono C (2004) Cyclooxygenase-2 expression and inhibition in atherothrombosis. Arterioscler Thromb Vasc Biol 24:246–255

31. Kawasaki T, Ozeki Y, Igawa T, Kambayashi J (2000) Increased platelet sensitivity to collagen in individuals resistant to low-dose aspirin. Stroke 31:591–595

32. Undas A, Brummel K, Musial J, Mann KG, Szczeklik A (2001) Pl(A2) polymorphism of beta(3) integrins is associated with enhanced thrombin generation and impaired antithrombotic action of aspirin at the site of microvascular injury. Circulation 104:2666–2672

33. Michelson AD, Furman MI, Goldschmidt-Clermont P, Mascelli MA, Hendrix C, Coleman L, Hamlington J, Barnard MR, Kickler T, Christie DJ, Kundu S, Bray PF (2000) Platelet GP IIIa Pl(A) polymorphisms display different sensitivities to agonists. Circulation 101:1013–1018

34. Cotter G, Shemesh E, Zehavi M, Dinur I, Rudnick A, Milo O, Vered Z, Krakover R, Kaluski E, Kornberg A (2004) Lack of aspirin effect: aspirin resistance or resistance to taking aspirin? Am Heart J 147:293–300

35. Gonzalez-Conejero R, Rivera J, Corral J, Acuna C, Guerrero JA, Vicente V (2005) Biological assessment of aspirin efficacy on healthy individuals: heterogeneous response or aspirin failure? Stroke 36:276–280

36. Catella-Lawson F, Reilly MP, Kapoor SC, Cucchiara AJ, DeMarco S, Tournier B, Vyas SN, FitzGerald GA (2001) Cyclooxygenase inhibitors and the antiplatelet effects of aspirin. N Engl J Med 345:1809–1817

37. Kurth T, Glynn RJ, Walker AM, Chan KA, Buring JE, Hennekens CH, Gaziano JM (2003) Inhibition of clinical benefits of aspirin on first myocardial infarction by nonsteroidal antiinflammatory drugs. Circulation 108:1191–1195

38. Lau WC, Gurbel PA (2006) Antiplatelet drug resistance and drug-drug interactions: Role of cytochrome P450 3A4. Pharm Res 23:2691–2708

39. Pulcinelli FM, Riondino S, Celestini A, Pignatelli P, Trifiro E, Di Renzo L, Violi F (2005) Persistent production of platelet thromboxane A2 in patients chronically treated with aspirin. J Thromb Haemost 3:2784–2789

40. Morrow JD, Hill KE, Burk RF, Nammour TM, Badr KF, Roberts LJ 2nd (1990) A series of prostaglandin F2-like compounds are produced in vivo in humans by a non-cyclooxygenase, free radical-catalyzed mechanism. Proc Natl Acad Sci USA 87:9383–9387

41. Freedman JE (2003) CD40-CD40L and platelet function: beyond hemostasis. Circ Res 92:944–946

42. Maclouf J, Folco G, Patrono C (1998) Eicosanoids and iso-eicosanoids: constitutive, inducible and transcellular biosynthesis in vascular disease. Thromb Haemost 79:691–705

43. Hurlen M, Seljeflot I, Arnesen H (2000) Increased platelet aggregability during exercise in patients with previous myocardial infarction. Lack of inhibition by aspirin. Thromb Res 99:487–494

44. Maree AO, Curtin RJ, Chubb A, Dolan C, Cox D, O'Brien J, Crean P, Shields DC, Fitzgerald DJ (2005) Cyclooxygenase-1 haplotype modulates platelet response to aspirin. J Thromb Haemost 3:2340–2345

45. Clarke TA, Waskell LA (2003) The metabolism of clopidogrel is catalyzed by human cytochrome P450 3A and is inhibited by atorvastatin. Drug Metab Dispos 31:53–59

46. Shankar H, Murugappan S, Kim S, Jin J, Ding Z, Wickman K, Kunapuli SP (2004) Role of G protein-gated inwardly rectifying potassium channels in P2Y12 receptor-mediated platelet functional responses. Blood 104:1335–1343

47. Ding Z, Kim S, Dorsam RT, Jin J, Kunapuli SP (2003) Inactivation of the human P2Y12 receptor by thiol reagents requires interaction with both extracellular cysteine residues, Cys17 and Cys270. Blood 101:3908–3914

48. Geiger J, Brich J, Honig-Liedl P, Eigenthaler M, Schanzenbacher P, Herbert JM, Walter U (1999) Specific impairment of human platelet P2Y(AC) ADP receptor-mediated signaling by the antiplatelet drug clopidogrel. Arterioscler Thromb Vasc Biol 19:2007–2011

49. Thebault JJ, Kieffer G, Lowe GD, Nimmo WS, Cariou R (1999) Repeated dose pharmacodynamics of clopidogrel in healthy subjects. Semin Thromb Hemost 25(Suppl 2):9–14

50. Thebault JJ, Kieffer G, Cariou R (1999) Single-dose pharmacodynamics of clopidogrel. Semin Thromb Hemost 25(Suppl 2):3–8

51. Savcic M, Hauert J, Bachmann F, Wyld PJ, Geudelin B, Cariou R (1999) Clopidogrel loading dose regimens: kinetic profile of pharmacodynamic response in healthy subjects. Semin Thromb Hemost 25(Suppl 2):15–19

52. Gurbel PA, Bliden KP (2003) Durability of platelet inhibition by clopidogrel. Am J Cardiol 91:1123–1125

53. Wiviott SD, Antman EM (2004) Clopidogrel resistance: a new chapter in a fast-moving story. Circulation 109:3064–3067

54. Lau WC, Gurbel PA, Watkins PB, Neer CJ, Hopp AS, Carville DG, Guyer KE, Tait AR, Bates ER (2004) Contribution of hepatic cytochrome P450 3A4 metabolic activity to the phenomenon of clopidogrel resistance. Circulation 109:166–171

55. Lau WC, Carville DG, Bates ER (2004) Clinical significance of the atorvastatin-clopidogrel drug-drug interaction. Circulation 110:e66–e67 author reply e66-67

56. Angiolillo DJ, Fernandez-Ortiz A, Bernardo E, Barrera Ramirez C, Sabate M, Fernandez C, Hernandez-Antolin R, Escaned J, Alfonso F, Macaya C (2004) Platelet aggregation according to body mass index in patients undergoing coronary stenting: should clopidogrel loading-dose be weight adjusted? J Invasive Cardiol 16:169–174

57. Samara WM, Bliden KP, Tantry US, Gurbel PA (2005) The difference between clopidogrel responsiveness and post-treatment platelet reactivity. Thromb Res 115:89–94

58. Fontana P, Remones V, Reny JL, Aiach M, Gaussem P (2005) P2Y1 gene polymorphism and ADP-induced platelet response. J Thromb Haemost 3:2349–2350

59. Angiolillo DJ, Fernandez-Ortiz A, Bernardo E, Alfonso F, Sabate M, Fernandez C, Stranieri C, Trabetti E, Pignatti PF, Macaya C (2004) PlA polymorphism and platelet reactivity following clopidogrel loading dose in patients undergoing coronary stent implantation. Blood Coagul Fibrinolysis 15:89–93

60. Angiolillo DJ, Fernandez-Ortiz A, Bernardo E, Ramirez C, Escaned J, Moreno R, Hernandez-Antolin R, Sabate M, Trabetti E, Pignatti PF, Macaya C (2004) 807 C/T Polymorphism of the glycoprotein Ia gene and pharmacogenetic modulation of platelet response to dual antiplatelet treatment. Blood Coagul Fibrinolysis 15:427–433

61. Born GV (1970) Observations on the change in shape of blood platelets brought about by adenosine diphosphate. J Physiol 209:487–511

62. Yardumian DA, Mackie IJ, Machin SJ (1986) Laboratory investigation of platelet function: a review of methodology. J Clin Pathol 39:701–712

63. Williams CE, Entwistle MB, Short PE (1985) Platelet function tests: a critical review of methods. Med Lab Sci 42:262–274

64. Michelson AD (2004) Platelet function testing in cardiovascular diseases. Circulation 110:e489–e493

65. Catella F, Healy D, Lawson JA, FitzGerald GA (1986) 11-Dehydrothromboxane B2: a quantitative index of thromboxane A2 formation in the human circulation. Proc Natl Acad Sci USA 83:5861–5865

66. Jilma B (2001) Platelet function analyzer (PFA-100): a tool to quantify congenital or acquired platelet dysfunction. J Lab Clin Med 138:152–163
67. Coleman JWJ, Simon JI (2004) Determination of individual response to aspirin therapy using the Accumetrics Ultegra RPFA-ASA system. Point Care 3:77–82
68. Gurbel PA, Bliden KP, Samara W, Yoho JA, Hayes K, Fissha MZ, Tantry US (2005) Clopidogrel effect on platelet reactivity in patients with stent thrombosis: results of the CREST Study. J Am Coll Cardiol 46:1827–1832
69. Gurbel PA, Bliden KP, Navickas I, Cohen E, Tantry US (2007) Post-coronary intervention recurrent ischemia in the presence of adequate platelet inhibition by dual antiplatelet therapy: what are we overlooking? J Thromb Haemost 5:2300–2301
70. DiChiara J, Bliden KP, Tantry US, Hamed MS, Antonino MJ, Suarez TA, Bailon O, Singla A, Gurbel PA (2007) The effect of aspirin dosing on platelet function in diabetic and nondiabetic patients: an analysis from the aspirin-induced platelet effect (ASPECT) study. Diabetes 56:3014–3019
71. Mehta SS, Silver RJ, Aaronson A, Abrahamson M, Goldfine AB (2006) Comparison of aspirin resistance in type 1 versus type 2 diabetes mellitus. Am J Cardiol 97:567–570
72. Feher G, Koltai K, Alkonyi B, Papp E, Keszthelyi Z, Kesmarky G, Toth K (2007) Clopidogrel resistance: role of body mass and concomitant medications. Int J Cardiol 120:188–192
73. Levine PH (1973) An acute effect of cigarette smoking on platelet function. A possible link between smoking and arterial thrombosis. Circulation 48:619–623
74. Mirkhel A, Peyster E, Sundeen J, Greene L, Michelson AD, Hasan A, Domanski M (2006) Frequency of aspirin resistance in a community hospital. Am J Cardiol 98:577–579
75. Lee PY, Chen WH, Ng W, Cheng X, Kwok JY, Tse HF, Lau CP (2005) Low-dose aspirin increases aspirin resistance in patients with coronary artery disease. Am J Med 118:723–727
76. Gum PA, Kottke-Marchant K, Poggio ED, Gurm H, Welsh PA, Brooks L, Sapp SK, Topol EJ (2001) Profile and prevalence of aspirin resistance in patients with cardiovascular disease. Am J Cardiol 88:230–235
77. Friend M, Vucenik I, Miller M (2003) Research pointers: Platelet responsiveness to aspirin in patients with hyperlipidaemia. BMJ 326:82–83
78. MacDonald TM, Wei L (2003) Effect of ibuprofen on cardioprotective effect of aspirin. Lancet 361:573–574
79. Lau WC, Waskell LA, Watkins PB, Neer CJ, Horowitz K, Hopp AS, Tait AR, Carville DG, Guyer KE, Bates ER (2003) Atorvastatin reduces the ability of clopidogrel to inhibit platelet aggregation: a new drug-drug interaction. Circulation 107:32–37
80. Neubauer H, Gunesdogan B, Hanefeld C, Spiecker M, Mugge A (2003) Lipophilic statins interfere with the inhibitory effects of clopidogrel on platelet functio006E – a flow cytometry study. Eur Heart J 24:1744–1749
81. Saw J, Steinhubl SR, Berger PB, Kereiakes DJ, Serebruany VL, Brennan D, Topol EJ (2003) Lack of adverse clopidogrel-atorvastatin clinical interaction from secondary analysis of a randomized, placebo-controlled clopidogrel trial. Circulation 108:921–924
82. Serebruany VL, Midei MG, Malinin AI, Oshrine BR, Lowry DR, Sane DC, Tanguay JF, Steinhubl SR, Berger PB, O'Connor CM, Hennekens CH (2004) Absence of interaction between atorvastatin or other statins and clopidogrel: results from the interaction study. Arch Intern Med 164:2051–2057
83. Mukherjee D, Kline-Rogers E, Fang J, Munir K, Eagle KA (2005) Lack of clopidogrel-CYP3A4 statin interaction in patients with acute coronary syndrome. Heart 91:23–26
84. Grotemeyer KH, Scharafinski HW, Husstedt IW (1993) Two-year follow-up of aspirin responder and aspirin non responder. A pilot-study including 180 post-stroke patients. Thromb Res 71:397–403
85. Antman EM, Cohen M, Bernink PJ, McCabe CH, Horacek T, Papuchis G, Mautner B, Corbalan R, Radley D, Braunwald E (2000) The TIMI risk score for unstable angina/non-ST elevation MI: A method for prognostication and therapeutic decision making. JAMA 284:835–842
86. Barnes GD, Li J, Kline-Rogers E, Vedre A, Armstrong DF, Froehlich JB, Eagle KA, Gurm HS (2007) Dual antiplatelet agent failure: a new syndrome or clinical nonentity? Am Heart J 154:732–735
87. Barragan P, Bouvier JL, Roquebert PO, Macaluso G, Commeau P, Comet B, Lafont A, Camoin L, Walter U, Eigenthaler M (2003) Resistance to thienopyridines: clinical detection of coronary stent thrombosis by monitoring of vasodilator-stimulated phosphoprotein phosphorylation. Catheter Cardiovasc Interv 59:295–302
88. Matetzky S, Shenkman B, Guetta V, Shechter M, Bienart R, Goldenberg I, Novikov I, Pres H, Savion N, Varon D, Hod H (2004) Clopidogrel resistance is associated with increased risk of recurrent atherothrombotic events in patients with acute myocardial infarction. Circulation 109:3171–3175
89. Cuisset T, Frere C, Quilici J, Barbou F, Morange PE, Hovasse T, Bonnet JL, Alessi MC (2006) High post-treatment platelet reactivity identified low-responders to dual antiplatelet therapy at increased risk of recurrent cardiovascular events after stenting for acute coronary syndrome. J Thromb Haemost 4:542–549

90. Lev EI, Patel RT, Maresh KJ, Guthikonda S, Granada J, DeLao T, Bray PF, Kleiman NS (2006) Aspirin and clopidogrel drug response in patients undergoing percutaneous coronary intervention: the role of dual drug resistance. J Am Coll Cardiol 47:27–33

91. Angiolillo DJ, Bernardo E, Sabate M, Jimenez-Quevedo P, Costa MA, Palazuelos J, Hernandez-Antolin R, Moreno R, Escaned J, Alfonso F, Banuelos C, Guzman LA, Bass TA, Macaya C, Fernandez-Ortiz A (2007) Impact of platelet reactivity on cardiovascular outcomes in patients with type 2 diabetes mellitus and coronary artery disease. J Am Coll Cardiol 50:1541–1547

92. Campbell CL, Smyth S, Montalescot G, Steinhubl SR (2007) Aspirin dose for the prevention of cardiovascular disease: a systematic review. JAMA 297:2018–2024

93. Topol EJ, Easton D, Harrington RA, Amarenco P, Califf RM, Graffagnino C, Davis S, Diener HC, Ferguson J, Fitzgerald D, Granett J, Shuaib A, Koudstaal PJ, Theroux P, Van de Werf F, Sigmon K, Pieper K, Vallee M, Willerson JT (2003) Randomized, double-blind, placebo-controlled, international trial of the oral IIb/IIIa antagonist lotrafiban in coronary and cerebrovascular disease. Circulation 108:399–406

94. Quinn MJ, Aronow HD, Califf RM, Bhatt DL, Sapp S, Kleiman NS, Harrington RA, Kong DF, Kandzari DE, Topol EJ (2004) Aspirin dose and six-month outcome after an acute coronary syndrome. J Am Coll Cardiol 43:972–978

95. Snoep JD, Hovens MM, Eikenboom JC, van der Bom JG, Huisman MV (2007) Association of laboratory-defined aspirin resistance with a higher risk of recurrent cardiovascular events: a systematic review and meta-analysis. Arch Intern Med 167:1593–1599

96. Hovens MM, Snoep JD, Eikenboom JC, van der Bom JG, Mertens BJ, Huisman MV (2007) Prevalence of persistent platelet reactivity despite use of aspirin: a systematic review. Am Heart J 153:175–181

97. Abaci A, Yilmaz Y, Caliskan M, Bayram F, Cetin M, Unal A, Cetin S (2005) Effect of increasing doses of aspirin on platelet function as measured by PFA-100 in patients with diabetes. Thromb Res 116:465–470

98. von Pape KW, Strupp G, Bonzel T, Bohner J (2005) Effect of compliance and dosage adaptation of long term aspirin on platelet function with PFA-100 in patients after myocardial infarction. Thromb Haemost 94:889–891

99. Tohgi H, Konno S, Tamura K, Kimura B, Kawano K (1992) Effects of low-to-high doses of aspirin on platelet aggregability and metabolites of thromboxane A2 and prostacyclin. Stroke 23:1400–1403

100. Gorelick PB, Weisman SM (2005) Risk of hemorrhagic stroke with aspirin use: an update. Stroke 36:1801–1807

101. Weil J, Colin-Jones D, Langman M, Lawson D, Logan R, Murphy M, Rawlins M, Vessey M, Wainwright P (1995) Prophylactic aspirin and risk of peptic ulcer bleeding. BMJ 310:827–830

102. Boneu B, Destelle G (1996) Platelet anti-aggregating activity and tolerance of clopidogrel in atherosclerotic patients. Thromb Haemost 76:939–943

103. Cadroy Y, Bossavy JP, Thalamas C, Sagnard L, Sakariassen K, Boneu B (2000) Early potent antithrombotic effect with combined aspirin and a loading dose of clopidogrel on experimental arterial thrombogenesis in humans. Circulation 101:2823–2828

104. Mehta SR, Yusuf S, Peters RJ, Bertrand ME, Lewis BS, Natarajan MK, Malmberg K, Rupprecht H, Zhao F, Chrolavicius S, Copland I, Fox KA (2001) Effects of pretreatment with clopidogrel and aspirin followed by long-term therapy in patients undergoing percutaneous coronary intervention: the PCI-CURE study. Lancet 358:527–533

105. Gurbel PA, Cummings CC, Bell CR, Alford AB, Meister AF, Serebruany VL (2003) Onset and extent of platelet inhibition by clopidogrel loading in patients undergoing elective coronary stenting: the Plavix Reduction Of New Thrombus Occurrence (PRONTO) trial. Am Heart J 145:239–247

106. Muller I, Seyfarth M, Rudiger S, Wolf B, Pogatsa-Murray G, Schomig A, Gawaz M (2001) Effect of a high loading dose of clopidogrel on platelet function in patients undergoing coronary stent placement. Heart 85:92–93

107. Knight CJ, Panesar M, Wilson DJ, Patrineli A, Chronos N, Wright C, Clarke D, Patel D, Fox K, Goodall AH (1998) Increased platelet responsiveness following coronary stenting. Heparin as a possible aetiological factor in stent thrombosis. Eur Heart J 19:1239–1248

108. Angiolillo DJ, Bernardo E, Ramirez C, Costa MA, Sabate M, Jimenez-Quevedo P, Hernandez R, Moreno R, Escaned J, Alfonso F, Banuelos C, Bass TA, Macaya C, Fernandez-Ortiz A (2006) Insulin therapy is associated with platelet dysfunction in patients with type 2 diabetes mellitus on dual oral antiplatelet treatment. J Am Coll Cardiol 48:298–304

109. Angiolillo DJ, Fernandez-Ortiz A, Bernardo E, Ramirez C, Sabate M, Banuelos C, Hernandez-Antolin R, Escaned J, Moreno R, Alfonso F, Macaya C (2004) High clopidogrel loading dose during coronary stenting: effects on drug response and interindividual variability. Eur Heart J 25:1903–1910

110. Kastrati A, von Beckerath N, Joost A, Pogatsa-Murray G, Gorchakova O, Schomig A (2004) Loading with 600 mg clopidogrel in patients with coronary artery disease with and without chronic clopidogrel therapy. Circulation 110:1916–1919

111. Gurbel PA, Bliden KP, Hayes KM, Yoho JA, Herzog WR, Tantry US (2005) The relation of dosing to clopidogrel responsiveness and the incidence of high post-treatment platelet aggregation in patients undergoing coronary stenting. J Am Coll Cardiol 45:1392–1396

112. von Beckerath N, Taubert D, Pogatsa-Murray G, Schomig E, Kastrati A, Schomig A (2005) Absorption, metabolization, and antiplatelet effects of 300-, 600-, and 900-mg loading doses of clopidogrel: results of the ISAR-CHOICE (Intracoronary Stenting and Antithrombotic Regimen: Choose Between 3 High Oral Doses for Immediate Clopidogrel Effect) Trial. Circulation 112:2946–2950

113. Patti G, Colonna G, Pasceri V, Pepe LL, Montinaro A, Di Sciascio G (2005) Randomized trial of high loading dose of clopidogrel for reduction of periprocedural myocardial infarction in patients undergoing coronary intervention: results from the ARMYDA-2 (Antiplatelet therapy for Reduction of MYocardial Damage during Angioplasty) study. Circulation 111:2099–2106

114. Cuisset T, Frere C, Quilici J, Morange PE, Nait-Saidi L, Carvajal J, Lehmann A, Lambert M, Bonnet JL, Alessi MC (2006) Benefit of a 600-mg loading dose of clopidogrel on platelet reactivity and clinical outcomes in patients with non-ST-segment elevation acute coronary syndrome undergoing coronary stenting. J Am Coll Cardiol 48:1339–1345

115. Smith SC Jr, Feldman TE, Hirshfeld JW Jr, Jacobs AK, Kern MJ, King SB III, Morrison DA, O'Neill WW, Schaff HV, Whitlow PL, Williams DO, Antman EM, Adams CD, Anderson JL, Faxon DP, Fuster V, Halperin JL, Hiratzka LF, Hunt SA, Nishimura R, Ornato JP, Page RL, Riegel B (2006) ACC/AHA/SCAI 2005 Guideline Update for Percutaneous Coronary Intervention–summary article: a report of the American College of Cardiology/American Heart Association Task Force on Practice Guidelines (ACC/AHA/SCAI Writing Committee to Update the 2001 Guidelines for Percutaneous Coronary Intervention). Circulation 113:156–175

116. Angiolillo DJ, Fernandez-Ortiz A, Bernardo E, Ramirez C, Sabate M, Jimenez-Quevedo P, Hernandez R, Moreno R, Escaned J, Alfonso F, Banuelos C, Costa MA, Bass TA, Macaya C (2005) Platelet function profiles in patients with type 2 diabetes and coronary artery disease on combined aspirin and clopidogrel treatment. Diabetes 54:2430–2435

117. Angiolillo DJ, Shoemaker SB, Desai B, Yuan H, Charlton RK, Bernardo E, Zenni MM, Guzman LA, Bass TA, Costa MA (2007) Randomized comparison of a high clopidogrel maintenance dose in patients with diabetes mellitus and coronary artery disease: results of the Optimizing Antiplatelet Therapy in Diabetes Mellitus (OPTIMUS) study. Circulation 115:708–716

118. Sugidachi A, Asai F, Ogawa T, Inoue T, Koike H (2000) The in vivo pharmacological profile of CS-747, a novel antiplatelet agent with platelet ADP receptor antagonist properties. Br J Pharmacol 129:1439–1446

119. Wiviott SD, Braunwald E, McCabe CH, Montalescot G, Ruzyllo W, Gottlieb S, Neumann FJ, Ardissino D, De Servi S, Murphy SA, Riesmeyer J, Weerakkody G, Gibson CM, Antman EM (2007) Prasugrel versus clopidogrel in patients with acute coronary syndromes. N Engl J Med 357:2001–2015

120. Storey RF, Newby LJ, Heptinstall S (2001) Effects of P2Y(1) and P2Y(12) receptor antagonists on platelet aggregation induced by different agonists in human whole blood. Platelets 12:443–447

121. Storey RF, Husted S, Harrington RA, Heptinstall S, Wilcox RG, Peters G, Wickens M, Emanuelsson H, Gurbel P, Grande P, Cannon CP (2007) Inhibition of platelet aggregation by AZD6140, a reversible oral P2Y12 receptor antagonist, compared with clopidogrel in patients with acute coronary syndromes. J Am Coll Cardiol 50:1852–1856

122. Wiviott SD, Antman EM, Winters KJ, Weerakkody G, Murphy SA, Behounek BD, Carney RJ, Lazzam C, McKay RG, McCabe CH, Braunwald E (2005) Randomized comparison of prasugrel (CS-747, LY640315), a novel thienopyridine P2Y12 antagonist, with clopidogrel in percutaneous coronary intervention: results of the Joint Utilization of Medications to Block Platelets Optimally (JUMBO)-TIM. Circulation 111:3366–3373

Index